Pediatric Critical Care Nutrition

Pediatric Critical Care Nutrition

Praveen S. Goday, MD, CNSC
Division of Pediatric Gastroenterology and Nutrition
Medical College of Wisconsin
Milwaukee, Wisconsin

Nilesh M. Mehta, MD
Division of Critical Care Medicine
Department of Anesthesiology, Perioperative and Pain Medicine
Boston Children's Hospital
Harvard Medical School
Boston, Massachusetts

Mc Graw Hill Education | Medical

New York Chicago San Francisco Athens London Madrid Mexico City
Milan New Delhi Singapore Sydney Toronto

Pediatric Critical Care Nutrition

1 2 3 4 5 6 7 8 9 0 CTP/CTP 18 17 16 15 14

ISBN 978-0-07-179852-5
ISBN 0-07-179852-8

This book was set in Minion Pro by MPS Limited.
The editors were Alyssa Fried and Brian Kearns.
The production supervisor was Rick Ruzycka.
Project management was provided by Shruti Chopra, MPS Limited.
The cover designer was Anthony Landi.
Image Credit: © Hans Berggren/Johnér Images/Corbis.
China Translation & Printing Services, Ltd. was printer and binder.

This book is printed on acid-free paper.

Library of Congress Cataloging-in-Publication Data

Pediatric critical care nutrition / [edited by] Praveen S. Goday, Nilesh M. Mehta.
p. ; cm.
Includes bibliographical references.
ISBN 978-0-07-179852-5 (alk. paper)—ISBN 0-07-179852-8 (alk. paper)
I. Goday, Praveen S., editor. II. Mehta, Nilesh M., editor.
[DNLM: 1. Child. 2. Infant. 3. Nutritional Support. 4. Child Nutritional Physiological Phenomena. 5. Critical Care. 6. Critical Illness. WS 115]
RJ48
618.92—dc23

2014027203

Goday

To my mother, for being my guiding light,
And to my father, for being hers.

Mehta

To Rheona, Sheil, and Manisha for your unconditional love and patience.
To my parents, for everything.
And to dietitians everywhere, who are the unsung champions.

Table of Contents

Contributors .... *ix*
Preface .... *xiii*

Section 1 Metabolic Alterations and Nutrients in the Critically ill Child

Chapter 1
The Acute Metabolic Response to Injury in Children 3

Chapter 2
Nutritional Assessment of the Critically ill Child 19

Chapter 3
Energy and Macronutrient Requirements in the Critically ill Child 33

Chapter 4
Micronutrient Requirements in the Critically ill Child 59

Chapter 5
Fluid, Electrolytes, and Acid–Base Physiology in Critically ill Children 71

Chapter 6
Drug–Nutrient Interactions 87

Section 2 Delivery of Nutrition Support to the Critically ill Child

Chapter 7
Parenteral Nutrition Support in the Critically ill Child 99

Chapter 8
Enteral Nutrition in the Critically ill Child 111

Chapter 9
Guidelines and Algorithms for Feeding the Critically ill 125

Section 3 Disease-related Nutrition Considerations

Chapter 10
Nutritional Support of the Critically ill Neonate 141

Chapter 11
Trauma and Traumatic Brain Injury 155

Chapter 12
Burns and Wound Healing 165

Chapter 13
Nutrition Management of Pediatric Patients Undergoing Liver Transplantation or Intestinal Transplantation 175

Chapter 14
Renal Failure 187

Chapter 15
Respiratory Failure 193

Chapter 16
Nutrition in Acute Liver Failure and Acute Pancreatitis 205

Chapter 17
Nutrition for the Infant or Child in the Cardiac Intensive Care Unit 217

Chapter 18
Nutritional Support of the Pediatric Surgical ICU Patient 227

Chapter 19
Immunonutrition 243

Chapter 20
Cancer and Hematopoietic Stem Cell Transplantation 257

Chapter 21
Nutrition in the Critically ill Obese Child 269

Chapter 22
Nutritional Support of Critically ill Children in Resource-Limited Settings 287

Chapter 23
Nursing Considerations in the Provision of Nutrition Support to the Critically ill Child 299

Index *311*

Contributors

Carol Okada, MD
Assistant Professor
Pediatric Critical Care Medicine
Children's Hospital Colorado
Aurora, Colorado

Carrie Smith, MS, RD, LD
Neonatal Dietitian
University of Cincinnati Medical Center
Cincinnati, Ohio

Christina J. Valentine MD, MS, RD
Assistant Professor/Neonatologist
The University of Cincinnati
Division of Neonatology, Perinatal, and Pulmonary Biology,
Cincinnati Children's Hospital Medical Center
Cincinnati, Ohio

Christopher Duggan MD, MPH
Senior Associate in Medicine, Center for Nutrition
Surgical Director of the Center for Advanced Intestinal Rehabilitation, Boston Children's Hospital
Associate Professor of Pediatrics, Harvard Medical School
Boston, Massachusetts

Diana Lerner, MD
Assistant Professor
Pediatric Gastroenterology and Nutrition
Medical College of Wisconsin
Milwaukee, Wisconsin

Enid E Martinez, MD
Division of Critical Care Medicine
Department of Anesthesiology, Perioperative and Pain Medicine, Boston Children's Hospital
Boston, Massachusetts

Eric Sparks, MD
Research Fellow
Department of Surgery and Center for Advanced Intestinal Rehabilitation
Boston Children's Hospital,
Boston, Massachusetts

Faraz Khan, MD
Research Fellow
Department of Surgery and Center for Advanced Intestinal Rehabilitation
Boston Children's Hospital
Boston, Massachusetts

Gil Hardy, PhD FRSC
Professor of Pharmaceutical Nutrition
Faculty of Medical and Health Sciences, University of Auckland, New Zealand

Heather E. Skillman, MS, RD, CSP, CNSC
Pediatric Critical Care Dietitian
Children's Hospital Colorado
Clinical Nutrition Department
Denver, Colorado

Heather Skillman, MS, RD, CSP, CNSC
Pediatric Critical Care Dietitian
Clinical Nutrition Department
Children's Hospital Colorado.
Aurora, Colorado

James D. Fortenberry MD, MCCM, FAAP
Professor, Department of Pediatrics, Division of Pediatric Critical Care Medicine
Emory University School of Medicine
Pediatrician in Chief
Children's Healthcare of Atlanta
Atlanta, Georgia

Jennifer A. McArthur, DO
Assistant Professor of Pediatrics
Division of Pediatric Critical Care
Medical College of Wisconsin
Milwaukee, Wisconsin

Jennifer N. Manzi, MSN, CPNP-AC/PC
Critical Care Pediatric Nurse Practitioner
Department of Pediatrics
Medical College of Wisconsin
Milwaukee, Wisconsin

Jeremy Fisher, MD
Research Fellow
Department of Surgery and Center for Advanced Intestinal Rehabilitation
Boston Children's Hospital
Boston, Massachusetts

Jessie M Hulst, MD, PhD
Pediatric Gastroenterology, Erasmus MC-Sophia Children's Hospital,
Rotterdam, The Netherlands

Jorge A. Coss-Bu, M.D
Associate Professor, Department of Pediatrics
Baylor College of Medicine
Associate Director of Research, Section of Critical Care Medicine
Texas Children's Hospital
Houston, Texas

Joy Lehman, PharmD, BCNSP
Specialty Practice Pharmacist,
The Ohio State University Wexner Medical Center
Department of Pharmacy
Columbus, Ohio

Katelyn Ariagno RD, LDN
Clinical Nutrition Specialist II, Critical Care Nutrition
GI/Center for Nutrition, Boston Children's Hospital
Boston, Massachusetts

Kathy Prelack, PhD, RD
Director, Clinical Nutrition
Shriners Hospitals For Children,
Boston, Massachusetts

Keith Thatch, MD
Clinical Assistant Professor, Division of Pediatric Surgery,
Department of Surgery,
University of Michigan
Ann Arbor, Michigan

Koen FM Joosten, MD, PhD
Department of Pediatrics, Pediatric Intensive Care
Erasmus MC-Sophia Children's Hospital,
Rotterdam, The Netherlands

Lauren Sorce RN, MSN, CPNP-AC/PC, FCCM
Pediatric Critical Care Nurse Practitioner, APN Manager
Division of Pediatric Critical Care
Ann and Robert H. Lurie Children's Hospital of Chicago
Chicago, Illinois

Lori J. Bechard, MEd, RD, LDN
Clinical Nutrition Specialist III
Center for Nutrition
Boston Children's Hospital
Boston, Massachusetts

Luise Marino RD, PhD
Chief Paediatric Dietitian
Department of Nutrition and Dietetics
University Hospital Southampton NHS Foundation Trust
Southampton, United Kingdom

Lynne Latten, BSc (Hons) RD
Advanced Paediatric Dietician
Dietetic Department
Alder Hey Children's NHS Foundation Trust
Liverpool, United Kingdom

Lyvonne N. Tume RN RSCN RNT Dip App Sci (Nurs), B Nurs, M Clin Nurs (Crit Care), PGDE, PhD
Senior Research Fellow PICU & CBU Research Lead
Alder Hey Children's NHS Foundation Trust and
University of Central Lancashire
Lancashire, United Kingdom

Maggie L. Dylewski, PhD, RD
Clinical Assistant Professor
Department of Molecular, Cellular, and Biomedical Sciences
University of New Hampshire
Durham, New Hampshire

Melissa S. Rice, DO
Fellow, Neonatal-Perinatal Medicine,
Division of Neonatology, Perinatal, and Pulmonary Biology,
Cincinnati Children's Hospital Medical Center
Cincinnati, Ohio

Nancy Krebs, MD, MS
Professor of Pediatrics
Head, Section of Nutrition
University of Colorado School of Medicine
Aurora, Colorado

Natalie Z. Cvijanovich, MD, FAAP
Associate Physician, Division of Critical Care
Children's Hospital of Oakland
Clinical Associate Professor
UCSF Pediatrics
Oakland, California

Nazima Pathan FRCPCH, PhD
Clinical Senior Lecturer
Department of Paediatric Intensive Care
Addenbrooke's Hospital
University of Cambridge
Cambridge, United Kingdom

Poyyapakkam R. Srivaths MD
Assistant Professor
Department of Pediatrics, Renal Section
Baylor College of Medicine
Houston, Texas

Renán A. Orellana, MD
Associate Professor of Pediatrics, Section of Critical Care Medicine,
Baylor College of Medicine
Attending Physician, Critical Care, Texas Children's Hospital
Houston, Texas

Renee Wieman, RD, CSP, LD, CNSD
Dietitian, Liver and Intestinal Transplantation
Cincinnati Children's Hospital Medical Center
Cincinnati, Ohio

Robert L. Sheridan, MD
Assistant Chief of Staff and Chief of Burn Surgery
Shriners Hospitals For Children,
Boston, Massachusetts

Sabina Siddiqui, MD
Clinical Lecturer, Division of Pediatric Surgery,
Department of Surgery,
University of Michigan
Ann Arbor, Michigan

Samir K. Gadepalli, MD, MBA
Clinical Lecturer,
Division of Pediatric Surgery,
Department of Surgery,
University of Michigan
Ann Arbor, Michigan

Samuel A. Kocoshis, MD
Professor of Pediatrics
University of Cincinnati College of Medicine
Director, Intestinal Transplantation and Intestinal Care Center
Cincinnati Children's Hospital Medical Center
Cincinnati, Ohio

Stacey L. Valentine, MD MPH, FAAP, FCCP
Assistant Professor, Department of Pediatrics, Division of Pediatric Critical Care Medicine
University of Massachusetts Children's Medical Center
Worcester, Massachusetts

Sunit Singhi, MBBS, MD, FIAP, FAMS, FISCCM, FCCM
Professor and Head Department of Pediatrics,
Head, Pediatric Emergency and Intensive Care Services
Advanced Pediatrics Centre
Post-Graduate Institute of Medical Education and Research
Chandigarh, India

Steven Werlin, MD
Professor
Pediatric Gastroenterology and Nutrition
Medical College of Wisconsin
Milwaukee, Wisconsin

Susan Hamilton RN, MS, CCRN, CWOCN
Pediatric Critical Care Clinical Nurse Specialist
Boston Children's Hospital
Boston, Massachusetts

Terezie Tolar Mosby, EdD, MS, RD, IBCLC, LDN
Clinical Nutritionist III
Clinical Nutrition Services
St. Jude Children's Research Hospital
Memphis, Tennessee

Theodoric Wong, BMedSc, MBBS, FRACP
Paediatric Gastroenterologist
Department of Gastroenterology and Clinical Nutrition, Birmingham Children's Hospital, Birmingham United Kingdom

Theresa A. Mikhailov, MD, PhD
Associate Professor of Pediatrics
Division of Pediatric Critical Care
Medical College of Wisconsin
Milwaukee, Wisconsin

Toni Petrillo-Albarano, MD, FCCM
Associate Professor, Department of Pediatrics, Division of Pediatric Critical Care Medicine
Emory University School of Medicine and Children's Healthcare of Atlanta
Atlanta, Georgia

Tom Jaksic, MD, PhD
W. Hardy Hendren Professor of Surgery
Harvard Medical School
Senior Associate and Vice-Chairman, Department of General Surgery, and Surgical Director of the Center for Advanced Intestinal Rehabilitation, Boston Children's Hospital
Boston, Massachusetts

Walter J. Chwals, MD, FCCM
Professor of Surgery and Pediatrics
Tufts University School of Medicine
Surgeon-in-Chief
Floating Hospital for Children
Boston, Massachusetts

William Manzanares, MD, PhD
Associate Professor
Department of Critical Care University Hospital (Hospital de Clínicas), Faculty of Medicina - Universidad de la República (UDELAR)
Montevideo, Uruguay

Preface

The provision of optimal nutrition to the critically ill child, to offset the catabolic effects of the illness or injury and to enhance clinical outcomes, is an important objective for healthcare providers. The last decade has seen a resurgence in interest in this area of critical care, with an increasing number of research publications and consensus documents. The field of critical care nutrition has evolved, and clear associations between bedside nutrient delivery and outcomes have been demonstrated. Nutrition delivery is no longer just supportive care, but it is now recognized as an important therapy with nutrients that can modulate disease. Despite the enthusiasm and the explosion in research on the subject, there are many unanswered questions, and the quest for best practices remains elusive, especially in the pediatric intensive care unit (PICU). The individual practitioner—the trainee, the intensivist, the dietitian, the nurse—is left with a number of practical questions on the nutritional management of the individual child in the PICU.

We are delighted to present the first edition of *Pediatric Critical Care Nutrition*, a comprehensive textbook that addresses nutrition therapy for the critically ill newborn infant and child. To our knowledge, this is the first and currently only available textbook on this subject. The book has been divided into three sections, with chapters that describe nutritional aspects of a variety of pediatric critical illnesses. The book includes contributions from some of the leading experts in this area from around the world. The authors represent a multidisciplinary group consisting of critical care physicians, critical care nurses, gastroenterologists, pediatric surgeons, dietitians, and pharmacists. Each author sees the critically ill child from a distinct vantage point based on their practice area and hence, provides a unique perspective. The chapters represent collaborations between authors from different institutions, regions, and specialties. We aimed for a book that is eminently readable, whether one chooses to read it from cover to cover or to focus on individual chapters. We have emphasized certain themes throughout this book, such as our belief in enteral nutrition as the best mode of nutrient delivery, screening for nutritional status, indirect calorimetry to accurately determine energy requirements, the role of a multidisciplinary team of nutrition champions, and the importance of studying the impact of nutrition therapy on clinical outcomes.

We believe that nutrition therapy has been ignored in the PICU, and it is time to emphasize its importance during critical illness and realize its potential impact on clinical outcomes. We hope that this book summarizes the important work done by several champions over the past decade, and that it will kindle an interest in researching the vast expanses of PICU nutrition knowledge that need to be explored. It is our sincere belief that by adopting and implementing the best practices in this book, hospitals and healthcare professionals can achieve safer care and make meaningful and long-lasting improvements to bedside nutrient delivery, with the ultimate aim of improving outcomes in the vulnerable child in the PICU. We also hope that this book will serve to encourage future research in this field so that we can continue to build on the strides that have already been achieved.

Finally, we would like to express our deep gratitude to all our authors for their time and tremendous contributions. Without them, this book would not have been possible. They are the true leaders and pioneers in our field, and we will continue to look to them for collaboration and guidance in the future.

SECTION 1

Metabolic Alterations and Nutrients in the Critically ill Child

CHAPTER 1

The Acute Metabolic Response to Injury in Children

Walter J. Chwals

■ OVERVIEW
■ NEUROENDOCRINE/AUTONOMIC NERVOUS SYSTEM RESPONSE
■ CYTOKINE RESPONSE
■ COUNTER-REGULATORY HORMONAL RESPONSE
AMS-Associated Anabolic Hormone Resistance
Metabolic Alterations Associated with Acute Metabolic Stress
Energy Metabolism Associated with Acute Metabolic Stress
Clinical Significance
■ OVERFEEDING ASSOCIATED WITH ACUTE METABOLIC STRESS
Pulmonary Pathophysiology
Hepatic Pathophysiology
Immune System Pathophysiology
■ SERIAL AMS RESPONSE ASSESSMENT
■ KEY POINTS
References

■ OVERVIEW

In response to a variety of injurious stimuli, such as trauma, sepsis, and acute inflammatory conditions, a series of metabolic changes occur that characterize the acute metabolic stress (AMS) response in humans (**Figs. 1-1A and 1-1B**). This response is basically stereotypical in nature in all patient populations (children and adults).[1-4] This response may vary to some degree with respect to the nature (e.g., sepsis, burn,) and severity of the insult, as well as factors that impact the endogenous metabolic reserve and/or reserve mobilization capacity (e.g., malnutrition, recent previous tissue injury, underlying systemic disease, age, pharmacologic intervention,) of the acutely injured host. In infants, especially those born prematurely, functional immaturity is a particularly important response-modifying variable.[5] Among the early features of the injury response is the release of cytokines, followed rapidly by important alterations in the hormonal environment. Increased counter-regulatory hormone concentrations are associated with insulin and growth hormone (GH) resistance. As a result of this response, a sequence of metabolic events is initiated that includes the catabolism of endogenous stores of protein, carbohydrate, and fat to provide essential substrate intermediates and energy necessary to fuel the ongoing response process. Amino acids from catabolized proteins flow to the liver where they provide substrate for the synthesis of acute-phase proteins and glucose (gluconeogenesis). Therefore, the AMS response represents a hypermetabolic,

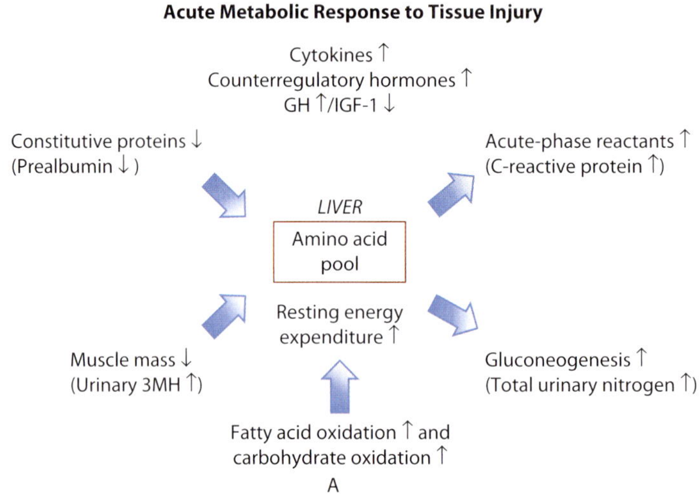

FIGURE 1-1. A Acute metabolic stress response to acute injury.

Reproduced with permission from Baker SS, Baker RD, Davis AM: Pediatric Nutritional Support Energy Metabolism. Jones & Bartlett; 2007

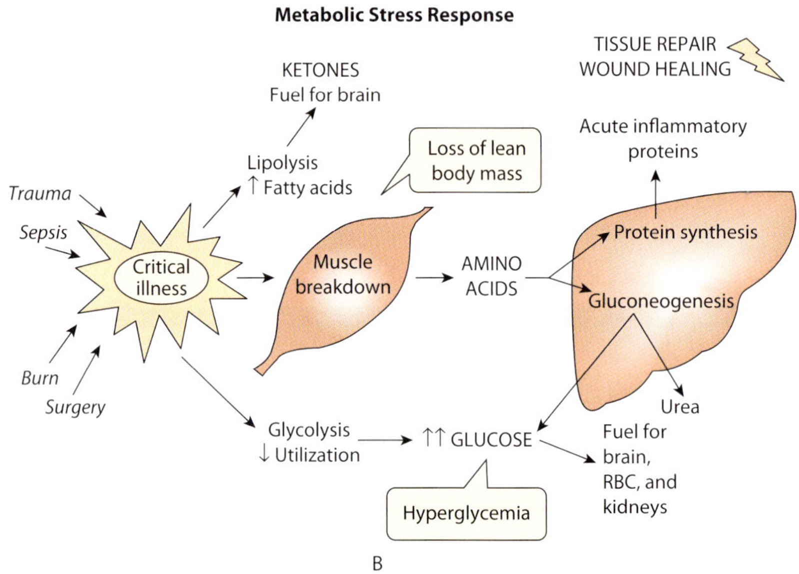

FIGURE 1-1. B GH, growth hormone; IGF-1, insulin-like growth factor I; U3MH, urinary 3-methyl histidine.

Reproduced with permission from Mehta N, Jaksic, T. The Critically ill Child. In: Duggan W, Walker., ed. Nutrition in Pediatrics. 4 ed. Hamilton, Ontario: B. C. Decker Inc.; 2008

hypercatabolic state that results in the loss of endogenous tissue stores with associated increases in glucose and free fatty acid (FFA) production and oxidation, increased energy expenditure, and increased protein turnover and breakdown. Growth, which is an anabolic process, is thought to be inhibited during periods of AMS. As the AMS response resolves, adaptive anabolic metabolism ensues to restore catabolic losses. In children, this phase is characterized by the resumption of somatic growth.

NEUROENDOCRINE/AUTONOMIC NERVOUS SYSTEM RESPONSE

Evolution of the stress response in mammals has resulted in the development of an intricate system of reflex neural injury-induced stimuli that trigger the central nervous system (CNS), causing alterations in the hypothalamic-anterior pituitary axes, including the adrenal (increased cortisol secretion), the somatotrophic (increased GH secretion), the thyrotrophic (decreased triiodothyronine [T_3] and increased reverse T_3 [rT_3] secretion), and the gonado-/lactotrophic (decreased testosterone, increased prolactin) axes.[3,6] The CNS also acts through the peripheral sympathetic nervous system to increase catecholamine secretion. Generally, these responses are directly proportional to the severity of the insult. In concert, these changes have a profound effect on cardiovascular tone, respiratory rate, immune and inflammatory reactions, and intermediate metabolism, initiating an intricate response cascade as described next.

■ CYTOKINE RESPONSE

The metabolic response to tissue injury is initiated by activation of the cytokine cascade. Cytokines are a group of proteins, glycoproteins, and peptides with short half-lives, which are synthesized by various tissue and white blood cell populations and have important and diverse cell-signaling functions. As a group, they have both pro-inflammatory and anti-inflammatory effects, as well as both stimulatory and suppressive immunoregulatory functions.[7,8] As such, the cytokine cascade acts as an essential homeostatic regulator during the AMS response. Regulatory response imbalances caused by an overwhelming insult and/or inadequate host metabolic/immunologic response capacity can undermine response homeostasis, leading to an increased risk of injury-induced morbidity and mortality.[9]

Tissue injury induces an early hyperinflammatory response, mediated principally by pro-inflammatory cytokines—initially tumor necrosis factor alpha (TNFα) and interleukin (IL)-1—followed shortly thereafter by IL-6 and IL-8.[3] These cytokines are produced by activated macrophages, monocytes, and endothelial cells, and their release triggers the up-regulation of anti-inflammatory cytokines such as IL-10.[10] The hepatic acute-phase response is primarily mediated by IL-6.[8] Furthermore, injury-induced cytokine release has been shown to promote catabolic metabolism by inhibiting the GH:insulin-like growth factor 1 (IGF-1) axis[11-15] (see "AMS-Associated Anabolic Hormone Resistance").

■ COUNTER-REGULATORY HORMONAL RESPONSE

Acute metabolic stress is characterized by substantial increases in serum concentrations of catecholamines, glucagon, and cortisol, which are referred to as counter-regulatory hormones because they oppose the anabolic effects of insulin. Serum concentrations of these metabolic stress-related hormones increase as a result of injury-induced cytokine release.[3,16]

Catecholamines are the primary agents of the hypermetabolic response.[3,17] They cause hyperglycemia by promoting hepatic glycogenolysis—causing conversions of skeletal muscle glycogen to lactate (which is then transported to the liver for conversion to glucose through the Cori cycle)—and by suppressing the pancreatic secretion of insulin. Catecholamines also induce lipolysis, which results in the mobilization of FFAs. Finally, catecholamines, in addition to glucagon and cortisol, induce hypermetabolism, which is associated with an increase in the basal metabolic rate.

Glucagon induces glycolysis and gluconeogenesis. These effects counteract the anabolic effects of insulin. Increased glycolysis results in increased serum lactate and alanine concentrations. These amino acids provide the substrate necessary for the endogenous regeneration of glucose (the Cori cycle and alanine cycle). These cycles are major contributors to altered carbohydrate metabolism during AMS.

Cortisol principally affects protein catabolism. It induces muscle proteolysis and promotes gluconeogenesis, although it also significantly contributes to hypermetabolism in synergy with catecholamines.[17] Glucocorticoids cause this muscle proteolysis associated with cytokine release, and they have been shown to be a predictor of protein breakdown and hypermetabolism in both acutely stressed adult and pediatric populations. The major amino acid sources for gluconeogenesis are alanine and glutamine from skeletal muscle and gut, respectively. Hepatic uptake of these amino acids is accelerated during AMS.[18] Like glucagon, cortisol also causes insulin resistance. Although insulin concentrations may be increased during AMS, its anabolic effects are inhibited. Serum cortisol levels have also been shown to predict survival in critically ill children.[19]

Much of what is currently understood concerning the metabolic response to injury is based on the study of healthy adult subjects who were administered a triple intravenous infusion of cortisol, glucagon, and epinephrine in concentrations reported in various acutely injured critical care populations.[17] This triple hormone infusion, compared with saline controls, resulted in significant hypermetabolism, glucose intolerance, hyperglycemia associated with hyperinsulinemia, insulin resistance, negative nitrogen balance, peripheral leukocytosis, and increased potassium excretion. Together, these counter-regulatory hormones demonstrated additive and synergistic interactions to generate an overall metabolic effect greater than that observed with individual hormone infusions. These hormone-induced changes included significant protein catabolism with resultant increases in protein breakdown and nitrogen excretion in association with stable protein synthesis rates. In concert with increased potassium excretion, these findings are associated with losses of lean tissue mass, specifically body cell mass (which constitutes the metabolically active tissue pool of the host)[20], observed in critically ill populations in proportion to injury severity.[3,17] When this study was repeated with the addition of octreotide to suppress serum insulin concentrations to levels nearer those observed in acutely injured patients, skeletal muscle protein breakdown and whole-body nitrogen losses were substantially accelerated, resulting in substantially greater negative nitrogen and potassium balances.[21] In total, all of the findings noted in this section are emblematic of the AMS-response–associated clinical profile in both critically ill children and adults.

AMS-Associated Anabolic Hormone Resistance

Throughout human existence, the metabolic response to acute injury and disease has been characterized by an associated decrease or absence of exogenous nutrient intake (anorexia). A predominant clinical feature of serious illness in children is feeding intolerance or a decreased willingness to feed. This phenomenon causes the body to rely on the mobilization of endogenous fuel stores for the provision of substrates and energy required during the period of AMS. Because normal anabolic metabolism, which essentially results in the uptake of substrates from the circulation and their deposition in tissue stores, is counterproductive in the face of increased demands for substrate mobilization (and because the advent of exogenous tube feeding and intravenous nutritional support have appeared too recently within the overall time frame of human development for evolutionary adjustment to occur), the attenuation of anabolic hormone effects in response to acute injury states represents an important teleological evolutionary compensatory mechanism. This mechanism is characterized by the suppression of, or resistance to, the anabolic effects of several key hormones.

Because the anabolic effects of these hormones depend on a variety of associated mechanisms and conditions, it is important when interpreting published studies to understand which of these mechanisms and associated conditions are altered in regard to "resistance"; for example:

- the nature of the injury insult (e.g., sepsis versus burn)
- the substrate pool affected (e.g., glucose versus protein)
- the body pool sampled (e.g., splanchnic, hepatic, peripheral muscle, or systemic circulatory beds)
- the timing of serum samples taken relative to the onset of injury
- the use of exogenous intervention (nutritional, hormonal, etc.)

Lack of attention to these details has led to considerable controversy, especially in relation to the nature of insulin resistance.[22-28]

Insulin is a potent anabolic hormone responsible for glycogen synthesis and the storage of carbohydrate, lipogenesis and the storage of fat, and net protein synthesis. Insulin stimulates glucose uptake into skeletal and cardiac muscle cells, suppresses hepatic glucose production and release, inhibits FFA release from adipose tissue, decreases proteolysis, and stimulates the process by which amino acids are incorporated into protein. Insulin and IGF-1 are essential hormones for somatic growth in infants and children. Insulin resistance is a condition in which adequate serum insulin levels do not appropriately stimulate the cellular uptake of glucose. Instead, glucose production, lipolysis, fatty acid oxidation, and proteolysis are all increased in association with decreased muscle glucose uptake. Both injury-induced oxidative stress[29] and increased FFA production during acute injury states[30] have been implicated as putative mechanistic factors contributing to insulin resistance. Normally, the rate of skeletal muscle glucose uptake is directly proportional to serum glucose concentrations (as determined by the rate of glucose production in the absence of exogenous glucose delivery) and is augmented by insulin. In response to tissue injury, however, glucose production increases despite normal, or even elevated, serum insulin concentrations, while the normal insulin-stimulated cellular uptake of glucose by skeletal muscle and adipose tissue is attenuated. While insulin levels in burned children have been shown to increase in proportion to severity, insulin resistance also increases.[3] Acute injury states in critically ill adults and children are thus characterized by hyperglycemia despite atypically high serum insulin concentrations.[3,17] Most of the glucose uptake during this period occurs in insulin-independent tissues (brain, erythrocytes, wound tissue), so peripheral glucose clearance (glucose utilization divided by plasma glucose) usually remains elevated.[31]

Early studies in patients with burns and other injuries demonstrated hyperglycemia in association with elevated serum insulin concentrations[24,25] that could not be reversed by the administration of exogenous insulin. Subsequent studies in septic adults and severely burned children have reported failure of exogenous insulin to suppress hepatic glucose production despite concomitant provision of exogenous glucose.[27,32] Reduced glucose-stimulated insulin secretion[33] and decreased insulin-stimulated whole-body oxidation of carbohydrate (relative to healthy controls) have been documented in septic adult patients.[28]

Conflicting data relative to whether glucose oxidation is appropriate to circulating insulin levels may, in part, be explained by the fact that pyruvate dehydrogenase activity is dependent on the nature of the injury or insult. The activity of this enzyme has been shown to be depressed by 2- to 3-fold in sepsis (thus reducing aerobic metabolism and glucose oxidation),[34,35] whereas activity in adult burn patients is increased by 300%.[32]

Because insulin is known to promote net protein anabolism, primarily by decreasing proteolysis, the protein breakdown observed in AMS states has been ascribed to insulin resistance.[36] However, despite the presence of proteolysis, the protein anabolic effect of insulin has been reported to be intact.[37] Furthermore, decreased leucine oxidation and improved nitrogen retention have been observed in hyperinsulinemic burned patients.[38] These findings suggest that exogenous insulin might be used to reverse or retard injury-induced protein catabolism. The exogenous provision of extremely large insulin doses (10 times higher than the range generally observed in injured patients) in severely burned adults has been shown to increase muscle protein synthesis (approximately 350% relative to that of control subjects), but without improvement in the rate of burn or wound healing compared with that of the control group.[39]

More recently, insulin-induced reduction in pro-inflammatory cytokine expression with decreased acute-phase and increased constitutive hepatic protein synthesis has been demonstrated in burned rats,[40] possibly due to reduced hepatic endoplasmic reticulum stress.[41,42] This anti-inflammatory effect associated with insulin administration has also been documented in critically ill children.[43,44] Moreover, randomized prospective evaluation of the use of insulin to treat injury-induced hyperglycemia has demonstrated decreased morbidity and mortality in both critically ill children and adults[44-46] (see "Overfeeding Associated with Acute Meta bolic Stress").

In health, the major actions of GH are to decrease protein catabolism and promote protein synthesis, promote fat mobilization and the conversion of FFAs to acetyl-coenzyme A, and decrease glucose oxidation while increasing glycogen deposition. However, the anabolic effects of GH, particularly as they relate to protein metabolism, result from the GH-stimulated synthesis and secretion, principally by the liver, of an extremely potent anabolic agent: IGF-1. Insulin-like growth factor I synthesis and activity is modulated by a specific group of IGF-1-binding proteins that either facilitate or suppress the synthesis and activity of IGF-1. Of these, IGF-binding protein (BP) 3 (IGFBP-3) is the predominant IGF-1 facilitator, and IGFBP-1 is the predominant suppressor. During AMS, the GH/IGF-1 axis is suppressed, in part due to injury-induced cytokine expression (notably of TNF-alpha, IL-1, and IL-6).[13-15] While GH levels rise, both serum IGF-1 and IGFBP-3 concentrations decrease and serum IGFBP-1 concentrations increase.[3,6,13,47] In this state, the substrate-mobilizing effects of GH dominate, resulting in increased lipolysis and fatty acid oxidation. These findings reflect anabolic GH resistance during AMS states. Serum GH concentrations increase and serum IGF-1 concentrations decrease in direct proportion to the severity of the injury or insult and can be used to predict clinical outcome.[3,18] Elevated GH levels with decreased IGF-1 levels have been shown to differentiate critically ill children with sepsis and septic shock from healthy subjects,[19] and to differentiate sepsis from trauma in critically ill adults.[48]

As noted earlier, recent studies suggest that acute injury-induced catabolism can be partially reversed by the administration of insulin. Along these lines, recombinant human GH (rhGH) administration in burned children has been shown to increase serum IGF-1 and IGFBP-3 concentrations in association with increased protein synthesis and nitrogen balance, improved recovery of catabolized lean body mass, and improved clinical outcome.[3,49] Also in burned children, rhGH (with propranolol) administration has been shown to stimulate hepatic constitutive protein synthesis while suppressing hepatic acute-phase protein synthesis, modulating cytokine expression, and increasing IGF-1 concentrations,[50] similar to catabolism-reversing effects observed in acute injury animal models following exogenous insulin administration.[40,41]

Metabolic Alterations Associated with Acute Metabolic Stress

As a consequence of counter-regulatory hormone release and anabolic hormonal resistance described earlier in association with acute injury, a series of important alterations of protein, carbohydrate, and lipid metabolism ensue, primarily involving the liver but also including the circulating constitutive protein pool, skeletal musculature, intestine, and adipose tissue reserves. This response is predominantly catabolic. The circulating proteins are most immediately affected, resulting in a precipitous decrease in serum-constitutive protein concentrations in direct proportion to the severity of the catabolic insult,[3,18,51] returning toward normal values as the AMS response subsides.[18,51-54] In terms of skeletal muscle, there is a precipitous and substantial increase in protein breakdown, while protein synthesis rates remain relatively stable, resulting in a negative net protein balance[3,17] and increased free amino acid concentrations.[55] Net protein balance equates to net nitrogen balance, which can be determined by measuring 24-hour total urinary nitrogen excretion and subtracting daily protein intake. Serial net nitrogen balance determinations reflect the magnitude and duration of the catabolic response to injury.[56,57] An increased amount of amino acids is mobilized—primarily alanine and glutamine from skeletal muscle and intestinal pools—and flows to the liver[58] to facilitate hepatic gluconeogenesis and the synthesis of acute-phase proteins. Hepatic protein synthesis is reprioritized away from the constitutive proteins, including albumin, prealbumin (transthyretin), transferrin, and retinol-binding protein, to instead synthesize acute-phase reactants during acute injury-response states.[59] As a result, serum acute-phase protein pool marker concentrations, such as C-reactive protein (CRP), increase while constitutive protein levels, such as prealbumin, remain depressed.[3,56]

Resolution of the AMS response is characterized by decreasing serum acute-phase protein concentrations in conjunction with increasing serum constitutive protein levels.[53,56,60] This response pattern is associated with a return of hepatic constitutive protein synthesis and resumption of anabolic metabolism.

Prominent alterations in glucose homeostasis are characteristic of the acute injury response, and hyperglycemia is its hallmark. The normal suppressive effect of exogenous glucose administration on endogenous glucose production is ablated during metabolic stress states.[31,61] Glucose production increases in direct proportion to the magnitude of the stress response, and production rates depend principally on epinephrine- and glucagon-driven glycogenolysis and cortisol-driven gluconeogenesis. Hepatic glycogen stores represent an immediately available endogenous resource, capable of lasting 2 to 3 days in well-nourished older children, down to several hours or less in stressed infants, particularly preterm babies, because the increase in energy requirements to support brain metabolism in these patients easily exhaust circulating glucose levels, thus impeding hepatic glycogen storage during nonstress periods.[62] Gluconeogenesis is de novo glucose production from noncarbohydrate precursors, most notably from lactate and alanine. Plasma glucose is taken up by the cell and undergoes glycolysis to form pyruvate, which can then (1) undergo decarboxylation to enter the Krebs cycle, (2) undergo reduction to form lactate, or (3) undergo transamination to form alanine. The fate of pyruvate is largely determined by pyruvate dehydrogenase complex activity, which is injury-type dependent (e.g., highly stimulated by burn injury and suppressed by sepsis).[32,34,35] There is a redundant process in which plasma glucose is taken up by a skeletal muscle cell, where it undergoes glycolysis to form lactate which then re-enters the bloodstream. This lactate is taken up by hepatocytes for use as a substrate for gluconeogenesis to resynthesize glucose, which is then returned to the bloodstream, thus repleting plasma glucose levels, and completing the Cori cycle. Alanine is the major amino acid precursor for gluconeogenesis, and while injury-induced skeletal muscle catabolism provides a wide variety of free amino acids to fuel gluconeogenesis, much of the alanine comes from the peripheral glycolytic breakdown of glucose.[63] Peripheral glycolysis yields pyruvate, which can either enter the Krebs cycle for complete oxidation or can be transaminated, using amino-group nitrogen derived from muscle valine, leucine, and isoleucine, to form alanine. Alanine is then transported to the liver where it is deaminated to re-form pyruvate, which then undergoes gluconeogenesis to regenerate plasma glucose. This redundant process is called the *alanine cycle* and is the reason why considerably more alanine is released from skeletal muscle than actually constitutes skeletal muscle protein. Nitrogen derived from the hepatic deamination of amino acids is predominantly used to synthesize urea, but can also be incorporated into ammonia and used to buffer ketone bodies in the urine.[64] Thus, total urinary nitrogen reflects muscle protein catabolism.

Injury-induced alterations in lipid metabolism are principally catecholamine driven, under the control of β_2-adrenergic stimulation, and include increased lipolysis and fatty acid oxidation proportional to the severity and duration of the insult, as well as the adequacy of endogenous adipose reserves to meet catecholamine-mediated demands. Free fatty acid production rates are independent of the rate of FFA oxidation and, during AMS, can substantially exceed oxidation rates. Approximately 50% of nonoxidized fatty acids undergo re-esterification with glycerol 3-phosphate under normal metabolic conditions, primarily in the liver. This lipid-recycling pathway is called the triglyceride–fatty acid cycle. During AMS, re-esterification percentage can be considerably greater due to increased lipolysis, suggesting that FFA availability can surpass energy needs.[65] While it was initially thought that glucose metabolism was limited by the rate of FFA release via lipolysis, it has instead been more recently proposed that FFA oxidation is largely limited by glucose availability at the site of oxidation.[66] Because FFA transport to liver and skeletal muscle is serum albumin dependent, and because malnutrition reduces adipose lipid stores, the degree of injury-associated protein catabolism and/or malnutrition can have a detrimental effect on FFA availability for energy metabolism during critical illness.

Energy Metabolism Associated with Acute Metabolic Stress

The assessment of energy expenditure has been widely used to characterize alterations in metabolism and to determine daily caloric requirements accompanying a variety of clinical states in both health and disease. Energy requirement can be partitioned into (1) maintenance metabolic needs (basal metabolic rate, activity, and heat loss to the environment) and (2) energy required for growth. A small amount of energy is also required to digest food and enable its conversion into the nutrients that the body needs. Energy requirements are age related and may be up to 3 to 4 times higher per unit of body weight for infants than for adults.[67] Energy requirements are also dependent on metabolic status and nutritional reserve, and can change rapidly in response to acute injury stimuli.

However, acute injury markedly alters pediatric energy needs. First, acute injury induces a catabolic response that is proportional to the magnitude, nature, and duration of the injury. Increased serum counter-regulatory hormone concentrations induce insulin and GH resistance. This results in the catabolism of endogenous stores of protein, carbohydrate, and fat to provide essential substrate intermediates and energy necessary to support the metabolic stress response. Approximately 30% to 35% of predicted energy requirements for healthy infants are needed for growth. These requirements diminish during childhood to approximately 10% for adolescents, finally approaching normal adult maintenance requirements in the late teenage period. Growth-related requirements are inversely proportional to gestational age and approach 50% in very-low-birth-weight babies. During the injury-induced catabolic response period, however, somatic growth cannot occur. Second, children treated in the intensive care setting are frequently sedated and their activity level is markedly reduced, further lowering energy needs. Third, the intensive care environment is temperature controlled and insensible energy losses are substantially reduced. This is especially true for children who are mechanically ventilated because, in addition to reduced energy needs for the work of breathing, these patients are ventilated with warmed, humidified air. This practice alone can reduce insensible losses by one-third. In concert, these factors result in substantial decreases in energy needs. Although increments in energy expenditure associated with the magnitude and duration of injury response per se have been documented, these positive values are substantially less than the reduction in daily needs due to inhibited growth, decreased activity, and decreased insensible heat losses.[68] Therefore, if calorie repletion based on the predicted requirements for healthy infants and children is administered during the acute phase of metabolic stress in critically ill infants, clinically significant overfeeding is likely.[56,69,70]

To account for these alterations in energy metabolism, caloric amounts equal to measured energy expenditure values or basal energy requirements should be provided. The significance of this therapeutic strategy is that it avoids the provision of calories and/or nutritional substrates in excess of the energy required to maintain the metabolic homeostasis of the injury response. Gender-based basal energy expenditure data are available in the publications of Talbot[71] and/or Schofield[72] for infants and children up to 18 years of age.

The value of indirect calorimetry in the intensive care setting lies in the fact that estimations of energy expenditure based on equations derived from other clinical criteria are notoriously inaccurate.[73-75] Although average measured energy expenditure (MEE) values in large series of patients tend to differentiate various degrees of injury, individual subjects can respond to similar injury states with widely diverse MEE values.[68,69,76] The actual MEE is frequently much less than predicted values based on the clinical grounds.[77] For this reason, predictive equations, even those specifically derived from pediatric populations, are significantly inaccurate (in approximately 75% of critically ill children) and most frequently overestimate the daily energy expenditure, which leads to excess caloric administration,[73] especially if an arbitrary incremental amount is added to account for metabolic stress.[77] During the course of the metabolic stress response, energy expenditure may change substantially in response to alterations in the insult (magnitude, duration, second injury or insult, etc.). For this reason, it is important to measure energy needs daily during the acute injury response period. Measurements can be carried out at bedside within 30 minutes or less, depending on patient stability.[69,77]

Pediatric energy expenditure after elective, complication-free surgical procedures does not increase substantially above measured baseline values.[78] The characteristics of injury metabolism will be present only during the acute stress response period. For surgical stress alone, this period is relatively short, generally less than 48 hours. For this reason, studies that attempt to evaluate surgically related acute stress changes during later post-injury periods are potentially flawed[79] and may introduce misleading conclusions. High response variability, in large part, may be attributable to substantial differences in the acute metabolic demands imposed by the underlying disease process (e.g., trauma, burns, sepsis) and the ability of the host to meet these demands (size and recruitability of host endogenous metabolic reserves).[3,5] In the final analysis, the most accurate way to currently manage nutritional resuscitation and avoid overfeeding during AMS is to measure energy expenditure daily and provide caloric repletion in exactly the MEE amount.[56]

Clinical Significance

Clinical Assessment of Injury Severity

Currently, adult injury severity analysis tools are still frequently used in critically ill children, notably in pediatric trauma patients. While a number of assessment instruments for determining injury severity have been developed specifically for children, metabolic parameters of injury response do not play a prominent role in currently available pediatric scoring systems.[80-85] As previously discussed, serum concentrations of acute-phase reactants, constitutive proteins, and blood glucose levels have been shown to reflect the magnitude and duration of the inflammatory, catabolic, and glycemic response to injury insult, respectively, in critically ill children.[3-5,18,51,52,54,68,86-88] As such, these metabolic response indices constitute a basis for injury severity analysis. A number of these studies have demonstrated a correlation between the patterns of metabolic response, based on *serial* monitoring of acute-phase and glycemic response parameters, and clinical outcome.[3,5,18,51,87] These findings support the development of acute injury scoring systems that incorporate such metabolic response indicators. As further substantiation of this concept, a modified Nutritional Index (NI) score utilizing serum acute-phase and constitutive protein metabolic stress response indices has recently been found to correlate well with injury-induced cytokine release and pediatric-adjusted injury severity scores.[86]

Relative to the way scoring systems are currently designed to be utilized, assessment tools—which are meant to be applied over a limited time interval, usually relying on a single evaluation of selected parameters at the onset of injury or upon admission to the intensive care unit—serve principally to delineate the magnitude of the insult and may describe the initial pathophysiologic status of the patient. They may even be used to predict outcome based on generally established trends, but provide little insight into the course of the individual patient response, which may be highly variable. In this regard, metabolic response markers, such as those previously discussed, can easily be serially monitored and thus provide a useful basis upon which to develop a dynamic injury assessment tool that could be applied on a daily basis to better characterize the evolving metabolic response to injury in critically ill children.[87-88] The putative value of this dynamic scoring system would be to more effectively adjust therapy to better address individual patient injury response status. As noted earlier, ample literature now exists to support the use of these metabolic response parameters, both to characterize the severity of injury or insult and to serve as a basis for the implementation of clinical therapeutic strategies.

OVERFEEDING ASSOCIATED WITH ACUTE METABOLIC STRESS

Overfeeding occurs during AMS, when the administration of calories or specific substrate exceeds the requirements to maintain metabolic homeostasis. These requirements, which vary according to the patient's age, state of health, and underlying nutritional status, are substantially altered during periods of injury-induced AMS. Excess nutritional delivery during this period can further increase the metabolic demands of acute injury.[89] Stress metabolism cannot be reversed by overfeeding during critical illness. Instead, overfeeding further increases the negative impact of metabolic stress by increasing hyperglycemia-associated risks and by augmenting the pulmonary and hepatic workload.[75,90] Excess caloric delivery has been shown to increase injury-associated morbidity and mortality in both pediatric and adult studies.[56,70,91-92] Younger children are particularly vulnerable in this regard. Therefore, it is important to ensure that calorie intake not exceed demand during the period of AMS in critically ill infants and children.

Pulmonary Pathophysiology

Excess caloric delivery, particularly excess carbohydrate administration, causes lipogenesis. Glucose administered in excess of maximum oxidation rates undergoes fat biosynthesis (lipogenesis), resulting in substantial increases in carbon dioxide production.[75,89,90,93-95] Since fatty acid oxidation is the predominant energy-generating pathway during acute injury response, excess lipid administration also promotes lipogenesis by reducing carbohydrate oxidation.[66] Pulmonary functional compromise results from the increased work of breathing due to excess carbon dioxide production.[75,89,91] This effect is harmful in critically ill postoperative children and can induce or prolong the requirement for mechanical ventilation and intensive care length of stay.[70] Preterm infants are especially vulnerable to the respiratory effects of overfeeding because of their immature pulmonary development and limited respiratory reserve.[75]

Hepatic Pathophysiology

Overfeeding also negatively affects hepatic morphology and function. Acute metabolic stress increases lipolysis and FFA oxidation. Counter-regulatory hormone-induced insulin resistance reduces the efficiency with which exogenous carbohydrate is metabolized. With excessive carbohydrate delivery, serum insulin, glucose, glucose oxidation, and fatty acid oxidation increase and lipogenesis remains high.[96] These metabolic events increase the hepatic workload and further predispose the liver to hepatic cellular injury, resulting in hepatic dysfunction.[56,89] Lipid overfeeding with long-chain triglyceride (LCT) formulations can inhibit the ability of the reticuloendothelial system of the liver to clear bacteria during acute injury states.[97] Decreased hepatic bacterial clearance is associated with increased bacterial sequestration in the lung, resulting in increased pulmonary neutrophil activation and the release of inflammatory mediators. Enteral replacement of LCT with medium-chain triglyceride (MCT), which is absorbed directly into the blood from the gut, preserves liver reticuloendothelial system function and reduces lung bacterial sequestration.[98] Parenteral lipid overfeeding heightens the risk of induced hepatic dysfunction, because standard lipid emulsions (e.g., Intralipid) contain high concentrations of linoleic acid. This omega-6 fatty acid and arachidonic acid precursor selectively stimulates the synthetic pathways of prostaglandins with high inflammatory activity, thus increasing inflammatory changes (steatosis, cholestasis, fibrosis) within the liver parenchyma.[99,100] In contrast, the use of lipid emulsions with omega-3 fatty acid (fish oil), which stimulates arachidonic acid pathways with lesser inflammatory activity, has been suggested as a strategy to improved or reverse parenteral nutrition-associated liver disease (PNALD).[101] This strategy may be particularly important in critically ill infants and children requiring long-term parenteral nutrition (e.g., with necrotizing enterocolitis, gastroschisis, short gut syndrome, etc.). Furthermore, the administration of even minimal amounts of enteral feedings can stimulate intestinal trophic hormone secretion, thus reducing the inflammatory effects of bacterial translocation and decreasing PNALD.[102]

Immune System Pathophysiology

As discussed previously (see "Acute Metabolic Stress Response"), the response to acute injury can itself result in hyperglycemia. Excess caloric delivery can result in an immunocompromised state by causing hyperglycemia. Deficiencies in white blood cell activation and function, including impaired granulocyte adhesion, chemotaxis and phagocytosis, decreased respiratory burst, and impaired intracellular killing, as well as decreased immunoglobulin function and complement fixation, have been demonstrated in vitro in direct association with hyperglycemia and have been shown to improve with glucose control.[103,104] Functional leukocyte abnormalities have been associated with sustained blood glucose levels greater than 200 mg/dL (11.1 mmol/L) and become more severe as serum levels increase. A number of studies have associated hyperglycemia with increased mortality and morbidity in critically ill adults and children.[46,49,70,105] Furthermore, exogenous insulin therapy to control blood glucose concentrations below 120 mg/dL (6.7 mmol/L) has been shown to improve morbidity and mortality in certain critically ill adults and children[44-46,49] in association with improved insulin sensitivity and mitochondrial oxidative capacity, a decreased inflammatory response, and decreased infection-related complications.[45,49]

Hyperglycemia can also result from excess caloric delivery from either parenteral or enteral routes. Parenteral nutrition is more typically associated with overfeeding-related hyperglycemia,[106] in part due to the absence of natural physiologic mechanisms, such as ileus and malabsorption, resulting in vomiting and diarrhea, which can help to protect the body against excessive caloric nutrition administered enterally. Overfeeding can be particularly harmful in critically ill patients during acute injury (catabolic) states where, in contrast to anabolic states, excess calories cannot be effectively deposited in storage compartments such as adipose tissue.[56,96] Thus, excess caloric delivery in this patient population can further increase injury-related hyperglycemia. Indirect calorimetric assessment in the adult intensive care setting has shown that, in the absence of serious burns, multiple trauma, or severe head injury, most patients have a resting energy expenditure of approximately 25 kcal/kg per day[107] and that if caloric delivery does not exceed this amount, overfeeding-associated hyperglycemia can be avoided.[108] Moreover, when energy delivery in adult patients substantially exceeds this amount, particularly parenteral delivery, hyperglycemia and infectious complications increase.[106,109-111]

Numerous studies have associated hyperglycemia with increased mortality and morbidity in critically ill adults and children.[44,46,70,87,105] Furthermore, some studies in adult and pediatric intensive care populations using insulin therapy have demonstrated significantly improved mortality and morbidity associated with tight glycemic control (blood glucose 80-110 mg/dL (4.4-6.1 mmol/L)).[44,46] This therapy has also resulted in higher rates of transient hypoglycemia that were substantially greater in enterally versus parenterally fed patients. Therapeutic glycemic target adjustment (<150 mg/dL (8.3 mmol/L) versus <110 mg/dL(6.1 mmol/L)), more accurate monitoring (point-of-care), parenteral nutrition, and appropriately applied algorithms have been shown to reduce insulin-induced hypoglycemia.[112]

SERIAL AMS RESPONSE ASSESSMENT

Nutrition assessment of critically ill infants must account for the acute metabolic impact due to injury severity and can be best accomplished clinically by serial measurement of (1) the visceral (or constitutive) protein pool, (2) the acute-phase protein pool, and (3) energy expenditure (see "Energy Metabolism Associated with Acute Metabolic Stress"). The variations of the injury response can thus be established on the basis of serial changes (response pattern) in the serum concentrations of CRP, an acute-phase protein pool marker, and prealbumin, a visceral protein pool marker.[3,18,68] Serum CRP and prealbumin concentrations are readily measured in most hospital clinical laboratories. Albumin should not be used because acute catabolic and anabolic changes, which occur in association with the evolving metabolic response to injury, have a smaller impact on overall serum levels of this visceral protein due to its substantially larger pool size and much longer endogenous serum half-life. Within 12 to 24 hours following injury, serum prealbumin levels fall, reflecting catabolism, and CRP levels rise because of hepatic reprioritization of protein synthesis in response to injury. During this acute metabolic injury response state, calories should be administered to match only MEE-established needs. If indirect calorimetry is unavailable, only basal metabolic needs should be administered.[71-72] Serum prealbumin and CRP levels are inversely related (i.e., serum prealbumin levels decrease and CRP levels increase with a magnitude proportional to injury severity and then return to normal as the acute metabolic response to injury resolves) and should be measured serially to establish the injury response pattern. Acute-phase protein changes have been shown to correlate well with glycemic response changes.[3,87] Serum blood glucose, prealbumin, and CRP concentrations have also been shown to be useful in predicting clinical outcome in critically ill children.[3,5,18,86,87] Furthermore, serum CRP concentrations have been shown to correlate well with MEE in this patient population.[88] Decreases in serum CRP values in conjunction with increases in serum prealbumin indicate resolution of the post-injury inflammatory (metabolic stress) response and cessation of catabolic metabolism.[3,18,75] In this regard, increasing serum prealbumin levels are particularly important, signifying the resumption of somatic growth (adaptive anabolic phase) at which time calories can be advanced to promote growth recovery.[52] This method provides a potentially useful guide to advance calorie delivery and optimize growth recovery without overfeeding infants during the acute phase of the metabolic response to injury.[56]

KEY POINTS

- The adaptive AMS response to injury in humans is stereotypical, but the hypermetabolic state is attenuated in children.
- The response is characterized by a cytokine-mediated increase in serum levels of counter-regulatory hormones with GH and insulin resistance.

- Endogenous protein breakdown during this response allows the release of free amino acids that are utilized for anti-inflammatory response, gluconeogenesis, and tissue repair.
- Sustained protein breakdown may result in significant loss of lean body mass during critical illness.
- Accurate assessment and provision of energy to match demand during acute stress is an important goal of critical care. Unintended underfeeding or overfeeding may be associated with poor outcomes.
- Adequate protein and energy intake, while unable to halt the protein breakdown, helps maintain protein balance and prevent lean body mass depletion during this period.

REFERENCES

1. Chang HR, Bistrian B. The role of cytokines in the catabolic consequences of infection and injury. *J Parenter Enteral Nutr*. 1998;22(3):156-166.
2. Hasselgren PO. Catabolic response to stress and injury: implications for regulation. *World J Surg*. 2000;24(12):1452-1459.
3. Jeschke MG, Chinkes DL, Finnerty CC, et al. Pathophysiologic response to severe burn injury. *Ann Surg*. 2008;248(3):387-401.
4. Wolfe RR. Sepsis as a modulator of adaptation to low and high carbohydrate and low and high fat intakes. *Eur J Clin Nutr*. 1999;53(1)(suppl):S136-S142.
5. Chwals WJ, Fernandez ME, Jamie AC, Charles BJ, Rushing JT. Detection of postoperative sepsis in infants using metabolic stress monitoring. *Arch Surg*. 1994;129(4):437-442.
6. Vanhorebeek I, Van den Berghe G. The neuroendocrine response to critical illness is a dynamic process. *Crit Care Clin*. 2006;22:1-15.
7. Ouyang W, Rutz S, Crellin NK, Valdez PA, Hymowitz SG. Regulation and functions of the IL-10 family of cytokines in inflammation and disease. *Annu Rev Immunol*. 2011;29:71-109.
8. Sander LE, Sackett SD, Dierssen U, et al. Hepatic acute-phase proteins control innate immune responses during infection by promoting myeloid-derived suppressor cell function. *J Exp Med*. 2010 5;207(7):1453-1464.
9. Proulx F, Joyal JS, Mariscalco MM, Leteurtre S, Leclerc F, Lacroix J. The pediatric multiple organ dysfunction syndrome. *Pediatr Crit Care Med*. 2009;10(1):12-22.
10. Reikerås O. Immune depression in musculoskeletal trauma. *Inflamm Res*. 2010;59(6):409-414.
11. Boisclair YR, Wang J, Shi J, Hurst KR, Ooi GT. Role of the suppressor of cytokine signaling-3 in mediating the inhibitory effects of interleukin-1beta on the growth hormone-dependent transcription of the acid-labile subunit gene in liver cells. *J Biol Chem*. 2000;275(6):3841-3847.
12. Wang P, Li N, Li JS, Li WQ. The role of endotoxin, TNF-alpha, and IL-6 in inducing the state of growth hormone insensitivity. *World J Gastroenterol*. 2002;8(3):531-536.
13. Lang CH, Fan J, Cooney R, Vary TC. IL-1 receptor antagonist attenuates sepsis-induced alterations in the IGF system and protein synthesis. *Am J Physiol*. 1996;270(3 Pt 1):E430-E437.
14. Delhanty PJ. Interleukin-1 beta suppresses growth hormone-induced acid-labile subunit mRNA levels and secretion in primary hepatocytes. *Biochem Biophys Res Commun*. 1998;243(1):269-272.
15. Samstein B, Hoimes ML, Fan J, Frost RA, Gelato MC, Lang CH. IL-6 stimulation of insulin-like growth factor binding protein (IGFBP)-1 production. *Biochem Biophys Res Commun*. 1996;228(2):611-615.
16. Michie HR, Spriggs DR, Manogue KR, et al. Tumor necrosis factor and endotoxin induce similar metabolic responses in human beings. *Surgery*. 1988;104:280-286.
17. PQ Bessey, JM Watters, TT Aoki, DW Wilmore. Combined hormonal infusion simulates the metabolic response to injury. *Ann Surg*. 1984;200(3):264-281.
18. Pons Leite H, Gilberto Henriques Vieira J, Brunow De Carvalho W, Chwals WJ. The role of insulin-like growth hormone and plasma proteins in surgical outcome of children with congenital heart disease. *Pediatr Crit Care Med*. 2001;2:29-35.
19. Onenli-Mungan N, Yildizdas D, Yapicioglu H, Topaloglu AK, Yüksel B, Ozer G. Growth hormone and insulin-like growth factor 1 levels and their relation to survival in children with bacterial sepsis and septic shock. *J Paediatr Child Health*. 2004;40(4):221-226.
20. Moore FD, Olesen KH, McMurray JD, Parker HV, Ball MR, Boyden CM. *The Body Cell Mass and Its Supporting Environment: Body Composition in Health and Disease*. W.B. Saunders (Phila.- Lond.), 1963.
21. Bessey PQ, Lowe KA. Early hormonal changes affect the catabolic response to trauma. *Ann Surg*. 1993;218(4):476-489;discussion 489-491.
22. Shangraw RE, Jahoor F, Miyoshi H, et al. Differentiation between septic and postburn insulin resistance. *Metabolism*. 1989;38(10):983-939.
23. Gump FE, Long C, Killian P, Kinney JM. Studies of glucose intolerance in septic injured patients. *J Trauma*. 1974;14:378-388.

24. Evans EI, Butterfield WJH. The stress response in the severely burned. *Ann Surg*. 1951;134:588-613.

25. Howard JM. Studies of the absorption and metabolism of glucose following injury. The systemic response to injury. *Ann Surg*. 1955;141:321-326.

26. White RH, Frayn KN, Little RA, Threlfall CJ, Stoner HB, Irving MH. Hormonal and metabolic responses to glucose infusion in sepsis by the hyperglycaemic glucose clamp technique. *J Parenter Enteral Nutr*. 1987;11:345-353.

27. Long CL, Kinney JN, Geiger JW. Nonsuppressability of gluconeogenesis by glucose in septic patients. *Metabolism*. 1976;25:193-201.

28. Henderson AA, Frayn KN, Galasko CS, et al. Dose-response relationships for the effects of insulin on glucose and fat metabolism in injured patients and control subjects. *Clin Sci (Colch)*. 1991;80:25-32.

29. Ceriello A, Motz E. Is oxidative stress the pathogenic mechanism underlying insulin resistance, diabetes, and cardiovascular disease? The common soil hypothesis revisited. *Arterioscler Thromb Vasc Biol*. 2004;24(5):816-823.

30. Roden M, Price TB, Perseghin G, et al. Mechanism of free fatty acid–induced insulin resistance in humans. *J Clin Invest*. 1996;97:2859-2865.

31. Wolfe RR, Durkot MJ, Allsop JR, Burke JF. Glucose metabolism in severely burned patients. *Metabolism*. 1979;28(10):1031-1039.

32. Wolfe RR, Jahoor R, Herndon DN, Miyoshi H. Isotopic evaluation of the metabolism of pyruvate and related substrates in normal adult volunteers and severely burned children: effect of dichloroacetate and glucose infusion. *Surgery*. 1991;110:54-67.

33. Dahn MS, Jacobs LA, Smith S, et al. The relationship of insulin production to glucose metabolism in severe sepsis. *Arch Surg*. 1985;120:166-172.

34. Vary TC. Sepsis-induced alterations in pyruvate dehydrogenase complex activity in rat skeletal muscle: effects on plasma lactate. *Shock*. 1996;6(2):89-94.

35. Vary TC, Siegel JH, Nakatani T, Sato T, Aoyama H. Regulation of glucose metabolism by altered pyruvate dehydrogenase activity. I. Potential site of insulin resistance in sepsis. *J Parenter Enteral Nutr*. 1986;10(4):351-355.

36. Frayn KN, Little RA, Stoner HB, Galasko CS. Metabolic control in non-septic patients with musculoskeletal injuries. *Injury*. 1984;16:73-79.

37. Brooks DC, Bessey PQ, Black PR, et al. Insulin stimulates branched chain amino acid uptake and diminished nitrogen flux from skeletal muscle of injured patients. *J Surg Res*. 1987;40:395-405.

38. Jahoor F, Shangraw RE, Miyoshi H, Wallfish H, Herndon DN, Wolfe RR. Role of insulin and glucose oxidation in mediating the protein catabolism of burns and sepsis. *Am J Physiol*. 1989;257:E323-E331.

39. Sakurai Y, Aarsland A, Herndon DN, et al. Stimulation of muscle protein synthesis by long-term insulin infusion in severely burned patients. *J Parenter Enteral Nutr*. 1994;18:214-218.

40. Klein D, Schubert T, Horch RE, Jauch KW, Jeschke MG. Insulin treatment improves hepatic morphology and function through modulation of hepatic signals after severe trauma. *Ann Surg*. 2004;240:340-349.

41. Jeschke MG, Kraft R, Song J, et al. Insulin protects against hepatic damage postburn. *Mol Med*. 2011;17(5-6):516-522.

42. Jeschke MG, Finnerty CC, Herndon DN, et al. Severe injury is associated with insulin resistance, endoplasmic reticulum stress response, and unfolded protein response. *Ann Surg*. 2012;255(2):370-378.

43. Jeschke MG, Klein D, Herndon DN. Insulin treatment improves the systemic inflammatory reaction to severe trauma. *Ann Surg*. 2004;239(4):553-560.

44. Vlasselaers D, Milants I, Desmet L, et al. Intensive insulin therapy for patients in paediatric intensive care: a prospective, randomised controlled study. *Lancet*. 2009;373:547-556.

45. Jeschke MG, Kulp GA, Kraft R, et al. Intensive insulin therapy in severely burned pediatric patients: a prospective randomized trial. *Am J Respir Crit Care Med*. 2010;182(3):351-359.

46. Van den Berghe G, Wouters P, Weekers F, et al. Intensive insulin therapy in critically ill patients. *N Engl J Med*. 2001 8;345(19):1359-1367.

47. Teng Chung T, Hinds CJ. Treatment with GH and IGF-1 in critical illness. *Crit Care Clin*. 2006;22(1):29-40, vi.

48. Pittoni G, Gallioi G, Zanello M, et al. Activity of GH/IGF-1 axis in trauma and septic patients during artificial nutrition: different behavior patterns? *J Endocrinol Invest*. 2002;25(3):214-223.

49. Fram RY, Cree MG, Wolfe RR, et al. Intensive insulin therapy improves insulin sensitivity and mitochondrial function in severely burned children. *Crit Care Med*. 2010;38(6):1475-1483.

50. Jeschke MG, Finnerty CC, Kulp GA, Przkora R, Mlcak RP, Herndon DN. Combination of recombinant human growth hormone and propranolol decreases hypermetabolism and inflammation in severely burned children. *Pediatr Crit Care Med*. 2008;9(2):209-216.

51. Chwals WJ, Fernandez ME, Jamie AC, Charles BJ. Relationship of metabolic indexes to postoperative mortality in surgical infants. *J Pediatr Surg*. 1993;28(6):819-822.

52. Tueting JL, Byerley LO, Chwals WJ. Anabolic recovery relative to degree of prematurity after acute injury in neonates. *J Pediatr Surg.* 1999;34(1):13-16;discussion 16-17.

53. Chwals WJ, Fernandez ME, Charles BJ, Schroeder LA, Turner CS. Serum visceral protein levels reflect protein-calorie repletion in neonates recovering from major surgery. *J Pediatr Surg.* 1992;27(3):317-320;discussion 320-321.

54. Briassoulis G, Zavras N, Hatzis T. Malnutrition, nutritional indices, and early enteral feeding in critically ill children. *Nutrition.* 2001;17(7-8):548-557.

55. Souba WW, Wilmore DW. Postoperative alteration of arteriovenous exchange of amino acids across the gastrointestinal tract. *Surgery.* 1983;94(2):342-350.

56. Chwals WJ. Overfeeding the critically ill child: fact or fantasy? *New Horiz.* 1994;2(2):147-155.

57. Mackenzie TA, Clark NG, Bistrian BR, Flatt JP, Hallowell EM, Blackburn GL. A simple method for estimating nitrogen balance in hospitalized patients: a review and supporting data for a previously proposed technique. *J Am Coll Nutr.* 1985;4(5):575-581.

58. Karinch AM, Pan M, Lin CM, Strange R, Souba WW. Glutamine metabolism in sepsis and infection. *J Nutr.* 2001; 131(9)(suppl):2535S-2538S.

59. Dickson PW, Bannister D, Schreiber G. Minor burns lead to major changes in synthesis rates of plasma proteins in the liver. *J Trauma.* 1987;27(3):283-286.

60. Davis CJ, Sowa D, Keim KS, Kinnare K, Peterson S. The use of prealbumin and C-reactive protein for monitoring nutrition support in adult patients receiving enteral nutrition in an urban medical center. *J Parenter Enteral Nutr.* 2012;36(2):197-204.

61. Shaw JH, Wolfe RR. Determinations of glucose turnover and oxidation in normal volunteers and septic patients using stable and radio-isotopes: the response to glucose infusion and total parenteral feeding. *Aust N Z J Surg.* 1986;56(10):785-791.

62. Chugani HT, Phelps ME, Mazziotta JC. Positron emission tomography study of human brain functional development. *Ann Neurol.* 1987;22(4):487-497.

63. Felig P. The glucose-alanine cycle. *Metabolism.* 1973;22(2):179-207.

64. Felig P, Marliss EB, Cahill GF Jr. Metabolic response to human growth hormone during prolonged starvation. *J Clin Invest.* 1971;50(2):411-421.

65. Wolfe RR, Herndon DN, Jahoor F, Miyoshi H, Wolfe M. Effect of severe burn injury on substrate cycling by glucose and fatty acids. *N Engl J Med.* 1987 13;317(7):403-408.

66. Wolfe RR. Metabolic interactions between glucose and fatty acids in humans. *Am J Clin Nutr.* 1998;67(3)(suppl): 519S-526S.

67. Holliday MA. Body composition and energy needs during growth. In: Falkner F, Tanner JM, eds. *Human Growth: A Comprehensive Treatise.* 2nd ed. (vol 2), Postnatal Growth Neurobiology. New York: Plenum;();1986:102-104.

68. Chwals WJ, Letton RW, Jamie A, Charles B. Stratification of injury severity using energy expenditure response in surgical infants. *J Pediatr Surg.* 1995;30:1161-1164.

69. Chwals WJ, Lally KP, Woolley MM, Mahour GH. Measured energy expenditure in critically ill infants and young children. *J Surg Res.* 1988;44:467-472.

70. Alaedeen DI, Walsh MC, Chwals WJ. Total parenteral nutrition-associated hyperglycemia correlates with prolonged mechanical ventilation and hospital stay in septic infants. *J Pediatr Surg.* 2006;41(1):239-244;discussion 239-244.

71. Talbot FB. Basal metabolism standards for children. *Am J Dis Child.* 1938;55:455-459.

72. Schofield WN. Predicting basal metabolic rate: new standards and review of previous work. *Hum Nutr Clin Nutr.* 1985;(1)(suppl):5-41.

73. De Wit B, Meyer R, Desai A, Macrae D, Pathan N. Challenge of predicting resting energy expenditure in children undergoing surgery for congenital heart disease. *Pediatr Crit Care Med.* 2010;11(4):496-501.

74. Framson_CM, LeLeiko NS, Dallal GE, Roubenoff R, Snelling LK, Dwyer JT. Energy expenditure in critically ill children. *Pediatr Crit Care Med.* 2007;8(3):264-267.

75. Letton RW, Chwals WJ, Jamie A, Charles B. Early postoperative alterations in infant energy use increase the risk of overfeeding. *J Pediatr Surg.* 1995;30(7):988-992;discussion 992-993.

76. Long CL, Schaffel N, Geiger JW, Schiller WR, Blakemore WS. Metabolic response to injury and illness: estimation of energy and protein needs from indirect calorimetry and nitrogen balance. *J Parenter Enteral Nutr.* 1979;3:452-456.

77. Mehta NM, Bechard LJ, Dolan M, Ariagno K, Jiang H, Duggan C. Energy imbalance and the risk of overfeeding in critically ill children. *Pediatr Crit Care Med.* 2011;12(4):398-405.

78. Shanbhogue RL, Lloyd DA. Absence of hypermetabolism after operation in the newborn infant. *MPEN J Parenter Enteral Nutr.* 1992;16:333-336.

79. Jones MO, Pierro A, Hammond P, Lloyd DA. The metabolic response to operative stress in infants. *J Pediatr Surgery.* 1993;28:1258-1263.

80. Graciano AL, Balko JA, Rahn DS, Ahmad N, Giroir BP. The Pediatric Multiple Organ Dysfunction Score (P-MODS): development and validation of an objective scale to measure the severity of multiple organ dysfunction in critically ill children. *Crit Care Med.* 2005;33(7):1484-1491.

81. Pollack MM, Patel KM, Ruttimann UE. PRISM III: an updated Pediatric Risk of Mortality score. *Crit Care Med.* 1996;24(5):743-752.

82. Zupancic JA, Richardson DK, Horbar JD, et al. Revalidation of the score for neonatal acute physiology in the Vermont Oxford Network. *Pediatrics.* 2007;119(1):e156-e163.

83. Shann F, Pearson G, Slater A, Wilkinson K. Paediatric index of mortality (PIM): a mortality prediction model for children in intensive care. *Intensive Care Med.* 1997;23(2):201-207.

84. Leteurtre S, Martinot A, Duhamel A, et al. Validation of the paediatric logistic organ dysfunction (PELOD) score: prospective, observational, multicentre study. *Lancet.* 2003 19;362(9379):192-197.

85. Bhal S, Tygai V, Kumar N, Sreenivas V, Puliyel JM. Signs of inflammation in children that can kill (SICK score): preliminary prospective validation of a new non-invasive measure of severity-of-illness. *J Postgrad Med.* 2006;52(2): 102-105.

86. Briassoulis G, Venkataraman S, Thompson A. Cytokines and metabolic patterns in pediatric patients with critical illness. *Clin Dev Immunol.* 2010:354047. doi: 10.1155/2010/354047. Epub 2010 May 16.

87. Brunengraber LN, Robinson AV, Chwals WJ. Relationship of serum C-reactive protein and blood glucose levels with injury severity and patient morbidity in a pediatric trauma population. *J Pediatr Surg.* 2009;44(5): 992-996.

88. Letton RW, Chwals WJ, Jamie A, Charles B. Neonatal lipid utilization increases with injury severity: recombinant human growth hormone versus placebo. *J Pediatr Surg.* 1996;31(8):1068-1072;discussion 1072-1074.

89. Askanazi J, Carpentier YA, Elwyn DH, et al. Influence of total parenteral nutrition on fuel utilization in injury and sepsis. *Ann Surg.* 1980;191(1):40-46.

90. Askanazi J, Nordenstrom J, Rosenbaum SH, et al. Nutrition for the patient with respiratory failure: glucose vs. fat. *Anesthesiology.* 1981;54(5):373-377.

91. Elwyn DH, Kinney JM, Jeevanandam M, Gump FE, Broell JR. Influence of increasing carbohydrate intake on glucose kinetics in injured patients. *Ann Surg.* 1979;190: 117-127.

92. Askanazi J, Carpentier YA, Elwyn DH, et al. Influence of total parenteral nutrition on fuel utilization in injury and sepsis. *Ann Surg.* 1980;191:40-46.

93. McGilvery RW. Fuel for breathing. *Am Rev Respir Dis.* 1979;119(2 Pt 2):85-88.

94. Bresson JL, Mariotti A, Narcy P, Ricour C, Sachs C, Rey J. Recovery of [13C]-bicarbonate as respiratory $13CO_2$ in parenterally fed infants. *Eur J Clin Nutr.* 1990; 44(1):3-9.

95. Van den Berg B, Stam H. Metabolic and respiratory effects of enteral nutrition in patients during mechanical ventilation. *Intensive Care Med.* 1988;14:206-211.

96. Wolfe RR. Substrate utilization/insulin resistance in sepsis/trauma. *Baillieres Clin Endocrinol Metab.* 1997;11(4):645-657.

97. Hirschberg Y, Pomposelli JJ, Mascioli EA, Bistrian BR, Blackburn GL. Effect of tracer and intravenous fat emulsion on the measurement of reticuloendothelial system function. *J Parenter Enteral Nutr.* 1990;14(5):463-466.

98. Sobrado J, Moldawer LL, Pomposelli JJ, et al. Lipid emulsions and reticuloendothelial system function in healthy and burned guinea pigs. *Am J Clin Nutr.* 1985;42(5): 855-863.

99. Tazuke Y, Teitelbaum D, Wasa M, Fukuzawa M, Iiboshi Y, Fujimoto J. Parenteral nutrition administration leads to specific alterations in the expression of adipocytokines and peroxisome proliferator-activated receptors in a rat model. *J Parenter Enteral Nutr.* 2011;35(3): 329-336.

100. Cober MP, Killu G, Brattain A, Welch KB, Kunisaki SM, Teitelbaum DH. Intravenous fat emulsions reduction for patients with parenteral nutrition-associated liver disease. *J Pediatr.* 2012;160(3):421-427.

101. Kalish BT, Le HD, Fitzgerald JM, et al. Intravenous fish oil lipid emulsion promotes a shift toward anti-inflammatory proresolving lipid mediators. *Am J Physiol Gastrointest Liver Physiol.* 2013;305(11):G818-G828.

102. Aynsley-Green A, Lucas A, Lawson GR, Bloom SR. Gut hormones and regulatory peptides in relation to enteral feeding, gastroenteritis, and necrotizing enterocolitis in infancy. *J Pediatr.* 1990;117(1 Pt 2):S24-S32.

103. McMahon MM, Bistrian BR. Host defenses and susceptibility to infection in patients with diabetes mellitus. *Infect Dis Clin North Am.* 1995;9:1-9.

104. Weekers F, Giulietti AP, Michalaki M, et al. Metabolic, endocrine, and immune effects of stress hyperglycemia in a rabbit model of prolonged critical illness. *Endocrinology.* 2003;144(12):5329-5338.

105. Hall NJ, Peters M, Eaton S, Pierro A. Hyperglycemia is associated with increased morbidity and mortality rates in neonates with necrotizing enterocolotis. *J Pediatr Surg.* 2004;39:6898-6901.

106. Rosmarin DK, Wardlaw GM, Mirtallo J. Hyperglycemia associated with high, continuous infusion rates of total parenteral nutrition dextrose. *Nutr Clin Pract.* 1996;11:151-157.

107. Hunter DC, Jaksic T, Lewis D, Benotti PN, Blackburn GL, Bistrian BR. Resting energy expenditure in critically ill patients: estimates versus measurement. *Br J Surg.* 1988;75:875-878.

108. McCowen KC, Friel C, Sternberg J, et al. Hypocaloric total parenteral nutrition: effectiveness in prevention of hyperglycemia and infectious complications—a randomized clinical trial. *Crit Care Med.* 2000;28:3606-3611.

109. Veterans Affairs Total Parenteral Nutrition Cooperative Study Group. Perioperative total parenteral nutrition in surgical patients. *N Engl J Med.* 1991;325:525-532.

110. Moore FA, Feliciano DV, Andrassy RJ, et al. Early enteral feeding, compared with parenteral, reduces postoperative septic complications. The results of a meta-analysis. *Ann Surg.* 1992;216(2):172-183.

111. Kudsk KA, Crose MA, Fabian TC, Minard G, et al. Enteral versus parenteral feeding. Effects on septic morbidity after blunt and penetrating abdominal trauma. *Ann Surg.* 1992;215:503-511.

112. Preissig CM, Rigby MR. Pediatric critical illness hyperglycemia: risk factors associated with development and severity of hyperglycemia in critically ill children. *J Pediatr.* 2009;155(5):734-739.

CHAPTER 2

Nutritional Assessment of the Critically ill Child

Koen FM Joosten and Jessie M Hulst

- MALNUTRITION IN THE CRITICALLY ILL CHILD
- CHALLENGES AND STRATEGIES TO DEFINING MALNUTRITION
- PRINCIPLES OF NUTRITIONAL ASSESSMENT
- ASSESSING AND SCREENING FOR MALNUTRITION, USING CLINICAL AND LABORATORY PARAMETERS
  - General Evaluation
  - Severity of illness Assessment and Risk for Malnutrition Assessment
  - Assessment of Body Composition
  - Laboratory Assessment
  - Energy Requirements
- IMPLICATIONS FOR CLINICAL PRACTICE
- KEY POINTS
  - References

MALNUTRITION IN THE CRITICALLY ILL CHILD

Critical illness greatly influences one's nutritional status; therefore, assessment of nutritional status should be an integral part of patient care. During a child's intensive care stay, however, attention is mostly focused on the primary medical problem, e.g., hemodynamic instability, serious infection, congenital anomaly, and nutritional status is often neglected.

Critically ill children are at high risk of developing nutritional deficiencies and altered nutritional status. Much more than adults, critically ill children are at high risk of clinical depletions because they have limited body reserves of fat and protein, higher energy expenditure, and increased energy requirements for growth and development.

Studies performed in the 1980s revealed that about 20% of the children admitted to a pediatric intensive care unit (PICU) were in poor nutritional state. Despite improvements in intensive care technology, feeding possibilities, and increased awareness of the significance of adequate nutritional support, the prevalence of malnutrition over the last 30 years still remains high—up to 45%.[1,2] The fact that the incidence has not decreased may be explained by certain developments in the care for critically ill children in recent years. As a result of these developments, more and more children with chronic disease or major congenital anomalies survive to an older age, and these children are more likely to be in poor nutritional state on admission to the PICU than are previously healthy children. One has also to take into account the high prevalence of underlying growth-affecting disease in those with acute malnutrition.[1]

The acute effects of malnutrition include poor wound healing, higher risk of infections due to poor immune defense, reduced gut function, longer dependency on mechanical ventilation, and longer hospital stays.[3] Considering that malnutrition might also jeopardize future growth and development,[4] it seems all important to identify on admission to the PICU those children with preexisting poor nutritional status and those at risk for developing malnutrition, with a view to tailoring their nutritional care.

With this specific aim in mind, we need to identify nutritional assessment tools that can easily be used in the intensive care setting, are patient friendly, are portable, and that have enough sensitivity/specificity to distinguish children with poor nutritional status from children with normal nutritional status.

CHALLENGES AND STRATEGIES TO DEFINING MALNUTRITION

Although both under- and overnutrition are forms of malnutrition, the term malnutrition used in the context of the PICU commonly refers to undernutrition. (Please see chapter 21 for details on care of the obese child in the PICU.) Malnutrition has been defined as a disorder of body composition characterized by macro- and/or micronutrient deficiencies and resulting from reduced nutrient intake or impaired metabolism. It describes a broad spectrum of clinical conditions ranging in severity from mild to very severe, which may result in reduced organ function, reduced body mass (muscle wasting and loss of subcutaneous fat), abnormal results in blood chemistry studies, and less favorable clinical outcomes.[5] In developed nations, malnutrition is generally secondary to disease and caused by inadequate dietary intake, increased metabolic demands, impaired absorption, or increased nutrient losses. Critically ill children may show a combination of these factors.[6] Malnutrition can be of the acute, chronic, or mixed type. Acute malnutrition is the type that usually occurs in critical illness, but children with underlying chronic diseases who are admitted to a PICU because of an acute illness can also present with chronic malnutrition. The recently released American Society for Parenteral and Enteral Nutrition (A.S.P.E.N.) definitions of pediatric malnutrition proposed a new classification of malnutrition based on its etiology: as illness related when it is secondary to disease/injury, as non-illness related when it is caused by environmental/behavioral factors, or both.[7] Various criteria based on anthropometry exist for classifying children as malnourished; these will be discussed in the section "Assessment of Body Composition" (see Table 2-2).

PRINCIPLES OF NUTRITIONAL ASSESSMENT

Nutritional assessment is defined as a structured way to establish the nutritional status and energy requirements of a child by objective measurements in relation to specific disease indications, whereby an adequate nutritional treatment can be developed and monitored. In general, a multidisciplinary setting is preferred, including physicians, dietitians, and nurses.

Different data must be interpreted together in order to perform a comprehensive nutritional assessment:

- General evaluation (including dietary and medical history and physical signs)
- Severity of illness assessment and determination of risk for malnutrition
- Assessment of body composition
- Measurement of nutrient balance
- Laboratory studies, including measurement of inflammatory activity, functional assessment, and estimation of energy requirements

The results of nutritional assessment in a critically ill patient reflect metabolic consequences of both undernutrition and the underlying disease. In this context, nutritional assessment and subsequent nutritional support are directed not only at treating malnutrition, but also at supporting the patient nutritionally and metabolically to prevent further physiologic deterioration while undergoing primary disease-directed therapy. Furthermore, in critically ill children, we must also aim at improving their nutritional status to maintain normal growth and development.

ASSESSING AND SCREENING FOR MALNUTRITION, USING CLINICAL AND LABORATORY PARAMETERS

Nutritional assessment is necessary to identify patients who have already developed or are at risk of developing protein energy malnutrition (PEM) to establish the degree of malnutrition and the risk of developing malnutrition-related complications, and to monitor the adequacy of nutritional support.[8] Accurate assessment of nutritional status in children is complicated by ongoing growth, changing energy needs, varying body composition, and disease.[9]

All critically ill children should undergo nutrition screening within 24 hours of admission. Currently, 5 screening tools are available for children admitted to the hospital: (1) the Nutrition Risk Score (NRS),[10] (2) the "pediatric nutritional risk score" (PNRS),[11] (3) the Screening Tool for the Assessment of Malnutrition in Paediatrics (STAMP),[12] (4) the Paediatric Yorkhill Malnutrition Score (PYMS),[13] and (5) the $STRONG_{kids}$ tool.[14] These scores have not yet been used for children admitted to the PICU. Children identified as malnourished or at risk for malnutrition should undergo more detailed nutrition assessment, ideally by a dietitian.

General Evaluation

A full medical and dietary history is necessary for an extensive nutritional assessment. Items such as food intake, anorexia, feeding problems, and underlying disease should be addressed. Critically ill children with a history of chronic disease may at admission show poor initial nutritional status and thus need extra attention. Physical signs of malnutrition usually do not appear until the malnutrition has been developing for some time and reached a severe stage, but the first impression of the child and subjective assessment of muscle and fat mass can help. Subjective global nutrition assessment (SGNA) is a clinical technique that assesses nutritional status based on features of the history and physical examination.[15,16]

Severity of illness Assessment and Risk for Malnutrition Assessment

Objective illness-severity scores are quite important in the overall nutritional assessment of a critically ill child during PICU admission. They provide insight into the degree of metabolic stress and help to determine the turning point from catabolism to anabolism in the course of disease. Several illness-severity scoring systems are available for use in children: the Pediatric Risk of Mortality Score (PRISM), the Pediatric Index of Mortality (PIM), and the Paediatric Logistic Organ Dysfunction (PELOD) score. Furthermore, changes in metabolic, endocrine, and inflammatory parameters over time might help to evaluate the severity of illness during PICU admission. At the moment, however, there is no universal scoring system for severity of disease in relation to nutritional assessment that can be used in daily practice.

Assessment of Body Composition

Currently, there is no consensus on the best method to assess body composition of children admitted to the PICU. Body composition can be assessed by classic anthropometry or by more sophisticated methods—e.g.; bioelectrical impedance analysis (BIA) and dual-energy x-ray absorptiometry (DEXA). Most of these newer methods have significant limitations in the intensive care unit, seeing that practical application is limited because of technical problems and that validated reference data are lacking. In general, results of body composition measurements may also be affected by the frequent alterations in the child's hydration status during the initial stages of critical illness.

Table 2-1 summarizes the practical and theoretical advantages and limitations of body composition measuring techniques for use in critically ill children.

Anthropometry

Classic anthropometry is the term describing the measurement of body weight, body length, and head circumference.

TABLE 2-1. Nutritional Assessment Techniques: Practical and Theoretical Advantages and Limitations for Use in Critically ill Children

Assessment Tool	What Is Assessed?	Advantages	Limitations
Subjective Global Nutrition Assessment (SGNA)	Identifies risk factors for malnutrition	• Good sensitivity and specificity • Good interobserver agreement • Validated in critically ill children	• Subjective • Depends on parental cooperation
Functional tests (skeletal muscle function)	Grip strength Respiratory muscle strength Response to electrical stimulation		• Not possible in neonates and young children • Relies on degree of patient cooperation • No standardized equipment and procedures • Interference of muscle relaxants and other drugs

(Continued)

■ **TABLE 2-1.** *(Continued)*

Assessment Tool	What Is Assessed?	Advantages	Limitations
Classic anthropometry (weight, height, head circumference)	Total body mass, growth (weight), Linear growth (length) Brain growth (HC)	• Reference standards available for all ages and both sexes	• Unreliable when edema is present • Special equipment necessary at the bedside
Knemometry knee heel length (KHL)	Short-term linear growth	• Sensitive to short-term changes	• Difficult in older children • No reference values available
Circumferences (MUAC, CC)	Body composition: indirect measure of somatic protein Indication of FM	• Reference standards available for all ages and both sexes	• Values may fall in the normal range in the presence of PEM • Unreliable when edema is present
Skin folds (TSF, SSF)	Body composition: Indication of FM	• Reference standards available for all ages and both sexes	• Large intra- and interobserver variability • Poor accuracy for individuals • Unreliable when edema is present • Equations are population specific
Bioelectrical impedance analysis (BIA)	Body composition Body water: estimation of FFM	• Noninvasive • Possible at the bedside • Quick and safe • Small interobserver variability	• No reference standards/equations for all ages • Equations mostly validated in healthy children • Assumes constant hydration of lean tissue; not useful in children with fluid imbalance problems • Influenced by many factors (e.g., skin temperature, prior food, body position)
DEXA	Body composition: FFM, FM, and BM	• Accurate • Low radiation dose • Not relying on equations	• Expensive • Technically difficult • Difficult to interpret when edema is present
Stable isotope studies	Body composition (deuterium-labeled water [^2H_2O]): TBW (FFM) Estimation of EE (doubly labeled water [$^2H_2{}^{18}O$])	• Few exclusion criteria • Very precise	• Invasive • Long-term assessment • Expensive and scarce • Not routinely possible
Indirect calorimetry	Estimation of EE/24 hr, RQ Accurate monitoring of energy needs	• Possible at the bedside • Can be used in mechanically ventilated patients • Noninvasive • Accounts for individual differences • Good follow-up tool of nutritional therapy	• Some exclusion criteria • Influenced by metabolic status, fever, activity, thermal effect of food • Expensive • Maintenance of equipment

BM, bone mass; CC, calf circumference; DEXA, dual x-ray absorptiometry; EE, energy expenditure; FM, fat mass; FFM, fat-free mass; HC, head circumference; L, length; LBM, lean body mass; MUAC, mid-upper arm circumference; RQ, respiratory quotient; SSF, subscapular skinfold thickness; TBW, total body water TSF, triceps skinfold thickness

Additional anthropometric measurements include limb circumferences, skinfold thicknesses, and measurements of limb lengths, e.g., lower leg length (knemometry). Age- and sex-specific reference data of anthropometric measures are widely available for both international and national use. Furthermore, growth references exist for various populations and diseases (e.g., Down syndrome preterm infants).

Diagnostic criteria for malnutrition using anthropometry

In order to diagnose acute malnutrition (wasting), different criteria have been proposed for weight-for-age (WFA) and weight-for-height (WFH). Length-for-age (LFA) or Height-for-age (HFA) usually serves to diagnose chronic malnutrition (stunting). An overview of the currently used criteria for defining malnutrition and failure to thrive in children based on anthropometry measurements are shown in Table 2-2[17,18]

For children with serious conditions and a high risk of malnutrition due to the primary disease or its treatment, the criteria for malnutrition screening at the population level, such as the Waterlow criteria or World Health Organization (WHO) criteria, may be too low in clinical practice.

Furthermore, there are several important problems involved with the use of anthropometry in critically ill children. These children tend to gain extra weight due to third spacing of fluid in acute metabolic stress, and standard anthropometric measurements may thus result in false-negative assessments. The individual child, however, may benefit from the initial assessment and follow-up over time.

Body weight is still the most important parameter for nutritional assessment of the critically ill child. However, weight is not easy to assess in this group, and changes in weight cannot be ascribed to growth only, because edema also plays an important role.

Body length is generally of limited value for nutritional assessment during PICU admission because linear growth changes over a short period of admission are minimal. Length measurements are nevertheless important in the initial assessment to obtain WFH indices and to evaluate chronic nutritional status. Length is also an important consideration in chronically critically ill children who spend prolonged periods of time in the PICU.

For newborn infants and children up to 24 months old, heel-to-knee measurement (knemometry) is a method for measuring short-term linear growth. It makes use of a handheld device that can be used inside

TABLE 2-2. Criteria for Acute Malnutrition, Chronic Malnutrition, and Failure to Thrive Based on Weight and Height Measurements[17,18]

Criteria for Acute Malnutrition
Weight-for-height SDS less than –2 [WHO[9]]
Weight for height less than 80% of median [Waterlow]
Weight-for-height less than 5th percentile [Tanner]
Body mass index SDS less than –2 [Cole]
% ideal body weight for height less than 80
Criteria for Chronic Malnutrition
Height-for-age SDS less than –2 SD (WHO)
Height for age less than 90% of median
Height for age HFA less than 5th percentile
Criteria for Failure to Thrive and Immediate Nutritional Intervention
Inadequate growth or weight gain for >1 mo in a child <2 y of age
Weight loss or no weight gain for >3 mo in a child >2 y of age
Change in weight for age >–1 SD in 3 mo for children <1 y of age on growth charts
Change in weight for height >–1 SD in 3 mo for children >1 y of age on growth charts
Decrease in height velocity 0.5–1 SD/y at <4 y of age and 0.25 SD/y at >4 y of age
Decrease in height velocity >2 cm from preceding year during early/mid-puberty

SDS, standard deviation score.

an incubator and is less interruptive than total body length measurements.

The measurement of head circumference (HC) is an important aspect of nutritional assessment in young children, as brain growth is highest in the first 4 years of life. In the PICU, this parameter is used predominantly in preterm and term neonates, but hardly in children outside this age group. Assessment of HC at admission could signal the presence of severe chronic malnutrition in the past, whereas serial measurements in neonates can help in detecting the development of malnutrition.

Anthropometric measurements that can provide information on fat mass (FM) and fat-free mass (FFM) include body circumferences (mid-upper arm, calf) and skinfold thickness. Mid-upper arm circumference (MUAC) is a measure of muscle, fat, and bone. It has served as an index of malnutrition in rapid nutritional surveys in which weight and length measurements were not feasible. Triceps skinfold (TSF) thickness is one of the most valuable anthropometric measures of nutritional status because (1) it is a good indicator of energy reserves; (2) it correlates well with total body fat stores; and (3) recent reference data are available for all age groups and from different countries. Combining the TSF measurement with MUAC enables one to estimate upper-arm muscle (muscle circumference = MUAC (cm) – (0.314*TSF (cm))) and fat stores. The latter correlate well with total body measures of FM and FFM. Furthermore, measuring arm muscle circumference is quite feasible—the arm is usually free of edema, and the outcome correlates with muscle wastage. Calf circumference was found to be useful for screening of nutritional status in healthy infants, but its utility in disease has not been well documented yet.

Bioelectrical impedance analysis Bioelectrical impedance analysis is a form of body composition analysis that is based on the physical principle that fat tissue has low electrical conductivity and high impedance relative to lean tissue (FFM). This is due to the much greater content of water and electrolytes in FFM. This technique consists of passing a sensation-free alternating current between electrodes on hands and feet to obtain total body impedance. Total body impedance combines resistance (R) and reactance (Xc) across tissues. These two measures can be converted with age-specific prediction equations to estimate body composition (total body water [TBW] or FFM). Several age-specific prediction equations of TBW and other body components, including length and mostly also weight and sex, derived from numerous small cross-sectional studies are available. There are almost as many different BIA equations in the literature as there are studies, denoting the population-specific character of these equations. Moreover, equations for neonates and young children are scarce.

For the population in the PICU, studies are limited. Bioelectrical impedance analysis was used to study changes in TBW in children <3 years post-cardiac surgery and was found to be valuable in researching the major water fluxes associated with cardiopulmonary bypass techniques.[19] Furthermore, BIA has been used in children on dialysis, and in one of these studies it was shown that BIA was more sensitive to body changes than the anthropometric measurements.[20,21]

The bioelectrical impedance vector analysis (BIVA) generated normal values of the bioelectrical impedance vector from birth to puberty in healthy children.[22,23] This method holds an advantage over the conventional BIA method in that no assumptions regarding body composition and models need be made.[22] Its application in children with altered body composition still needs to be tested.

One of the limitations of BIA is the need for a constant hydration condition. Certain pathophysiological factors may interfere with TBW and make this technique difficult to use in patients who present with abnormal hydric distribution.

Although BIA has not been investigated in critically ill children, it has potential value, as it can be carried out easily, quickly, and safely at the patient's bedside, and may show less interobserver variation than do traditional anthropometric measurements.

Dual energy x-ray absorptiometry Dual energy x-ray absorptiometry provides a method to assess three body components: bone mass, FM, and FFM. Because of their varying densities, these tissues attenuate the energy beams or dual photons differentially as they pass through. Dual energy x-ray absorptiometry causes extremely low radiation exposure and yields precise body composition in infants and children within a few minutes. However, large errors may be anticipated in children with abnormal hydration status because attenuation of water is similar to that of FFM. Nevertheless, DEXA has a wide application for assessing bone mineral content and body composition in preterm and term neonates,[24] as well as patients with cystic fibrosis; Crohn disease; anorexia nervosa; severe neuromuscular disease; and chronic liver, cardiac, and renal disease.[9] Compared with bioelectrical and anthropometric methods of body composition assessment, DEXA has the added advantage of being independent of sample-based equations. A portable DEXA device would be necessary in the PICU setting.

Muscle function tests Muscle function tests such as grip strength, respiratory muscle strength, and the response of specific muscles to electrical stimulation are used nowadays for evaluating nutritional status. It has been shown that skeletal muscle function can be altered rapidly by undernutrition.[25] These tests do not apply very well to the PICU patient below 6 years of age, but deserve to be investigated, however, in older children.

Research tools Many other methods, such as isotope studies, total body potassium, neutron activation analysis, ultrasonography, computed tomography scanning, and magnetic resonance imaging, have been developed to accurately estimate the body composition of children.[26,27] Data on the use of these methods in critically ill children are lacking. So far, these methods have shown practical and logistical limitations in a nonresearch clinical setting, but they are important as gold standards to which easier methods can be evaluated against.

Total body water and consequently FFM can be estimated by dilution methods using stable isotopes of water (deuterium, ^{18}O) that are ingested or infused. They can safely and effectively measure TBW volumes in infants and children.[28] Protein status can be accurately measured using an amino acid labeled with a stable isotope (e.g., ^{13}C leucine).[29] Routine use of stable isotope studies is difficult, however, since the analyses require mass spectrometers, which are not available in most hospitals for these purposes.

Laboratory Assessment

In general, laboratory tests are only of relative importance in nutritional assessment, e.g., all values can be normal in a malnourished child. Selected laboratory tests, however, may be useful to identify nutritional deficiencies before clinical findings are evident, and may be helpful to monitor clinical recovery from malnutrition, but practically all of these tests are affected by inflammation and cannot be relied upon in the PICU (Table 2-3).

Visceral Proteins

Synthesis of visceral proteins is inhibited in the acute phase of trauma and sepsis. In the recovery phase, however, the liver will return to produce visceral proteins, which are needed for repair of injured tissue and in children for somatic growth. Various parameters and indices can describe protein status. Proteins with a short biologic half-life, such as prealbumin (t1/2 = 2 days) and retinol-binding protein (t1/2 = 10 hours), are more suited to predict changes in acute nutritional status than are albumin (t1/2 = 20 days) and transferrin (t1/2 = 8 days), which have longer

TABLE 2-3. Clinical Use and Limitations of Laboratory Parameters in Nutritional Assessment of Critically ill Children

	Clinical Use	Limitations
BIOCHEMICAL		
Albumin	• Valuable as a prognostic indicator • Useful for long-term assessments	• Affected by many other factors present in ICU patients (e.g., infusion of fluids, capillary leak syndrome) • Long t1/2 (15-20 d): levels reflect chronic rather than acute protein depletion
Prealbumin	• Short t1/2 (2-3 d) and small body pool: sensitive in evaluating acute changes in nutritional (protein and energy) adequacy	• Influenced by liver, renal, and inflammatory disease
Transferrin	• More sensitive than albumin in reflecting protein depletion	• Long t1/2 (8 d): more reflective of chronic changes in nutritional status. • Influenced by iron status, liver, and inflammatory disease
Retinol-binding protein	• Short t1/2 (12 h) • Decreases rapidly with PEM	• Low plasma concentrations • Shows minimal changes in short-term nutritional repletion • Influenced by liver, renal, and inflammatory disease

(Continued)

TABLE 2-3. (Continued)

	Clinical Use	Limitations
Urinary nitrogen excretion	• Marker of protein metabolism • Estimates daily protein losses with reasonable accuracy	• Many factors affecting: adequacy of collection, diuretics, renal function, and protein intake
Muscle metabolites (urine 3-methylhistidine/ urine creatinine)	• Reflects muscle mass and loss • Correlates with FFM assessed by anthropometry	• Influenced by renal function and protein intake • Not reliable as marker of body composition in conditions in which accelerated rates of protein degradation occur
CRP	• Reflects illness severity/acute metabolic response and inflammation	• Not a direct measure of nutritional status
ENDOCRINE		
IGF-1	• Small body pool and short t1/2 (2-8 h): sensitive in evaluating acute changes in nutritional (protein and energy) adequacy	• Not a routine laboratory assessment
Thyroid hormones: TSH, T_3, rT_3, T_3/rT_3 ratio	• Possible parameter for signaling return to anabolism • Related to severity of illness	• Not a direct measure of nutritional status
Glucose/insulin ratio	• Possible parameter for signaling return to anabolism	• Not a direct measure of nutritional status

CRP, C-reactive protein; IGF-1, insulin-like growth factor 1; FFM, fat-free mass; PEM, protein energy malnutrition; T_3, triiodothyronine; TSH, thyroid-stimulating hormone; rT_3, reverse T_3. Note: As discussed in the text, practically all of these tests are affected by inflammation and cannot be relied upon in the PICU population.

half-lives. Clinical studies in critically ill infants and preterm infants showed prealbumin and retinol-binding protein to be the most suitable proteins to evaluate protein nutritional status and protein-energy adequacy.[30,31] Moreover, in growing preterm infants, changes in prealbumin occurred 1 week before changes in anthropometric measurements.

Various acute-phase proteins rise after serious injury or sepsis in association with a drop in visceral proteins. The measurement of a visceral protein as a nutritional index should, therefore, at least be complemented by a C-reactive protein (CRP) measurement as an indicator of the presence of an acute-phase response, aiding in the interpretation of sequential easurements.[32] Chwals et al used levels of pre-albumin and CRP in combination with total urinary nitrogen excretion and values obtained with indirect calorimetry as guidelines for infant metabolic monitoring during acute stress.[33] Nutritional intake was increased when serial measurements of these metabolic parameters demonstrated a resolution of the acute-phase response.

Total Urinary Nitrogen and Nitrogen Balance

Acute metabolic stress will intensify protein breakdown and urinary nitrogen loss. Since urinary excretion is, in fact, the predominant (>90%) mechanism of nitrogen removal, measuring urinary nitrogen excretion is sufficient. Patients with uremia and/or renal failure will also experience important gastrointestinal and skin losses. Furthermore, infants after digestive tract surgery may have increased fecal nitrogen losses, as well as losses via nasogastric tubes, enterostomies, and wound drains. Daily assessment of nitrogen intake and nitrogen excretion (nitrogen balance) has been used in studies of critically ill children, newborn infants, and infants after surgical procedures to estimate needs, to assess nutritional therapy, and to follow metabolic status and the capacity to synthesize protein. Protein need is calculated from urinary nitrogen excretion using the formula protein (g/kg per day) = 6.25 × urinary urea nitrogen excretion.[34] An adjustment can be made for the 10% to 20% of other urinary nitrogen loss such as ammonia, creatinine, and uric and amino acids. A 24-hour urinary collection is preferred, but is not always easy in clinical practice; a 6-hr collection or 12-hr collection (preterm neonates) may be sufficient.

Micronutrients

Certain micronutrients have antioxidant properties and a role during critical illness. A complex system of special enzymes, their cofactors (selenium, zinc, iron, and manganese), sulfhydryl group donors (glutathione), and vitamins (E and C) form a defense system to counter the oxidant stress seen in the acute phase of injury or illness.[35] Critically ill patients may have variable deficiencies of micronutrients in the course of the disease. Because hypocalcemia, hypomagnesemia, and hypophosphatemia commonly occur in the critically ill, it is essential to determine their levels. Low plasma levels of selenium and zinc will be present as well, but in daily practice, it might be difficult to perform laboratory measurements of these micronutrients.[36] In prolonged critical illness it might be vital to assess levels of vitamins and carnitine sequentially, as decreased nutrient intakes and increased requirements may easily lead to a deficiency state.[37-39]

Endocrine Methods

Endocrine parameters might be used to signal the turning point from catabolism to anabolism in critically ill children and thereby help in optimizing individual nutritional support.

Insulin sensitivity Initial screening for hypo- and hyperglycemia should be performed in all critically ill children. Both low and high blood glucose levels worsen outcome and should be treated; however, there is ongoing debate over how tight serum glucose levels should be controlled. In a randomized controlled study of young children undergoing heart surgery, tight glycemic control did not significantly change the infection rate, mortality, length of stay, or measures of organ failure.[40] Hyperglycemia with high plasma insulin concentrations is the result of insulin insensitivity that occurs during stress. Both insulin resistance and (relative) β-cell dysfunction play a role in the occurrence of hyperglycemia in critically ill children. The gold standard for quantifying insulin sensitivity in vivo is the hyperinsulinemic euglycemic clamp technique. This is a complex and invasive technique, and therefore not easily applied in studies with critically ill children. The search for uncomplicated and inexpensive quantitative tools to evaluate insulin sensitivity has led to the development of other assessments. The fasting glucose-to-insulin ratio and homeostasis model assessment (HOMA) of insulin resistance also have been proven to be useful estimates of insulin sensitivity in critical illness. There is a good correlation between estimates of insulin resistance derived from HOMA and from the hyperinsulinemic euglycemic clamp. The assessment of β-cell function is difficult because the β-cell response to secretory stimuli is complex. There is no gold standard for β-cell function. The HOMA method for assessing β-cell function (HOMA-%B) is based on measurements of fasting insulin or C-peptide concentration to calculate prehepatic insulin secretion in relation to blood glucose levels. So far, methods to quantify insulin sensitivity are used in the research setting and not for bedside use in the PICU. Although it has been applied in many centers, based on results from adult populations, routine strict glycemic control in the PICU should not be considered as standard care until the results of ongoing multicenter studies are available.

Thyroid hormones Critical illness causes multiple alterations in the thyroid axis, both in adults and in children. Described as the "low T_3 syndrome," the "euthyroid sick syndrome," or "nonthyroidal illness," this syndrome combines a low serum triiodothyronine (T_3) level with an increased reverse T_3 (rT_3) concentration and a normal or low thyroxine (T_4) level, all with a normal functioning thyroid gland. This syndrome is generally thought not to produce hypothyroidism, but rather to constitute an adaptation aimed at preventing protein catabolism and lowering energy requirements. In critically ill children with meningococcal sepsis, it was shown that levels of rT_3, T_3, and rT_3/T_3 ratio showed a quick return to normalization, indicating that these levels might be used to prelude anabolism.[41] In a group of critically ill children, it was shown in the first week after admission that an increase in T_3 and T_3/rT_3 ratio and a decrease in rT_3 were significantly associated with a decrease in CRP levels, indicating the influence of inflammation on the anabolic response.[42] Measurement of thyroid hormones in the PICU might be useful to determine the return of anabolic function.

Insulin-like growth factor The anabolic hormone insulin-like growth factor 1 (IGF-1) is often propagated as a marker of nutritional status, as its short half-life allows rapid responses to alterations in nutritional status and because changes in IGF-1 reflect the changes in nitrogen balance and the severity of the nutritional insult. In healthy children or children with a chronic disease, IGF-1 concentrations are regulated by energy and protein intakes and are related to anthropometric parameters of nutritional status. Studies among critically ill children show conflicting results, however, on the relationship between IGF-1 concentration and nutritional status.[43,44] The IGF-1 concentration can be expected to increase when the acute stress response has come to a halt and increase further when the nutritional status improves. Studies in critically ill children in which IGF-1 levels are assessed over a prolonged period in relation to other nutritional indices and nutritional therapy are lacking. Such studies are needed to assess the utility of IGF-1 in screening for malnutrition.

Energy Requirements

Measuring Energy Expenditure

Measuring energy expenditure allows for a more accurate monitoring of the child's varying energy needs during the course of critical illness. In the research setting, total and resting energy expenditure can be estimated by using the following methods: indirect calorimetry, doubly labeled water (DLW), whole-body calorimetry, thermic effect of food assessment, and heart rate monitoring. The DLW method is mostly used in research settings and evaluates energy expenditure (EE) over a longer period. Since the results are not readily available, its use to estimate EE and adjust energy intake in clinical practice is of limited value and restricted to the research setting. Measuring EE by indirect calorimetry is well applicable clinically, in the intensive care unit, and more accurate than estimating individual EE from standard prediction equations.

Indirect calorimetry Indirect calorimetry provides noninvasive, reliable, repeatable, and affordable measurements of actual EE—i.e., resting EE (REE) in nonventilated children and total daily EE (TDEE) in ventilated children. Quantification of EE is also important for diagnostics in the critically ill child because it can reveal hyper- or hypometabolic conditions directly related to the individual prognosis. The greatest asset of indirect calorimetry is its potential in designing a nutrition regimen that exactly meets a patient's energy requirements while avoiding the complications of overfeeding.[45]

Several factors commonly present in the PICU population that might affect measured EE and must be taken into account when interpreting the outcome, e.g., fever can increase EE, and sedatives can decrease EE.[46]

The second parameter obtained from indirect calorimetry, the respiratory quotient (RQ), may help in evaluating substrate utilization and/or nutritional support and in determining overfeeding and underfeeding.[34,47] Fat oxidation results in an RQ of 0.7, whereas protein and carbohydrate oxidation result in RQs of 0.83 and 1.0, respectively. Net lipogenesis is shown by an RQ >1.0, which is indicative of overfeeding. However, it is not clear if the RQ should be used to guide adequacy of nutrition support for individual patients, and at least 2 studies suggest caution in its application in the adult and pediatric ICU.[47,48]

Indirect calorimetry is being widely used as a clinical and research tool to determine energy requirements. In most PICUs, however, its routine use is hampered by limited space at the bedside, the cost of the metabolic cart, and the lack of trained staff to operate and maintain these devices. In addition, several criteria need to be fulfilled before accurate indirect calorimetry measurements can be performed, some of which are described here:

- Regular and correct calibration of the calorimeter
- A sufficient period of measurement to achieve steady state VO_2 and VCO_2 levels
- Endotracheal tube leakage <10%
- Inspired oxygen fraction (FiO_2) stable and below 60%
- Steady hemodynamic, respiratory, and metabolic states to ensure that respiratory gas exchange is equivalent to tissue gas exchange

Estimating EE In clinical practice, the use of equations based on weight and sex to estimate REE (e.g., Schofield equation)[49] can be helpful to guide nutritional support. None of these equations will predict EE with acceptable precision for use in the individual, especially in disease states. Nevertheless, in the absence of equipment to measure EE, equations such as the Schofield equation may be used to calculate REE and aid the initial energy prescription (Table 2-4).

IMPLICATIONS FOR CLINICAL PRACTICE

It is important to include a form of routine nutritional assessment in the daily care of critically ill children. This will allow us to identify those children at nutritional risk on admission and those children with deteriorating nutritional status during admission. This does not mean that a full nutritional assessment—anthropometry, laboratory parameters, and metabolic monitoring—should be performed in all children admitted to an ICU. In **Fig. 2-1**,

TABLE 2-4. Calculation of Resting Energy Expenditure (kcal) According to Schofield Equation Based on Age and Weight[49]

Age	Boys	Girls
0-3 y	60.9 × (kg) − 54	61.0 × (kg) − 51
3-10 y	22.7 × (kg) + 495	22.5 × (kg) + 499
10-18 y	17.5 × (kg) + 651	12.2 × (kg) + 746

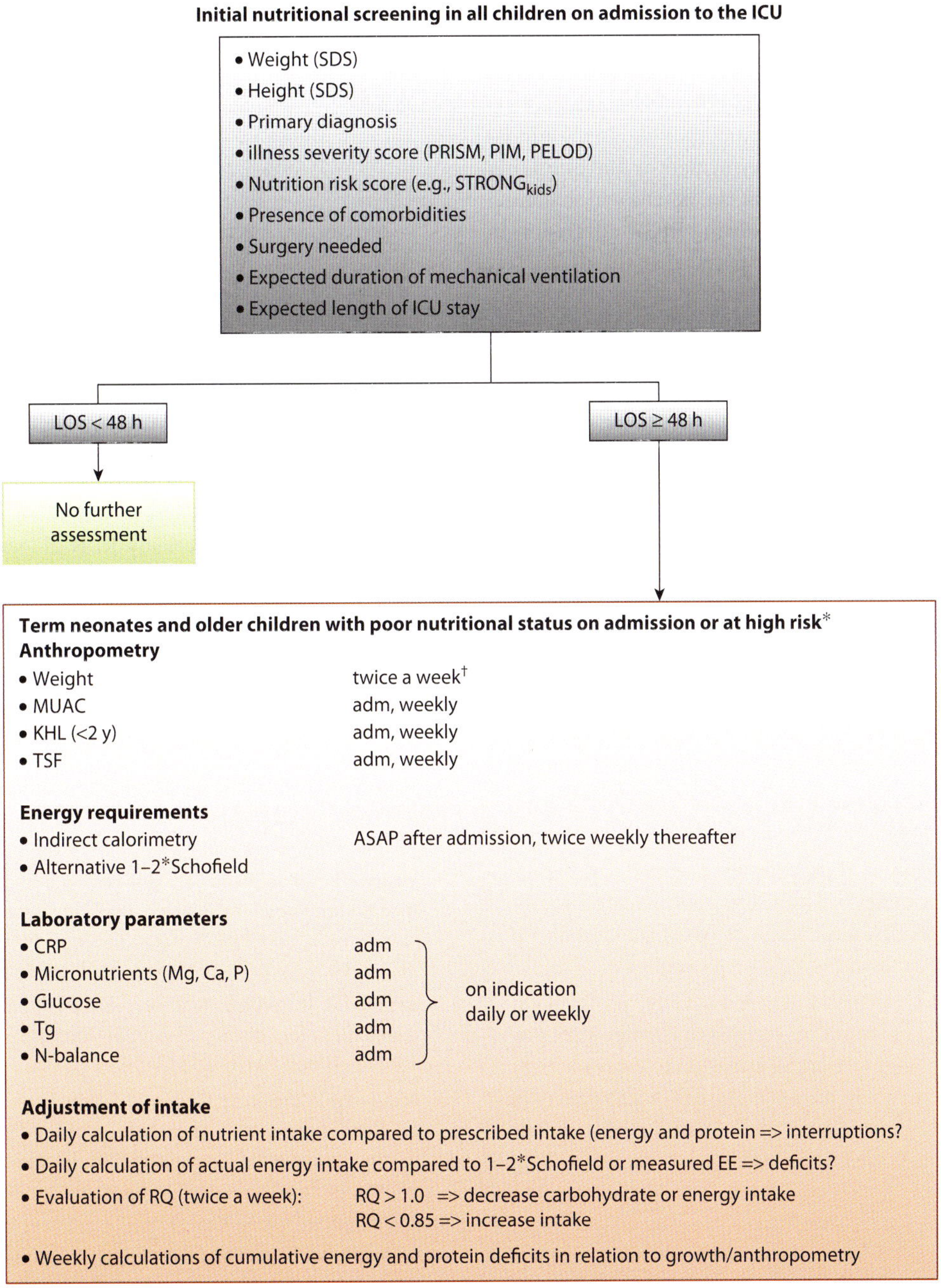

SDS standard deviation score; PRISM pediatric risk of mortality; PIM pediatric index of mortality; PELOD pediatric logistic organ dysfunction; ICU intensive care unit; LOS length of stay; MUAC mid-upper arm circumference; KHL knee-heel length; TSF triceps skinfold; adm admission; CRP c-reactive protein; Tg triglyceride; N-balance nitrogen balance; RQ respiratory quotient; adm, admission; ASAP, as soon as possible; CC, calf circumference; CRP, C-reactive protein; EE, energy expenditure; KHL, knee-heel length; LOS, length of stay; MUAC, mid-upper arm circumference; PELOD, Pediatric Logistic Organ Dysfunction Score; PIM, Pediatric Index of Mortality; PRISM, Pediatric Risk of Mortality; RQ, respiratory quotient; SDS, standard deviation score; Tg, triglycerides; TSF, triceps skinfold.

FIGURE 2-1. Standard Nutritional Assessment in the PICU Population
**Poor nutritional status: weight-for-age SDS or height-for-age; SDS or weight-for-height; SDS < −2; risk groups: prolonged expected PICU stay, prolonged duration of mechanical ventilation, children undergoing surgery, children with underlying growth-affecting disease such as children with major congenital malformations, cardiac anomalies, cystic fibrosis, inflammatory bowel disease, human immunodeficiency virus infection (see text for details); †depending on age of the child.*

we propose an algorithm for performing a nutritional assessment in routine clinical practice based on the current literature. It consists of a simple initial screening on admission aimed at identifying children at nutritional risk. This initial screening should be incorporated in the admission procedure and can be performed by the attending nurse and/or physician. In addition, nutritional screening should be repeated regularly during PICU admission in order to monitor changes in nutritional status, diagnoses, or conditions that might put the child at nutritional risk, and to monitor the efficacy of nutritional support.

The indirect calorimetry measurements must be interpreted as soon as possible in order to establish the child's minimal energy needs. Later measurements must be evaluated during the daily clinical rounds along with the data on actual intake. Furthermore, the differences between prescribed and delivered nutrition must be evaluated and energy imbalance determined and acted upon when necessary.

KEY POINTS

- The reported prevalence of malnutrition in the PICU remains high.
- Screening tools help identify hospitalized children who are at increased risk of nutritional deterioration.
- Assessment of nutritional status should be an integral part of patient care in the PICU.
- Body composition can be assessed by classic anthropometry or by more sophisticated methods—e.g., BIA and DEXA. Most of these methods are unreliable in the PICU environment.
- Indirect calorimetry, where available, allows accurate determination of energy requirement in critically ill patients. Careful attention to daily nutrient balance may help prevent cumulative imbalances of energy and protein, as well as associated morbidities in the critically ill child.

REFERENCES

1. Hulst J, Joosten K, Zimmermann L, et al. Malnutrition in critically ill children: from admission to 6 months after discharge. *Clin Nutr*. 2004;23(2):223-232.
2. de Souza Menezes F, Leite HP, Koch Nogueira PC. Malnutrition as an independent predictor of clinical outcome in critically ill children. *Nutrition*. 2012;28(3):267-270. PubMed PMID: 21872433. Epub 2011/08/30.
3. Heyland DK, MacDonald S, Keefe L, Drover JW. Total parenteral nutrition in the critically ill patient: a meta-analysis. *JAMA*. 1998;280(23):2013-2019. PubMed PMID: 9863853.
4. Lucas A, Morley R, Cole TJ. Randomised trial of early diet in preterm babies and later intelligence quotient. *BMJ*. 1998;317(7171):1481-1487. PubMed PMID: 9831573.
5. *Guidelines for Detection and Management of Malnutrition. A Report by the Malnutrition Advisory Group*. Elia M, ed. Maidenhead: BAPEN; 2000.
6. Corish CA, Kennedy NP. Protein-energy undernutrition in hospital in-patients. *Br J Nutr*. 2000;83(6):575-591. PubMed PMID: 10911765.
7. Mehta NM, Corkins MR, Lyman B, et al. Defining pediatric malnutrition: a paradigm shift toward etiology-related definitions. *J Parenter Enteral Nutr*. 2013;37(4):460-481. PubMed PMID: 23528324. Epub 2013/03/27.
8. Klein S, Kinney J, Jeejeebhoy K, et al. Nutrition support in clinical practice: review of published data and recommendations for future research directions. Summary of a conference sponsored by the National Institutes of Health, American Society for Parenteral and Enteral Nutrition, and American Society for Clinical Nutrition. *Am J Clin Nutr*. 1997;66(3):683-706. PubMed PMID: 9280194.
9. Khoshoo V. Nutritional assessment in children and adolescents. *Curr Opin Pediatr*. 1997;9(5):502-507. PubMed PMID: 9360831.
10. Reilly HM, Martineau JK, Moran A, Kennedy H. Nutritional screening—evaluation and implementation of a simple Nutrition Risk Score. *Clin Nutr*. 1995;14(5):269-273. PubMed PMID: 16843942. Epub 1995/10/01.
11. Secker DJ, Jeejeebhoy KN. Subjective Global Nutritional Assessment for children. *Am J Clin Nutr*. 2007;85(4):1083-1089. PubMed PMID: 17413109.
12. McCarthy H, Dixon M, Crabtree I, Eaton-Evans MJ, McNulty H. The development and evaluation of the Screening Tool for the Assessment of Malnutrition in Paediatrics (STAMP) for use by healthcare staff. *J Hum Nutr Diet*. 2012;25(4):311-318. PubMed PMID: 22568534. Epub 2012/05/10.
13. Gerasimidis K, Keane O, Macleod I, Flynn DM, Wright CM. A four-stage evaluation of the Paediatric Yorkhill Malnutrition Score in a tertiary paediatric hospital and a district general hospital. *Br J Nutr*. 2010;104(5):751-576. PubMed PMID: 20398432. Epub 2010/04/20.
14. Hulst JM, Zwart H, Hop WC, Joosten KF. Dutch national survey to test the STRONG(kids) nutritional risk screening tool in hospitalized children. *Clin Nutr*. 2010;29(1):106-111. PubMed PMID: 19682776.

15. Vermilyea S, Slicker J, El-Chammas K, et al. Subjective global nutritional assessment in critically ill children. *J Parenter Enteral Nutr*. 2013;37(5):659-666. PubMed PMID: 22730117. Epub 2012/06/26.
16. Secker DJ, Jeejeebhoy KN. Subjective Global Nutritional Assessment for children. *Am J Clin Nutr*. 2007;85(4):1083-1089. PubMed PMID: 17413109. Epub 2007/04/07.
17. Joosten KF, Hulst JM. Malnutrition in pediatric hospital patients: current issues. *Nutrition*. 2011;27(2):133-137. PubMed PMID: 20708380. Epub 2010/08/17.
18. Joosten KF, Hulst JM. Prevalence of malnutrition in pediatric hospital patients. *Curr Opin Pediatr*. 2008;20(5):590-596. PubMed PMID: 18781124.
19. Maehara T, Novak I, Wyse RK, Elliot MJ. Perioperative monitoring of total body water by bioelectrical impedance in children undergoing open heart surgery. *Eur J Cardiothorac Surg*. 1991;5(5):258-264; discussion 65. PubMed PMID: 1859666.
20. Foster BJ, Leonard MB. Measuring nutritional status in children with chronic kidney disease. *Am J Clin Nutr*. 2004;80(4):801-814. PubMed PMID: 15447884. Epub 2004/09/28.
21. Edefonti A, Picca M, Damiani B, et al. Prevalence of malnutrition assessed by bioimpedance analysis and anthropometry in children on peritoneal dialysis. *Perit Dial Int*. 2001;21(2):172-179. PubMed PMID: 11330562. Epub 2001/05/02.
22. Piccoli A, Fanos V, Peruzzi L, et al. Reference values of the bioelectrical impedance vector in neonates in the first week after birth. *Nutrition*. 2002;18(5):383-387. PubMed PMID: 11985941.
23. De Palo T, Messina G, Edefonti A, et al. Normal values of the bioelectrical impedance vector in childhood and puberty. *Nutrition*. 2000;16(6):417-424. PubMed PMID: 10869896.
24. Lafeber HN. Nutritional assessment and measurement of body composition in preterm infants. *Clin Perinatol*. 1999;26(4):997-1005. PubMed PMID: 10572733.
25. Russell DM, Leiter LA, Whitwell J, Marliss EB, Jeejeebhoy KN. Skeletal muscle function during hypocaloric diets and fasting: a comparison with standard nutritional assessment parameters. *Am J Clin Nutr*. 1983;37(1):133-138. PubMed PMID: 6849274.
26. Lukaski H. Methods for the assessment of human body composition: traditional and new. *Am J Clin Nutr*. 1987;46:537-556.
27. Ellis KJ. Human body composition: in vivo methods. *Physiol Rev*. 2000;80(2):649-680. PubMed PMID: 10747204.
28. Schoeller DA, van Santen E, Peterson DW, Dietz W, Jaspan J, Klein PD. Total body water measurement in humans with 18O and 2H labeled water. *Am J Clin Nutr*. 1980;33(12):2686-2693. PubMed PMID: 6776801.
29. Van Goudoever JB, Sulkers EJ, Halliday D, et al. Whole-body protein turnover in preterm appropriate for gestational age and small for gestational age infants: comparison of [15N]glycine and [1-(13)C]leucine administered simultaneously. *Pediatr Res*. 1995;37(4 Pt 1):381-388. PubMed PMID: 7596675.
30. Chwals WJ, Fernandez ME, Charles BJ, Schroeder LA, Turner CS. Serum visceral protein levels reflect protein-calorie repletion in neonates recovering from major surgery. *J Pediatr Surg*. 1992;27(3):317-320; discussion 320-21.
31. Polberger SK, Fex GA, Axelsson IE, Raiha NC. Eleven plasma proteins as indicators of protein nutritional status in very low birth weight infants. *Pediatrics*. 1990;86(6):916-921.
32. Manning EM, Shenkin A. Nutritional assessment in the critically ill. *Crit Care Clin*. 1995;11(3):603-634. PubMed PMID: 7552973.
33. Chwals WJ. Metabolism and nutritional frontiers in pediatric surgical patients. *Surg Clin North Am*. 1992;72(6):1237-1266. PubMed PMID: 1440155.
34. Joosten KF, Verhoeven JJ, Hazelzet JA. Energy expenditure and substrate utilization in mechanically ventilated children. *Nutrition*. 1999;15(6):444-448.
35. Mehta NM, Duggan CP. Nutritional deficiencies during critical illness. *Pediatr Clin North Am*. 2009;56(5):1143-1160. PubMed PMID: 19931068. Epub 2009/11/26.
36. Carcillo JA, Dean JM, Holubkov R, et al. The randomized comparative pediatric critical illness stress-induced immune suppression (CRISIS) prevention trial. *Pediatr Crit Care Med*. 2012;13(2):165-173. PubMed PMID: 22079954. PubMed Central PMCID: 3302948. Epub 2011/11/15.
37. Seear M, Lockitch G, Jacobson B, Quigley G, MacNab A. Thiamine, riboflavin, and pyridoxine deficiencies in a population of critically ill children. *J Pediatr*. 1992;121(4):533-538. PubMed PMID: 1403385.
38. Shenkin A. Micronutrients in the severely-injured patient. *Proc Nutr Soc*. 2000;59(3):451-456. PubMed PMID: 10997673.
39. Proulx F, Lacroix J, Qureshi IA, Nadeau D, Gauthier M, Lambert M. Acquired carnitine abnormalities in critically ill children. *Eur J Pediatr*. 1997;156(11):864-869. PubMed PMID: 9392402.
40. Agus MS, Steil GM, Wypij D, et al. Tight glycemic control versus standard care after pediatric cardiac surgery.

N Engl J Med. 2012;367(13):1208-1219. PubMed PMID: 22957521. PubMed Central PMCID: 3501680. Epub 2012/09/11.

41. Joosten KF, de Kleijn ED, Westerterp M, et al. Endocrine and metabolic responses in children with meningoccocal sepsis: striking differences between survivors and nonsurvivors. *J Clin Endocrinol Metab.* 2000;85(10):3746-3753. PubMed PMID: 11061534.
42. Hulst JM, van Goudoever JB, Visser TJ, Tibboel D, Joosten KF. Hormone levels in children during the first week of ICU admission: is there an effect of adequate feeding? *Clin Nutr.* 2006;25(1):154-162. PubMed PMID: 16297504. Epub 2005/11/22.
43. Leite HP, Fisberg M, Vieira JGH, De Carvalho WB, Chwals WJ. The role of insulin-like growth factor 1, growth hormone, and plasma proteins in surgical outcome of children with congenital heart disease. *Pediatr Crit Care Med.* 2001;2(1):29-35.
44. Balcells J, Moreno A, Audi L, Roqueta J, Iglesias J, Carrascosa A. Growth hormone/insulin-like growth factors axis in children undergoing cardiac surgery. *Crit Care Med.* 2001;29(6):1234-1238.
45. Brandi LS, Bertolini R, Calafa M. Indirect calorimetry in critically ill patients: clinical applications and practical advice. *Nutrition.* 1997;13(4):349-358.
46. McClave SA, McClain CJ, Snider HL. Should indirect calorimetry be used as part of nutritional assessment? *J Clin Gastroenterol.* 2001;33(1):14-19. PubMed PMID: 11418784.
47. Hulst JM, van Goudoever JB, Zimmermann LJ, et al. Adequate feeding and the usefulness of the respiratory quotient in critically ill children. *Nutrition.* 2005;21(2):192-198. PubMed PMID: 15723748. Epub 2005/02/23.
48. McClave SA, Lowen CC, Kleber MJ, McConnell JW, Jung LY, Goldsmith LJ. Clinical use of the respiratory quotient obtained from indirect calorimetry. *J Parenter Enteral Nutr.* 2003;27(1):21-26. PubMed PMID: 12549594. Epub 2003/01/29.
49. Schofield WN: Predicting basal metabolic rate, new standards and review of previous work. *Hum Nutr: Clin Nutr.* 1985;39C:5-40.

CHAPTER 3

Energy and Macronutrient Requirements in the Critically ill Child

Renán A. Orellana and Jorge A. Coss-Bu

- ENERGETIC DERANGEMENTS DURING CRITICAL ILLNESS
- METHODS TO MEASURE ENERGY NEEDS
  - Gas Exchange Measurement
  - Tracer Methodology
  - Reversed Fick Equation
- METHODS TO ESTIMATE CALORIC REQUIREMENTS
  - Reference Values for Pediatric Patients
  - Correction Factors
  - Predictive Equations
- ENERGY PROVISION IN THE CRITICALLY ILL
  - Enteral Nutrition
  - Parenteral Nutrition
  - Clinical Considerations for Energy Expenditure Assessment in the Critically ill Child
  - Nutritional Support in the Obese Child
  - Malnutrition and Chronic illness
  - Hypermetabolism and Hypometabolism
- PROTEIN AND AMINO ACID REQUIREMENTS IN PEDIATRIC CRITICAL ILLNESS
  - Alterations in Protein and Amino Acid Metabolism During Critical illness in Pediatrics
  - Assessment of Protein and Amino Acid Turnover in the Critically ill Child
  - Nitrogen Balance
  - Tracer Methodologies
  - Prescription and Provision of Protein and AA in the Critically ill Child
- KEY POINTS
  - References

ENERGETIC DERANGEMENTS DURING CRITICAL ILLNESS

The metabolic response to tissue injury and the stress of critical illness is a cascade of events supported by an intricate, complex network of mediators, cytokines, growth factors, and hormones that significantly alter energy requirements.[1] The initial response after injury is manifested by a decrease in energy expenditure (the ebb phase), lasting 2 to 3 days and aimed at the preservation of energy; this is followed by the flow phase, which is characterized by an increase in energy expenditure and a catabolic response that varies in duration, depending of the nature of the initial insult.[2] Critically ill patients are characterized by alterations in the metabolism of carbohydrates, proteins, and lipids. During critical illness, typical alterations include increased secretion of cortisol, glucagon, and catecholamines; decreased secretion of insulin-like growth factor 1 (IGF-1); and resistance to the combined effects of insulin and growth hormone[3] and growth hormone alone.[4]

METHODS TO MEASURE ENERGY NEEDS

Accurate measurement of energy requirements, when available, must be used to guide energy prescription during critical illness. Energy expenditure may be measured by indirect calorimetry, tracer dilution studies or by the reverse Fick method.

Gas Exchange Measurement – Indirect Calorimetry

Indirect calorimetry (IC) is the method by which metabolic rate and substrate utilization are estimated from respiratory gas exchange measurements and urinary nitrogen excretion. Indirect calorimetry measures minute-to-minute whole-body oxygen consumption (VO_2) and carbon dioxide production (VCO_2). The gas exchange method provides both VO_2 and VCO_2 by measuring the absolute amounts of O_2 and CO_2 in inspired and expired gas. Accurate measurements of inspired as well as expired gas volumes are necessary for this testing, and are potential sources of error. The Haldane transformation is applied to prevent the need to measure both inspired and expired volumes, and hence decreases the potential for error, as follows: (1) $VO_2 = [(1 - FEO_2 - FECO_2)/(1 - FIO_2) \times FIO_2] - (FEO_2 \times VE)$, where FEO_2 is expired oxygen concentration, FIO_2 is inspired oxygen concentration, $FECO_2$ is expired CO_2 concentration, and VE is expired minute ventilation; (2) $VCO_2 = VE\ (FECO_2) - VI\ (FICO_2)$. Then, the VO_2 and VCO_2 values are converted to a caloric equivalent based on equations developed by Weir: $REE = [VO_2\ (3.941) + VCO_2\ (1.11)] \times 1440$.[5] These values can be used to calculate the substrate oxidation rates by the Consolazio formulas once total urinary nitrogen is measured in a 24-hr urine collection.[6] Gas exchange reflects the composition of oxidized substrates—1 kcal energy requires 0.236, 0.214, and 0.199 liters of oxygen for protein, lipid, and carbohydrate oxidation, producing 0.190, 0.151, and 0.199 liters of carbon dioxide as a byproduct, respectively.[7] It is important to mention that the use of IC and urinary nitrogen allows the calculation of "net" oxidation rates for carbohydrates, protein, and fat.

The VCO_2/VO_2 ratio is known as the respiratory quotient (RQ), and its value is constant and specific for each substrate; however, RQ is adimensional and is unable to give any details about absolute values of VO_2 and VCO_2, whose values are influenced by the cardiopulmonary function.[8] It is well known that the conversion of glucose to fat elevates the RQ and reflects the proportion of substrate utilization in the body. The nonprotein RQ (npRQ) represents the ratio of glucose and fat utilization by excluding the participation of protein, and varies in value from 0.70 to 1.0, with values >1.0 indicating net fat biosynthesis from glucose (lipogenesis). Studies of critically ill children have shown that changes in the metabolic condition, or excessive energy intake in the form of glucose, modify the npRQ value. Two studies in critically ill patients have concluded that RQ should not be used to finely adjust the nutrition support regimen.[9,10]

The correct interpretation of IC results implies an understanding of the assumptions and technical considerations of this methodology. Recent advances in technology and the availability of precise and portable metabolic carts have made IC practical at the bedside even in critically ill patients on mechanical ventilatory support. However, there are several sources of error and many technical difficulties in applying this methodology in the intensive care unit, including (1) model of calculation and assumptions, (2) calorimetric factors used, (3) leak around the endotracheal tube, (4) inspired oxygen concentration above 0.60, (5) use of high levels of positive end expiratory pressure (PEEP), (6) unstable gas analyzers, (7) inability to reach steady state, (8) human factors, etc.[11-13] The duration of the test is important in relation to the achievement of steady state, defined as a coefficient of variation less than 10% for VO_2 and VCO_2, and as a reflection of a 24-hr energy expenditure equivalent by IC test. Studies in mechanically ventilated adults and children have suggested that the use of an abbreviated IC protocol of 3 to 5 minutes' duration may be enough to achieve steady state and obtain reasonable accuracy;[11,13] although in most cases, the energy expenditure result from a 30-min IC test is preferred as a surrogate for a 24-hr test result.[14,15]

In healthy individuals, total energy expenditure (TEE) can be partitioned into three main components: basal metabolic rate (BMR), thermogenesis, and physical work. Basal metabolic rate represents 60% to 70% of TEE, while thermogenesis represents 10%, and physical work accounts for 20% to 30% of TEE.[16] During conditions of stress, the proportions of these components vary depending of the severity of the insult, management strategies in the pediatric intensive care unit (PICU), amount of substrate intake, and physical activity. Diet-induced thermogenesis (DIT) refers to the amount of energy required to absorb, process, and store nutrients and accounts for an increase in energy expenditure with respect to post-absorptive state.[16] Energy supply greater than 2 to 3 times the resting energy expenditure gives rise to a DIT that increases from 10% up to 20%, with resultant increases in VO_2 and VCO_2 and higher ventilatory and cardiocirculatory demands on the patient;[17] therefore, it is important not to supply excessive calories in relation to measured energy expenditure or BMR during the acute phase of the injury or surgical stress.

The potential clinical applications of IC in critically ill patients can be summarized as follows: (1) assessment of energy expenditure in patients who fail to adequately respond to estimated nutritional needs; (2) assessment of energy expenditure in patients with single or multiple organ dysfunction who need prolonged ICU care and artificial nutritional support; (3) assessment of the effects induced by artificial nutrition on the cardiocirculatory and respiratory systems in mechanically ventilated patients with acute and chronic respiratory failure; and (4) monitoring of VO_2 while weaning from mechanical ventilation.[18] Recently, Mehta et al suggested indications for targeted measurement of resting energy expenditure (REE) in the PICU that are included in the American Society of Parenteral and Enteral Nutrition (A.S.P.E.N) Clinical Guidelines for the Nutrition and Support of the Critically ill Child.[19] In summary, IC has allowed an increased understanding of how energy is utilized during critical illness; this has yet to be translated into improving patient outcomes. Studies examining the role of a simplified IC technique, its role in optimizing nutrient intake, its ability to prevent overfeeding or underfeeding in selected subjects, and the cost–benefit analyses of its application in the PICU are needed.[20]

Other methods used to measure energy expenditure in humans include direct calorimetry, isotope dilution, 24-hr heart rate measurements, and activity monitors.[21,22] Direct calorimetry measures heat dissipation, and in a steady-state condition under resting conditions, heat loss is identical to heat production. Indirect calorimetry measures heat production based on respiratory gas exchange and measures REE. Total energy expenditure takes into account physical activity and can be measured using the doubly labeled water (DLW) technique. The isotope dilution technique uses stable isotopes (^2H_2O, $H_2{}^{18}O$, $NaH^{13}CO_3$) to measure energy expenditure.

Tracer Methodology

The DLW method was developed about 50 years ago and is based on the differences in turnover rates of ^2H_2O and $H_2{}^{18}O$ in body water. After equilibration, both ^2H and ^{18}O are lost as water, whereas only ^{18}O is lost by respiration as carbon dioxide. The difference in the rate of turnover of the two isotopes can be used to calculate VCO_2. Assuming a mean RQ (i.e., VCO_2/VO_2) of 0.85, the energy expenditure can then be calculated from VO_2 and VCO_2. The DLW technique has been validated against IC and is now considered a gold standard for measurements of TEE under free-living conditions. Sources of error are analytical errors in the mass spectrometric determination of isotopic enrichment, biological variations in the isotope enrichment, isotopic fractionation during formation of carbon dioxide and during vaporization of water, the calculation of total body water, and the assumption or calculation of the 24-hr RQ.[23] The use of the DLW method is not possible in the critically ill child because of the fluid shifts and imbalances, which restrict the use of this method to the outpatient setting.

The carbon dioxide production during respiration has long been used as an index of substrate oxidation and energy expenditure. The isotopic dilution technique allows the ^{13}C from infused labeled bicarbonate ($NaH^{13}CO_3$) tracer to be diluted by metabolically produced carbon dioxide. By measuring the extent of isotopic dilution in expired air or blood, VCO_2 rates can be estimated. The assessment of energy expenditure must involve knowledge of the amount of energy released per liter of carbon dioxide produced, or the energy equivalents of CO_2 (E $EqCO_2$), which constitutes the food quotient, which serves as a surrogate for RQ under conditions of nutrient balance.[24,25] Two important concerns in relying on this technique relate to (1) errors in quantifying the tracer dose (or infusion rate) of labeled bicarbonate and (2) the possibility that the labeled bicarbonate does not adequately trace total CO_2 formed in the mitochondria.[26] Another limitation is the need to know accurately the labeled bicarbonate correction factor(s) required for the physiological condition investigated (recovery factor). Sy et al [27] published average values of fractional recovery rate of bicarbonate of 0.63, 0.69, and 0.70 in critically ill children receiving a mixture of glucose and electrolytes intravenously, enteral feeds, and total parenteral nutrition, respectively. In a study by Kingdon et al,[28] the mean fractional recovery rate of bicarbonate in a group of 11 spontaneously breathing, continuously fed, very-low-birth-weight infants was 0.95. The results of these studies emphasize the importance of measuring the fractional recovery rate of bicarbonate for a given study population rather than assuming a value based on adult studies.

In summary, isotopic tracer techniques and IC should be considered complementary techniques, in particular, since the tracer techniques require the measurement of carbon dioxide production obtained by IC. However, it should be kept in mind that the assessment of substrate oxidation by IC may involve large errors, especially over a short period. By using IC, energy expenditure (heat production) is calculated with substantially less error than substrate oxidation rates.[12,29]

Reversed Fick Equation

In critically ill patients who have thermodilution pulmonary catheters in place, it is possible to measure VO_2 and VCO_2 by measuring cardiac output (CO) and arteriovenous oxygen and CO_2 content differences using the Fick method. The method uses the reversed Fick equation: VO_2 Fick = CO × [(SaO_2 – SvO_2) × Hb × 0.0134 + (paO_2 – pvO_2) × 0.003], where CO is cardiac output (L/min), Hb is hemoglobin concentration (g/L), SaO_2 and SvO_2 are measured arterial and mixed venous hemoglobin oxygen saturations (%), and PaO_2 and PvO_2 are arterial and mixed venous oxygen tensions (torr).[30] There are methodological concerns regarding the accuracy and precision of the Fick method in the measurement of VO_2, including: (1) underestimation of whole-body VO_2 because it does not include the oxygen consumption of the bronchial and Thebesian circulation;[31,32] (2) it may not reflect actual fluctuations and trends in VO_2 in the early post-injury phase;[33] and (3) when this method is used to calculate both oxygen delivery and VO_2, the formulas for both are mathematically linked.[34]

Several studies in critically ill adults have concluded that IC is the preferred noninvasive method to measure VO_2 compared to the Fick method.[30,35-39] Currently, the use of this method in critically ill children is limited because the indications to place a thermodilution catheter are rare, there are technical difficulties in placing this catheter in infants and small children, and in recent years metabolic monitors have become available that are more accurate and easier to use at the bedside.

METHODS TO ESTIMATE CALORIC REQUIREMENTS

Critically ill children in the PICU differ in their energy needs from healthy children in terms of underlying metabolism and growth, comorbidities, and preexisting energy reserve, and therefore, it is difficult to estimate energy needs in this population.[40] In addition, frequent monitoring of their energy expenditure is necessary to accommodate any variations throughout the course of illness.[41] In the absence of metabolic equipment to measure energy needs in the PICU, caution should be used when reference values are used to estimate energy needs in this population.

Reference Values for Pediatric Patients

The BMR reference values appropriate for children include the Harris-Benedict; the Food Agricultural Organization, the World Health Organization, and the United Nations University (FAO/WHO/UNU); the Talbot; and the Schofield equations. The Harris-Benedict equation[42] (Harris-Benedict 1919), one of the most widely used to estimate BMR, was based on measurements made on 97 infants <8 days of age and 239 individuals >16 years of age. This equation has never been validated in children. The FAO/WHO/UNU equations were based on data derived from 6,100 individuals under a variety of conditions and represent BMR.[43] Talbot published guidelines in 1938 for the estimation of BMR based on measurements made in children, and these values were based on studies performed by the author combined with ones previously published in the literature.[44] The Schofield equations[45] were based on data from the FAO/WHO/UNU report with some additional data (Table 3-1). It is important to mention that the use of these reference values in critically ill children could lead to underfeeding or overfeeding because of the variability of the metabolic state of patients during their stay in the PICU.[46] A recent study by Kyle et al[47] found that in a cohort of 240 critically ill children admitted to the PICU for more than 48 hours, on average, a cumulative negative caloric balance was accrued during the first 8 days of admission to the PICU when Schofield equations were used as a reference value to assess energy needs.

Correction Factors

The use of stress and activity factors in addition to the BMR reference values has been reported to overestimate and underestimate energy needs in critically ill children.[48-52] In a study by Coss-Bu et al[48] of 55 critically ill children on mechanical ventilation, the use of Harris-Benedict and Talbot methods with correction factors of 1.3 and 1.5 to estimate energy needs was found to have significant differences when compared to measured energy expenditure by IC, reinforcing the concept that IC should be used as the only reliable strategy to measure energy needs in this population of patients.

TABLE 3-1. Prediction Equations

Equation	Gender	Age	Basal Metabolic Rate Estimate
Harris-Benedict[42]		Infants	[22.1 + (31.05 × Wt) + (11.6 × Ht)
	Female		[665.0955 + (9.5634 × Wt) + (1.8496 × Ht) − (4.6756 × age)
	Male		[66.473 + (13.7516 × Wt) + (5.0033 × Ht) − (6.755 × age)
FAO/WHO/UNU[43]	Female	0-3 y	[(61 × Wt) − 51]
		3-10 y	[(22.5 × Wt) + 499]
		10-18 y	[(12.2 × Wt) + 746]
	Male	0-3 y	[(60.9 × Wt) − 54]
		3-10 y	[(22.7 × Wt) + 495]
		10-18 y	[(17.5 × Wt) + 651]
Schofield[45]	Female	0-3 y	[(16.252 × Wt) + (10.232 × Ht) − 413.5]
		3-10 y	[(16.969 × Wt) + (1.618 × Ht) + 371.2]
		10-18 y	[(8.365 × Wt) + (4.65 × Ht) + 200.0]
		18-30 y	[(13.623 × Wt) + (2.83 × Ht) + 98.2]
	Male	0-3 y	[(0.167 × Wt) + (15.174 × Ht) − 617.6]
		3-10 y	[(19.59 × Wt) + (1.303 × Ht) + 414.9]
		10-18 y	[(16.25 × Wt) + (1.372 × Ht) + 515.5]
		18-30 y	[(15.057 × Wt) − (0.1 × Ht) + 705.8]

FAO, Food and Agriculture Organization; WHO, World Health Organization; UNU, United Nations University. Basal Metabolic Rate estimate in kcal/day; Weight (WT) in kg; Height (Ht) in cm.

Predictive Equations

The use of regression equations based on multiple variables (sex, weight, height, body temperature, heart rate, inotrope dose, sepsis, days of admission to the ICU, minute ventilation, etc.) has been reported in both adults and children admitted to the ICU[53-56] and has shown to be more accurate than reference values when compared to measured energy expenditure by IC. However, these equations were derived from healthy populations and are, therefore, often inaccurate when applied to critically ill children, resulting in unintended underfeeding or overfeeding. Caution should be exercised when using predictive equations because of the dynamic nature of the metabolic condition of critically ill patients.

ENERGY PROVISION IN THE CRITICALLY ILL

During acute illness, the aim should be to provide energy as close as possible to the measured REE in order to avoid energy deficits.[57] There is inconclusive evidence that caloric restriction offers an advantage to overcome critical illness, while excessive calories are associated with hyperglycemia and worse outcomes. Once accurate determination of the energy goal has been made, the optimal delivery route needs to be determined for individual patients.

Enteral Nutrition

Enteral nutrition (EN) should be the feeding method of choice in critically ill children because it replicates the normal pattern of nutrient consumption required for circulation and hormonal homeostasis, maintains and improves gastrointestinal integrity, and reduces the incidence of multiorgan failure.[19,58-60] Early EN appears to be well tolerated in the general PICU population and is associated with early attainment of nutritional goals.[61] The impact of early EN and optimal energy balance on clinical outcomes might be most relevant in children with preexisting malnutrition, who cannot afford further nutritional worsening during the course of the acute illness.[62]

Please see chapter 8 for details on EN in the critically ill child.

Parenteral Nutrition

Enteral nutrition is preferable to parenteral nutrition (PN), but if the EN route is contraindicated or not tolerated, PN should be considered as soon as the patient has been stabilized.[63] If EN is partially tolerated or advanced slowly but does not cover energy and protein needs, then supplemental PN should be considered based on age-appropriate guidelines for PN.[60,64,65] It has been suggested that PN is not associated with increased mortality rates, yet it does show an increase in the incidence of infections.[60,66] In a recent multicenter study by Goday et al,[67] the authors retrospectively reviewed a total of 2,069 children that received no EN for the first 4 days of admission to the PICU and concluded that early PN was strongly associated with higher mortality, as well as with longer duration of mechanical ventilation and PICU length of stay. Since infants, and particularly PICU patients, are highly dependent on substrate availability to maintain growth, have lower protein reserves, and have been shown to be at risk of malnutrition, PN may be initiated as soon as clinically feasible. In pediatric critically ill patients, current recommendations agree on beginning total parenteral nutrition (TPN) if EN has failed or is contraindicated.[19,63] If low-volume EN is started and is inadequate to cover nutritional needs, supplemental PN should continue and be gradually decreased as EN is advanced until full volume of enteral feeds covering nutritional requirements is achieved.[68] A more detailed account of PN in critically ill children is provided in chapter 7.

Clinical Considerations for Energy Expenditure Assessment in the Critically ill Child – Targeted Indirect Calorimetry

To accurately account for the dynamic alterations in energy metabolism during critical illness, measured REE via IC remains the gold standard to determine energy needs in this population. This is supported by recent A.S.P.E.N) guidelines[19] suggesting that IC measurements be obtained when possible in pediatric patients with suspected metabolic alterations or malnutrition. These guidelines recommend that special attention should be given to any imbalance between energy intake and expenditure to prevent over- and underfeeding in this population,[69,70] given the potential for adverse consequences.

The most recent nutritional guidelines for the critically ill child by A.S.P.E.N.[19] suggested that IC could have a role in a select group of patients in the PICU, where inaccuracy in estimated REE is related to clinical suspicion of hypermetabolism or hypometabolism (Table 3-2). In a study by Mehta et al,[46] IC measurements were performed in critically ill children admitted to a multidisciplinary PICU and concluded that targeted IC on selected high-risk patients

TABLE 3-2. Criteria for High Risk for Metabolic Alterations and Candidates for Targeted Indirect Calorimetry per American Society for Parenteral and Enteral Nutrition (A.S.P.E.N)

1. Underweight (BMI <5th percentile for age) or at risk for overweight (BMI >85th percentile for age) or overweight (BMI >95th percentile)
2. Children with >10% weight gain or loss during PCU stay
3. Failure to consistently meet prescribed caloric goals (for >5 days)
4. Failure to wean or need to escalate respiratory support
5. Need for muscle relaxants for >7 days
6. Neurological trauma (traumatic, hypoxic, and/or ischemic) with evidence of dysautonomia
7. Oncologic diagnoses (including children with stem cell or bone marrow transplant)
8. Children with thermal injury
9. Children requiring mechanical ventilatory support for >7 days
10. Children suspected to be severely hypermetabolic (status epilepticus, hyperthermia, systemic inflammatory response syndrome, dysautonomic storms, etc.) or hypometabolic (hypothermia, hypothyroidism, pentobarbital or midazolam coma, etc.)
11. Any patient with ICU length of stay >4 weeks may benefit from indirect calorimetry to assess adequacy of nutrient intake

BMI, body mass index; ICU, intensive care unit.
Reproduced with permisison from Mehta NM, Compher C; A.S.P.E.N Board of Directors. A.S.P.E.N Clinical Guidelines: nutrition support of the critically ill child. *J Parenter Enteral Nutr*. 2009;33(3):260-76

may prevent cumulative excesses and deficits in energy balance. Most recently, Kyle et al[40] performed a prospective study in 150 critically ill children to determine the number of patients who would meet criteria for IC during the first week of stay in the PICU according to the A.S.P.E.N 2009 guidelines for targeted IC. The authors found that 3 out of 4 patients were candidates for targeted IC and approximately one-third had ≥2 indications. These results emphasize the need for future studies to determine the cost-benefit ratios of performing IC in critically ill children. Given the flux of energy requirements during the course of critical illness, it is also recommended that repeated measurement of IC be performed on a timely basis.[19]

Nutritional Support in the Obese Child

Calculation of nutritional requirements in obese critically ill patients is controversial in both adults and children. Caloric restriction has been proposed for critically ill obese adults.[71] In the absence of evidence to support it, diet and caloric restriction has no place when feeding a critically ill obese pediatric patient;[72] however, overfeeding should be avoided.[51,73] Critically ill obese pediatric patients are at risk of overfeeding because calculations of BMR yield higher requirements due to larger body weight and the wide variability in body composition among obese patients.[72] Moreover, energy needs estimations vary considerably between measured and predicted resting metabolic rate by various equations and tables.[74,75] Substituting an adjusted body weight leads to underestimated resting metabolic rate, and adding stress correction factors leads to overfeeding.[76] Therefore, calculating energy needs based on actual weight, without adjusting for the degree of metabolic stress, is recommended to avoid overfeeding.[76] Frankenfield et al found that measurement of REE in obese adults by IC remains the most accurate way to estimate energy needs.[77] Critically ill obese children should be carefully monitored for tolerance of glucose and protein, and energy delivery and nutrient intake should be adjusted accordingly. Patients must also be monitored for prediabetic conditions and hyperglycemia. Protein and fat should not be restricted in critically ill obese pediatric patients.[78,79] With increasing incidence of obesity among children, the need for clinical studies is required to be able to develop evidence-based recommendations for the nutritional support of critically ill obese children. The nutritional management of the obese child in the PICU is discussed in detail in chapter 21 of this book.

Malnutrition and Chronic illness

Malnutrition has been shown to affect patient outcomes and represents a continuous spectrum ranging from marginal nutrient status to severe metabolic and functional alterations, with different degrees of relative alterations of body weight and body composition.[80] Previous studies have reported a prevalence of malnutrition ranging from 15% to 30% in hospitalized children,[81,82] while the prevalence of malnutrition in critically ill children has been reported from 16% to 45%.[47,83-85]

The presence of a chronic condition makes the patient more likely to become malnourished, and this risk is accentuated upon admission to the PICU. The report by Kyle UG et al[47] of 240 children admitted to the PICU showed that patients with chronic diagnoses were significantly more likely to exhibit moderate or severe chronic malnutrition compared to patients without chronic diagnoses. A recent study by de Souza et al[83] of 385 children admitted to the PICU showed that almost half of the patients were malnourished on admission, and malnutrition was associated with longer length of mechanical ventilation and length of PICU stay, but not with mortality. Two recent studies have reported nutritional support practices in critically ill children with acute kidney injury (AKI) and in children receiving chronic renal replacement therapy (CCRT).[84,86] The study by Kyle et al[84] of 167 children admitted to the PICU found that a third of the children with AKI had acute malnutrition and were more likely to be malnourished compared to the children with no AKI; also, AKI patients were more likely to be fasted and to receive less than 90% of BMR compared to patients without AKI. The report by Castillo et al[86] of 174 children receiving CRRT found that mortality for patients with weight <3rd percentile was greater compared to children with weight >3rd percentile and that the risk of mortality doubled in patients with malnutrition. Hence, careful consideration of energy needs in these populations is paramount.

Hypermetabolism and Hypometabolism

The metabolic response to injury, surgery, and trauma is proportional to the severity and duration of the stress, resulting in the catabolism of endogenous stores of protein, carbohydrate, and fat in order to provide substrate and energy to support the metabolic stress response. The traditional concept is that the critically ill patient exhibits a hypermetabolic response preceded by an initial phase of conservation of energy.

Critically ill children have been reported to have, on average, a hypermetabolic condition,[41,48,87] while other authors have reported, on average, a normal metabolic state[88-90] or a tendency toward decreased energy expenditure.[27,46,91-94] The aggregate result of all these reports of measured energy expenditure by IC results in an average metabolic index (measured energy expenditure/predicted BMR) of 1.02±0.1 (SD), indicating, on average, a normal metabolic condition. Children with burns (at least 60% body surface area [BSA])[52,95] have been reported to be hypermetabolic, with an average metabolic index of 1.37±0.21 (SD). The importance of measuring energy needs with IC in this heterogeneous population of critically ill children is it avoids the likelihood of unintended underfeeding and overfeeding.[40,46,48,87,96,97] Several authors have reported measured energy expenditure in postsurgical infants and neonates using indirect calorimetry and tracer methodology .[50,98-101] The results of these studies suggest that postsurgical infants and neonates do not show increased energy expenditure and, therefore, the routine administration of excessive calories is not recommended in this population.[98]

In summary, energy needs of critically ill children are variable and often difficult to estimate. Commonly used equations may be inaccurate and must be used with caution. Both underfeeding and overfeeding may be prevalent in the PICU, with an undesirable impact on clinical outcomes. Indirect calorimetry is recommended as the gold standard for determining energy expenditure in this population.

PROTEIN AND AMINO ACID REQUIREMENTS IN PEDIATRIC CRITICAL ILLNESS

Proteins are folded, three-dimensional macromolecules constituted by diverse amino acids (AA). Amino acids cannot be stored and for that reason must be partitioned between incorporation into protein or oxidation.[102] In normal conditions, dietary protein provides the AA requirements, which are frequently measured and expressed based on their nitrogen content. Nitrogen constitutes 16% of the weight of a protein, and thus a factor of 6.25 is used to convert grams of nitrogen to grams of protein.

Normally, body protein is continuously degraded and resynthesized, a process known as protein turnover. When energy intake is insufficient to satisfy the metabolic demands, body proteins are catabolized from tissues and oxidized to produce energy. Amino acids released from the protein structure may be reutilized for accretion of tissue protein, or may perform intracellular or physiologic functions. In adults, AA released from the breakdown of endogenous proteins are recycled inefficiently; catabolized; and the nitrogen disposed in skin, urine, and feces. Nitrogen losses drive further dietary AA needs for the net accretion and maintenance of body protein. In children, maintenance protein and AA needs must also include fractional needs required for growth. Protein intake must be adjusted based on the conversion rate of dietary protein to body proteins, or the biological value of protein after absorption.[103] In pediatric patients, the efficiency with which dietary protein is used for growth is 58% from 0.5 to 13 years of age and 43% from 14 to 18 years.[104]

Lean body mass (LBM) accounts for the largest protein reserve in the body. Skeletal muscle mass accounts for a major component of the LBM, and may vary across ages, gender, and body sizes from 30% to 45% of human body weight.[105-107] Circulating proteins, such as visceral proteins, acute-phase reactants, hemoglobin, leucocytes, and immunoglobulins, constitute a smaller and unmeasured compartment of the body protein reserve. When caloric expenditure is adequate, the aim is to achieve a balance between protein and AA intake, protein turnover, and nitrogen loss. This ensures maintenance of LBM and protein homeostasis, as well as growth of the lean mass component for children.[108]

Infants and children differ from adults in their need for a continuous supply of nutrients to maintain growth, even when faced with a critical illness. In contrast to adults, pediatric patients in periods of rapid growth have better utilization of dietary protein and AA released from endogenous protein breakdown.[109] Whole-body protein turnover and muscle breakdown are highest in the neonatal period when tissues are maturing and the growth rates are at their highest.[103,110,111] In infants and children, an influx of AA to the tissues from the diet rapidly stimulates protein synthesis.[109,112,113] For infants and pediatric patients, accretion of skeletal muscle mass is a dominant component of growth, since the majority of their mass increase occurs in skeletal muscle.[108] Rapid growth in the neonatal animal occurs, in large part, due to very high protein synthesis rates in skeletal muscle, which are extremely sensitive to stimulation by insulin and AA.[114,115] In healthy neonates, muscle protein degradation is not affected in response to this anabolic stimulation;[116] this highly anabolic response is reduced as the infant matures;[117] and in adults, protein consumption primarily reduces whole-body protein breakdown with only a moderate change in protein synthesis.[103,110,118]

Alterations in Protein and Amino Acid Metabolism During Critical illness in Pediatrics

Critical illness is associated with catabolism of body protein due to several mechanisms, including starvation, immobility, stress, and inflammation.[119] Patients in the PICU, especially those with a longer stay, may have depleted or low protein reserves. This is a particularly challenging group, with mortality and morbidity associated with chronic illness and the risk of nutritional deterioration.[120,121] Suboptimal macronutrient intake in the PICU has been associated with higher mortality.[122] Mechanical ventilation, organ transplantation, exogenous steroids, sedatives, immunosuppression, organ dysfunction, and life support devices (dialysis, extracorporeal support) cause prolongation of the catabolic state. With time, such conditions create a cumulative nitrogen deficit.[123] In addition to protein requirements to sustain LBM and growth, PICU patients need a protein intake to supplement their daily nitrogen loss, recover their cumulative protein deficit from their ICU stay, and reverse a chronic state of protein deficiency, sometimes defined as "catch-up growth," induced by their chronic ailments.[124]

Nitrogen Shuttle and Metabolic Partitioning

Figure 3-1B illustrates compartmental protein kinetics during critical illness in the absence of dietary protein. Injury, sepsis, and inflammation induce protein breakdown from endogenous protein stores, and the skeletal muscle releases AA and nitrogen to the systemic circulation to supply AA for whole-body protein metabolism.[125-127] This response is driven by stress hormones, neural mediators, and cytokines, and it is not reversed by providing exogenous protein. Circulating plasma AA are cleared from the circulation for oxidation and energy production, gluconeogenesis, fuel and substrate for immune cells and enterocytes, and to supply the hepatic needs for nitrogen to synthesize acute-phase reactants. If not enough energy is provided, AA may be channelized for oxidation to produce energy.[126,127] Therefore, circulating plasma AA concentrations are lower in patients with critical illness.[126,128] Whole-body protein synthesis is increased due to high protein synthesis in the liver and immune cells. If dietary protein is not provided, the splanchnic bed does not receive AA from absorbed protein and the synthesis of visceral protein such as albumin and prealbumin decreases and intestinal epithelial breakdown occurs.[129,130]

Critically ill children have a high protein turnover due to increased whole-body protein synthesis and breakdown.[124,131] In contrast to the net increase in whole-body protein synthesis during inflammation, skeletal muscle protein synthesis decreases and protein degradation

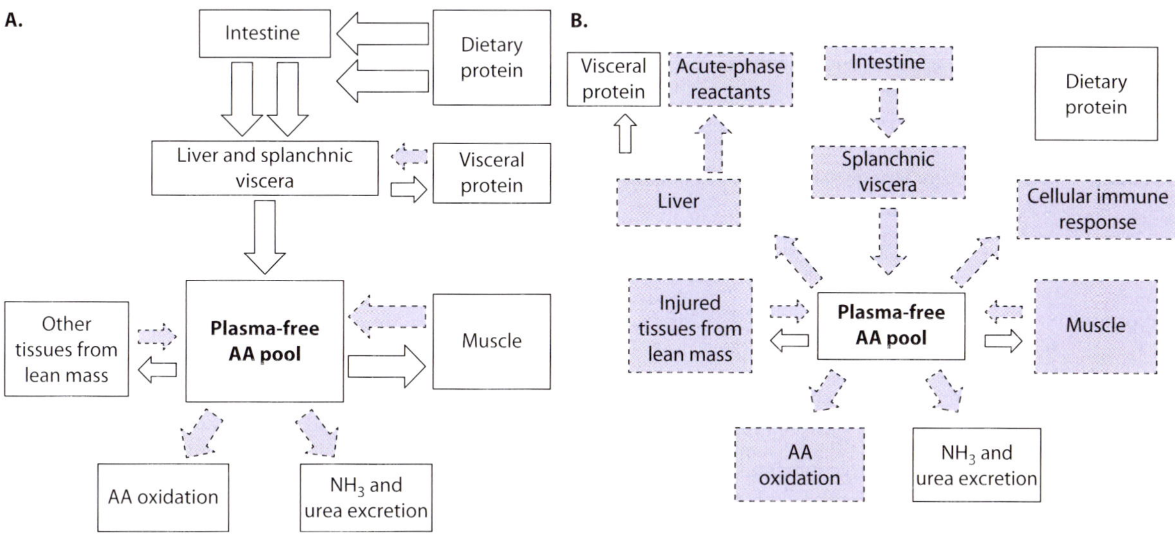

FIGURE 3-1. Schematic representation of the compartmental model used to study whole-body protein kinetics in normal conditions (**A**), and during critical illness/inflammation when fasting (**B**). Red indicates pathways toward catabolism, while blue follows contributions toward protein and AA intake and attrition. In healthy neonates, muscle protein turnover is high, and their anabolic drive toward synthesis is very sensitive to stimulation, such that muscle protein breakdown may not be worsened by a catabolic insult, and muscle protein synthesis rates may still remained elevated compared to adults. This response dampens as the organism matures.

increases to decrease utilization and release and to shuttle AA and nitrogen to visceral tissues and immune cells.[124,132] Partitioning in protein metabolism also occurs, as different organ systems may have specific AA requirements or certain AA may exert particular functions in critical illness, as shown in Table 3-3A.

TABLE 3-3A. Potential Physiologic Roles of Essential and Nonessential Amino Acids in Pediatric Critical illness

	Physiologic or Metabolic Function
EAA	Must be provided exogenously. Close to one-third of protein requirement in infancy and about one-tenth in adulthood.
Histidine	Protein methylation; histamine precursor. Supplier of around 25% of EAA; limiting for hemoglobin and myofibrillar protein synthesis.
Isoleucine	Synthesis of glutamine and alanine; BCAA balance.
Leucine	Direct activation of muscle protein synthesis; interorgan metabolism of nitrogen and carbon; HMB precursor (muscle anabolism and immune modulation); component of acute-phase reactants; BCAA balance.
Lysine	Regulation of NO and collagen synthesis; protein methylation. Carnitine precursor.
Methionine	Precursor of cystein, taurine, homocysteine, and phospholipids. Methylation of DNA and thus gene expression; acetyl choline synthesis; NO metabolism; redox balance.
Phenylalanine	Synthesis of tyrosine; neurological development and function.
Threonine	Synthesis of intestinal mucin: intestinal integrity and function; immune function.
Tryptophan	Precursor of neurotransmitters, niacin and melatonin; inhibits production of inflammatory cytokines and superoxide immune function.
Valine	Synthesis of glutamine and alanine; balance among BCAA.
BCAA	Leucine, isoleucine, and valine. Constitute about one-third of EAA in muscle. Provision suggested in liver failure.
NEAA	Can be synthesized endogenously.
Alanine	Major nitrogen shuttle for gluconeogenesis; precursor of coenzyme A and pantothenic acid; constituent of 3-methylhistidine.
Asparagine	Cell metabolism and physiology; regulation of gene expression and immune function; ammonia detoxification.
Citrulline	Antioxidant; precursor for arginine synthesis; osmoregulation; ammonia detoxification; nitrogen reservoir. Nonprotein α –AA.
Ornithine	Ammonia detoxification; syntheses of proline, glutamate, and polyamines; mitochondrial integrity; wound healing. Nonprotein α –AA.
Serine	Gluconeogenic substrate; protein phosphorylation for intracellular signaling; synthesis of cysteine, purine, pyrimidine, ceramide, and phosphatidylserine; antioxidant; neurotransmitter; activation of NMDA receptors.
Homocysteine	Recycling from methionine. Oxidant; prothrombotic, especially when coexisting with vitamin B deficiencies; inhibition of NO synthesis. Nonprotein α –AA.

BCAA, branched-chain amino acids; EAA, essential amino acids; NEAA, nonessential amino acids; AA, amino acids; HMB, β-hydroxy-β-methylbutyrate; NO, nitric oxide; NMDA, NMDA: *N*-methyl-D-aspartate.

TABLE 3-3B. Potential Physiologic Roles of Conditionally Essential Amino Acids in Pediatric Critical illness

	Physiologic or Metabolic Function
Conditionally EAA	AA that normally can be synthesized endogenously, but become deficient or insufficient under certain conditions, such as critical illness and pediatrics, and therefore must be provided exogenously.
Arginine	Direct activation of tissue protein synthesis; nitric oxide precursor; regulation of hormone secretion; regulation of gene expression and immune function; nitrogen reservoir; methylation of proteins (epigenetics). Needs enteral provision in preterm infants and newborns due to immature gut metabolism.
Glutamine	Major fuel for rapidly proliferating cells, lymphocytes, and enterocytes; nitrogen reservoir and shuttle; regulation of protein turnover, gene expression, and immune function; inhibition of apoptosis.
Proline	Maintenance of intestinal integrity; collagen structure and function; DNA synthesis; lymphocyte proliferation.
Glycine	May be CEAA in preterm infants and newborns due to small amount in milk. Calcium influx; inhibitory neurotransmitter in CNS; NMDA receptors; sleep; constitution of heme proteins.
Cysteine	Transport of sulfur; taurine precursor. Needs provision in preterm infants and newborns due to immature synthesis from precursors.
Tyrosine	Protein phosphorylation, nitrosation, precursor of vasoactive amines and neurotransmitters; regulation of immune response. Needs enteral provision in preterm infants and newborns due to immature synthesis from precursors.
Taurine	Functional AA not incorporated into proteins. Antioxidant; osmoregulation; organ development; anti-inflammation.
Carnitine	Functional AA not incorporated into proteins. Enteral formulas may be insufficient for its synthesis in infants. Transport of long-chain fatty acids into mitochondria for oxidation; storage of energy as acetylcarnitine; antioxidant.

CEAA, conditionally essential amino acids; AA, amino acids; CNS, central nervous system; NMDA, *N*-methyl-D-aspartate.

The sustained imbalance between muscle protein synthesis and protein degradation eventually lead to muscle atrophy and loss of LBM, which is associated with growth failure in children.[133,134] In critically ill adults, more than 14% of total body protein can be lost over 3 weeks, achieving maximal loss rate in the first 10 days,[135] estimating 3% to 4% of muscle fiber cross-sectional area loss per day.[105]

Intracellular Protein Turnover in Critical illness

In skeletal muscle, as well as in most cells, the cellular protein mass is maintained by a balance between protein synthesis and degradation, as shown in Figure 3-2. In animal models and humans, protein synthesis occurs through activation of a signaling pathway that stimulates translation of messenger RNA (mRNA) into protein. Translation involves activation of the mammalian target of rapamycin (mTOR), which stimulates mRNA binding to the 43S ribosomal complex; eIF2B, which stimulates the binding of the initiator methionyl-tRNA (met-tRNAi) to form the 43S preinitiation complex; and dephosphorylation of the eukaryotic elongation factor 2 (eEF2) for elongation of the peptide chain, as shown in Figure 3-2.[136,137] High protein synthesis rates in the neonatal animal are due to an enhanced translational process that declines as the animal develops because of decreased translation activation and a reduced abundance of the signaling proteins.[117,138] Sepsis and systemic inflammation impair the efficiency of translation of mRNA into protein in muscle, while in the liver, they increase protein synthesis by activating the translational machinery.[136,139]

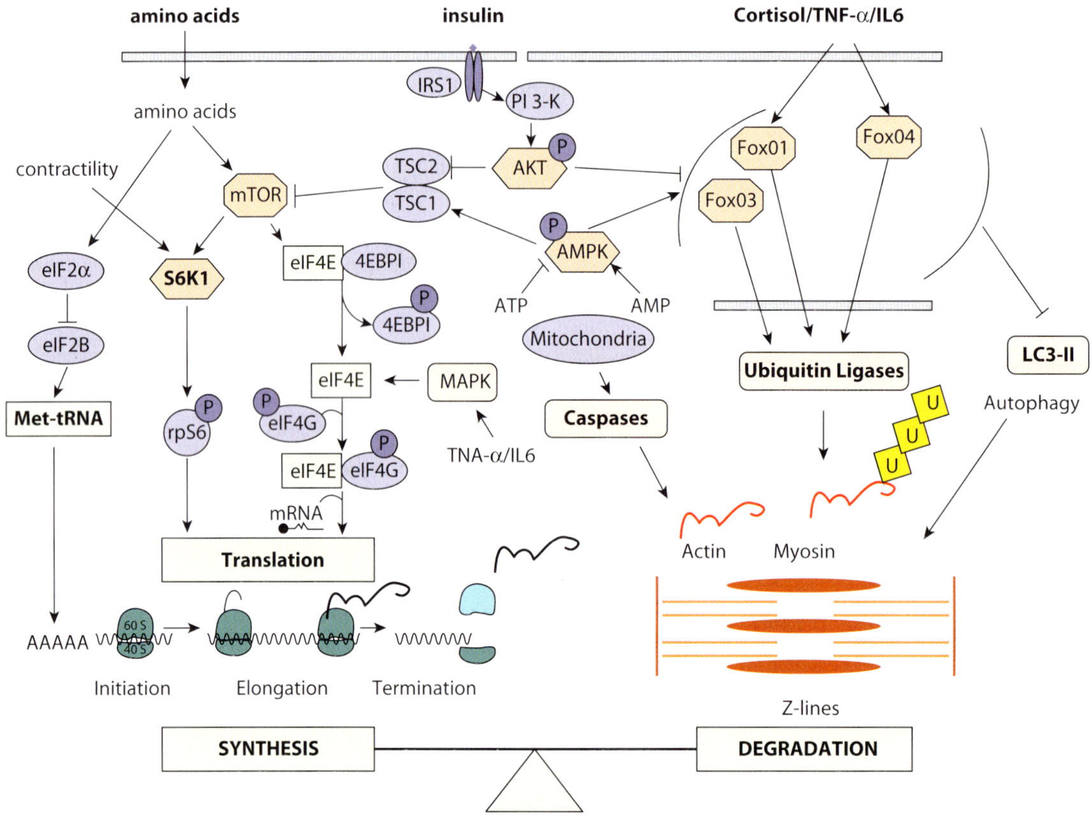

FIGURE 3-2. Schematic representation of the sequence of molecular events that lead to protein balance in tissues, cells, and organs. Muscle is the major protein reservoir in the body. In muscle, protein synthesis is regulated by amino acids, hormones, and contractility, and such events promote mRNA translation into protein. The regulation of protein degradation involves myofibrillar degradation by caspases, activation of the ubiquitin-proteasome system, and autophagy. AA degraded from muscle can be released into the free AA pool or reutilized by skeletal muscle. Inflammation and stress stimulate, suppress, or modulate synthesis and degradation pathways differently, depending on the role of the tissue or cell during critical illness.

As shown in Figure 3-2, protein degradation in skeletal muscle is controlled by signals that are also involved in translation.[140] Caspase-3 is a protease that facilitates the destruction of intact muscle fibers to release monomeric contractile proteins such as actin and myosin for degradation by the ubiquitin-proteasome system into AA.[141] Caspase-3 activity is inhibited by protein kinase B (PKB, also known as Akt), an insulin-signaling protein. 5′-AMP-activated protein kinase (AMPK), a sensor of cellular energy, is activated in the presence of energy starvation and limits mTOR inhibition and protein synthesis and increases the expression of the E3 ubiquitin ligases, muscle atrophy F-box (MAFbx, atrogin1), and muscle RING finger 1 (MuRF1), which have been associated with activation of the ubiquitin-proteasomal system.[142,143]

Protein Catabolism and Anabolic Resistance

Critical illness may induce a catabolic response and a loss of lean body mass that may be unresponsive to exogenous nutrient support, in contrast to simple starvation.[133] Even when AA are provided, insulin resistance, the effects of stress, cortisol, cytokines, and alterations in growth hormone may limit an adequate response to protein provision. Injury, sepsis, and inflammation diminish the anabolic response to hormones and nutrients that stimulate protein deposition in the major protein reservoir, skeletal muscle.[135,136]

Insulin is crucial for skeletal muscle protein deposition, as it stimulates protein synthesis, inhibits muscle protein degradation, and improves energy homeostasis.[144] In critical illness, insulin stimulates skeletal muscle protein synthesis and inhibits muscle protein degradation,[145,146] but has failed to attenuate whole-body proteolysis when provided at higher-than-physiological concentrations.[147,148] Systemic inflammation and circulating cytokines such as tumor necrosis factor α (TNF-α) have shown to decrease whole-body protein metabolism responsiveness to insulin during critical illness.[149-151] However, assessment of the response of protein metabolism to insulin at the whole-body level may not reflect the beneficial effects of insulin in muscle, since insulin does not affect visceral protein synthesis,[130] which is highly elevated due to elevated protein synthesis in the liver in response to systemic inflammation.[146,152] In addition, the beneficial effects of insulin on whole-body protein metabolism are permissive for protein synthesis and suppressive for protein breakdown only with adequate availability of AA,[132,148,149] and in skeletal muscle are also related to glucose and energy homeostasis,[134,153] stimulation of translation that leads to protein synthesis,[154] modulation of protein degradation,[134,148] and intrinsic anti-inflammatory effects.[155]

Other important mediators that cause protein catabolism in pediatric critical illness are the mediators of the stress response. Corticosteroids cause insulin resistance, hyperglycemia, net release of glutamine from muscle,[126] decrease in translation initiation, and enhancement of protein degradation in muscle.[156] Although the adrenergic system actions of epinephrine and norepinephrine on energy metabolism are usually associated with catabolic processes, evidence suggests that catecholamines may have an anabolic effect on skeletal muscle protein metabolism.[157] Critical illness is associated with complex alterations in the growth hormone (GH)/IGF axis, acquired GH resistance, reduced levels of IGF-1, and a decreased anabolic response to GH administration. However, in prolonged critical illness, patients are no longer overtly GH resistant.[135]

Functional Role of AA

Potential functional roles of plasma AA in critical illness are described in Table 3-3. Seventy-five percent of the body's nitrogen requirement is supplied by 5 amino acids: branched-chain AA (leucine, isoleucine, valine), threonine, and lysine.[158] Several AA have been used to improve outcomes in intensive care, mostly in adults. However, AA metabolism and requirements are affected by development.

AA are intrinsically anabolic and can stimulate a marked rise in muscle protein synthesis even in the face of basal insulin.[148] In critical illness, Ala, Glu, Gln, and Asp can act as gluconeogenic substrates, shuttling nitrogen from peripheral skeletal muscle to the circulating AA pool. Glutamine is a major component in muscle protein, shuttling about one-third of all AA nitrogen.[159] Glutamine also serves as fuel for enterocytes and cellular immune response. Arginine is a precursor of nitric oxide, creatine, agmatine, and other polyamines, and modulates protein anabolism,[160,161] but some of its effects may be affected by development. In adults, citrulline released from the small intestine is converted into arginine, primarily in the kidneys, while in neonates, citrulline from the intestine is utilized locally for arginine synthesis.[162] Leucine, and its metabolite β-hydroxy-β-methylbutyrate, exert a primary anabolic effect in skeletal muscle and have been used to stimulate nitrogen retention.[163,164] Parenteral branched-chain AA (BCAA) have been used to improved outcomes in critical illness without success.[127] Arginine, glutamine, and leucine are insulin secretagogues.[162]

To date, A.S.P.E.N does not recommend the use of specific AA therapies in pediatric critical care due to lack of proven efficacy.[19] Even though certain AA may modulate a specific cellular or physiologic effect, AA imbalances may also be detrimental for metabolic homeostasis. All 20 protein AA and their metabolites are required for normal cell physiology and function.[162] More studies are needed to understand the use of AA for specific therapeutic targets to modulate pediatric critical illness physiology.[124]

Assessment of Protein and Amino Acid Turnover in the Critically ill Child

Critical illness is a rapidly changing physiologic state in which protein requirements, utilization, and balance are evolving in accordance to the progression of the acute physiologic alterations.[165] Clinical examination, weight-for-height, body mass index (BMI), historically charted weight velocity, and anthropometry may help to detect risk factors for protein depletion, such as cachexia, limited muscle bulk, the presence of edema, obesity, and stunted growth.[57] Routine methods to assess body protein stores do not reflect the evolving protein and AA needs of a pediatric critically ill patient. Fat deposition may determine weight gain in chronically ill children in response to nutrition support without restitution of LBM.[166] Skinfold thickness to measure body composition is inaccurate in children with severe neurologic impairment.[167] Body mass index does not discriminate between alterations in LBM and body fat in pediatric patients with chronic inflammatory conditions.[166] Pediatric patients have rapid fat accumulation during the first year of life,[108] and in the presence of excess body fat, BMI may obscure deficits of LBM.[168-170]

Body Composition

Estimations of body composition to assess whole-body protein reserves have shown that clinically undetected decreases in LBM may exist despite preserved BMI.[170] Body composition estimates have been used to detect protein reserves and assess the response to nutritional interventions in critically ill patients.[171] Muscle and LBM correlate with disease severity, respiratory function, inflammation, and clinical outcomes during pediatric and adult illness.[170,172,173] In normal adult subjects, changes in diet may result in changes in body composition within 7 days.[171,174] In contrast to adults, neonatal and pediatric patients have high rates of protein turnover and accretion of skeletal muscle, the largest component and contributor to weight gain and body mass during periods of rapid growth.[106,114] Moreover, expansion of the fat mass compartment occurs rapidly during infancy, thus obscuring evaluations of LBM.[108,168,169] Accordingly, estimations of LBM and body fat determination in pediatric critically ill patients with prolonged PICU or chronic illness can provide valuable information for patient assessment.[171]

Body composition techniques, such as dual-energy x-ray absorptiometry (DEXA), computed tomography, and magnetic resonance imaging, provide information related to tissue density or volume of the protein compartments, but lack practicality or validation in the PICU.[57,175,176] Air-displacement plethysmography,[177] bioelectrical impedance analysis, and the use of tracer dilution with stable isotopes may allow measurement of body composition in select critically ill children, in the absence of major fluid shifts. These methods need further validation in the PICU setting.

Circulating Proteins, Amino Acids, and Degradation Markers

Visceral proteins are circulating proteins that are synthetized by the liver in response to AA, and their circulating levels have been used to evaluate nutritional status.[130] These include plasma albumin, prealbumin, and retinol-binding protein. However, none of the visceral proteins reflect losses or gains in total body protein, as 35% to 45% of the body mass resides in muscles. Therefore, protein wasting may occur despite adequate visceral protein concentrations.[57,176] The presence of capillary leak and hemoconcentration from third-space fluid shifts limits the interpretation of plasma concentration of serum proteins, and thus plasma proteins with a lower half-life, such as prealbumin and retinol-binding protein, are better indicators of acute changes in the formation of a de novo plasma pool of proteins in response to dietary protein than proteins with a longer half-life such as albumin.[176,178]

Acute-phase reactants, such as plasma C-reactive protein (CRP), help evaluate whether the liver preferentially makes acute-phase reactants rather than normal visceral proteins in response to nutrition support.[129,179] In inflammatory states, anabolism and catabolism are driven by the systemic inflammatory response, and not just by the appropriate availability of macronutrients.[133,180,181] Low prealbumin levels, despite provision of the calculated protein requirements, may occur in the presence of elevated plasma CRP.[182] In normal conditions, blood urea nitrogen (BUN) decreases during starvation and increases during dehydration,[176] renal insufficiency, in the presence of excessive dietary protein, or in the presence of blood in the gastrointestinal (GI) tract. However, in the PICU patient, circulating BUN can also be affected by the presence of decreased muscle mass, high protein utilization, and AKI.

Plasma AA concentrations are lower in patients with critical illness.[126,128] Amino acid profiles have been studied in the postsurgical and critically ill adult patient, and they appear to be highly variable and difficult to interpret due to the phase and intensity of the injury response; prior existing nutritional, metabolic, and hemodynamic status; and the characteristics of the nutritional therapy provided.[126]

3-methylhistidine (3-MH) is a component of the myofibrils that is liberated when the muscle structure is damaged or degraded, and it has been linked to proteolysis and muscle degradation in humans.[183,184] 3-methylhistidine released from muscle is not metabolized and is excreted in the urine.[185] Hence, levels of 3-MH may provide an indirect measure of skeletal muscle breakdown. Although 3-MH was initially studied in urine, plasma concentrations can also be used.[183] Similarly, full-length (42 kDa) α-actin is a product of myofibrillar degradation that is released when the muscle structure is damaged or degraded, and has been linked with muscle damage during injury in animals.[186,187] Some investigators have advocated that the cleaved fraction of α-actin (14 kDa) may be used as an accurate tool to assess muscle protein degradation in humans.[187-189]

Estimation of Whole-Body and Organ Protein and AA Kinetics

Critical illness evolves, and protein requirements, utilization, and balance also change in accordance to the evolution of the acute physiologic alterations.[165] Continuous adjustments of protein, nitrogen, and AA needs require a sound understanding of this dynamic state of protein flux during the course of illness.

Nitrogen Balance

The hypercatabolic state of injury or sepsis has been characterized by a marked negative nitrogen balance.[87,97,132,190] Adequacy of nitrogen intake is calculated and compared to nitrogen losses in urine, stool, skin, and other fluids, such as dialysate and thoracic or abdominal drainage, to assure equality to losses or retention.[191-193] Maintaining positive protein balance has been used as a surrogate measure of LBM preservation, but it does not evaluate protein or AA utilization, quality of intake, or protein reserves. Whole-body nitrogen utilization is affected by energetic deficits, and protein can be oxidized for energy in catabolic conditions.[87] In addition, adequate amounts of energy are needed to effectively utilize the supplemented protein. During sepsis in adults, variable increases in nitrogen intake improved nitrogen balance.[97,132] When protein and energy are supplied during critical illness, whole-body protein synthesis rates are increased without affecting protein breakdown. Therefore, improvement in protein balance at the expense of higher protein synthesis[97] may occur despite resulting ongoing losses of body protein.[194] In this regard, achieving protein balance may not prevent loss of LBM or skeletal muscle mass in adults.[195]

Nitrogen balance has significant limitations to assess protein metabolism in the ICU. The rapidly changing physiology and nutritional interventions during the acute phase in the critically ill do not allow a steady state of nitrogen intake or loss immediately following the 24-hr period of nitrogen loss estimation.[165] In addition, measurements of nitrogen loss through urinary excretion are difficult to compare among published evidence,[196] where nitrogen excretion and balance, illness severity, and age are highly variable.[97,196] Protein balance studies require standardization in the method used to estimate nitrogen in the biologic samples and require dedicated personnel to perform and interpret them.[196] Excretion of urea is highly variable in critical illness, and measurement of total urinary nitrogen is more accurate.[87,196]

Total urinary nitrogen losses have been reported between 170 and 347 $mg \cdot kg^{-1} \cdot d^{-1}$ in critically ill children.[97] Enterally fed infants with low severity of illness may require protein intake of >1.5 g/kg/day and energy intake >57 kcal/kg/day to achieve positive nitrogen balance, but a protein intake of 2.8 g kg/day with higher severity of illness.[97,196]

Tracer Methodologies

By labeling AA with molecules that can be traced, isotope techniques follow interorgan and systemic movement of the labeled AA, their metabolic fate, their interaction with hormones and body substances, and the degree of incorporation into tissue protein or fluids. Most studies in humans use stable isotopes and measure protein kinetics at the whole-body level. In animal models or tissue biopsy, the incorporation of the labeled molecule into tissue can be traced while manipulating substrate and hormonal relations. Tracer methodologies can be used to determine the extraction of the tracee by organs or splanchnic or limb beds, or to establish whole-body protein balance in relation to insulin, protein prescription, and synthesis of specific proteins in healthy and ill neonates, children, and adolescents.

The indicator AA technique has been used to determine specific AA requirements in children. It assumes that AA cannot be stored and must be partitioned between incorporation into protein or oxidation. With increasing intake of the limiting AA, oxidation of the indicator AA will decrease, reflecting increasing incorporation into protein. Once the requirement is met for the limiting AA, there will be no further change in the oxidation of the indicator AA.[102]

Tracer methodologies have significant limitations to assess protein metabolism in the ICU. While these methods are very accurate to measure protein kinetics, they are expensive and require specialized equipment and expertise to understand and perform the studies. The use of a specific AA as a tracee to interpret whole-body protein kinetics may be potentially altered by the metabolic fate and the characteristics of such specific AA and thus, the proper indicator must be chosen. For pediatric patients, the applicability of this method is limited further by the need to provide exogenous substances to pediatric patients and the inability to obtain tissue in infants and children due to its cost and invasiveness.

Prescription and Provision of Protein and AA in the Critically ill Child

The estimated protein requirements in grams/kg/day in the critically ill child should be based upon an understanding of protein metabolism, as most recommendations are based on expert opinion.[19] Protein requirements in critically ill children recommended by A.S.P.E.N are higher than protein recommendations for healthy children recommended by WHO.[165,197] This is because protein recommendations by WHO cover requirements needed for age-appropriate growth and development in healthy children, but they do not cover the increased needs driven by critical illness.[19,194]

Even though provision of adequate protein requirements to maintain nitrogen balance may not prevent whole-body catabolism and loss of skeletal muscle mass,[194,195] early administration of protein- and energy-enriched formula in critically ill infants has shown to promote protein balance by increasing protein synthesis without adverse effects.[198] The effects of excessive dietary protein have not been studied extensively, and the findings are equivocal.[199] In infants, empiric increase of enteral protein provision above requirements has been well tolerated without increased amino acid oxidation and urea formation.[111] Even when provided with the appropriate estimated requirements, the critically ill may lose more protein than they are able to assimilate.[194]

Enteral Protein Delivery

Enteral delivery of protein is the preferred way to provide protein to replenish the AA pool during critical illness. Figure 3-3A shows the effect of enteral feeding on AA kinetics during critical illness. Enteral delivery of protein may allow enteric and portal AA delivery to the liver and splanchnic bed. In this regard, not all the dietary protein reaches the plasma AA pool (Figures 3-1A and 3-3A). Thirty percent to fifty percent of essential amino acids (EAA) in the diet may be catabolized by the small intestine in first-pass metabolism for enteral utilization by the enterocyte[162] and splanchnic extraction.[111] In noncritically ill conditions, portal rather than arterial AA are preferentially used for hepatic protein synthesis of visceral protein after enteral feeding.[130]

Therefore, when calculating enteral feeding in the pediatric critically ill patient, it is safe and necessary to increase protein delivery above the age-appropriate estimated requirements for children.[165,197] Nitrogen balance in critically ill infants has been achieved within the first days after admission to the PICU by increasing enteral protein above dietary reference levels using a protein–energy-enriched formula, but not with a standard infant formula, and this intervention was well tolerated.[111]

The type of protein provided enterally to the critically ill child may affect tolerance, absorption, and utilization. Fast proteins, such as whey, are rapidly digested and absorbed and quickly induce an anabolic drive, possibly from their high leucine content.[200,201] Conversely, slow proteins such as casein have a longer enteric transit time, allowing a less robust but more sustained AA delivery to the AA pool.[201] In this regard, slow proteins will require more digestion and may promote the use of the derived AA toward energy precursors, inducing a smaller anabolic response than fast proteins.[201] The use of fast proteins or enteral formulas with predigested protein in the form of dipeptides or AA may be better tolerated in the critically ill due to the risk of impaired digestion. However, a combination of both types of protein may be beneficial for the recovery phase, when feasible.[200]

Continuous enteral tube feeding is frequently used in the ICU setting due to better tolerance to small enteral volumes, the use of transpiloric feeding, and with hopes to reduce bronchial aspiration. Continuous enteral delivery lacks the pulsatile effect that a rapid rise in AA provides.[116] In neonatal animal studies, intermittent boluses of protein have improved feeding efficiency by inducing a greater stimulatory effect on skeletal muscle protein synthesis than continuous feeding.[116]

Parenteral Protein Delivery

Parenteral protein is delivered to critically patients while awaiting readiness of the GI tract to tolerate dietary protein. Protein is provided as AA solutions, which can be designed with several profiles, based on their composition of branched-chain, sulfur, or EAA. Free AA mixtures provide 17% less protein substrate than does whole protein.[202] Moreover, the conventional factor 0.16 to convert AA nitrogen to its protein equivalent does not apply to free AA mixtures.[202] Infant parenteral solutions containing more essential AA are recommended.[203] Currently, we lack evidence-based recommendations to design an ideal, target-oriented parenteral AA composition for the critically ill child.

Figure 3-3B shows the effect of parenteral protein delivery on AA kinetics during critical illness. Parenteral protein bypasses the splanchnic extraction of a meal-derived AA, replenishing the plasma AA pool, but limiting enteral cells from surface substrate. Visceral protein synthesis is less responsive to parenteral than enteral protein. Intravenous AA bypass the splanchnic uptake and are presented to the liver through the portal venous circulation in lower concentrations.[130] Portal rather than arterial AA are preferentially used for hepatic protein synthesis.[130] Moreover, parenteral delivery of AA also lacks the anabolic pulsatile effect of a protein bolus meal, as parenteral nutrition is provided continuously throughout the day. However, parenteral nutrition is associated with a higher risk of mortality in mechanically ventilated children.[122]

Protein–Energy Interactions

The ideal caloric proportion (50% to 60% of calories from carbohydrates, 25% to 35% from protein, and 10% to 25% from fat) is most commonly appropriate, but such partitioning should be adjusted if an increased protein need arises. In order to avoid overfeeding, calories provided

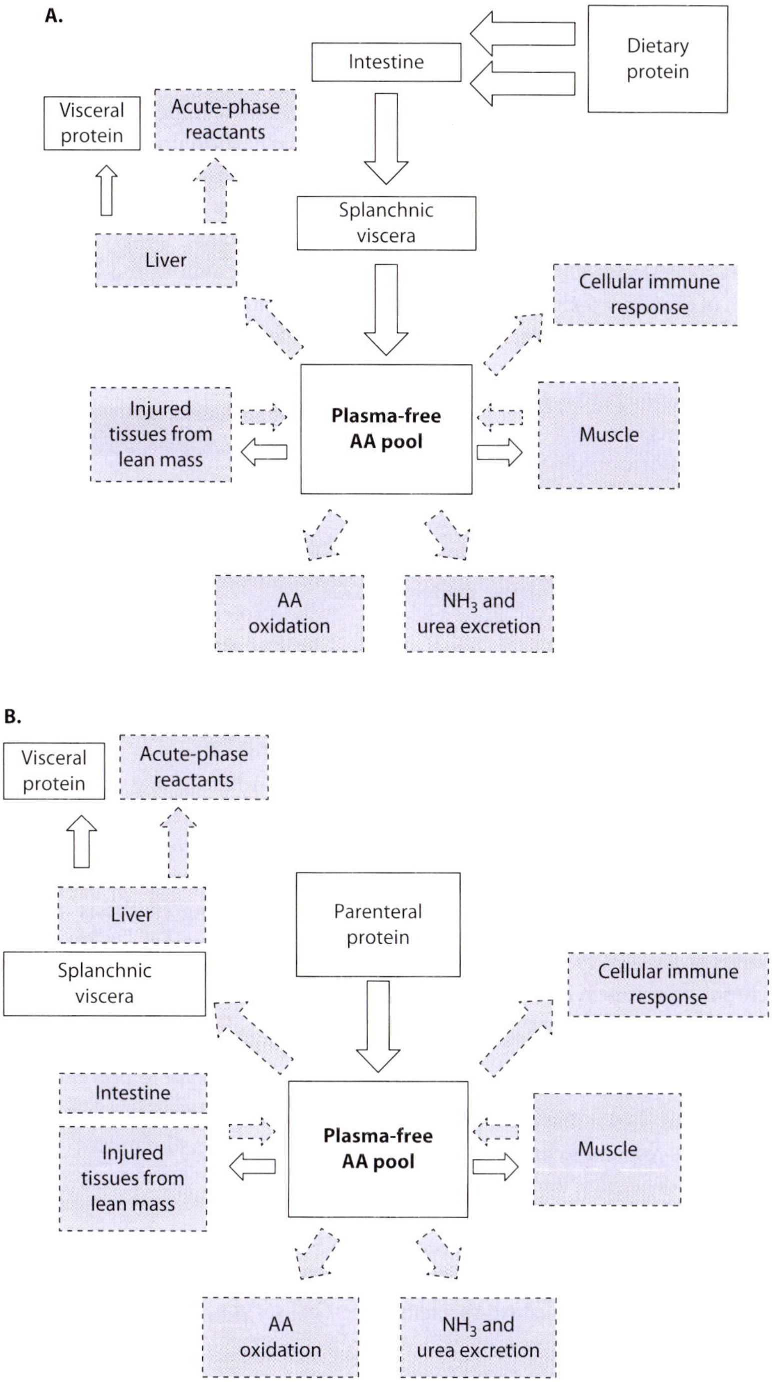

FIGURE 3-3. Schematic representation of the compartmental model used to study whole-body protein kinetics during critical illness/inflammation when supported with enteral (**A**) and parenteral protein (**B**). Red indicates pathways toward catabolism, while blue follows contributions toward protein and AA intake and attrition. Critical illness and inflammation drive the metabolic response despite provision of protein and AA. Parenteral protein bypasses the portal circulation and accesses the free AA pool directly.

from protein should be included in the predictions of nutrition requirements and in the calculation of the nutrition prescription.[204]

The calculation of calorie-to-nitrogen ratio, whether total or nonprotein calories, was historically proposed to appraise specific enteral formulas, but supports the concept of providing adequate caloric intake when high protein is provided.[57] In critical illness, the recommended calorie-to-nitrogen ratio has been suggested around 130-150 kcal/gram of nitrogen (1 gram of protein = 6.25 grams of nitrogen). This recommendation was based on expert opinion. For healthy active young men, a calorie-to-nitrogen ratio of 382:1 has been shown to promote nitrogen balance.[194]

For intensive care patients, protein underfeeding is more pronounced than caloric underfeeding.[47,84,126] Currently, patients in the PICU receive less than 50% of estimated caloric and protein requirements in the first 10 days of ICU care.[47,119,122] Protein underfeeding during critical illness exaggerates the cumulative protein deficit, which is most notable in infants with low reserves of LBM.[122] Metabolic utilization rate of macronutrients, dynamic changes in protein requirements, variation in nutrition practice, and cumulative deficits should be considered when providing protein support during critical illness. The underfed patients may benefit from safely increasing protein and energy intakes.[111,123,194]

Proteostasis in the Critically ill Child

Scientific developments will provide new insight into protein metabolism and adaptation to stress. Early studies on protein metabolism in natives of Papua New Guinea revealed human adaptation to chronic low protein intake with maintenance of appropriate health.[205] These concepts have been widened by our understanding of metabolic adaptation and plasticity, nutriogenomics,[206] metabolomics, and epigenetics.[162] Recently, it has been shown that during conditions of protein starvation, cells respond to the stress of AA deprivation by sensing the AA deficiency, leading to modulation of global protein synthesis to save energy expenditure through translation reprogramming to maintain metabolic homeostasis[206] In the future, advances in molecular and AA biology may offer promising targets to modulate the protein metabolic response during critical illness.

In pediatric critical care, the global evaluation of outcome in nutrition therapy is inherently difficult. Critically ill children with chronic protein malnutrition and depleted or low protein reserves[47,84,120,122] due to chronic diseases may have different AA requirements to achieve homeostasis.[102,162] Further studies are required to recognize adequate protein and AA requirements and prescription for high-risk infants and children in the PICU. Comprehensive understanding of protein metabolism and metabolic partitioning in the critically ill child emphasizes the need to individualize protein support therapy toward achievement of proteostasis (protein metabolic homeostasis) rather than simply balancing nitrogen expenditure.[207,208] Eventually, the goal of nutrition therapy is to optimize protein delivery and modulate protein catabolism, with the aim to prevent the loss of LBM and muscle function during critical illness.

KEY POINTS

- The metabolic stress response to injury, surgery, or illness is characterized by variable energy requirement and profound protein catabolism. The goal of nutrition therapy is to provide optimal energy and protein to offset these demands and facilitate healing and growth.
- A sound understanding of energy and protein metabolism during illness must guide macronutrient prescription.
- In contrast to starvation, the protein catabolism in critical illness cannot be eliminated with exogenous caloric provision. However, adequate macronutrient provision may help offset protein losses by increasing synthesis and thereby maintaining protein balance.
- The objectives of macronutrient intake during critical illness include prevention of underfeeding and overfeeding of calories and provision of enough protein to prevent loss of lean body mass.
- Indirect calorimetry, where available, should be used as the gold standard for assessing energy needs.

REFERENCES

1. Barton RG. Nutrition support in critical illness. *Nutr clin Pract: Off Paentre Enteral Nutr.* 1994;9(4):127-139.
2. Weissman C, Kemper M, Askanazi J, Hyman AI, Kinney JM. Resting metabolic rate of the critically ill patient: measured versus predicted. *Anesthesiology.* 1986;64(6):673-679.
3. Shangraw RE, Jahoor F, Miyoshi H, et al. Differentiation between septic and postburn insulin resistance. *Metab: Clin Exp.* 1989;38(10):983-989.

4. Jenkins RC, Ross RJ. Acquired growth hormone resistance in adults. *Bailliere's Clin Endocrinol Metab.* 1998;12(2): 315-329.
5. Weir JB. New methods for calculating metabolic rate with special reference to protein metabolism. *J Physiol* 1949;109(1-2):1-9.
6. Conzolazio CF, Pecora LJ. *The Computation of Metabolic Balances.* New York: McGraw-Hill, Blakiston Division; 1963.
7. Frayn KN. Calculation of substrate oxidation rates in vivo from gaseous exchange. *J Appl Physiol: Respir, Environ Exerc Physiol.* 1983;55(2):628-634.
8. Silberman H, Silberman AW. Parenteral nutrition, biochemistry and respiratory gas exchange. *J Parenter Enteral Nutr.* 1986;10(2):151-154.
9. Hulst JM, van Goudoever JB, Zimmermann LJ, et al. Adequate feeding and the usefulness of the respiratory quotient in critically ill children. *Nutrition.* 2005;21(2): 192-198.
10. McClave SA, Lowen CC, Kleber MJ, McConnell JW, Jung LY, Goldsmith LJ. Clinical use of the respiratory quotient obtained from indirect calorimetry. *J Parenter Enteral Nutr.* 2003;27(1):21-26.
11. McClave SA, Spain DA, Skolnick JL, et al. Achievement of steady state optimizes results when performing indirect calorimetry. *J Parenter Enteral Nutr.* 2003;27(1):16-20.
12. Schutz Y. On problems of calculating energy expenditure and substrate utilization from respiratory exchange data. *Zeitschrift fur Ernahrungswissenschaft.* 1997;36(4):255-262.
13. Smallwood CD, Mehta NM. Accuracy of abbreviated indirect calorimetry protocols for energy expenditure measurement in critically ill children. *J Parenter Enteral Nutr.* 2012;36(6):693-699.
14. Smyrnios NA, Curley FJ, Shaker KG. Accuracy of 30-minute indirect calorimetry studies in predicting 24-hour energy expenditure in mechanically ventilated, critically ill patients. *J Parenter Enteral Nutr.* 1997;21(3):168-174.
15. White MS, Shepherd RW, McEniery JA. Energy expenditure measurements in ventilated critically ill children: within- and between-day variability. *J Parenter Enteral Nutr.* 1999;23(5):300-304.
16. Jequier E, Acheson K, Schutz Y. Assessment of energy expenditure and fuel utilization in man. *Annu Rev Nutr.* 1987;7:187-208.
17. Radrizzani D, Iapichino G. Nutrition and lung function in the critically ill patient. *Clin Nutr.* 1998;17(1):7-10.
18. Brandi LS, Bertolini R, Calafa M. Indirect calorimetry in critically ill patients: clinical applications and practical advice. *Nutrition.* 1997;13(4):349-358.
19. Mehta NM, Compher C. A.S.P.E.N. Clinical Guidelines: nutrition support of the critically ill child. *J Parenter Enteral Nutr.* 2009;33(3):260-276.
20. Mehta NM. Nutrient Metabolism and nutrition therapy during critical illness. In: Mosby, ed. *Pediatric Critical Care* 4th ed. Saint Louis: Mosby; 2011:1073-1088.
21. Murgatroyd PR, Shetty PS, Prentice AM. Techniques for the measurement of human energy expenditure: a practical guide. *Int J Obes Relate Metab Disord: J Int Assoc Stud Obes.* 1993;17(10):549-568.
22. Schutz Y. The basis of direct and indirect calorimetry and their potentials. *Diabetes/Metab Rev.* 1995;11(4):383-408.
23. Muller MJ, Bosy-Westphal A. Assessment of energy expenditure in children and adolescents. *Curr Opin Clin Nutr Metab Care.* 2003;6(5):519-530.
24. Elia M. Energy equivalents of CO2 and their importance in assessing energy expenditure when using tracer techniques. *Am J Physiol.* 1991;260(1 Pt 1):E75-88.
25. Elia M, Fuller NJ, Murgatroyd PR. Measurement of bicarbonate turnover in humans: applicability to estimation of energy expenditure. *Am J Physiol.* 1992;263(4 Pt 1):E676-687.
26. Kien CL. Isotopic dilution of CO2 as an estimate of CO2 production during substrate oxidation studies. *Am J Physiol.* 1989;257(2 Pt 1):E296-298.
27. Sy J, Gourishankar A, Gordon WE, et al. Bicarbonate kinetics and predicted energy expenditure in critically ill children. *Am J Clin Nutr.* 2008;88(2):340-347.
28. Kingdon CC, Mitchell F, Bodamer OA, Williams AF. Measurement of carbon dioxide production in very low birth weight babies. *Arch Dis Child. Fetal Neonate Ed.* 2000;83(1):F50-55.
29. Tappy L, Schneiter P. Measurement of substrate oxidation in man. *Diabetes Metab.* 1997;23(5):435-442.
30. Epstein CD, Peerless JR, Martin JE, Malangoni MA. Comparison of methods of measurements of oxygen consumption in mechanically ventilated patients with multiple trauma: the Fick method versus indirect calorimetry. *Crit Care Med.* 2000;28(5):1363-1369.
31. Light RB. Intrapulmonary oxygen consumption in experimental pneumococcal pneumonia. *J Appl Physiol.* 1988;64(6):2490-2495.
32. Nunn JF. Pulmonary oxygen consumption. *Intensive Care Med.* 1996;22(4):275-276.
33. Carlsson M, Nordenstrom J, Hedenstierna G. Clinical implications of continuous measurement of energy expenditure in mechanically ventilated patients. *Clin Nutr.* 1984;3(2):103-110.

34. Archie JP Jr. Mathematic coupling of data: a common source of error. *Ann Surg.* 1981;193(3):296-303.
35. Brandi LS, Grana M, Mazzanti T, Giunta F, Natali A, Ferrannini E. Energy expenditure and gas exchange measurements in postoperative patients: thermodilution versus indirect calorimetry. *Crit Care Med.* 1992;20(9):1273-1283.
36. Marson F, Auxiliadora Martins M, Coletto FA, Campos AD, Basile-Filho A. Correlation between oxygen consumption calculated using Fick's method and measured with indirect calorimetry in critically ill patients. *Arquivos Brasileiros de Cardiologia.* 2004;82(1):77-81, 72-76.
37. Ogawa AM, Shikora SA, Burke LM, Heetderks-Cox JE, Bergren CT, Muskat PC. The thermodilution technique for measuring resting energy expenditure does not agree with indirect calorimetry for the critically ill patient. *J Parenter Enteral Nutr.* 1998;22(6):347-351.
38. Schneeweiss B, Druml W, Graninger W, et al. Assessment of oxygen-consumption by use of reverse Fick-principle and indirect calorimetry in critically ill patients. *Clin Nutr.* 1989;8(2):89-93.
39. Walsh TS, Hopton P, Lee A. A comparison between the Fick method and indirect calorimetry for determining oxygen consumption in patients with fulminant hepatic failure. *Crit Care Med.* 1998;26(7):1200-1207.
40. Kyle UG, Arriaza A, Esposito M, Coss-Bu JA. Is indirect calorimetry a necessity or a luxury in the pediatric intensive care unit? *J Parenter Enteral Nutr.* 2012;36(2):177-182.
41. Framson CM, LeLeiko NS, Dallal GE, Roubenoff R, Snelling LK, Dwyer JT. Energy expenditure in critically ill children. *Pediatr Crit Care Med: J Soc Crit Care Med World Fed Pediatr Intensive Crit Care Sic.* 2007;8(3):264-267.
42. Harris JA, Benedict FG. Standard basal metabolism constants for physiologists and clinicians. In: Washington CIPo, ed. *A Biometric Study of Basal Metabolism in Man.* Philadelphia: JB Lippincott; 1919:223-250.
43. Energy and protein requirements. Report of a joint FAO/WHO/UNU Expert Consultation. *WHO Organ Tech Rep Ser.* 1985;724:1-206.
44. Talbot FB. Basal metabolism standards for children. *Am J Dis Child.* 1938;55:455.
45. Schofield WN. Predicting basal metabolic rate, new standards and review of previous work. *Hum Nutr. Clin Nutr.* 1985;39(1)(suppl):1:5-41.
46. Mehta NM, Bechard LJ, Leavitt K, Duggan C. Cumulative energy imbalance in the pediatric intensive care unit: role of targeted indirect calorimetry. *J Parenter Enteral Nutr.* 2009;33(3):336-344.
47. Kyle UG, Jaimon N, Coss-Bu JA. Nutrition support in critically ill children: underdelivery of energy and protein compared with current recommendations. *J Acad Nutr Diet.* 2012;112(12):1987-1992.
48. Coss-Bu JA, Jefferson LS, Walding D, David Y, Smith EO, Klish WJ. Resting energy expenditure in children in a pediatric intensive care unit: comparison of Harris-Benedict and Talbot predictions with indirect calorimetry values. *Am J Clin Nutr.* 1998;67(1):74-80.
49. Havalad S, Quaid MA, Sapiega V. Energy expenditure in children with severe head injury: lack of agreement between measured and estimated energy expenditure. *Nutr Clin Pract: Off Pub Am Soc Parenter Enteral Nutr.* 2006;21(2):175-181.
50. Letton RW, Chwals WJ, Jamie A, Charles B. Early postoperative alterations in infant energy use increase the risk of overfeeding. *J Pediatr Surg.* 1995;30(7):988-992; discussion 992-983.
51. Mehta NM, Bechard LJ, Dolan M, Ariagno K, Jiang H, Duggan C. Energy imbalance and the risk of overfeeding in critically ill children. *Pediatr Crit Care Med: J Soc Crit Care Med World Fed Pediatr Intensive Crit Care Soc* 2011;12(4):398-405.
52. Suman OE, Mlcak RP, Chinkes DL, Herndon DN. Resting energy expenditure in severely burned children: analysis of agreement between indirect calorimetry and prediction equations using the Bland-Altman method. *Burns: J Int Soc Burn Inj.* 2006;32(3):335-342.
53. Frankenfield DC, Omert LA, Badellino MM, et al. Correlation between measured energy expenditure and clinically obtained variables in trauma and sepsis patients. *J Parenter Enteral Nutr.* 1994;18(5):398-403.
54. Pierro A, Jones MO, Hammond P, Donnell SC, Lloyd DA. A new equation to predict the resting energy expenditure of surgical infants. *J Pediatr Surg.* 1994;29(8):1103-1108.
55. Swinamer DL, Grace MG, Hamilton SM, Jones RL, Roberts P, King EG. Predictive equation for assessing energy expenditure in mechanically ventilated critically ill patients. *Crit Care Med.* 1990;18(6):657-661.
56. White MS, Shepherd RW, McEniery JA. Energy expenditure in 100 ventilated, critically ill children: improving the accuracy of predictive equations. *Crit Care Med.* 2000;28(7):2307-2312.
57. Orellana RA, Kyle UG, Coss-Bu JA. Nutritional Assessment and Feeding in the ICU. In: Stockwell JA, Preissig CM, eds. *Comprehensive Critical Care: Pediatric.* Mount Prospect, IL: Society of Critical Care Medicine; 2012:931-948.
58. Adams S, Dellinger EP, Wertz MJ, Oreskovich MR, Simonowitz D, Johansen K. Enteral versus parenteral

nutritional support following laparotomy for trauma: a randomized prospective trial. *J Trauma.* 1986;26(10): 882-891.

59. McClave SA, Lukan JK, Stefater JA, et al. Poor validity of residual volumes as a marker for risk of aspiration in critically ill patients. *Crit Care Med.* 2005;33(2):324-330.
60. Singer P, Berger MM, Van den Berghe G, et al. ESPEN Guidelines on Parenteral Nutrition: intensive care. *Clin Nutr.* 2009;28(4):387-400.
61. Chellis MJ, Sanders SV, Webster H, Dean JM, Jackson D. Early enteral feeding in the pediatric intensive care unit. *J Parenter Enteral Nutr.* 1996;20(1):71-73.
62. Skillman HE, Mehta NM. Nutrition therapy in the critically ill child. *Curr Opinion Crit Care.* 2012;18(2):192-198.
63. Heyland DK, Dhaliwal R, Drover JW, Gramlich L, Dodek P. Canadian clinical practice guidelines for nutrition support in mechanically ventilated, critically ill adult patients. *J Parenter Enteral Nutr.* 2003;27(5):355-373.
64. Heidegger CP, Darmon P, Pichard C. Enteral vs. parenteral nutrition for the critically ill patient: a combined support should be preferred. *Curr Opinion Crit Care.* 2008;14(4):408-414.
65. McClave SA, Martindale RG, Vanek VW, et al. Guidelines for the Provision and Assessment of Nutrition Support Therapy in the Adult Critically ill Patient: Society of Critical Care Medicine (SCCM) and American Society for Parenteral and Enteral Nutrition (A.S.P.E.N). *J Parenter Enteral Nutr.* 2009;33(3):277-316.
66. Peter JV, Moran JL, Phillips-Hughes J. A metaanalysis of treatment outcomes of early enteral versus early parenteral nutrition in hospitalized patients. *Crit Care Med.* 2005;33(1):213-220; discussion 260-211.
67. Goday PS, Mikhailov TA, Kuhn EM. Early parenteral nutrition is associated with significantly higher mortality in critically ill children. *J Parenter Enteral Nutr.* 2013 2013;37(1):140.
68. McClave SA, Heyland DK. The physiologic response and associated clinical benefits from provision of early enteral nutrition. *Nutr Clin Pract: Off Pub Am Soc Parenter Enteral Nutr.* 2009;24(3):305-315.
69. Hardy CM, Dwyer J, Snelling LK, Dallal GE, Adelson JW. Pitfalls in predicting resting energy requirements in critically ill children: a comparison of predictive methods to indirect calorimetry. *Nutr Clin Pract: Off Pub Am Soc Parenter Enteral Nutr.* 2002;17(3):182-189.
70. Reid CL. Nutritional requirements of surgical and critically-ill patients: do we really know what they need? *The Proceedings of the Nutrition Society.* 2004;63(3):467-472.
71. McClave SA, Kushner R, Van Way CW III, et al. Nutrition therapy of the severely obese, critically ill patient: summation of conclusions and recommendations. *J Parenter Enteral Nutr.* 2011;35(5)(suppl):88S-96S.
72. Lazzer S, Bedogni G, Lafortuna CL, et al. Relationship between basal metabolic rate, gender, age, and body composition in 8,780 white obese subjects. *Obesity.* 2010;18(1):71-78.
73. Alberda C, Gramlich L, Jones N, et al. The relationship between nutritional intake and clinical outcomes in critically ill patients: results of an international multicenter observational study. *Intensive Care Med.* 2009;35(10):1728-1737.
74. Lazzer S, Boirie Y, Bitar A, et al. Assessment of energy expenditure associated with physical activities in free-living obese and nonobese adolescents. *Am J Clin Nutr.* 2003;78(3):471-479.
75. Maffeis C, Zaffanello M, Pinelli L, Schutz Y. Total energy expenditure and patterns of activity in 8-10-year-old obese and nonobese children. *J Pediatr Gastroenterol Nutr.* 1996;23(3):256-261.
76. Stucky CC, Moncure M, Hise M, Gossage CM, Northrop D. How accurate are resting energy expenditure prediction equations in obese trauma and burn patients? *J Parenter Enteral Nutr.* 2008;32(4):420-426.
77. Frankenfield D, Roth-Yousey L, Compher C. Comparison of predictive equations for resting metabolic rate in healthy nonobese and obese adults: a systematic review. *J Am Diet Assoc.* 2005;105(5):775-789.
78. Aggett PJ, Haschke F, Heine W, et al. Committee report: childhood diet and prevention of coronary heart disease. ESPGAN Committee on Nutrition. European Society of Pediatric Gastroenterology and Nutrition. *J Pediatr Gastroenterol Nutr.* 1994;19(3):261-269.
79. Daniels SR. Lipid concentrations in children and adolescents: it is not all about obesity. *Am J Clin Nutr.* 2011;94(3):699-700.
80. Waterlow JC. Classification and definition of protein-calorie malnutrition. *Br Med J.* 1972;3(5826):566-569.
81. Pawellek I, Dokoupil K, Koletzko B. Prevalence of malnutrition in paediatric hospital patients.*Clin Nutr.* 2008;27(1):72-76.
82. Hendricks KM, Duggan C, Gallagher L, et al. Malnutrition in hospitalized pediatric patients: current prevalence. *Arch Pediatr Adolesc Med.* 1995;149(10):1118-1122.
83. de Souza Menezes F, Leite HP, Koch Nogueira PC. Malnutrition as an independent predictor of clinical outcome in critically ill children. *Nutrition.* 2012;28(3):267-270.

84. Kyle UG, Akcan-Arikan A, Orellana RA, Coss-Bu JA. Nutrition Support among Critically ill Children with AKI. *Clin J Am Soc Nephrol.* 2013. *CJASN.* 2013.

85. Pollack MM, Wiley JS, Holbrook PR. Early nutritional depletion in critically ill children. *Crit Care Med.* 1981;9(8):580-583.

86. Castillo A, Santiago MJ, Lopez-Herce J, et al. Nutritional status and clinical outcome of children on continuous renal replacement therapy: a prospective observational study. *BMC Nephrol.* 2012;13:125.

87. Coss-Bu JA, Jefferson LS, Walding D, David Y, Smith EO, Klish WJ. Resting energy expenditure and nitrogen balance in critically ill pediatric patients on mechanical ventilation. *Nutrition.* 1998;14(9):649-652.

88. Chwals WJ, Lally KP, Woolley MM, Mahour GH. Measured energy expenditure in critically ill infants and young children. *J Surg Res.* 1988;44(5):467-472.

89. Vazquez Martinez JL, Martinez-Romillo PD, Diez Sebastian J, Ruza Tarrio F. Predicted versus measured energy expenditure by continuous, online indirect calorimetry in ventilated, critically ill children during the early postinjury period. *Pediatr Crit Care Med: J soc Crit Care Med World Fed Pediatr Intensive Crit Care Soc.* 2004;5(1):19-27.

90. Verhoeven JJ, Hazelzet JA, van der Voort E, Joosten KF. Comparison of measured and predicted energy expenditure in mechanically ventilated children. *Intensive Care Med.* 1998;24(5):464-468.

91. Oosterveld MJ, Van Der Kuip M, De Meer K, De Greef HJ, Gemke RJ. Energy expenditure and balance following pediatric intensive care unit admission: a longitudinal study of critically ill children. *Pediatr Crit Care Med: J soc Crit Care Med World Fed Pediatr Intensive Crit Care Soc.* 2006;7(2):147-153.

92. Selby AM, McCauley JC, Schell DN, O'Connell A, Gillis J, Gaskin KJ. Indirect calorimetry in mechanically ventilated children: a new technique that overcomes the problem of endotracheal tube leak. *Crit Care Med.* 1995;23(2):365-370.

93. Taylor RM, Cheeseman P, Preedy V, Baker AJ, Grimble G. Can energy expenditure be predicted in critically ill children? *Pediatr Crit CAre Med: J Soc Crit Care Med World Fed Pediatr Intensive Crit Care Soc.* 2003;4(2):176-180.

94. van der Kuip M, de Meer K, Oosterveld MJ, Lafeber HN, Gemke RJ. Simple and accurate assessment of energy expenditure in ventilated paediatric intensive care patients. *Clin Nutr.* 2004;23(4):657-663.

95. Liusuwan RA, Palmieri TL, Kinoshita L, Greenhalgh DG. Comparison of measured resting energy expenditure versus predictive equations in pediatric burn patients. *J Burn Care Rehabil.* 2005;26(6):464-470.

96. Askanazi J, Rosenbaum SH, Hyman AI, Silverberg PA, Milic-Emili J, Kinney JM. Respiratory changes induced by the large glucose loads of total parenteral nutrition. *JAMA.* 1980;243(14):1444-1447.

97. Coss-Bu JA, Klish WJ, Walding D, Stein F, Smith EO, Jefferson LS. Energy metabolism, nitrogen balance, and substrate utilization in critically ill children. *Am J Clin Nutr* 2001;74(5):664-669.

98. Jaksic T, Shew SB, Keshen TH, Dzakovic A, Jahoor F. Do critically ill surgical neonates have increased energy expenditure? *J Pediatr Surg.* 2001;36(1):63-67.

99. Turi RA, Petros AJ, Eaton S, et al. Energy metabolism of infants and children with systemic inflammatory response syndrome and sepsis. *Annals of Surgery.* 2001;233(4):581-587.

100. Garza JJ, Shew SB, Keshen TH, Dzakovic A, Jahoor F, Jaksic T. Energy expenditure in ill premature neonates. *J Pediatr Surg.* 2002;37(3):289-293.

101. Alaedeen DI, Queen AL, Leung E, Liu D, Chwals WJ. C-Reactive protein-determined injury severity: length of stay predictor in surgical infants. *J Pediatr Surg.* 2004;39(12):1832-1834.

102. Elango R, Ball RO, Pencharz PB. Indicator amino acid oxidation: concept and application. *J Nutr.* 2008;138(2):243-246.

103. Protein. In: Kleinman RE, ed. *Pediatric Nutrition Handbook.* 6th ed. Washington DC.: American Academy of Pediatrics; 2009:325-342.

104. *Dietary Reference Intakes for Energy, Carbohydrate, Fiber, Fat, Fatty Acids, Cholesterol, Protein, and Amino Acids (Macronutrients).* National Academies Press; 2005.

105. Jespersen JG, Nedergaard A, Reitelseder S, et al. Activated protein synthesis and suppressed protein breakdown signaling in skeletal muscle of critically ill patients. *PLoS One.* 2011;6(3):e18090.

106. Jordan PN, Hall KD. Dynamic coordination of macronutrient balance during infant growth: insights from a mathematical model. *Am J Clin Nutr.* 2008;87(3):692-703.

107. Kyle UG, Genton L, Slosman DO, Pichard C. Fat-free and fat mass percentiles in 5225 healthy subjects aged 15 to 98 years. *Nutrition.* 2001;17(7-8):534-541.

108. Butte NF, Hopkinson JM, Wong WW, Smith EO, Ellis KJ. Body composition during the first 2 years of life: an updated reference. *Pediatr Res.* 2000;47(5):578-585.

109. Thivierge MC, Bush JA, Suryawan A, et al. Positive net movements of amino acids in the hindlimb after overnight food deprivation contribute to sustaining the elevated anabolism of neonatal pigs. *J Appl Physiol.* 2008;105(6):1959-1966.

110. Waterlow JC, Jackson AA. Nutrition and protein turnover in man. *Br Med J.* 1981;37(1):5-10.

111. de Betue CT, van Waardenburg DA, Deutz NE, et al. Increased protein-energy intake promotes anabolism in critically ill infants with viral bronchiolitis: a double-blind randomised controlled trial. *Arch Dis Child.* 96(9):817-822.

112. Denne SC, Kalhan SC. Leucine metabolism in human newborns. *Am J Physiol Endocrinol Metab.* 1987;253 (6 Pt 1):E608-E615.

113. Denne SC, Rossi EM, Kalhan SC. Leucine kinetics during feeding in normal newborns. *Pediatr Res.* 1991;30(1):23-27.

114. Davis TA, Fiorotto ML. Regulation of muscle growth in neonates. *Curr Opin Clin Nutr Metab Care.* 2009; 12(1):78-85.

115. Davis TA, Suryawan A, O'Connor PMJ, et al. Insulin and amino acids independently stimulate translation initiation in neonatal muscle. *Faseb J.* 2001;15(4):A268-A268.

116. El-Kadi SW, Suryawan A, Gazzaneo MC, et al. Anabolic signaling and protein deposition are enhanced by intermittent compared with continuous feeding in skeletal muscle of neonates. *Am J Physiol Endocrinol Metab.* 15;302(6):E674-686.

117. Davis TA, Suryawan A, Orellana RA, Nguyen HV, Fiorotto ML. Postnatal ontogeny of skeletal muscle protein synthesis in pigs. *J Anim Sci.* 2008;86(1)(suppl):E13-E18.

118. Matthews DE. Observations of branched-chain amino acid administration in humans. *J Nutr.* Jun 2005;135 (6 Suppl):1580S-1584S.

119. Rogers EJ, Gilbertson HR, Heine RG, Henning R. Barriers to adequate nutrition in critically ill children. *Nutrition.* 2003;19(10):865-868.

120. Typpo KV, Petersen NJ, Petersen LA, Mariscalco MM. Children with chronic illness return to their baseline functional status after organ dysfunction on the first day of admission in the pediatric intensive care unit. *J Pediatr.* 2010;157(1):108-113.

121. Edwards JD, Houtrow AJ, Vasilevskis EE, et al. Chronic conditions among children admitted to U.S. pediatric intensive care units: their prevalence and impact on risk for mortality and prolonged length of stay. *Crit Care Med.* 2012;40(7):2196-2203.

122. Mehta NM, Bechard LJ, Cahill N, et al. Nutritional practices and their relationship to clinical outcomes in critically ill children—an international multicenter cohort study. *Crit Care Med.* 40(7):2204-2211.

123. Hulst JM, van Goudoever JB, Zimmermann LJ, et al. The effect of cumulative energy and protein deficiency on anthropometric parameters in a pediatric ICU population. *Clin Nutr.* 2004;23(6):1381-1389.

124. Pierro A, Eaton S. Metabolism and nutrition in the surgical neonate. *Sem Pediatr Surg.* 2008;17(4):276-284.

125. Hasselgren PO, Fischer JE. Sepsis: stimulation of energy-dependent protein breakdown resulting in protein loss in skeletal muscle. *World J Surg.* 1998;22(2):203-208.

126. Hoffer LJ, Bistrian BR. Appropriate protein provision in critical illness: a systematic and narrative review. *Am J Clin Nutr.* 2012;96(3):591-600.

127. De Bandt JP, Cynober L. Therapeutic use of branched-chain amino acids in burn, trauma, and sepsis. *J Nutr.* 2006;136(1)(suppl):308S-313S.

128. Druml W, Heinzel G, Kleinberger G. Amino acid kinetics in patients with sepsis. *Am J Clin Nutr.* 2001;73(5):908-913.

129. Schreiber G, Howlett G, Nagashima M, et al. The acute phase response of plasma protein synthesis during experimental inflammation. *J Biol Chem.* 1982;257(17): 10271-10277.

130. Verbruggen SC, Schierbeek H, Coss-Bu J, Joosten KF, Castillo L, van Goudoever JB. Albumin synthesis rates in post-surgical infants and septic adolescents; influence of amino acids, energy, and insulin. *Clin Nutr.* 2011;30(4):469-477.

131. van Waardenburg DA, Deutz NE, Hoos MB, et al. Assessment of whole body protein metabolism in critically ill children: can we use the [15N] glycine single oral dose method? *Clin Nutr.* 2004;23(2):153-160.

132. Verbruggen SC, Coss-Bu J, Wu M, et al. Current recommended parenteral protein intakes do not support protein synthesis in critically ill septic, insulin-resistant adolescents with tight glucose control. *Crit Care Med.* 2011;39(11):2518-2525.

133. Evans WJ, Morley JE, Argiles J, et al. Cachexia: a new definition. *Clin Nutr.* 2008;27(6):793-799.

134. Wolfe RR. Regulation of skeletal muscle protein metabolism in catabolic states. *Curr Opin Clin Nutr Metab Care.* 2005;8(1):61-65.

135. Teng Chung T, Hinds CJ. Treatment with GH and IGF-1 in critical illness. *Crit Care Clin.* 2006;22(1): 29-40, vi.

136. Lang CH, Frost RA, Vary TC. Regulation of muscle protein synthesis during sepsis and inflammation. *Am. J Physiol Endocrinol Metab.* 2007;293(2):E453-E459.

137. Suryawan A, Jeyapalan AS, Orellana RA, Wilson FA, Nguyen HV, Davis TA. Leucine stimulates protein synthesis in skeletal muscle of neonatal pigs by enhancing mTORC1 activation. *Am J Physiol Endocrinol Metab.* 2008;295(4):E868-875.

138. Suryawan A, Nguyen HV, Bush JA, Davis TA. Developmental changes in the feeding-induced activation of the insulin-signaling pathway in neonatal pigs. *Am J Physiol Endocrinol Metab.* 2001;281(5):E908-E915.

139. Orellana RA, Suryawan A, Kimball SR, et al. Insulin signaling in skeletal muscle and liver of neonatal pigs during endotoxemia. *Pediatr Res.* 2008;64(5):505-510.

140. Glass DJ. Skeletal muscle hypertrophy and atrophy signaling pathways. *Int J Biochem Cell Biol.* 2005;37(10):1974-1984.

141. Du J, Wang X, Miereles C, et al. Activation of caspase-3 is an initial step triggering accelerated muscle proteolysis in catabolic conditions. *J Clin Invest.* 2004;113(1): 115-123.

142. Orellana RA, Suryawan A, Wilson FA, et al. Development aggravates the severity of skeletal muscle catabolism induced by endotoxemia in neonatal pigs. *Am J Physiol Regul Integr Comp Physiol.* 302(6):R682-690.

143. McKinnell IW, Rudnicki MA. Molecular mechanisms of muscle atrophy. *Cell.* 2004;119(7):907-910.

144. Dioguardi FS. Wasting and the substrate-to-energy controlled pathway: a role for insulin resistance and amino acids. *Am J Cardiol.* 2004;93(8A):6A-12A.

145. Biolo G, clan Fleming RY, Wolfe RR. Physiologic hyperinsulinemia stimulates protein synthesis and enhances transport of selected amino acids in human skeletal muscle. *J Clin Invest.* 1995;95(2):811-819.

146. Gore DC, Wolf SE, Sanford AP, Herndon DN, Wolfe RR. Extremity hyperinsulinemia stimulates muscle protein synthesis in severely injured patients. *Am J Physiol Endocrinol Metab.* 2004;286(4):E529-E534.

147. Whyte MB, Jackson NC, Shojaee-Moradie F, et al. Metabolic effects of intensive insulin therapy in critically ill patients. *Am J Physiol Endocrinol Metab.* 298(3): E697-E705.

148. Greenhaff PL, Karagounis LG, Peirce N, et al. Disassociation between the effects of amino acids and insulin on signaling, ubiquitin ligases, and protein turnover in human muscle. *Am J Physiol Endocrinol Metab.* 2008;295(3):E595-E604.

149. Dhar A, Castillo L. Insulin resistance in critical illness. *Curr Opin Pediatr.* 2011;23(3):269-274.

150. Hotamisligil GS, Peraldi P, Budavari A, Ellis R, White MF, Spiegelman BM. IRS-1-mediated inhibition of insulin receptor tyrosine kinase activity in TNF-alpha- and obesity-induced insulin resistance. *Science.* 1996;271(5249):665-668.

151. Das UN. Current advances in sepsis and septic shock with particular emphasis on the role of insulin. *Med Sci Monit.* 2003;9(8):RA181-RA192.

152. Bruins MJ, Deutz NE, Soeters PB. Aspects of organ protein, amino acid and glucose metabolism in a porcine model of hypermetabolic sepsis. *Clin Sci (Lond).* 2003;104(2):127-141.

153. del Aguila LF, Claffey KP, Kirwan JP. TNF-alpha impairs insulin signaling and insulin stimulation of glucose uptake in C2C12 muscle cells. *Am J Physiol.* 1999;276 (5 Pt 1):849-855.

154. Orellana RA, Kimball SR, Suryawan A, et al. Insulin stimulates muscle protein synthesis in neonates during endotoxemia despite repression of translation initiation. *Am J Physiol Endocrinol Metab.* 2007;292(2):E629-E636.

155. Perseghin G, Petersen K, Shulman GI. Cellular mechanism of insulin resistance: potential links with inflammation. *Int J Obes Relat Metab Disord.* 2003;27(3) (suppl):S6-11.

156. Hu Z, Wang H, Lee IH, Du J, Mitch WE. Endogenous glucocorticoids and impaired insulin signaling are both required to stimulate muscle wasting under pathophysiological conditions in mice. *J Clin Invest.* 2009;119(10):3059-3069.

157. Navegantes LC, Migliorini RH, do Carmo Kettelhut I. Adrenergic control of protein metabolism in skeletal muscle. *Curr Opin Clin Nutr Metab Care.* 2002;5(3): 281-286.

158. Young VR, Bier DM. Amino acid requirements in the adult human: how well do we know them? *J Nutr.* 1987;117(8):1484-1487.

159. Demling R. The use of anabolic agents in catabolic states. *J Burns Wounds.* 2007;6:e2.

160. Beale RJ, Sherry T, Lei K, et al. Early enteral supplementation with key pharmaconutrients improves Sequential Organ Failure Assessment score in critically ill patients with sepsis: outcome of a randomized, controlled, double-blind trial. *Crit Care Med.* 2008;36(1):131-144.

161. Argaman Z, Young VR, Noviski N, et al. Arginine and nitric oxide metabolism in critically ill septic pediatric patients. *Crit Care Med.* 2003;31(2):591-597.

162. Wu G. Amino acids: metabolism, functions, and nutrition. *Amino Acids.* 2009;37(1):1-17.

163. Kovarik M, Muthny T, Sispera L, Holecek M. Effects of beta-hydroxy-beta-methylbutyrate treatment in different types of skeletal muscle of intact and septic rats. *J Physiol Biochem.* 2010;66(4):311-319.

164. Wilson FA, Suryawan A, Gazzaneo MC, Orellana RA, Nguyen HV, Davis TA. Stimulation of muscle protein synthesis by prolonged parenteral infusion of leucine is dependent on amino acid availability in neonatal pigs. *J Nutr.* 2010;140(2):264-270.

165. World Health O. *Protein and Amino Acid Requirements in Hum Nutr.* Geneva: WHO press

166. King SJ, Nyulasi IB, Strauss BJ, Kotsimbos T, Bailey M, Wilson JW. Fat-free mass depletion in cystic fibrosis: associated with lung disease severity but poorly detected by body mass index. *Nutrition.* 2010;26(7-8):753-759.

167. Rieken R, van Goudoever JB, Schierbeek H, et al. Measuring body composition and energy expenditure in children with severe neurologic impairment and intellectual disability. *Am J Clin Nutr.* 94(3):759-766.

168. Ellis KJ. Human body composition: in vivo methods. *Physiol Rev.* 2000;80(2):649-680.

169. Ellis KJ, Shypailo RJ, Abrams SA, Wong WW. The reference child and adolescent models of body composition. A contemporary comparison. *Ann N Y Acad Sci.* 2000;904:374-382.

170. Engelen MP, Schroder R, Van der Hoorn K, Deutz NE, Com G. Use of body mass index percentile to identify fat-free mass depletion in children with cystic fibrosis. *Clin Nutr.* 31(6):927-933.

171. Plank LD, Hill GL. Similarity of changes in body composition in intensive care patients following severe sepsis or major blunt injury. *Ann N Y Acad Sci.* 2000;904: 592-602.

172. Ionescu AA, Evans WD, Pettit RJ, Nixon LS, Stone MD, Shale DJ. Hidden depletion of fat-free mass and bone mineral density in adults with cystic fibrosis. *Chest.* 2003;124(6):2220-2228.

173. Thomson MA, Quirk P, Swanson CE, et al. Nutritional growth retardation is associated with defective lung growth in cystic fibrosis: a preventable determinant of progressive pulmonary dysfunction. *Nutrition.* 1995;11(4):350-354.

174. Muller MJ, Lagerpusch M, Enderle J, Schautz B, Heller M, Bosy-Westphal A. Beyond the body mass index: tracking body composition in the pathogenesis of obesity and the metabolic syndrome. *Obes Rev.* 13 Suppl 2: 6-13.

175. Feferbaum R, Delgado AF, Zamberlan P, Leone C. Challenges of nutritional assessment in pediatric ICU. *Curr Opin Clin Nutr Metab Care.* 2009;12(3):245-250.

176. Kleinman RE. Assessment of Nutritional Status. *Pediatric Nutrition Handbook*; vol 6. Washington DC: American Academy of Pediatrics; 2009:559-576.

177. Rosendale RP, Bartok CJ. Air-displacement plethysmography for the measurement of body composition in children aged 6-48 months. *Pediatr Res.* 71(3):299-304.

178. Hulst JM, van Goudoever JB, Zimmermann LJ, Tibboel D, Joosten KF. The role of initial monitoring of routine biochemical nutritional markers in critically ill children. *J Nutr Biochem.* 2006;17(1):57-62.

179. Delgado AF, Okay TS, Leone C, Nichols B, Del Negro GM, Vaz FA. Hospital malnutrition and inflammatory response in critically ill children and adolescents admitted to a tertiary intensive care unit. *Clinics. (Sao Paulo).* 2008;63(3):357-362.

180. Cerra FB, Benitez MR, Blackburn GL, et al. Applied nutrition in ICU patients. A consensus statement of the American College of Chest Physicians. *Chest.* 1997;111(3):769-778.

181. Hulst J, Joosten K, Zimmermann L, et al. Malnutrition in critically ill children: from admission to 6 months after discharge. *Clin Nutr.* 2004;23(2):223-232.

182. Briassoulis G, Venkataraman S, Thompson A. Cytokines and metabolic patterns in pediatric patients with critical illness. *Clin Dev Immunol.* 2010;2010:354047.

183. Rathmacher JA, Nissen SL. Development and application of a compartmental model of 3-methylhistidine metabolism in humans and domestic animals. *Adv Exp Med Biol.* 1998;445:303-324.

184. Vesali RF, Klaude M, Thunblad L, Rooyackers OE, Wernerman J. Contractile protein breakdown in human leg skeletal muscle as estimated by [2H3]-3-methylhistidine: a new method. *Metabolism.* 2004;53(8):1076-1080.

185. Rathmacher JA, Nissen SL, Paxton RE, Anderson DB. Estimation of 3-methylhistidine production in pigs by compartmental analysis. *J Anim Sci.* 1996;74(1):46-56.

186. Martinez-Amat A, Boulaiz H, Prados J, et al. Release of alpha-actin into serum after skeletal muscle damage. *Br J Sports Med.* 2005;39(11):830-834.

187. Workeneh BT, Mitch WE. Review of muscle wasting associated with chronic kidney disease. *Am J Clin Nutr.* 91(4):1128S-1132S.

188. Mitch WE, Goldberg AL. Mechanisms of muscle wasting. The role of the ubiquitin-proteasome pathway. *N Engl J Med.* 1996;335(25):1897-1905.

189. Workeneh BT, Rondon-Berrios H, Zhang L, et al. Development of a diagnostic method for detecting increased muscle protein degradation in patients with catabolic conditions. *J Am Soc Nephrol.* 2006;17(11): 3233-3239.

190. Coss-Bu JA, Jefferson LS, Levy ML, Walding D, David Y, Klish WJ. Nutrition requirements in patients with toxic epidermal necrolysis. *Nutr Clin Pract: Off Pub Am Soc Parenter Enteral Nutr.* 1997;12(2): 81-84.

191. Maxvold NJ, Smoyer WE, Custer JR, Bunchman TE. Amino acid loss and nitrogen balance in critically ill

children with acute renal failure: a prospective comparison between classic hemofiltration and hemofiltration with dialysis. *Crit Care Med.* 2000;28(4):1161-1165.

192. Zappitelli M, Goldstein SL, Symons JM, et al. Protein and calorie prescription for children and young adults receiving continuous renal replacement therapy: a report from the Prospective Pediatric Continuous Renal Replacement Therapy Registry Group. *Crit Care Med.* 2008;36(12):3239-3245.

193. Zappitelli M, Juarez M, Castillo L, Coss-Bu J, Goldstein SL. Continuous renal replacement therapy amino acid, trace metal and folate clearance in critically ill children. *Intensive Care Med.* 2009;35(4):698-706.

194. Kreymann G, Delegge MH, Luft G, Hise ME, Zaloga GP. The ratio of energy expenditure to nitrogen loss in diverse patient groups—a systematic review. *Clin Nutr.* 2012;31(2):168-75.

195. Paddon-Jones D, Sheffield-Moore M, Urban RJ, et al. Essential amino acid and carbohydrate supplementation ameliorates muscle protein loss in humans during 28 days bedrest. *J Clin Endocrinol Metab.* 2004;89(9): 4351-4358.

196. Bechard LJ, Parrott JS, Mehta NM. Systematic review of energy and protein intake on protein balance in critically ill children. *J Pediatr.* 2012;161(2):333-339.

197. World Health O. *Energy and Protein Requirements.* Geneva: WHO;1985. 724.

198. van Waardenburg DA, de Betue CT, Goudoever JB, Zimmermann LJ, Joosten KF. Critically ill infants benefit from early administration of protein and energy-enriched formula: a randomized controlled trial. *Clin.Nutr.* 2009;28(3):249-255.

199. IOM FaNB. Dietary Reference Intakes for Energy, Carbohydates, Fiber, Fat, Fatty Acids, Cholesterol, Protein, and Amino Acids. *Protein and Amino Acids.* Washington, DC.: National Academies Press; 2006:689-768.

200. Tang JE, Moore DR, Kujbida GW, Tarnopolsky MA, Phillips SM. Ingestion of whey hydrolysate, casein, or soy protein isolate: effects on mixed muscle protein synthesis at rest and following resistance exercise in young men. *J Appl Physiol.* 2009;107(3):987-992.

201. Pennings B, Boirie Y, Senden JM, Gijsen AP, Kuipers H, van Loon LJ. Whey protein stimulates postprandial muscle protein accretion more effectively than do casein and casein hydrolysate in older men. *Am J Clin Nutr.* 93(5):997-1005.

202. Hoffer LJ. How much protein do parenteral amino acid mixtures provide? *Am J Clin Nutr.* 2011;94(6):1396-1398.

203. Verbruggen S, Sy J, Arrivillaga A, Joosten K, van Goudoever J, Castillo L. Parenteral amino acid intakes in critically ill children: a matter of convenience. *J Parenter Enteral Nutr.* 2010;34(3):329-340.

204. Skipper A, Tupesis N. Is there a role for nonprotein calories in developing and evaluating the nutrient prescription? *Nutr Clin Pract.* 2005;20(3):321-324.

205. Fujita Y, Okuda T, Rikimaru T, et al. Studies of nitrogen balance in male highlanders in Papua New Guinea. *J Nutr.* Apr 1986;116(4):536-544.

206. Liu B, Qian SB. Translational regulation in nutrigenomics. *Adv Nutr.* 2(6):511-519.

207. Hoffer LJ. Protein requirement of school-age children. *Am J Clin Nutr.* 2012;95(3):777; author reply 777-778.

208. Singer P. Toward protein-energy goal-oriented therapy? *Crit Care.* 2009;13(5):188.

CHAPTER 4

Micronutrient Requirements in the Critically ill Child

Theodoric Wong and Gil Hardy

- INTRODUCTION
- TRACE ELEMENTS
  - Zinc (Zn)
  - Selenium (Se)
  - Chromium (Cr)
  - Copper (Cu)
  - Manganese (Mn)
  - Iron (Fe)
- VITAMINS
- FAT-SOLUBLE VITAMINS
  - Vitamin A
  - Vitamin D
  - Vitamin E
  - Vitamin K
- WATER-SOLUBLE VITAMINS
  - Thiamine (Vitamin B_1)
  - Riboflavin (Vitamin B_2)
  - Niacin
  - Pantothenic Acid (Vitamin B_5)
  - Pyridoxine (Vitamin B_6)
  - Cyanocobalamin (Vitamin B_{12})
  - Ascorbic Acid (Vitamin C)
  - Folic Acid
  - Biotin
  - Choline
- KEY POINTS
  - References

INTRODUCTION

Inflammation and the generation of free radicals is the hallmark pathology of critical illness. Micronutrients with antioxidant properties have received much attention due to their role in these reactions. Reactive oxygen species, produced by leukocyte aerobic metabolism and free radical generation from nitric oxide metabolism, facilitate the release of nuclear transcription factor kappa B (NFκB). Cytoplasmic NFκB translocates to the nucleus, where it binds to DNA and increases acute-phase mediators like tumor necrosis factor α (TNFα), interleukin 2 (IL-2), and IL-2 receptors. Micronutrients such as selenium act to down-regulate NFκB.[1,2] Micronutrient deficiency may be due to suboptimal premorbid intake; redistribution from the circulation to tissues; and excessive losses from the kidneys, gastrointestinal (GI) tract, skin, and drains. Iron, selenium, zinc, vitamin D, and water-soluble vitamins are decreased in critical illness, whereas copper and manganese levels may be increased. Administration of micronutrients during illness is an area of great interest. Trace elements and vitamins that support antioxidant function—particularly high-dose parenteral selenium, alone or in combination with other antioxidants—are reportedly safe and may be associated with a reduction in mortality in critically ill patients.[2] Studies investigating the role of supplementation with selenium, vitamin E, and vitamin C in the critically ill have shown promising results, although there are still a number of unanswered questions.[3] Systematic reviews and meta-analyses in adults have shown that micronutrient supplementation may be associated with a decrease in overall mortality and specifically 28-day mortality. Decreased mortality seems to be mainly associated with combination products rather than any single micronutrient. However, supplementation does not affect infectious complications or length of stay in the intensive care unit (ICU) or hospital. The majority of trials have reported no adverse effects from micronutrients, with the exception of one study, which reported a worse outcome in patients with severe acute pancreatitis.[4]

TRACE ELEMENTS

Current daily recommendations for pediatric trace elements and vitamins are provided in Table 4-1[5] and Table 4-2, respectively, for reference, and the commoner manifestations of deficiency states are shown in Table 4-3. A brief description of the role of individual micronutrients and a summary of the literature related to their supplementation during pediatric illness are provided in this chapter.

Zinc (Zn)

Zinc is important during critical illness, mainly because of two properties: (1) it is a component of metallothioneins, which act as free radical scavengers (and, hence, are important as anti-inflammatory and antioxidant agents); and (2) it is a component of transcription factors and metalloproteinases that aid in keratinocyte migration during wound healing.[6] In view of these properties, most of the evidence for zinc supplementation in the critically ill comes from studies of patients following sepsis and burns.

Plasma Zinc Levels in the Critically ill

In a recent UK survey, only 18% of adult ICUs tested plasma zinc levels routinely.[7] Unlike most other trace elements, zinc has no functional reserve or store. When intake is insufficient and demand for zinc is high, tissue zinc is conserved by a reduction/cessation of growth and a decrease in its excretion.[5,8] In addition, decreased plasma zinc levels have been observed in a number of different settings. These include situations of increased losses (burns), increased cellular turnover (bone marrow

TABLE 4-1. Suggested Daily Pediatric Parenteral Trace Element Provision

	Zinc (mcg/kg)	Copper (mcg/kg)	Chromium (mcg/kg)	Iodine (mcg/kg)	Manganese (mcg/kg)	Selenium (mcg/kg)	Iron (mcg/kg)
Preterm infant <3 kg	400	20	0.05-0.2	30	Monitoring required	5-7 [15]	200-4000
Term infant 3-10 kg	250	20	0.2	0-1	Monitoring required	2	50-100
Child 10-40 kg	50	20	0.2	0-1	Monitoring required	2	50-100
	Zinc (mcg)	**Copper (mcg)**	**Chromium (mcg)**	**Iodine (mcg)**	**Manganese (mcg)**	**Selenium (mcg)**	**Iron (mcg)**
Adolescent >40 kg	2000-5000	200-500	5-15	No recommendations	50-100	30-60	1000
Adult	2500-5000	300-500	10-15	Not defined	60-100	20-60	1000

Reproduced with permission from Wong T. Parenteral trace elements in children: clinical aspects and dosage recommendations, Curr Opin Clin Nutr Metab Care 2012;15(6):649-656

TABLE 4-2. Summary Recommendations for Vitamins in Pediatric Critical Care

	DRI for Oral Intake		Daily Parenteral Dose	
Vitamins	Infants	Children	Infants	Children
Vitamin A	400-500 (RAE[1]) mcg/kg	400-500 mcg/kg	150-300 mcg/kg	150 mcg
Vitamin D	10-15 mcg	10-15 mcg	0.8 mcg/kg	10 mcg
Vitamin E	4-5 α-TE[2] mg	6-7 α-TE mg	2.8-3.5 mg/kg	7 mg
Vitamin K	2.0-2.5 mcg	30-55 mcg	10 mcg/kg	200 mcg
Vitamin B_1 (Thiamine)	0.2-0.3 mg	0.5-0.6 mg	0.35-0.5 mg/kg	1.2 mg
Vitamin B_2 (Riboflavin)	0.3-0.4 mg	0.5-0.6 mg	0.15-0.2 mg/kg	1.45 mg
Niacin	2-4 mg	6-8 mg	4.0-6.8 mg/kg	17 mg
Pantothenic Acid	1.7-1.8 mg	2-3 mg	1.0-2.0 mg/kg	5 mg
Vitamin B_6 (Pyridoxine)	0.1-0.3 mg	0.5-0.6 mg	0.15-0.2 mg/kg	1.0 mg
Folic Acid	65-80 mcg	150-200 mcg	56 mcg/kg	140 mcg
Vitamin B_{12} (Cyanocobalamin)	0.4-0.5 mcg	0.9-1.2 mcg	0.3 mcg/kg	1.0 mcg
Vitamin C (Ascorbic Acid)	40-50 mg	15-25 mg	15-25 mg/kg	80 mg
Biotin	5 mcg	8-12 mcg	5.0-8.0 mcg/kg	20 mcg
Choline	125-150 mg	200-250 mg	125-150 mg	200-250 mg

[1]RAE, retinol activity equivalents, I RAE = 1 mcg of retinol; RAE from plant sources calculated based on 12 mcg β-carotene.
[2]α-TE, c-tocopherol equivalents; DRI, Dietary Reference Intakes.

transplantation), and increased production of acute-phase reactants (inflammation/sepsis).[9] Low plasma zinc in critically ill children has also been reported in association with lymphopenia.[10] The mechanism for this has yet to be elucidated.

Although earlier studies in adults with burn injury did not show a significant drop in plasma zinc levels,[11] subsequent studies have established it is a common observation[12] that has also been found in children. Cunningham et al.[13] found decreased plasma zinc in severely burned children despite supplementation with parenteral zinc. The mechanism of the low plasma zinc has been attributed to a redistribution of zinc from muscle and skin to liver and bone marrow, initially as an acute response[14] and high urinary losses,[11,15,16] although poor premorbid zinc intake cannot be excluded. Zinc moves into tissues with rapid cell proliferation and intense acute-phase protein synthesis.[11] This is mediated via IL-6 and induction of metallothionein and zinc transporter expression.[17] Nonsurvivors, in particular, seem to have increased expression of two isoforms of metallothionein.[18] This raises further questions into how septic shock triggers genomic-level alterations in zinc homeostasis and affects survival.

Low serum zinc concentrations are associated with severity of illness.[17] In a prospective study that included 20 children with at least 1 organ failure or an unadjusted pediatric risk of mortality III score >5 admitted to the pediatric intensive care unit (PICU), all patients had low plasma zinc levels on admission.[19] Furthermore, patients with a lower plasma zinc level on day 3 of admission

TABLE 4-3. Symptoms Seen in Deficiency States of Trace Elements and Vitamins

Fat-soluble vitamins	
Vitamin A	Ocular manifestations: night blindness, dry eyes, poor growth, papillary hyperkeratosis, and impaired resistance to infections
Vitamin D	Rickets (enlargement of costochondral junctions, cranial bossing, persistently open anterior fontanelle, bowed legs, and epiphyseal enlargement)
Vitamin E	Hemolytic anemia in the newborn, hyporeflexia and spinocerebellar, and retinal degeneration
Vitamin K	Prolonged bleeding and hemorrhagic manifestations
Water-soluble vitamins	
Thiamine (vitamin B_1)	**Peripheral neuropathy, cardiac failure, lactic acidosis**
Riboflavin (vitamin B_2)	Cheilosis, glossitis, corneal vascularization, and photophobia
Niacin	Pellagra: diarrhea, dermatitis, dementia
Pyridoxine (vitamin B_6)	Microcytic anemia, seizures
Vitamin B_{12}	Megaloblastic anemia, neurological changes
Folate	Megaloblastic anemia
Vitamin C	**Scurvy, petechial hemorrhages, bleeding gums**
Trace elements	
Iron	Microcytic anemia, irritability
Zinc	**Hypogonadism, growth failure, diarrhea, decreased taste acuity, hair loss, and skin rash**
Chromium	Glucose intolerance
Copper	**Neutropenia, anemia, neurological manifestations**
Selenium	**Myalgia, cardiomyopathy**

Deficiencies that may be more commonly apparent during care in the intensive care unit are shown in bold.[31]

were associated with 2 or more organ failures. An inverse correlation with C-reactive protein (CRP) and the degree of organ failure at day 3 of the study was also reported. Possible etiologies such as decreased albumin (which binds zinc in the circulation) and increased urinary losses have been suggested.[20] Amino acid infusions and hyperglycemia may also increase urinary zinc losses through proximal renal tubule secretion.[17]

Effect of Zinc Supplementation in the Critically ill

At present, there are no reports of the effects of isolated zinc supplementation in critically ill children. Low plasma zinc has been found in burns, despite supplementation with doses that are 300% above the recommended daily amount (RDA)[21] and in adults may persist for up to 2 to 3 months.[12] One explanation for the persistently low plasma zinc levels is the large exudative losses from the skin where wound zinc concentration exceeded plasma concentrations.[21,22] Barbosa et al. showed that supplementation of zinc, together with vitamin E and vitamin C, in children decreased lipid peroxidation and time needed for wound healing (5.3 vs. 7.5 days in the nonsupplemented group).[23] In adults, delayed wound healing and infections were seen more than a month after injury in nonsupplemented burn patients despite the fact that no signs of trace element deficiency were present at the time of supplementation.[12] A combination product containing zinc and other trace elements modulated pulmonary infections and decreased length of hospital stay in burn patients.[24] In a recent double-blinded comparative effectiveness trial, children in the PICU were randomized to receive either supplementation with zinc, selenium, glutamine, and metoclopramide or whey protein.[25] The primary endpoint was time to development of nosocomial sepsis or infection. The study showed no difference in the outcome between the groups. In a subgroup of children in this study who were immunocompromised (9% of the cohort), supplementation with a combination of zinc, selenium, glutamine, and metoclopramide was associated with a reduction in the rate of nosocomial infection/sepsis.

Recommendations for Zinc Supplementation in the Critically ill Child

Agarwal et al.[20] have recommended enteral zinc intake of 25 mg per day or a parenteral dose of 50 mcg/kg per day in children with major burns, but the basis for this recommendation is unclear. Children weighing 10 to 40 kg would require a parenteral dose of 50 mcg/kg per day for their daily requirement, but this does not take into account additional requirements of burn patients.[5]

Otherwise, there is insufficient evidence for extra supplementation of zinc in the critically ill child. There appears to be a therapeutic window for zinc supplementation, as adult patients supplemented with more than 30 mg/d of parenteral zinc have been shown to have increased IL-6 and inflammatory response.[26] When enteral supplementation of zinc is being considered, competition with copper and iron for absorption may lead to deficiencies of the latter elements as an unintended consequence.

Selenium (Se)

Selenium's role in glutathione peroxidase (GPx) which inhibits proinflammatory cytokines up-regulated by NFκB, has made it an attractive pharmaconutrient.

Even though up to 50% of plasma selenium is found as selenoprotein P,[27] plasma selenium level reflects dietary intake rather than selenium stores or bioavailability, and may be a good reflection of short-term changes in selenium status. As selenium levels drop during the first weeks of life, selenium-dependent enzyme activity in tissue and body fluids may be a better measure of selenium status than serum selenium in the neonatal period.[28]

Plasma Selenium Levels in the Critically ill

Plasma selenium is lower in critically ill patients due to inflammation[29] and cannot be solely relied upon as a marker of selenium status.[10] Erythrocyte selenium concentration might be an alternative test of selenium status.[29] In adults, low selenium in the critically ill correlates directly with disease severity, as well as with morbidity and mortality.[30] Like other micronutrients, reduced plasma measurements may reflect redistribution of selenoproteins to the tissues and/or increased losses. Similarly, urinary selenium losses are associated with urinary nitrogen losses, which signifies catabolism and injury severity.[17]

Selenium Supplementation

There is some promising evidence for selenium monotherapy in critically ill adults, with possible reduction in infections and a trend toward reduced mortality in patients with systemic inflammatory response syndrome (SIRS), severe sepsis, or septic shock.[31] However, a recent meta-analysis of phase III clinical trials did not show clear benefit of selenium supplementation in these cohorts.[32,33] A Cochrane review by Darlow et al.[34] showed that high doses of selenium supplements may be able to reduce some complications (such as sepsis) in preterm neonates, but most of the evidence comes from a country where selenium levels were unusually low. Moreover, selenium was supplemented parenterally at doses ranging from 1.5 mcg/kg per day to 7 mcg/kg per day and in various forms (selenious acid, sodium selenate, and sodium selenite). Supplementation in critically ill adults often includes an initial bolus dose over 30 minutes, followed by daily infusions for up to 14 days.[17]

Because the major route of selenium excretion is via the kidneys, a decrease in parenteral selenium supplementation is recommended in patients with renal impairment.[35]

Chromium (Cr)

The role of chromium as a regulator of insulin action and hence glucose metabolism might be important in the critically ill.[36,37] Up to 75% of critically ill nondiabetic children may have persistent hyperglycemia.[38] Plasma chromium can be reduced in acute illnesses,[39] probably due to increased urinary losses from metabolic stress, trauma, or ascorbic acid deficits.[17] Although not all of these children will have chromium deficiency–related hyperglycemia, a therapeutic trial of intravenous chromium over several days might be beneficial, especially if inadequate intake is suspected.[40] Chromic chloride at 0.2 mcg/kg per day (daily pediatric parenteral requirement)[5] can be given unless there are other contraindications such as renal failure, as chromium is excreted via urine.[36,41] In addition, excessive amounts of chromium have been found to accumulate in the livers of patients on long-term parenteral nutrition (PN),[36] and their chromium provision will need to be revised when they become critically ill.

Copper (Cu)

Copper is a component of several metalloenzymes, mainly oxidases, hydroxylases, and superoxide dismutases. The liver is the key organ involved in maintaining plasma copper levels. Like zinc, copper is mainly stored in enterocytes as metallothionein and is lost with intestinal cell turnover every 2 to 3 days. Copper is absorbed in the ileum and largely excreted in the bile.

Berger et al. reported that plasma copper levels were normal in critically ill patients on continuous venovenous hemodiafiltration (CVVHDF),[42] but ceruloplasmin, the major copper-carrying protein in blood, is an acute-phase protein and is increased during inflammation and critical illness.[17]

Supplementation is not usually warranted unless copper deficiency is suspected. Excessive losses through biliary drains, high-output stomas, or burns may quickly lead to a deficiency characterized by a microcytic, hypochromic anemia that is unresponsive to iron therapy, poor wound healing, and osteoporosis,[43-46] with neutropenia being one of the earliest manifestations of copper deficiency.[44] Recent studies have found no correlation between cholestasis and serum copper levels,[47] nor copper toxicity or worsening of liver disease in cholestatic infants with supplementation of 20 mcg/kg per day.[46,48] Although there is poor correlation between hepatic tissue copper levels and serum copper levels,[49] patients with biliary obstruction should have their supplementation reduced or stopped in this circumstance with frequent monitoring.[50,51] Pediatric copper-balance studies have not been reported, but the available literature suggests that infants and children on PN should receive 20 mcg/kg per day, with a maximum up to 0.3 mg/d.[46] Decreased copper recovery in patients with a jejunostomy or exterior biliary drainage may require an increased provision of 10 to 15 mcg/kg per day of copper, depending on the amount of stomal losses.[35]

Manganese (Mn)

Manganese (Mn) is a nonspecific enzyme activator. It is a component of the metalloenzymes superoxide dismutase and pyruvate carboxylase, which play a significant role in antioxidant protection and energy metabolism. Manganese concentrations are typically elevated in critically ill patients, mainly due to manganese being a contaminant in intravenous products.[52,53] Urinary losses appear to be greater in patients with functioning kidneys on continuous venovenous hemofiltration (CVVH) and CVVHDF, which may also be due to contamination in the dialysate.[17]

Earlier studies have shown that bilirubin infusions in manganese-loaded animals can cause cholestasis,[54] and as the biliary tract is the major route of excretion, manganese provision needs to be revised in patients with biliary obstruction or hepatobiliary dysfunction.[55] Furthermore, hepatic dysfunction and cholestasis are suspected risk factors for increased manganese accumulation in the brain.[52] In addition, it is important to understand that it may take 5 to 6 months for elevated manganese levels in the blood to normalize after discontinuation of therapy.[52] There is currently no evidence for manganese supplementation during critical illness unless a true deficiency has been identified.

Iron (Fe)

Iron is an essential component of heme proteins such as hemoglobin, myoglobin, and cytochrome P450. The main manifestation of iron deficiency is anemia, although initial symptoms are nonspecific and can include lethargy, tachycardia, dizziness, and headache.

Anemia in the critically ill is not an uncommon phenomenon; the two main factors are inflammation and iron deficiency. Low serum iron and high ferritin levels are typical for critically ill patients, and this profile is indicative of inflammation. Anemia found in this setting has been termed "anemia of inflammation."[56] Inflammation-related IL-1 secretion stimulates ferritin synthesis, which is independent of iron stores, and so, despite a profile that might signify iron overload, iron deficiency might be present.[57] Reviewing the serum iron and transferrin saturation might be a better guide to iron deficiency in this circumstance.

VITAMINS

The following recommendations are largely updated from our previous review on micronutrient deficiencies in intestinal failure[58] and subsequent literature.[59]

Serum levels of some vitamins decrease with the inflammatory response,[60] but vitamins B_1, B_2, B_{12}, and folate are not affected by inflammation. Decreased levels of these vitamins may represent a true deficiency when observed in patients with inflammatory bowel disease (IBD) from losses through high-output GI fistulas or with diarrhea. Refeeding of upper GI secretions into the jejunum, either via a nasojejunal tube or jejunostomy,[61] will facilitate uptake of fat-soluble vitamins that require bile and pancreatic secretions for optimal absorption.[62] Most water-soluble vitamins are absorbed easily from the proximal GI tract, and deficiencies may be seen in patients with relatively short lengths of jejunum or residual ileum. Fat-soluble vitamins are absorbed in the mid- and distal ileum, as digestion of fat by bile and pancreatic lipase is required. If the terminal ileum is missing, then these vitamins plus B_{12} become depleted. In conditions where fat malabsorption can occur, such as pancreatic insufficiency and bile loss, deficiency of fat-soluble vitamins is common.

Drug–nutrient and other complex interactions between vitamins and/or trace elements during compounding, storage, and administration of PN admixtures can substantially reduce the amounts of individual vitamins delivered to the pediatric patient. Protection from air and sunlight can minimize many chemical losses,[63] but it may also be necessary to compensate for vitamin losses with an increased dosage.

FAT-SOLUBLE VITAMINS

Vitamin A

Vitamin A (retinol) comprises a number of beta-ionone derivatives of beta-carotene, the most biologically active of which is all-trans-retinol. It is required for vision, bone development, and immune function. Supplementation of excess vitamin E may antagonize vitamin A function. There is considerable epidemiological evidence of an important relationship between vitamin A and iron metabolism. Recent animal data confirm that vitamin A deficiency may inhibit release of iron from the liver and adversely affect iron homeostasis.[64] Since postoperative patients exhibit decreased levels of vitamin A and septic patients excrete high levels in the urine, it is important to ensure that both vitamin A and iron are supplemented in the critically ill child. Retinol is highly sensitive to daylight, undergoing rapid degradation by more than 90% during infusion if no precautions are taken.[65] It is, therefore, essential to cover the PN container with a light-protecting overwrap when infusing in daylight. Pediatric dosage recommendations for vitamin A supplementation are 150 to 300 mcg/kg per day, as summarized in Table 4-2.

Vitamin D

Ergocalciferol (vitamin D_2) and cholecalciferol (D_3) have similar sterol-like structures. They are considered to be biologically equivalent in humans, but 25-hydroxyvitamin D_3 (25-OH-D) is the form measured to determine vitamin D status. Hypovitaminosis D is generally present at serum levels <20 ng/mL and is common in critically ill children, especially in those with heart disease. Thus, serum levels should be routinely monitored in the critically ill child and maintained at 30 to 100 ng/mL by daily supplementation at 0.8 mcg/kg (see Table 4-2).[66] Vitamin D is required for bone synthesis, immunomodulation, and cardiovascular function. Diseases such as Crohn disease, or any malabsorption syndrome, will interfere with vitamin D absorption in the GI tract[67] Small-bowel absorption of calcium is dependent upon an adequate supply of vitamin D. It regulates induction of proteins that enable the gut enterocytes to transport calcium into plasma. Calcium losses combined with insufficient vitamin D can lead to hypocalcemia, osteomalacia, and increased risk of fractures. Hypovitaminosis D is associated with alterations in glucose and lipid metabolism, and increases the risk of osteoporosis, heart disease, and rickets. It has also been associated with higher levels of illness severity, infection, septic shock, and mortality in adults. The inverse association of vitamin D levels with septic shock may be partly due to fluid resuscitation, but pre-PICU dietary supplementation of vitamin D can protect against deficiency.[68] An Australian study reported hypovitaminosis D in one-third (34.5%) of children on admission to PICU. This is lower than adults in the ICU, but higher than the 18% prevalence in healthy American children. A correlation between vitamin D levels and ionized calcium has been observed, but no association was seen between vitamin D deficiency and mortality.[69] Similarly, in the United States, a 31% prevalence of vitamin D deficiency in infants and 46% depletion in children in a PICU have been reported.[68] The capacity to synthesize vitamin D from sunlight is likely to be reduced during long-term hospitalization, but bioavailability studies in children have suggested that vitamin D status can be maintained during long-term home parenteral nutrition (HPN).[70] However, losses may be incurred in PN admixtures: Gillis et al.[71] reported significant cholecalciferol depletion from non-fat-containing PN bags during simulated administration, speculating that binding to the plastic bag and administration set occurs. In contrast, no losses were reported during vitamin D infusion in a lipid emulsion, which may have a protective effect.[72] Nevertheless, light protection of PN systems is always advisable.[58]

Vitamin E

Vitamin E (tocopherol) deficiencies are rare, but absorption of vitamin E requires adequate biliary and pancreatic function. A serum ά-tocopheral:cholesterol ratio < 2.47 mg/g is consistent with deficiency,[73] and repletion should be at a dosage up to 3.5 mg/kg (Table 4-2). Moreover, vitamins E and C are synergistic, so a deficiency of the latter in postoperative patients also decreases vitamin E function.[74,75] The 4 tocopherol isomers (the usual artificial sources of vitamin E) have variable biological activity but are relatively stable after addition to PN mixtures, at least when light protected.[76] Exposure to daylight causes degradation by a photo-oxidative reaction in the presence of oxygen. This can account for losses amounting to 30% to 50% during administration.[71] Some lipid emulsions also contain alpha-tocopherol and may be partially light protective.

Vitamin K

Vitamin K has an important role in bone health, blood clotting, and regulation of several enzymatic reactions. However, ingested vitamin K in the form of phylloquinone is poorly absorbed. Antimicrobial drugs that alter the intestinal flora responsible for synthesis of vitamin K may also cause depletion. Measurement of phylloquinone in serum is a useful indicator of vitamin K status, whereas the international normalized ratio (INR) is an insensitive method.[77] Plasma levels of PIVKA-II (proteins induced by vitamin K absence) are a sensitive method of assessing subclinical vitamin K deficiency. The natural form of the vitamin is also present in relatively high levels in soybean oil lipid emulsions, while the synthetic derivative used in some additives is a mixture of cis and trans isomers, but contains more than 80% of the natural trans isomer. The U.S. Food and Drug Administration (FDA) has recommended that parenteral multivitamin products should provide 150 mcg/d, but nutrition support teams (NSTs) need to be aware that this amount could be almost doubled from the lipid emulsion content when considering supplementation.[78] Vitamin K is stable in PN mixtures during storage for at least 20 days at 4°C, but losses may occur from daylight exposure.

WATER-SOLUBLE VITAMINS

Thiamine (Vitamin B_1)

Thiamine diphosphate (cocarboxylase), employed in many parenteral multivitamin products, is the coenzyme form of vitamin B_1. Most malnourished patients are thiamine deficient, and without concurrent supplementation, as indicated in Table 4-2, large carbohydrate loads will trigger thiamine deficiency. Thiamine is rapidly consumed in glycolysis and can cause lactic acidosis with impaired glucose metabolism. Thus, when levels become depleted, pyruvate cannot be decarboxylated and cannot enter the Krebs cycle. This leads to failed synthesis of adenosine triphosphate and an energy deficit,[79] resulting in hypotension, tachycardia, and severe metabolic acidosis that does not respond well to bicarbonate therapy. Other symptoms include altered mental status, diplopia, vomiting, and abdominal pain.

Riboflavin (Vitamin B_2)

Riboflavin has numerous roles as a coenzyme in critical oxidation reduction reactions. Deficiency symptoms are nonspecific and include nausea, vomiting, abdominal pain, weight loss, and fatigue, but can be easily reversed by supplementation at the doses indicated in Table 4-2 through its beneficial effect on mitochondrial function.[62]

Niacin

Nicotinamide, or niacin, the physiologically active form of the vitamin, is the amide derivative of nicotinic acid and the form of the vitamin found in plasma and tissues. Vitamin C; copper; zinc; iron; and the amino acids leucine, methionine, and especially tryptophan are all involved in the metabolism of nicotinamide. Requirements are directly related to dietary tryptophan and energy intake, and are increased when pyridoxine (vitamin B_6) and riboflavin (vitamin B_2) deficiencies are present.[62]

Recommended dosages range from 5 to 6 mg/d for infants and 9 to 12 mg/d for older children. Preterm babies can be given doses between 380 and 5500 mcg/kg per day. The amount of tryptophan usually included in pediatric PN admixtures, together with the nicotinamide in commercially available multivitamin products, provides a good proportion of daily requirements.[59,80]

Pantothenic Acid (Vitamin B_5)

Pantothenic acid is a key component of coenzyme A, and is essential for many acetylation reactions, especially the tricarboxylic acid cycle. Deficiencies are rare in humans, and diarrhea is the only reported evidence of any toxicity.[62] Only the D (+) enantiomer of this vitamin has biological activity, and it is usually provided as the alcohol, D-pantothenyl alcohol (dexpenthanol), which is the form incorporated into the various multivitamin preparations used for routine PN supplementation, at daily doses ranging from 2 mg for infants up to 10 mg for older children (Table 4-2).

Pyridoxine (Vitamin B_6)

Pyridoxine plays an essential role in maintenance of brain function, where many key enzymatic reactions are dependent upon adequate levels of B_6. Pyridoxal-5-phosphate is also involved in lipid metabolism. The intravenous pediatric dose is normally between 4 and 10 mg/d (Table 4-2).

Cyanocobalamin (Vitamin B_{12})

Cyanocobalamin is a complex molecule, comprising 4 pyrrole groups joined in a large ring with a cobalt atom attached to a cyanide group. The vitamin requirement is similar for adults and children, but malabsorption, gastrectomy, or terminal ileum resection may lead to vitamin B_{12} deficiency, which alters intestinal mucosal cell morphology and intestinal cell wall transport function. Typically, patients at greatest risk for B_{12} deficiency include those with a history of surgical resection greater than 15 to 45 cm of ileum as infants. Loss of the ileum (>100 cm) is metabolically much more significant than loss of the jejunum, since it is the site of absorption of intrinsic factor-bound B_{12}. Nitrous oxide administration during anesthesia and use of proton pump inhibitors (PPIs) or H_2 receptor antagonists can also interfere with B_{12} metabolism.[81,82] Vitamin B_{12} deficiency is associated with megaloblastic anemia and potentially irreversible neurocognitive complications. Detecting increased levels of methylmalonic acid is often used for diagnosis of deficiency states, as serum vitamin B_{12} assays are less precise. Patients with vitamin B_{12} deficiency secondary to ileal resection will not respond to oral supplementation and should be treated with daily intranasal administration of the vitamin. Vitamin B_{12} levels have been shown to correlate with Acute Physiology and Chronic Health Evaluation (APACHE) II score (in adults), and in a study where 95% of patients had a diagnosis of SIRS, an increase of serum vitamin B_{12} was recorded for those patients who did not survive beyond 90 days in ICU.[83] Since the symptoms of vitamin B_{12} deficiency may be masked by high folate intake, careful monitoring is imperative so as to avoid neurological complications. Recommended doses are shown in Table 4-2.

Ascorbic Acid (Vitamin C)

Scurvy is the best-known manifestation of severe vitamin C deficiency, but in the critically ill, vitamin C depletion is also associated with poor wound healing and decreased vitamin A function. Ascorbate is an important antioxidant and a cofactor for several enzymes involved in the synthesis of carnitine, dopamine, serotonin, and the metabolism of cholesterol. Nevertheless, there is no clear indicator of inadequate vitamin C status. A serum level less than 20 mmol/L has been advocated, but plasma concentrations will be altered by inflammation.[84] The U.S. Dietary Reference Intakes (DRI) recommends 75 mg/d for females and 90 mg/d for males, increasing to 200 mg/d for parenteral use.[59] A parenteral dosage of 100 to 150 mg/d has been standard European practice,[85] but PN supplementation requires care. Ascorbic acid is the least stable vitamin in solution. The compound reacts directly with oxygen to form dehydroascorbic acid, which in turn is rapidly hydrolyzed to 2,3-diketogluconic acid. This reaction is catalyzed by heavy metals, in particular, copper and iron. The final stage of the degradation pathway leads to oxalate formation, which is toxic. Both the rate and extent of losses of ascorbic acid in PN mixtures depend on the quantity of oxygen present during storage and administration. Losses due to this process can be prevented by multilayered plastic bags, which are largely impermeable to oxygen, and mixtures prepared in such containers may be assigned extended shelf-lives.[86] Some initial loss of ascorbic acid after addition to a PN mixture is inevitable, but the reaction with dissolved oxygen will be complete within a few hours and can be compensated for by increasing the recommended dose (Table 4-2).

Folic Acid

Folic acid is a B-complex vitamin consisting of a pteridine molecule linked through a methylene bridge to p-aminobenzamide, which is bonded to glutamic acid. This structure enables folate to function as a coenzyme in single-carbon (methylene) transfers for the metabolism of amino acids and nucleic acids. Folate intake may have been limited by special diets or its uptake reduced by interference from certain medications. Continuous renal replacement therapy (CRRT) may also affect nutrition status. In a study of 15 children (mean age 7.7 yrs) receiving CVVHD, selenium balances were negative and serum folate concentrations decreased significantly, supporting the suggestion that standard pediatric folate supplementation (Table 4-2) may not be adequate during replacement therapy.[87]

Biotin

Biotin is important for carboxylase enzymes involved with carbohydrate and fat metabolism. Deficiencies are rare in the critically ill, but symptoms include dermatitis, conjunctivitis, alopecia, and paresthesia. A scaly, red rash, often confused with that seen with zinc deficiency or essential fatty acid deficiency, can develop around the eyes, nose, mouth, or genital area. However, insufficient information precludes making firm recommendations for doses above the level of 20 mcg/d for children (Table 4-2). Data on the stability of biotin in PN mixtures are sparse.

Choline

Choline is a quaternary amine salt synthesized from methionine. It is not actually a vitamin, but is required to be supplemented in infant enteral formulas in the United States. No parenteral product is currently available, but dosage recommendations have been made[59] (Table 4-2).

KEY POINTS

- Critically ill patients have variable deficiencies of micronutrients during the course of illness.
- Thiamine, vitamin C, zinc, copper, and selenium are the most common micronutrient deficiencies seen in adults with critical illness.
- A high degree of clinical suspicion is required to anticipate, diagnose, and treat micronutrient deficiencies during critical illness.
- A systematic approach to assessing micronutrients is essential to prevent complications due to deficiencies in calcium, magnesium, phosphorus, zinc, selenium, and multivitamins.
- In the future, there may be a role for routine supplementation of certain micronutrients during critical illness.

REFERENCES

1. Berger MM, Shenkin A. Update on clinical *micronutrient supplementation studies in the critically ill. Curr Opin Clin Nutr Metab Care*. 2006;9(6):711-716.
2. Hardy G, Hardy IJ, Manzanares W. Selenium supplementation in the critically ill. Nutr Clin Practice. 2012:12; 21-33.
3. Atkinson M, Worthley LI. Nutrition in the critically ill patient: part II. Parenteral nutrition. *Crit Care Resusc*. 2003;5(2):121-136.
4. Visser J, Labadarios D, Blaauw R. Micronutrient supplementation for critically ill adults: a systematic review and meta-analysis. *Nutrition*. 2011;27(7-8):745-758.
5. Wong T. Parenteral trace elements in children: clinical aspects and dosage recommendations. *Curr Opin Clin Nutr Metab Care*. 2012;15(6):649-656.
6. Berger MM. Zinc: a key pharmaconutrient in critically ill patients? *J Parenter Enteral Nutr*. 2008;32(5):582-584.
7. Duncan A, Dean P, Simm M et al. Zinc supplementation in intensive care: results of a UK survey. *J Crit Care*. 2012;27(1)102.e1-6.
8. King, JC. Assessment of zinc status. *J. Nutr*. 1999;120(11)(suppl):1474-1479.
9. Berger MM, Shenkin A. Trace element requirements in critically ill burned patients. *J Trace Elem Med Biol*. 2007;21(1)(suppl):44-48.
10. Heidemann SM et al. Baseline serum concentrations of zinc, selenium, and prolactin in critically ill children. *Pediatr Crit Care Med*. 2013. Feb 7 (ahead of print).
11. Shakespeare PG. Studies on the serum levels of iron, copper and zinc and the urinary excretion of zinc after burn injury. *Burns Incl Therm Inj*. 1982;8(5):358-364.
12. Berger MM et al. Trace element supplementation after major burns increases burned skin trace element concentrations and modulates local protein metabolism but not whole-body substrate metabolism. *Am J Clin Nutr*. 2007;85(5):1301-1306.
13. Cunningham JJ et al. Zinc and copper status of severely burned children during TPN. *J Am Coll Nutr*. 1991;10(1):57-62.
14. Ding HQ et al. Oxidative stress and metallothionein expression in the liver of rats with severe thermal injury. *Burns*. 2002;28(3):215-221.
15. Fell GS et al. Urinary zinc levels as an indication of muscle catabolism. *Lancet*. 1973;1(7798):280-282.
16. Boosalis MG et al. Increased urinary zinc excretion after thermal injury. *J Lab Clin Med*, 1991;118(6):538-545.
17. Boullata JI. Trace elements in critically ill patients. *J Infus Nurs*. 2013;36(1):16-23.
18. Wong HR et al. Genome-level expression profiles in pediatric septic shock indicate a role for altered zinc homeostasis in poor outcome. *Physiol Genomics*. 2007;30(1):146-155.
19. Cvijanovich NZ et al. Zinc homeostasis in pediatric critical illness. *Pediatr Crit Care Med*. 2009;10(1):29-34.
20. Agarwal A et al. Trace elements in critical illness. *J Endocrin Metab*. 2011;1(2):57-63.
21. Voruganti VS et al. Impaired zinc and copper status in children with burn injuries: need to reassess nutritional requirements. *Burns*. 2005;31(6):711-716.
22. Larson DL et al. Zinc deficiency in burned children. *Plast Reconstr Surg*. 1970;46(1):13-21.
23. Barbosa E et al. Supplementation of vitamin E, vitamin C, and zinc attenuates oxidative stress in burned children: a randomized, double-blind, placebo-controlled pilot study. *J Burn Care Res*. 2009;30(5):859-866.

24. Berger MM et al. Trace element supplementation modulates pulmonary infection rates after major burns: a double-blind, placebo-controlled trial. *Am J Clin Nutr.* 1998;68(2):365-371.
25. Carcillo JA et al. The randomized comparative pediatric critical illness stress-induced immune suppression (CRISIS) prevention trial. *Pediatr Crit Care Med.* 2012;13(2):165-173.
26. Braunschweig CL et al. Parenteral zinc supplementation in adult humans during the acute phase response increases the febrile response. *J Nutr.* 1997;127(1):70-74.
27. Ashton K et al. Methods of assessment of selenium status in humans: a systematic review. *Am J Clin Nutr.* 2009;89(6):2025S-2039S.
28. Loui A et al. Selenium status in term and preterm infants during the first months of life. *Eur J Clin Nutr.* 2007;62(3):349-355.
29. Stefanowicz FA et al. Erythrocyte selenium concentration as a marker of selenium status. *Clin Nutr.* 2013 (Jan 16 (ahead of print).
30. Forceville X et al. Effects of high doses of selenium, as sodium selenite, in septic shock: a placebo-controlled, randomized, double-blind, phase II study. *Crit Care.* 2007;11(4):R73.
31. Singer P, Berger MM, Van den Berghe G, et al. ESPEN guidelines on parenteral nutrition: intensive care. *Clin Nutr.* 2009:28:387-400.
32. Stawicki SP et al. Current evidence from phase ill clinical trials of selenium supplementation in critically ill patients: why should we bother? *Mini Rev Med Chem.* 2007;7(7):693-699.
33. Avenell A et al. *Selenium supplementation for critically ill adults. Cochrane Database Syst Rev.* 2008. Oct 8 (online publication).
34. Darlow BA, Austin NC. Selenium supplementation to prevent short-term morbidity in preterm neonates. *Cochrane Database Syst Rev.* 2011. Feb 16 (published online).
35. Greene HL et al. Guidelines for the use of vitamins, trace elements, calcium, magnesium, and phosphorus in infants and children receiving total parenteral nutrition: report of the Subcommittee on Pediatric Parenteral Nutrient Requirements from the Committee on Clinical Practice Issues of the American Society for Clinical Nutrition. *Am J Clin Nutr.* 1988;48(5):1324-1342.
36. Moukarzel A. Chromium in parenteral nutrition: too little or too much? *Gastroenterology.* 2009;137(5)(suppl):S18-S28.
37. Krebs NF, Hambidge KM. Trace elements. In: *Nutrition in Pediatrics*, Duggan CW, Watkins JB,Walker WA, eds. Hamilton, Canada: BC Decker Inc;2009:67-82.
38. Faustino EV, Apkon M. Persistent hyperglycemia in critically ill children. *J Pediatr.* 2005;146(1):30-34.
39. Pekarek R et al. Relationship between serum chromium concentrations and glucose utilisation in normal and infected subjects. *Diabetes.* 1975;24:350-353.
40. Via M et al. Chromium infusion reverses extreme insulin resistance in a cardiothoracic ICU patient. *Nutr Clin Pract.* 2008;23(3):325-328.
41. Nutrient needs and feeding of premature infants. Nutrition Committee, Canadian Paediatric Society. *CMAJ.* 1995;152(11):1765-1785.
42. Berger MM et al. Copper, selenium, zinc, and thiamine balances during continuous venovenous hemodiafiltration in critically ill patients. *Am J Clin Nutr.* 2004;80(2):410-416.
43. Spiegel JE and Willenbucher RF. Rapid development of severe copper deficiency in a patient with Crohn's disease receiving parenteral nutrition. *J Parenter Enteral Nutr.* 1999;23(3):169-172.
44. Cordano A. Clinical manifestations of nutritional copper deficiency in infants and children. *Am J Clin Nutr.* 1998;67(suppl):1012-1016.
45. Shike M. Copper in parenteral nutrition. *Bull NY Acad Med.* 1984;60(2):132-143.
46. Shike M. Copper in parenteral nutrition. *Gastroenterology.* 2009;137(5)(suppl):S13-S17.
47. McMillan NB et al. Correlation of cholestasis with serum copper and whole-blood manganese levels in pediatric patients. *Nutr Clin Pract.* 2008;23(2):161-165.
48. Frem J et al. Copper supplementation in parenteral nutrition of cholestatic infants. *J Pediatr Gastroenterol Nutr.* 2010;50(6):650-654.
49. Blaszyk H et al. Hepatic copper in patients receiving long-term total parenteral nutrition. *J Clin Gastroenterol.* 2005;39(4):318-320.
50. Hurwitz M et al. Copper deficiency during parenteral nutrition: a report of four pediatric cases. *Nutr Clin Pract.* 2004;19(3):305-308.
51. Shike M et al. Copper metabolism and requirements in total parenteral nutrition. *Gastroenterology.* 1981;81:290-297.
52. Hardy G. Manganese in parenteral nutrition: who. when, and why should we supplement? *Gastroenterology.* 2009;137(5)(suppl):S29-S35.
53. Pluhator-Murton MM et al. Trace element contamination of total parenteral nutrition. 1. Contribution of component solutions. *J Parenter Enteral Nutr.* 1999;23(4):222-227.
54. Witzleben CL. Bilirubin as a cholestatic agent. Physiologic and morphologic observations. *Am J Pathol.* 1971;62(2):181-194.

55. Hambidge KM et al. Plasma manganese concentrations in infants and children receiving parenteral nutrition. *J Parenter Enteral Nutr.* 1989;13(2):168-171.

56. Heming N, Montravers P, Lasocki S. Iron deficiency in critically ill patients: highlighting the role of hepcidin. *Crit Care.* 2011;15(2):210.

57. Pieracci FM, Barie PS. Diagnosis and management of iron-related anemias in critical illness. *Crit Care Med.* 2006;34(7):1898-1905.

58. Hardy G. Micronutrient deficiencies in intestinal failure. In: *Clinical Management of Intestinal Failure.* Duggin C, Gura K, Jaksic T, eds. New York, NY: CRC Press; 2011: 283-299.

59. Vanek VW et al. A.S.P.E.N. position paper: recommendations for changes in commercially available parenteral multivitamin and multi-trace element products. *Nutr Clin Pract.* 2012;27(4):440-491.

60. Galloway P, McMillan DC, Sattar N. Effect of the inflammatory response on trace element and vitamin status. *Ann Clin Biochem.* 2000;37(Pt 3):289-297.

61. Sriram K, Sridhar K. Gastroduodenal decompression and simultaneous nasoenteral nutrition: "extracorporeal gastrojejunostomy." *Nutrition.* 1996;12(6):440-441.

62. Sriram K, Lonchyna VA. Micronutrient supplementation in adult nutrition therapy: practical considerations. *J Parenter Enteral Nutr.* 2009;33(5):548-562.

63. Hardy G, Menendez AM, Manzanares W. Trace element supplementation in parenteral nutrition: pharmacy, posology, and monitoring guidance. *Nutrition.* 2009;25 (1-2):1073-1084.

64. Jiang S et al. Vitamin A deficiency aggravates iron deficiency by upregulating the expression of iron regulatory protein-2. *Nutrition.* 2012;28(3):281-287.

65. Allwood MC, Plane JH. The wavelength-dependent degradation of vitamin A exposed to ultraviolet light. *Int J Pharmaceutics.* 1986;31:1.

66. DeLuca HF. Vitamin D and the parenteral nutrition patient. *Gastroenterology.* 2009;137(5)(suppl):S79-91.

67. Cantorna MT. Vitamin D and its role in immunology: multiple sclerosis, and inflammatory bowel disease. *Prog Biophys Mol Biol.* 2006;92(1):60-64.

68. Madden K et al. Vitamin D deficiency in critically ill children. *Pediatrics.* 2012;130(3):421-428.

69. Rippel C et al. Vitamin D status in critically ill children. *Intensive Care Med.* 2012;38(12):2055-2062.

70. Davis AT et al. Plasma vitamin and mineral status in home parenteral nutrition patients. *J Parenter Enteral Nutr.* 1987;11(5):480-485.

71. Gillis J, Jones G, and Pencharz Delivery of vitamins A, D, and E in total parenteral nutrition solutions. *J Parenter Enteral Nutr.* 1983;7(1):11-14.

72. Dahl GB, Jeppsson RI, and Tengborn HJ. Vitamin stability in a TPN mixture stored in an EVA plastic bag. *J Clin Hosp Pharm.* 1986;11(4):271-279.

73. Louw JA et al. Blood vitamin concentrations during the acute-phase response. *Crit Care Med.* 1992;20(7): 934-941.

74. Thurnham DI et al. The use of different lipids to express serum tocopherol: lipid ratios for the measurement of vitamin E status. *Ann Clin Biochem.* 1986;23(Pt 5): 514-520.

75. Agarwal N et al. Effect of surgery on serum antioxidant vitamins. *J Parenter Enteral Nutr.* 1966;20(suppl):32S.

76. McGee CD et al. Selenium and vitamin E stability in parenteral solutions. *J Parenter Enteral Nutr.* 1985;9(5): 568-570.

77. Shearer MJ. Vitamin K in parenteral nutrition. *Gastroenterology.* 2009;137(5)(suppl):S105-S118.

78. Singh H, Duerksen DR. Vitamin K and nutrition support. *Nutr Clin Pract.* 2003;18(5):359-365.

79. Manzanares W and Hardy G. Thiamine supplementation in the critically ill. *Curr Opin Clin Nutr Metab Care.* 2011;14(6):610-617.

80. Chen MF, Boyce, HW, Jr and Triplett L. Stability of the B vitamins in mixed parenteral nutrition solution. *J Parenter Enteral Nutr.* 1983;7(5):462-464.

81. Schilling RF. Is nitrous oxide a dangerous anesthetic for vitamin B12-deficient subjects? *JAMA.* 1986;255(12): 1605-1606.

82. Marian M, Sacks G. Micronutrients and older adults. *Nutr Clin Pract.* 2009;24(2):179-195.

83. Sviri S et al. Increased Vitamin B12 levels are associated with mortality in critically ill medical patients. *Clin Nutr.* 2012;31(1):53-59.

84. Berger MM. Vitamin C requirements in parenteral nutrition. *Gastroenterology.* 2009;137(5)(suppl):S79-91.

85. Shenkin A. Trace elements and vitamins in enteral and parenteral nutrition. In: Sobotka L, ed. Basics in Clinical Nutrition ESPEN (European Society for Clinical Nutrition and Metabolism). Prague: Galen; 2004.

86. Allwood MC et al. The stability of ascorbic acid in TPN mixtures stored in a multilayered bag. *Clin Nutr.* 1992;11(5):284-288.

87. Zappitelli M et al. Continuous renal replacement therapy amino acid, trace metal and folate clearance in critically ill children. *Intensive Care Med.* 2009;35(4):698-706.

CHAPTER 5

Fluid, Electrolytes, and Acid–Base Physiology in Critically ill Children

Stacey L. Valentine
Toni Petrillo-Albarano
James D. Fortenberry

■ FLUID MANAGEMENT
Fluid Homeostasis
Body Water Distribution and the Intracellular and Extracellular Compartments
Maintenance Parenteral Fluid Requirements
■ ELECTROLYTE COMPOSITION FOR PARENTERAL FORMULATIONS
Sodium
Potassium
Calcium
Magnesium
Phosphorus
■ ACID–BASE PHYSIOLOGY AND ASSOCIATED DISORDERS
Acid–Base Terminology and Mechanisms
Quantification of Acid–Base Status
Diagnosis and Management of Acid–Base Disorders
■ KEY POINTS
References

■ FLUID MANAGEMENT

Fluid management is essential in caring for the critically ill child and can be challenging, given the alteration of normal fluid and electrolyte physiology in critical illness.

Fluid Homeostasis

Fluid and electrolyte derangements are common in critically ill children and either can be related to the patient's underlying disease or can be a consequence of therapy. Estimating fluid and electrolyte needs in the critically ill child requires an understanding of normal basal metabolism as well as knowledge of fluid homeostasis. Furthermore, the derangements that occur in critical illness must be appreciated in order to adapt fluid and electrolyte management appropriately. It is important to note that many of the principles that guide fluid and electrolyte management in children are based on normal physiologic principles, which can be severely altered in critical illness.

Body Water Distribution and the Intracellular and Extracellular Compartments

Total body water (TBW) accounts for 50% to 80% of body weight and varies by gender and age.[1-4] Water is largely distributed into the intracellular fluid (IFC) compartment and the extracellular fluid (ECF) compartment. The ICF compartment comprises approximately two-thirds of TBW, or 40% of total body weight, while the ECF compartment comprises approximately one-third of TBW, or 20% of total body weight. The ECF is further divided into interstitial fluid and plasma.[2-4] The ECF decreases over time in infants, reaching 30% at 1 year of age, and approaching 20%, or adult values, in early childhood. The ICF volume remains relatively constant throughout infancy to adulthood.[1-2]

The ICF and ECF space each have a primary solute that is generally restricted to that compartment by a semipermeable membrane. This primary solute helps regulate the osmolality of the compartment and the movement of water between spaces. The primary solute in the ICF compartment is potassium (K^+), while the primary solute in the ECF is sodium (Na^+). Potassium (K^+) and magnesium (Mg^+) are the major cations in the ICF, while proteins and organic phosphates are the major anions. The primary cation in the ECF is sodium (Na^+), while the major anions are (Cl) and (HCO_3^-).[1-2]

Lastly, TBW content is inversely correlated with adipose tissue content and decreases with age. Total body water accounts for 75% of body weight in the term infant. By 6 months of age, TBW content decreases to 65%, and by 1 year of age, TBW approaches 60% of body weight.[1-4] On average, males have slightly higher TBW (as a percentage of body weight) than females, which is attributed to the slightly higher percentage of adipose tissue in females. Understanding the relationship between TBW content and weight and the electrolyte components in each space are important when calculating fluid deficits.

Maintenance Parenteral Fluid Requirements

The estimates for parenteral fluid requirements are based on the understanding of normal basal metabolism; to achieve homeostasis, fluid intake must balance fluid losses. Fluid losses primarily consist of insensible losses and urine output. Evaporative losses account for approximately two-thirds of insensible losses, approximating 30 mL/100 kcal/day, while respiratory losses account for the remaining one-third, approximating 15 mL/100 kcal/day.[3-6] Sensible losses, which are primarily composed of urinary losses, account for approximately 55 mL/100 kcal/day. In 1957, Holliday and Segar calculated the maintenance water requirements for children based on normal metabolism and estimates from water evaporation (heat dissipation) and caloric expenditure (heat production).[7] Accounting for the net water production from oxidative metabolism, a 10-kg child has a net insensible loss of 34 mL/kg/day and a urinary loss of 66 mL/kg/day. As shown in Table 5-1, Holliday and Segar[7] estimated maintenance water requirements of an infant/child using the following formula: 100 mL/kg/day for each of the first 10 kg, 50 mL/kg/day for each additional 1 kg from 11 to 20 kg, and 20 mL/kg/day for each subsequent kilogram over 20 kg.

It is important to note that this model was based on healthy children and does not take into account the insensible losses and energy expenditure in the critically ill child. The loss from the respiratory tract is minimal in the mechanically ventilated child, while evaporative losses increase with increasing body temperature. Therefore, in the critically ill child, fluid must be titrated based on factors such as decreased fluid excretion in renal failure and elevated antidiuretic hormone (ADH) states, as well as decreased insensible losses in the mechanically ventilated patient.[4]

Special Considerations in the Critically Ill Child

The prescription of intravenous (IV) fluids should be carefully considered in all critically ill patients, taking into account the disease state, current electrolytes, glucose, body weight, and fluid balances.[4] Holliday and Segar established the tool for prescribing maintenance parenteral fluids in healthy children, which needs to be individualized to each child, with the primary goal to maintain adequate end-organ perfusion while minimizing pulmonary edema. The Surviving Sepsis Guidelines published in 2012 by Dellinger and colleagues recommend early fluid resuscitation in the critically ill child with hypovolemic shock using 20 mL/kg boluses of isotonic fluids, up

TABLE 5-1. Water Requirements for Maintenance Fluids

Body Weight (kg)	Water Requirements (ml/day)
0-10 kg	100 ml/kg/day
11-20 kg	1000 ml + 50 ml/kg for each kg > 10 kg
>20 kg	1500 ml + 20 ml/kg for each kg > 20 kg

to 40 to 60 mL/kg, with the goal to reverse hypotension; increase urine output; and attain normal capillary refill, peripheral pulses, and level of consciousness without inducing hepatomegaly or rales. In the child who develops signs of fluid overload, hepatomegaly, or rales, fluids should be tailored and inotropes administered to reverse hypotension.[8]

Further consideration must be given to fluid management in the critically ill child with respiratory failure. Mechanically ventilated children are at risk for developing acute lung injury (ALI) and its more severe form, acute respiratory distress syndrome (ARDS). The goal of fluid administration in critically ill patients with ARDS is to maintain intravascular volume to ensure adequate end-organ perfusion while minimizing extravascular lung water and pulmonary edema. Guidelines for fluid management in mechanically ventilated children are extrapolated from adult studies on ALI and ARDS. In 2006, the ARDS Network found a significant reduction in the duration of mechanical ventilation ($p < 0.001$), length of stay (LOS) in the intensive care unit (ICU) ($p < 0.001$), and oxygenation index in patients with ALI exposed to a conservative versus liberal fluid strategy.[9] Similarly, both prospective and retrospective studies have shown that increasing fluid balance in children with ALI is associated with worse outcomes.[10-18] In 2012, a multicenter retrospective cohort study of 168 children with ALI revealed that increasing fluid balance at day 3 was independently associated with fewer ventilator-free days.[11] This association between increasing fluid balance and increased duration of mechanical ventilation was similarly shown in studies by Flori and Arikan.[12-13] Fluid requirements must be carefully altered in the child with respiratory failure to maintain intravascular volume status while avoiding pulmonary edema. The electrolyte composition of IV fluids for critically ill children must have equal consideration.[19,20]

ELECTROLYTE COMPOSITION FOR PARENTERAL FORMULATIONS

Holliday and Segar established the tool for prescribing maintenance parenteral fluids in healthy children.[4] The electrolyte composition of maintenance parenteral fluids is calculated based on estimates for sodium of 2 to 3 mmol/100 kcal/day and potassium 1 to 2 mmol/100 kcal/day. These estimates were originally calculated from the sodium and potassium concentration of cow's milk and breast milk and represent normal electrolyte hemeostasis.[1-2] Using these assumptions, hypotonic IV solutions are often recommended; however, hypotonic IV fluids can cause hyponatremia in children with altered electrolyte needs or increased ADH states. Hospital-acquired hyponatremia has been observed in children where hypotonic fluids were prescribed. In these children, ADH levels were greater than expected for their degree of hyponatremia.[4]

Sodium

Dysnatremias are one of the most common electrolyte abnormalities in patients in the ICU.[21-22] Although these abnormalities can be related to the disease process, selection of IV fluids can also be a contributor. Changes in serum [Na^+] generally reflect changes in water balance despite total body Na^+ levels being high, low, or even normal.[23] Sodium equilibrium is directly related to serum osmolality, and water will shift from the compartment with lower osmolality to that of higher osmolality to maintain osmotic equilibrium.

Hyponatremia

Hyponatremia, defined as a serum [Na^+] of less than 135 mEq/L, has been reported to occur in up to 40% of ICU patients and is more common in women and children.[4] Hyponatremia can occur from Na^+ loss, water excess, or both. To assess the cause of hyponatremia, it is useful to first categorize the serum osmolarity as hypo-, iso-, or hyperosmolar. Hypo-osmolar hyponatremia is the most common cause of hyponatremia in critically ill patients.[24,25] Hypo-osmolar hyponatremia is then further subdivided into hypovolemic, hypervolemic, and isovolemic hypo-osmolar hyponatremia based on the overall extracellular fluid status.

Hypovolemic hypo-osmolar hyponatremia is often caused by both volume and Na^+ loss. Gastrointestinal (GI) losses from vomiting and diarrhea are one of the most common offenders in pediatric hypovolemic hypo-osmolar hyponatremia. Blood loss from hemorrhage, surgical drain outputs, nasogastric suctioning, and insensible skin losses from burns or excessive sweating can also contribute. Likewise, other causes include excessive diuretic use (e.g., furosemide) and cerebral salt wasting, which is seen in patients with traumatic brain injury or brain tumors.[18] Isovolemic hypo-osmolar hyponatremia in critically ill patients is most commonly caused by inappropriate secretion of antidiuretic hormone (despite normal plasma volume) . Syndrome of inappropriate antidiuretic hormone (SIADH) can be associated with intracranial lesions, such as brain tumors, brain abscesses, or subdural hematomas, or an inflammatory processes, such as meningitis, systemic lupus erythematosus, severe pneumonia, or tuberculosis. In order to diagnose SIADH, one must have a low serum osmolarity and a high urine osmolarity with high urine [Na^+]. Hypervolemic hypo-osmolar hyponatremia often results from both an excess of free water and total body Na^+; however, the excess water is disproportionate to the excess Na^+ and results in hyponatremia. Congestive heart failure, renal failure, cirrhosis, and nephrotic syndrome all fit into this category.

Management of hyponatremia is focused on symptoms. While [Na^+] below 130 mEq/L should be addressed, most patients are not symptomatic until [Na^+] levels drop below 130 mEq/L. Initial signs of hyponatremia are often vague: nausea, vomiting, restlessness, and headache. When serum [Na^+] drops below the low 120s, symptoms increase and can include altered mental status (AMS), seizures, respiratory failure, cerebral edema, and even death. In critically ill, sedated patients, these symptoms may not be apparent. In the patient with isovolemic hypo-osmolar hyponatremia, water restriction can be used to correct the disturbance. In patients with hypervolemic hypo-osmolar hyponatremia, fluid and Na^+ restriction should occur, often in conjunction with loop diuretics. Treatment of the underlying condition should be optimized, and in some cases may necessitate the use of extracorporeal ultrafiltration.

Severe symptomatic hyponatremia (AMS, seizures, etc.), regardless of the cause, should receive correction with hypertonic saline to bring serum [Na^+] levels above 120 mEq/L. Once the [Na^+] levels rise above 120 mEq/L, the Na^+ deficit should be calculated and replaced. One can calculate the sodium deficit using the following equation: Na^+ deficit = TBW × (140 – serum Na^+), where TBW for infants equals 0.7 × (weight in kg), and for children greater than a year, 0.6 × (weight in kg). It is important to note that this formula only calculates the deficit and does not account for maintenance needs, and most recommend correction by no more than 8 to 12 mEq/L in a 24-hr period. Correction that is too quick can result in irreversible osmotic central nervous system demyelination (central pontine myelinolysis).

Hypernatremia

Critically ill patients are at risk for developing hypernatremia ($Na^+ > 145$ mEq/L). Hypernatremia may result from GI losses from vomiting and diarrhea; excessive water losses from fever, drains, or wounds; or renal losses via osmotic diuresis from glucose or mannitol.[2] In these instances, serum osmolality and urine osmolality are high. In the hospitalized patient, excess Na^+ may also be seen with the use of sodium bicarbonate infusions used to correct metabolic acidosis or large volumes of normal saline for fluid resuscitation. Determining urine [Na^+] is helpful in differentiating Na^+ overload from excessive fluid loss; if the Na^+ level is high, then Na^+ overload is likely the culprit. Acute diabetes insipidus (DI), central or nephrogenic, can also cause hypernatremia. Central DI is more common and is caused by a deficiency in vasopressin secretion. It can be associated with neurological insult from entities like traumatic brain injury, hypoxic ischemic encephalopathy, and brain tumors, as well as leukemia or lymphoma. Conversely, nephrogenic DI is caused by a relative resistance to the effects of vasopressin in the kidney and can be induced by a metabolic derangement, such as hypokalemia and hypercalcemia, or drugs such as amphotericin B.[7] Patients with DI typically have elevated serum [Na^+] and serum osmolality levels; however, the urine osmolality is not as high as expected, since there is a defect in the ability to concentrate the urine. To differentiate central DI from nephrogenic DI, one can administer exogenous vasopressin. In central DI, the urine osmolality should increase by at least 50% from baseline.[24]

The signs and symptoms of hypernatremia are very similar to those of hyponatremia and can include restlessness, irritability, nausea, vomiting, fatigue, seizure, and coma. If serum osmolality increases significantly, there is a risk of intraparenchymal hemorrhage and venous thrombosis.[19] Management of hypernatremia is based on etiology and symptoms. As with hyponatremia, large shifts in the serum Na^+ are generally not well tolerated and, therefore, the Na^+ should not be corrected more than 1 to 2 mEq/L/hr to prevent cerebral edema. As a rule, approximately half the fluid deficit is repleted over the first 24 hours and the remaining deficit over the 48 hours.

The water deficit can be calculated in one of two ways:

1. The expected change in serum [Na^+] levels after a liter of a given concentration of fluid can be calculated using the following equation:

   Change in serum [Na^+] = (Infusate [Na^+] – serum [Na^+])/(TBW + 1)

   So, for example, if the infusate was normal saline, the [Na^+] would equal 154 mEq/L and TBW is 0.6 × (weight in kg).

2. Alternatively, the water deficit can be calculated using the following equation:

   Water deficit (Liters) = TBW × (1 – [140 mEq/L/serum [Na^+]])

In unusual cases of hypernatremia caused by excessive administration of Na^+, one should review the type and quantity of fluids being delivered and consider options to limit the Na^+ delivery. This should include mixing compatible drips in dextrose rather than saline. In cases of central DI, fluid replacement and administration of exogenous vasopressin are generally required. For cases of nephrogenic DI, one should correct metabolic derangements and look for causative agents. The administration of thiazide diuretics may also be beneficial.

Potassium

Potassium is the most abundant intracellular cation and plays a significant role in many physiologic functions. It is especially important in the resting membrane potential of muscle and nerve cells. The regulation of K^+ in and out of the cell is largely limited by the activity of the sodium-potassium-adenosine triphosphate pump (Na^+, K^+-ATPase). The activity of this pump can be affected by many factors, including insulin, glucagon, catecholamines, acid–base status, and intracellular K^+ levels.[23]

Hypokalemia

Hypokalemia can occur due to inadequate intake; however, abnormalities are much more likely to occur due to an increase in losses or a shift in K^+ from the extracellular space to the intracellular space. Some losses may be obvious, as those seen with excessive vomiting, diarrhea, or nasogastric losses. However, many of the interventions that regularly occur in the ICU setting may also contribute to potassium depletion. For example, loop diuretics cause inhibition of Na^+ reabsorption in the loop of Henle, leading to an increased sodium load in collecting ducts—potassium then is excreted as sodium is reabsorbed. In addition, several medications, including amphotericin B, aminoglycosides, and corticosteroids, may play a role in K^+ depletion. Likewise, hypokalemia may also be exacerbated by magnesium deficiency, rendering it refractory to treatment until the magnesium deficiency is corrected. One theory is that low levels of intracellular magnesium inhibit renal outer medullary potassium channel (ROMK) function, leading to an increase in K^+ efflux and wasting.[26] Moreover, in ill patients, hypokalemia can be a result of shifts of extracellular potassium into the intracellular space. Insulin, beta agonists, catecholamines, and metabolic alkalosis can all contribute to this shift.

Hypokalemia results in hypopolarization of cell membranes. Therefore, symptoms of hypokalemia are generally related to impaired muscular contraction. These symptoms may be mild (muscle cramping, vomiting), moderate (ileus, weakness), or severe (cardiac dysrhythmias and arrest). When levels begin to decrease, electrocardiographic (EKG) changes may become apparent. These can include ST segment depression, flattening of the T wave, and presence of U waves. Levels below 2.5 mEq/L are critical and warrant urgent treatment.

Treatment for hypokalemia should be aimed at correcting the underlying cause and driven by the K^+ level and clinical condition. In the nonemergent settings, either oral potassium supplements or supplementation via IV fluids and/or parenteral nutrition (PN) may be sufficient. Correction of severe hypokalemia via PN supplementation is not recommended. Parenteral nutrition should be started after severe hypokalemia has been corrected. In severe hypokalemia, a bolus of IV K^+ may be necessary. For children, the dose ranges between 0.3 mEq/kg and 1 mEq/kg, with a maximum single dose of 40 mEq. The rate of the infusion should not exceed 0.5 mEq/kg/hr. This is generally given as potassium chloride, but depending on the clinical situation, may be given as potassium phosphate or acetate. Careful consideration must be used in children with concomitant renal failure, and if potassium supplements need to be given, one should consider starting with 50% of the normal dosage. If K^+ is being administered through peripheral access, it should be diluted. Likewise, dextrose-containing vehicles should be avoided if possible, as they may trigger insulin release and worsen the hypokalemia. And, as noted earlier, correction of hypomagnesemia is imperative if present.

Hyperkalemia

Hyperkalemia can occur due to increased intake, extracellular shifts, or decreased elimination. Renal insufficiency is a common contributor in ICU patients due to impaired potassium excretion. Conditions that lead to rhabdomyolysis, such as heat stroke, trauma, or extensive burns, can lead to an increase in endogenous potassium release. Hyperkalemia can also occur in the initial treatment of some cancers; the rapid breakdown of cancer cells causes a release of intracellular potassium from the dying cells. Likewise, acidosis will lead to shifts of the K^+ from the intracellular to extracellular space. In addition, several drugs commonly used in the ICU setting can lead to hyperkalemia. One of the most obvious is the K^+ sparing diuretics. One of the not-so-obvious are the nonsteroidal drugs, which decrease renal tubular flow and renin release, resulting in impaired excretion.[19] Beta blockers, alpha agonists, angiotensin-converting enzyme (ACE) inhibitors, and immune modulators such as cyclosporine and tacrolimus can also contribute to hyperkalemia.

Patients are often asymptomatic until levels rise significantly. Early signs may include muscle twitching and weakness. If left unchecked, serious dysrhythmias can occur. Electrocardiographic changes initially include peaked T waves, prolongation of the QT interval, and widening of the QRS complex. If this goes untreated, refractory ventricular fibrillation may occur, which can be difficult to correct.

Aggressive treatment of hyperkalemia is critical. Because pseudohyperkalemia can occur with hemolysis or contamination of the blood sample with the intravenous fluid (IVF) being administered, one should confirm the lab value prior to action. Mild hyperkalemia may be monitored while trying to eliminate the inciting cause. Obviously, one should reduce or remove K^+ from IVF or hyperalimentation. However, if the potassium levels are critical, immediate treatment may be required. If cardiac instability is present (i.e., EKG changes), an injection of calcium should be given to stabilize the cell membrane. Either calcium chloride (20 mg/kg with a maximum single dose of 1 gram) or calcium gluconate (100 mg/kg with a maximum single dose of 2 grams) can be used. Next, a combination of insulin and glucose should be administered. The general recommended dose is 1 gram of dextrose/kg of body weight and insulin 0.1 unit/kg. In addition, some recommend albuterol nebulization and loop diuretics. Although sodium bicarbonate is often administered, the data on its usage are equivocal and it generally should not be given as a first-line treatment.[21-22] With the exception of furosemide, none of these therapies cause K^+ removal, but merely shift the potassium from one space to another. Therefore, one should consider dialysis or sodium polystyrene sulfonate, an enteral cation exchange resin.

Calcium

Calcium (Ca^{2+}) availability is regulated by parathyroid hormone (PTH), vitamin D, and calcitonin. It plays a role in neuromuscular activity, contractility of the heart and smooth muscle, coagulation, and bone metabolism. Approximately half the serum calcium is bound to albumin, rendering it inactive. The unbound, or ionized, calcium is the active form, and in critically ill patients, who are often hypoalbuminemic, may be a better reflection of functional status.[6] Acidosis affects the binding of Ca^{2+} to the plasma proteins and can cause shifts in levels of ionized calcium; acidosis will increase concentrations of ionized calcium, and alkalosis will decrease its availability.

Hypocalcemia

Hypocalcemia is a frequent occurrence in the ICU setting. One study reported that close to 50% of critically ill children had abnormal serum calcium levels, and almost 20% had low ionized levels.[19] Many inciting factors can contribute to low levels. Citrate, which is used as a preservative agent in packed red blood cells (RBCs), will cause chelation. It is postulated that in sepsis, interleukin-1 (IL-1) causes an increase in intracellular calcium, which can suppress PTH, resulting in decreased levels. Other disease processes that affect the functioning of the PTHs, like DiGeorge syndrome, can lead to hypocalcemia. In addition, commonly used drugs can play a role in the development of hypocalcemia. Aminoglycosides may potentiate hypomagnesemia, which, in turn, can suppress PTH. Steroids can increase intestinal reabsorption and promote increased urinary secretion. Loop diuretics can increase renal excretion of calcium. Likewise, calcium levels and phosphorous levels are closely linked and regulated. Generally, when the level of one ion is increased, the other decreases; therefore, hypocalcemia will occur in processes that cause hyperphosphatemia, such as in tumor lysis syndrome.

There are generally few signs of mild hypocalcemia. In moderate cases, one can see muscle cramping or twitching. Severe hypocalcemia leads to tetany, which can manifest as stridor, laryngospasm, or even apnea. Cardiovascular side effects of hypocalcemia include hypotension, poor myocardial contractility, and prolonged QT syndrome. Emergency treatment for symptomatic hypocalcemia is IV calcium repletion with calcium chloride or calcium gluconate. Since alterations in both magnesium and phosphorus can lead to hypocalcemia, one should check levels if experiencing refractory hypocalcemia.

Hypercalcemia

Hypercalcemia is fairly uncommon in the hospitalized child. It can be seen in certain malignancies, vitamin D intoxication, hyperparathyroidism, and with certain drugs like the thiazides or lithium. The most common cause of hypercalcemia in the critically ill child is likely immobilization resulting in excessive bone resorption.

Symptoms of hypercalcemia are often vague: nausea, vomiting, weakness, and lethargy. In severe cases, myocardial depolarization can be impacted, leading to bradycardia or ventricular fibrillation. If the kidneys are functioning, the most effective treatment is to increase renal excretion. Renal excretion of calcium is linked to urinary excretion of sodium; therefore, delivering increased sodium to the kidneys will promote increased excretion. This can be accomplished through boluses of normal saline and loop diuretics. In patients with renal failure, dialysis may be necessary. In severe, life-threatening hypercalcemia, ethylene diamine tetra-acetate (EDTA) can also be used. Ethylene diamine tetra-acetate will cause calcium chelation and increase excretion. However, it should be used with caution, as it can lead to renal insufficiency. While biphosphonates are potent inhibitors of bone resorption and are often used to treat chronic hypercalcemia, they are of little use in the acute treatment, as effects are not generally seen for a few days.

Magnesium

Magnesium is the second most abundant cation in the intracellular space. It plays an important role in several enzymatic functions, such as muscle contractility, DNA synthesis, protein synthesis, and carbohydrate metabolism. It is especially important in the transfer of phosphorus in the formation of adenosine triphosphate (ATP). Regulation appears to be controlled by intestinal absorption and renal excretion.

Hypomagnesemia

Hypomagnesemia is often related to increased losses or poor intake/absorption.[27] Certainly, malnutrition and starvation can result in decreased levels of magnesium. Conditions such as diarrhea, Crohn disease, and celiac disease affect resorption from the GI tract and can also result in magnesium deficiency. Many drugs (loop diuretics, osomotic diuretics, aminoglycosides, antineoplastic drugs) increase renal wasting and can result in low magnesium levels.

Hypomagnesemia can manifest in several ways. With mild deficiencies, the symptoms are generally vague and include nausea, anorexia, weakness, paresthesias, and central nervous system irritability. Severe deficiencies can lead to life-threatening cardiac dysrhythmias, seizures, coma, and even death. Symptomatic hypomagnesemia should be repleted with IV magnesium—generally, with magnesium sulfate. Replacement can be initiated at 40 to 50 mg/kg to a maximum of 2 grams for a single dose. It should be remembered that an abrupt elevation in the plasma magnesium concentration will cause up to 50% of the infused magnesium to be excreted in the urine. Furthermore, magnesium uptake by the cells is slow, and repletion requires sustained correction of the hypomagnesemia. Thus, magnesium either should be given as a continuous infusion or will require consistent IV or oral dosing to ensure correction.

Hypermagnesemia

High levels of magnesium are rather infrequent. It can be seen with renal insufficiency or with iatrogenic/inadvertent excessive administration. Symptoms include nausea, vomiting, and decreased deep tendon reflexes. With increased severity, it can cause respiratory depression, hypotension, and dysrhythmias. When levels are high, one should discontinue exogenous administration. If there are neuromuscular or cardiac complications, IV calcium should be given.

Phosphorus

Phosphorus is the major anion in the intracellular space. Most of the body's phosphorus exists in the bone. Its existence is generally balanced in concert with calcium levels. Its main function is energy generation, mostly through its involvement in ATP synthesis. However, it also plays an important role in glucose utilization, glycolysis, and 2,3-diphosphoglycerate (2,3-DPG) synthesis. 2,3-diphosphoglycerate is necessary for oxygen release from hemoglobin and delivery of oxygen to the tissues. Levels of phosphorus are regulated by GI resorption, renal excretion, and by PTH. Increased secretion of PTH causes phosphorus to be reabsorbed from the bone and GI tract; however, it also increases renal excretion. The increase of PTH results in an overall net loss, as renal excretion is more efficient than the resorption.

Hypophosphatemia

The effects of low levels of phosphorus can be very serious given the significant role phosphorus plays in energy production. Hypophosphatemia can result from malnutrition, refeeding syndrome, and the use of diuretics and antacids. Hypophosphatemia is also seen with sepsis and catecholamine release. Cytokines such as interleukin-6 (IL-6) could potentially affect transcellular shifts of phosphorus.[21] Hypophosphatemia results in poor contractility of both cardiac and skeletal muscle. This can result in decreased cardiac function and ineffective skeletal muscle movement. In the respiratory system, this might equate to inadequate chest wall and diaphragm function and subsequent respiratory failure and/or inability to wean from the ventilator. In addition, if 2,3-DPG is significantly impaired, tissue hypoxia will occur. Low levels of phosphorus also lead to immunosuppression due to its effect on phagogytosis and lymphyocyte activity.[21] Hypophosphatemia can also affect platelet aggregation and lead to more profound bleeding in trauma or postsurgical patients. In critically ill patients or those with severe deficits, IV phosphorous replacement is recommended. It can be given as either sodium or potassium phosphate.

Hyperphosphatemia

The most common cause of hyperphosphatemia in critically ill patients is renal insufficiency; however, high levels must be interpreted cautiously, as high levels are not necessarily indicative of total body stores. Hyperphosphatemia can also result from laxative use, acidosis, hemolysis, rhabdomyolysis, and tumor lysis syndrome. The most significant clinical concern is the resultant hypocalcemia that occurs due to an increase in calcium phosphorus binding. Treatment is generally phosphorus binders. These can include aluminum hydroxide, magnesium hydroxide, calcium acetate, and calcium carbonate.

ACID–BASE PHYSIOLOGY AND ASSOCIATED DISORDERS

An appropriate acid–base milieu is essential for normal cellular function of the child.[22] An acid can be defined as a substance that can donate H^+ ions, and a base as a substance that can accept H^+ ions.[29] Two classes of acids are physiologically important: carbonic acid (H_2CO_3) and noncarbonic acids. Metabolism of carbohydrates and fats generates carbon dioxide (CO_2), which combines with water to generate carbonic acid. The lung plays an essential role in acid–base regulation via removal of CO_2. Noncarbonic acids are derived from the metabolism of proteins and are excreted by the kidney. Extracellular pH is normally regulated between 7.35 and 7.45 by chemical buffering and by respiratory and renal regulatory mechanisms. Disturbances of this balance can frequently occur in critically ill or injured children, often serving as a marker of an underlying disorder, but acid–base disturbances may in themselves require monitoring and treatment in the pediatric intensive care unit (PICU). Assessment and treatment of acid–base imbalances thus requires an understanding of terminology, insight into buffer systems, and recognition of the compensatory interactions involved in maintaining balance.

The terms *acidosis* and *alkalosis* refer to the states that result in a given acid–base disturbance. The pH scale is used by convention to describe acid–base disturbances in the body. The pH of arterial blood is the negative logarithm of the H^+ concentration. pH and $[H^+]$ are inversely related. An increase in $[H^+]$ is defined by a decreasing pH, while a decrease in $[H^+]$ is defined by an increasing pH. Normal limits of arterial pH of 7.35 correspond to an $[H^+]$ of 45 nEq/L, and 7.45 corresponds to an $[H^+]$ of 35 nEq/L. *Acidemia* refers to an arterial pH <7.35 (H^+ concentration above 45 nEq/L), while *alkalemia* refers to an arterial pH >7.45 (H^+ concentration below 35 nEq/L).

Primary acid–base disorders are further classified as either metabolic or respiratory. A primary deviation of plasma bicarbonate concentration (HCO_3^-) from the normal range leads to a metabolic acidosis or alkalosis. A respiratory acidosis or alkalosis results from a primary abnormality in the arterial carbon dioxide tension ($PaCO_2$). Secondary compensatory mechanisms attempt to restore the extracellular pH back to normal. Secondary respiratory compensation to a primary metabolic acid–base disturbance by an alteration in minute ventilation to change $PaCO_2$ occurs within minutes and is usually complete within 12 to 24 hours (although arterial pH is not fully restored to a normal pH). Conversely, secondary metabolic compensation by the kidney to a primary respiratory acidosis may require 3 to 5 days for compensation.[24] Most acid–base disturbances are *simple acid–base disorders*, with a primary disruption producing a physiologic compensatory response, but mixed acid–base disorders can also result from more than one primary disturbance.

Acid–Base Terminology and Mechanisms

A buffer is defined as any substance that can absorb or donate H^+ ions and thereby diminish the effects on the pH of a solution. The inherent tendency of a particular acid to dissociate or ionize determines the degree to which it can act as a buffer, denoted by the ionization constant, pK. The most effective buffers have pKs that approximate the physiologic range of pH. The most important buffer pairs in blood are carbonic acid/bicarbonate (H_2CO_3/HCO_3^-), phosphate ($H_2PO_4^-/HPO_4^{2-}$), and certain proteins, e.g., hemoglobin.[30] The most important buffer system is the H_2CO_3/HCO_3^- system:

$$CO_2 + H_2O \leftrightarrow H_2CO_3 \leftrightarrow H^+ + HCO_3^-$$

Carbonic anhydrase catalyzes the conversion of carbonic acid to CO_2 and H_2O. When chemical buffering is not sufficient to maintain normal pH, either metabolic or respiratory compensation occurs. Changes in pH, therefore, result entirely from changes in the respiratory response and the subsequent effect on volatile acids ($PaCO_2$), changes in the metabolic response, and the subsequent effect on nonvolatile acids (hydrochloric, sulfuric, lactic acids), or changes in nonvolatile weak acids (chemical buffers).

Respiratory Compensation – Volatile Acids (CO_2)

CO_2 is transported through the arterial blood primarily as bicarbonate (80% to 90%) following combination in the RBC membrane with water to form carbonic acid, dissociation to HCO_3^- and H^+, buffering of H^+ by hemoglobin, and leaving the RBC. CO_2 is then excreted in the lungs by a reversal of this process to diffuse freely into the alveolar space. Changes in the arterial or cerebrospinal fluid pH stimulate central medullary and carotid body chemoreceptors to regulate minute ventilation. Maximal compensatory response to a severe metabolic acidosis can decrease $PaCO_2$ to a lower limit of 10 to 12 mm Hg. Conversely, minute ventilation slows and $PaCO_2$ generally increases to approximately 50 mm Hg to compensate for a metabolic alkalosis with plasma bicarbonate concentrations of 35 mEq/L or greater, but response generally does not exceed 65 mm Hg with normal lung function.

Metabolic Compensation and Nonvolatile Acids/Strong Ion Difference

Nonvolatile acids are also produced by cellular metabolism, and their resultant effect on acid–base homeostasis is controlled by the kidney. The metabolism of sulfur-containing amino acids, such as cysteine and methionine, to sulfuric acid provides the major source of nonvolatile acids, but other sources include phosphoric acid, uric acid, lactic, and keto acids. Excretion occurs together with the regeneration of HCO_3^-. In addition, the kidneys filter large amounts of circulating plasma HCO_3^- with almost complete reabsorption with sodium in the proximal tubule. Metabolic compensation for respiratory volatile acid effects occurs via the kidney. Volume contraction also increases proximal HCO_3^- reabsorption by resetting the glomerulotubular balance upward and increasing the fractional rate of Na^+ and HCO_3^- reabsorption. Hypokalemia increases the rate of bicarbonate reabsorption as well, probably by raising intracellular H^+ concentration. Thus, correcting hypokalemia may be necessary to correct a metabolic alkalosis, particularly in children with volume contraction.

Metabolic contribution to acid–base homeostasis is based on the presence of strong anions and cations. Ion strength is based on the tendency of an ion to dissociate in aqueous solutions. Strong ions are always free and remain charged because they do not combine with other ions. Strong cations, which include sodium (Na^+), potassium (K^+), calcium (Ca^{++}), and magnesium (Mg^{++}), outnumber strong anions (predominantly chloride [Cl^-] and lactate) in blood plasma. The concentration difference between the sum of all strong anions and strong cations is defined as the strong ion difference (SID). If other *unmeasured* anions are excluded, the apparent SID (SIDa) can be estimated by the following:

$$SIDa = (Na^+ + K^+ + Ca^{++} + Mg^{++}) - (Cl^- + lactate)$$

Because of electrical neutrality, plasma cannot be charged, and the SID difference is balanced by negative charges, primarily from CO_2 and from weak acids (A^-). Thus, SID – ($CO_2 + A^-$) = 0 or SID = $CO_2 + A^-$. This measure is known as the effective SID (SIDe), where A^- can be estimated by the following formula:

$$A^- = 2 \times (\text{albumin, g/dL}) + 0.5 \times (\text{phosphorus, g/dL})$$

Strong ion difference drives water dissociation and with it, the generation of H^+ ions; as SID increases, H^+ decreases and pH increases. Strong ion difference in healthy humans is typically between 40 and 42 mEq/L, but can be significantly decreased with critical illness, resulting in a rapid decline in pH.

Nonvolatile Weak Acid Buffers

In contrast to strong ions, weak nonvolatile acids (or anions) exist as either charged (dissociated) or uncharged forms in vivo. Weak acids can be forced to combine with other ions and thus lose their charge. HCO_3^- is the most important weak acid in the buffer system, as it can readily combine with another weak ion, H^+, to form H_2CO_3, which dissociates into CO_2 and water. Weak acids serve as a buffer to take up protons within the human physiologic plasma pH range.

Quantification of Acid–Base Status

Three different methods can be used to quantify acid–base disorders, based on assessing HCO_3^- concentration in the context of $PaCO_2$, standard base excess (BE) supplemented by anion gap (AG) determination, or strong ion gap (SIG) based on the SID. The first approach has been the most commonly accepted one. As discussed earlier, the bicarbonate-carbonic acid pair provides the primary buffer system for extracellular fluid. The relationship between this buffer pair and $PaCO_2$ is defined by the Henderson-Hasselbalch equation, in which $pH = pK + \log [HCO_3^-]/0.03 \times PaCO_2$. Thus, an increase in $PaCO_2$ will lead to a decrease in pH and later a compensatory increase in $[HCO_3^-]$. An alternative expression of buffering capacity in whole blood can be performed by calculation of the BE:

$$BE = -1.2 \times (24 - \text{measured bicarbonate concentration})$$

However, the plasma bicarbonate–carbon dioxide system only accounts for approximately 75 percent of the buffer action of blood. Buffering is also provided by hemoglobin, phosphates, and plasma proteins, particularly albumin. Use of the Siggaard-Andersen nomogram utilizes pH, $PaCO_2$, and HCO_3^- to calculate a BE that takes into account the remaining buffer systems. Positive BE signifies metabolic alkalosis, and negative BE implies metabolic acidosis. Standard base excess (SBE) represents the base excess of whole blood together with the surrounding interstitial fluid, comprising total extracellular fluid (ECF).

Calculation of BE and SBE does not allow determination between types of metabolic acidosis, for which AG is more useful. Anion gap is based on the principle of electroneutrality: The net ionic charge in a given solution is zero. In extracellular fluid, sodium is the primary cation and is balanced primarily by the strong cation Cl^- and the weak cation bicarbonate. The difference between these measured ions normally exists due to the presence of unmeasured anions (sulfates, lactate, and ketoacids), but primarily due to phosphates and negatively charged proteins such as albumin. The AG is the difference between measured cations and anions, represented by the equation:

$$AG = [Na^+ + K^+] - [Cl^- + HCO_3^-]$$

Under normal conditions, the AG is equal to 12 ± 4 mEq/L. Potassium is often omitted from the calculation because of its low extracellular concentration. Because albumin is the major anion in the blood, for every 1 g/dL decrease in serum albumin, the anion gap will decrease by approximately 2 to 3 mEq/L. As hypoalbuminemia is relatively common in critically ill children, a correction factor of AG for albumin concentration can be used:[31]

$$AG_{corr} = AG + 0.25 \times (40\ g/L - \text{observed albumin})$$

Strong ion gap refers to the difference between the SIDa and the SIDe: SIG = SIDa − SIDe. In contrast to AG, a normal SIG is zero. Strong ion gap does not change with changes in pH or in albumin concentration, but AG can be significantly altered by abnormal albumin or phosphate concentrations. Thus, AG is an estimate of the sum of SIG plus weak acids (A^-), where A^- can be estimated as previously described. The SID and SIG concepts are helpful conceptually, but AG is more commonly used in clinical practice for assessment and management.

Diagnosis and Management of Acid–Base Disorders

Awareness of the acid–base physiology and a stepwise approach will facilitate management of in-blood gas and electrolyte disturbances in critically ill children.[32] Based on the primary etiology, acid–base disorders are classified as respiratory, metabolic, or mixed.

Respiratory Acidosis

A primary respiratory acidosis is due most commonly to a decreased CO_2 clearance (e.g., alveolar hypoventilation) and less commonly to increased CO_2 production. The arterial pH will acutely decrease by 0.08 units for every 10 mm Hg increase in $PaCO_2$. Chronic renal compensation through proximal reabsorption of filtered HCO_3^- and excretion of H^+ as ammonia generally occurs within 12 to 24 hours, such that the $[HCO_3^-]$ increases by 0.3 mEq/L for each 1 mm Hg increase in $PaCO_2$ to a maximal increase of approximately 45 mEq/L.[26] Similarly, pH will decrease by 0.03 units for each 10 mm Hg increase in $PaCO_2$. The bone provides additional buffering of chronic respiratory acidosis as calcium phosphates and carbonates, and thus osteoporosis is a common finding in children with chronic lung disease. Chronic respiratory acidosis also results in chloride depletion due to increased chloride excretion by the kidney and a shift of chloride ions into the RBC (in exchange for bicarbonate), which usually takes place over 3 to 5 days, and also necessitates adequate chloride supplementation during correction of the chronic respiratory acidosis to prevent posthypercapnic alkalosis.

The clinical implications of respiratory acidosis depend largely upon the acuity of the event, as well as the degree of hypoxemia that is present. Treatment of respiratory acidosis is directed at the underlying ventilatory cause.[33]

The role of sodium bicarbonate ($NaHCO_3$) in the treatment of acute respiratory acidosis is not well defined. Administration of $NaHCO_3$ has several theoretical disadvantages. CO_2 freely and rapidly diffuses across the blood–brain barrier, while HCO_3^- does not, leading to the potential for worsening intracellular pH in the brain, cardiomyocytes, and other cells, leading to further cellular damage and dysfunction.[34-37] Additional concerns include the potential for transient $PaCO_2$ increase, displacement of the oxyhemoglobin dissociation curve, acute intracellular shift of potassium, and calcium binding to serum proteins. Given the absence of significant clinical benefit and the potential inherent risks, the routine administration of $NaHCO_3$ in the clinical setting of primary respiratory acidosis is probably not justified.

Respiratory Alkalosis

Respiratory alkalosis most commonly occurs in children due to tachypnea secondary to anxiety, pain, agitation, or fever. Hypoxemia can induce a hyperventilatory response in association with parenchymal lung disease, congestive heart failure, pulmonary edema (of any etiology), or pulmonary thromboembolism. Neurogenic causes to consider included increased intracranial pressure due to major head trauma, infection, or tumor. Respiratory alkalosis could also arise from either deliberate or unintentional overventilation in a child with respiratory failure. The initial fall in $PaCO_2$ is titrated by a mild decrease in arterial HCO_3^- (a decrease by approximately 0.2 mEq/L for every 1 mm Hg decrease in $PaCO_2$), which occurs rapidly, and the pH will increase by 0.08 units for each 10 mm Hg decrease in $PaCO_2$. The compensatory response to a chronic respiratory alkalosis by the kidneys usually occurs within 2 to 4 days via decreased tubular reabsorption of HCO_3^-, resulting in an increase in pH by 0.03 units for each 10 mm Hg decrease in $PaCO_2$. Respiratory alkalosis leads to acute decreased serum potassium, phosphate, and ionized calcium.[38] Clinical manifestations include AMS, confusion, and seizures (due to the effects of hypocarbia on cerebral perfusion), tachycardia, arrhythmias, muscle cramping, and muscle spasms. Treating the underlying cause is the therapeutic approach to respiratory alkalosis.

Metabolic Acidosis

Primary metabolic acidosis is generally caused by loss of HCO_3^- (from GI or renal sources), an increase in endogenous acid production, decreased excretion of endogenous acids, or accumulation of exogenous acids from toxins. The lungs respond to an acute metabolic acidosis with increased minute ventilation. The expected compensatory decrease in PaCO2 may be determined using the Winters equation: $PaCO_2 = 1.5 \times [HCO_3^-] + 8 \pm 2$. If the observed and calculated (i.e., expected) PaCO2 differ, then a mixed acid–base disorder is present. The etiology of metabolic acidosis can be generally characterized by the AG.

TABLE 5-2. Causes of High Anion Gap Metabolic Acidosis: MUDPILES

M =	METHANOL
U =	UREMIA
D =	DIABETIC KETOACIDOSIS (DKA)
P =	PARALDEHYDE
I =	IRON, ISONIAZID, OR INBORN ERRORS OF METABOLISM
L =	LACTIC ACIDOSIS
E =	ETHYLENE GLYCOL
S =	SALICYLATES

Elevated AG acidosis Elevated AG acidosis is due to either the retention of endogenous acids or the addition of exogenous acids and has a variety of causes that are easily recalled by the classic mnemonic *MUDPILES* (Table 5-2). Lactic acidosis is by far the most common type of high AG acidosis in the PICU. Ketoacidosis may develop with starvation (i.e., free fatty acids are metabolized to ketoacids rather than being used for triglyceride formation), but more commonly develop during diabetic ketoacidosis (DKA). Starvation is usually associated with a mild metabolic acidosis, while DKA is commonly associated with profound metabolic acidosis. Inborn errors of metabolism (i.e., endogenous organic acids) also are associated with an elevated AG.

The normal arterial lactate concentration is 1.0 ± 0.5 mmol/L, representing equilibrium between production and consumption during normal metabolism.[39] Several studies have examined the correlation between lactic acidosis and subsequent outcome in both children and adults with critical illness from myriad causes,[39,40] The initial lactate level, as well as the change in lactate over time, predict outcome in children with septic shock[41,42] and low cardiac output syndrome following cardiopulmonary bypass.[43,44] Hyperlactatemia thus appears to be a useful indicator of poor tissue perfusion, and serial measurement may provide a more useful assessment tool.

Severe metabolic acidosis (pH<7.20) can produce decreased cardiac output, decreased systemic vascular resistance, increased susceptibility to ventricular arrhythmias, increased pulmonary vascular resistance, and decreased responsiveness to both endogenous and exogenous catecholamines[39]; effects of moderate acidosis are uncertain. Furthermore, there is evidence to suggest that acidosis may have protective effects in critical illness.[45,46] Treatment of metabolic acidosis is, therefore, determined primarily by its etiology. In general, the focus of treating an increased AG acidosis should be on treating the underlying cause of the increased acid accumulation. Sodium bicarbonate could be harmful in children with DKA and is, therefore, contraindicated in this setting.[47] Theoretical concerns exist for treating lactic acidosis with sodium bicarbonate. Acidosis shifts the oxyhemoglobin dissociation curve to improve oxygen delivery at the tissue level; by shifting the oxyhemoglobin dissociation curve back to the left, correction of acidosis with bicarbonate could theoretically worsen oxygen delivery to hypoxic tissues. Controlled trial evidence is lacking to suggest either a benefit or harmful effect of sodium bicarbonate in treating metabolic acidosis in either children or adults with shock. Therefore, small, titrated doses of sodium bicarbonate to achieve a pH >7.15 to 7.20 in children with shock should be considered in concert with attempts to improve oxygen delivery and minimize oxygen consumption.

Non-AG acidosis A metabolic acidosis in the presence of a normal AG suggests loss of HCO_3^- (usually via the kidneys or GI tract) or rapid dilution of the ECF, with a proportional increase of chloride. Common causes of a normal AG, hyperchloremic metabolic acidosis (Table 5-3) include diarrhea (diarrheal fluid contains a high concentration of HCO_3^- relative to plasma) and renal tubular acidosis (RTA). Renal tubular acidosis results from failure of bicarbonate reabsorption/regeneration (i.e., decreased H^+ secretion) in the distal tubule (type 1, or distal RTA), bicarbonate wasting in the proximal tubule (type 2, or proximal RTA), or aldosterone deficiency with decreased clearance of potassium (type 4, distal or hyperkalemic RTA). Certain diuretics can also induce the hyperchloremic acidotic state by inhibiting proximal sodium bicarbonate absorption (acetazolamide) or distal reabsorption (spironolactone). Dilutional acidosis can also occur, with large-volume ECF expansion, such as during resuscitation of shock with non-HCO_3^--containing fluids such as normal saline (154 mEq/L of sodium and chloride).[48-50] For this reason, use of Ringer's lactate solution (Na^+ 130 Eq/L, Cl^- 109mEq/L, K^+ 4 mEq/L, and lactate 28 mEq/L) could be a recommended alternative for use during resuscitation. The lactate is generally metabolized by the liver and does not typically contribute to lactic acidosis.

Metabolic Alkalosis

Metabolic alkalosis is maintained when the kidneys fail to compensate by excreting excess HCO_3^- due to volume contraction, low glomerular filtration, or associated depletion of chloride or potassium. It is typically accompanied by an elevated $PaCO_2$ due to compensatory alveolar hypoventilation. The appropriate compensatory increase in $PaCO_2$ may be calculated by:

$$PaCO_2 = 0.7\ \Delta\ [HCO_3^-].$$

Conditions can either be temporary and corrected by chloride replacement (*chloride responsive*) or those in which hormonal mechanisms produce ongoing acid and chloride losses that are not effectively corrected by chloride (*chloride resistant*).[51] Chloride-responsive causes (characterized by low urine chloride concentration) include GI losses from vomiting or excessive nasogastric suction, renal losses from loop diuretics, and as compensation for chronic hypercarbia. These states are exacerbated by volume contraction and/or hypokalemia, which both augment distal H^+ secretion. Chloride-resistant causes (characterized by a high urine chloride concentration) can be related to mineralocorticoid excess from hyperaldosteronism, acetate in PN, use of diuretics, exogenous alkali loads related to massive citrated blood transfusions, or citrated sodium in replacement solutions for continuous renal replacement therapies.

Treatment of metabolic alkalosis is based on etiology. Chloride-responsive disorders benefit from replacement of chloride through normal saline infusion, though potassium chloride can also provide a dual replacement benefit. Ammonium chloride can be helpful if liver disease is not present. Discontinuation of diuretics may also be helpful. If ongoing diuresis is desired, the carbonic anhydrase inhibitor acetazolamide may be effective. Treatment of chloride-resistant states is directed at treating mineralocorticoid excess. Agents blocking distal tubular sodium reabsorption, restriction of sodium intake, and potassium supplementation are used to treat primary hyperaldosteronism, and ACE inhibitors or discontinuation of exogenous corticosteroids are used for secondary hyperaldosteronism.

TABLE 5-3. Causes of Normal Anion Gap (Hyperchloremic) Metabolic Acidosis [Modified from Fortenberry et al.]

BICARBONATE LOSS

GASTROINTESTINAL

- DIARRHEA
- EXTERNAL PANCREATIC OR SMALL-BOWEL DRAINAGE
- URETEROSIGMOIDOSTOMY, JEJUNAL LOOP, ILEAL LOOP
- DRUGS
  - CALCIUM CHLORIDE (ACIDIFYING AGENT)
  - MAGNESIUM SULFATE (DIARRHEA)
  - CHOLESTYRAMINE (BILE ACID DIARRHEA)

RENAL

- HYPOKALEMIA
  - PROXIMAL RENAL TUBULAR ACIDOSIS (RTA) (TYPE 2)
  - DISTAL (CLASSIC) RTA (TYPE 1)
- HYPERKALEMIA
  - GENERALIZED DISTAL NEPHRON DYSFUNCTION (TYPE 2 RTA)
    - – MINERALOCORTICOID DEFICIENCY
    - – MINERALCORTICOID RESISTANCE
    - – DECREASED SODIUM DELIVERY TO DISTAL NEPHRON
    - – TUBULOINTERSTITIAL DISEASE
    - – AMMONIUM EXCRETION DEFECT

DRUG-INDUCED HYPERKALEMIA (WITH RENAL INSUFFICIENCY)

- POTASSIUM-SPARING DIURETICS (AMILORIDE, TRIAMTERENE, SPIRONOLACTONE)
- TRIMETHOPRIM
- PENTAMIDINE
- ANGIOTENSIN-CONVERTING ENZYME INHIBITORS
- NONSTEROIDAL ANTI-INFLAMMATORY DRUGS
- CYCLOSPORINE

OTHER

- ACID LOADS (AMMONIUM CHLORIDE, PARENTERAL NUTRITION)
- LOSS OF POTENTIAL BICARBONATE: KETOSIS WITH KETONE EXCRETION
- DILUTIONAL ACIDOSIS (RAPID SALINE ADMINISTRATION)
- HIPPURATE

CATION EXCHANGE RESINS

Modified with permission from Wheeler DS, Wong HR, Shanley TP ed: Pediatric Critical Care Medicine: Basic Science and Clinical Evidence. Spriinger-Verlag London; 2007

TABLE 5-4. Systematic Approach to Analysis of Acid-Base Disorders [Modified from Fortenberry et al.]

1. Interpret the arterial pH to determine whether an acidemia or alkalemia present:

   if pH > 7.45, an alkalemia is present

   if pH < 7.35, an acidemia is present

2. Determine whether the primary disturbance is respiratory or metabolic in origin:

   respiratory acidosis: ↓ pH, ↑ $paco_2$

   respiratory alkalosis: ↑ pH, ↓ $paco_2$

   metabolic acidosis: ↓ pH, ↑ $[hco_3^-]$

   metabolic alkalosis: ↑ pH, ↓ $[hco_3^-]$

3. Calculate anion gap ($AG = [Na^+] - [HCO_3^- + Cl^-]$). correct for hypoalbuminemia if indicated.

   Generally, an anion gap >10 mEq/l suggests the presence of a metabolic acidosis, while an anion gap >20 mEq/l is always associated with a metabolic acidosis. Review causes of elevated anion gap metabolic acidosis to determine most likely causes.

4. Using the formulas listed in the chapter, determine whether the degree of compensation is appropriate. if it is not, then a mixed acid–base disorder is likely.

5. Calculate the delta anion gap: delta gap = (calculated AG – normal AG), i.e., (AG_{calc} – 12). For every 1 mEq/l increase in the calculated anion gap, there should be a 1 mEq/l decrease in $[HCO_3^-]$:

   If the $[HCO_3^-]$ is lower than predicted by this relationship, a normal anion gap (hyperchloremia) metabolic acidosis is also present.

   If the $[HCO_3^-]$ is higher than predicted by this relationship, a metabolic alkalosis is also present.

6. Measure urine pH and urine electrolytes if a metabolic alkalosis is present.

Modified with permission from Wheeler DS, Wong HR, Shanley TP ed: Pediatric Critical Care Medicine: Basic Science and Clinical Evidence. Spriinger-Verlag London; 2007

Mixed Acid–Base Disorders

Salicylate ingestions classically produce both a respiratory alkalosis (via direct stimulation of the respiratory centers in the brain) and a metabolic acidosis (elevated AG). Normal compensatory response to a primary acid–base disorder is not considered a mixed acid–base disorder. Proper analysis and interpretation of acid–base disorders requires a systematic approach (Table 5-4).[28,52,53]

KEY POINTS

- Accurate estimation of fluid and electrolyte needs is crucial in caring for the critically ill child and requires an understanding of basal metabolism and fluid homeostasis.
- The goal of fluid administration in critically ill patients with ARDS is to maintain intravascular volume to ensure adequate end-organ perfusion while minimizing extravascular lung water and pulmonary edema.
- Increasing fluid balance is associated with worse outcomes in adults and children with ALI.
- Dysnatremias, particularly hypo-osmolar hyponatremia, are the most common electrolyte abnormalities in patients in the intensive care unit. Awareness as well a systematic approach to determining the etiology (disease related and iatrogenic) and a proactive intervention strategy will help decrease morbidity from severe hyponatremia in the PICU.
- Assessment and treatment of acid-base imbalance in the critically ill child requires an understanding of terminology, insight into the buffer systems, and recognition of the compensatory interactions involved in maintaining balance.

REFERENCES

1. Roberts KB. Fluid and electrolytes: parenteral fluid therapy. *Pediatr Rev*. 2001;22:380-387.
2. Kliegman RM, Stanton, BF, Geme JW, Schor NF, Behrman RE, eds. *Nelson Textbook of Pediatrics*, 19th ed., Philadelphia, PA: Elsevier Saunders; 2011:chaps 52-55.
3. Roberts KE. Pediatric fluid and electrolyte balance: critical care case studies. *Crit Care Nurs Clin North Am*. 2005; 17:361-73.
4. Choong K, Bohn D. Maintenance parenteral fluids in the critically ill child. *J Pediatr*. 2007;83:S3-S10.
5. Simmons CF, Ichikawa I. External balance of water and electrolytes. In: Ichikawa I, ed. *Pediatric Textbook of Fluids and Electrolytes*. Baltimore, MD: Williams & Wilkins; 1990.
6. Feld LG, Kaskel FJ, Schoeneman MJ. The approach to fluid and electrolyte therapy in pediatrics. *Adv Pediatr*. 1988; 35:497-535.
7. Holliday MA, Segar ME. The maintenance need for water in parenteral fluid therapy. *Pediatrics*. 1957;19:823-832.
8. Dellinger RP, Levy MM, Carlet JM, et al. Surviving Sepsis Campaign: international guidelines for management of severe sepsis and septic shock: 2008. *Crit Care Med*. 2008; 36:296-327.
9. Wiedemann HP, Wheeler AP, Bernard GR, et al. Comparison of two fluid-management strategies in acute lung injury. *N Engl J Med*. 2006;354:2564-2575.
10. Randolph AG, Forbes PW, Gedeit RG, et al. Pediatric Acute Lung Injury & Sepsis Investigators (PALISI) Network: Cumulative fluid intake minus output is not associated with ventilator weaning duration or extubation outcomes in children. *Pediatr Crit Care Med*. 2005;6:642-647.
11. Valentine SL, Sapru A, Higgerson RA, et al on behalf of the Pediatric Acute Lung Injury and Sepsis Investigator's (PALISI) Network and the Acute Respiratory Distress Syndrome Clinical Research Network (ARDSNet). Fluid balance in critically ill children with acute lung injury. *Crit Care Med*. 2012;40:2883-2889.
12. Flori HR, Church G, Liu KD, et al. Positive fluid balance is associated with higher mortality and prolonged mechanical ventilation in pediatric patients with acute lung injury. *Crit Care Res Pract*. 2011;2011:854142.
13. Arikan AA, Zappitelli M, Goldstein SL, et al. Fluid overload is associated with impaired oxygenation and morbidity in critically ill children. *Pediatr Crit Care Med*. 2012;13:253-258.
14. Willson D, Thomas N, Tamburro R, et al. The relationship of fluid administration to outcome in the pediatric calfactant in acute respiratory distress syndrome (CARDS) trial. *Pediatr Crit Care Med*. 2013:In press.
15. Sutherland SM, Zappitelli M, Alexander SR, et al. Fluid overload and mortality in children receiving continuous renal replacement therapy: the prospective pediatric continuous renal replacement therapy registry. *Am J Kidney Dis*. 2010;55:316-325.
16. Goldstein SL, Somers MJ, Baum MA, et al. Pediatric patients with multi-organ dysfunction syndrome receiving continuous renal replacement therapy. *Kidney Int*. 2005; 67:653-658.
17. Foland JA, Fortenberry JD, Warshaw BL, et al. Fluid overload before continuous hemofiltration and survival in critically ill children: a retrospective analysis. *Crit Care Med*. 2004;32:1771-1776.
18. Goldstein SL, Currier H, Graf CD, et al. Outcome in children receiving continuous venovenous hemofiltration. *Pediatrics*. 2001;107:1309-1312.
19. Khilnani P. Electrolyte abnormalities in critically ill children. *Crit Care Med*. 1992;20:241-250.
20. Perkin RM, Levin DL. Common fluid and electrolyte problems in the pediatric intensive care unit. *Pediatr Clin N Am*. 1980;27:567-586.
21. Sedlacek M, Schoolwerth AC, Remillard BD. Electrolyte disturbances in the intensive care unit. *Semin in Dialysis*. 2006;19:496-501.
22. Lee JW. Fluid and electrolyte disturbances in critically ill patients. *Electrolyte Blood Press*. 2010;8:71-82.
23. Kraft MD, Btaiche IF, Sacks GS et al. Treatment of electrolyte disorders in adult patients in the intensive care unit. *Am J Health-Syst Pharm*. 2005;62:1663-1682.
24. Bagshaw SM, Townsend DR, McDermid RC. Disorders of sodium and water balance in hospitalized patients. *Can J Anesth*. 2009;56:151-167.
25. Adler SM, Verbalis JG. Disorders of body water homeostasis in critical illness. *Endocrinol Metab Clin N Am*. 2006;35:873-894.
26. Huang C, Kuo E. Mechanism of hypokalemia in magnesium deficiency. *J Am Soc Nephrol*. 2007;18:2649-2652.
27. Workman ML. Magnesium and phosphorus the neglected electrolytes. *AACN Clin Issues*. 1992;3:655-663.
28. Fortenberry JD, Hebbar K, Wheeler D. Acid-base balance. In: Wong H, Wheeler D, eds. *Pediatric Critical Care*. Springer, 2007.
29. Story DA. Bench-to-bedside review: a brief history of clinical acid-base. *Crit Care*. 2004;8:253-258.
30. Adrogue HE, Adrogue HJ. Acid-base physiology. *Respir Care*. 2001;46:328-341.

31. Durward A, Mayer A, Skellett S, et al. Hypoalbuminaemia in critically ill children: incidence, prognosis, and influence on the anion gap. *Arch Dis Child.* 2003;88:419-422.

32. Fencl V, Jabor A, Kazda A, Figge J. Diagnosis of metabolic acid-base disturbances in critically ill patients. *Am J Respir Crit Care Med.* 2000;162:2246-2251.

33. Epstein SK, Singh N. Respiratory acidosis. *Respir Care.* 2001;46:366-383.

34. Berenyi KJ, Wolk M, Killip T. Cerebrospinal fluid acidosis complicating therapy of experimental cardiopulmonary arrest. *Circulation.* 1975;52:319-324.

35. Steenbergen C, Deleeuw G, Rich T, Williamson JR. Effects of acidosis and ischemia on contractility and intracellular pH of rat heart. *Circ Res.* 1977;41:849-858.

36. Clancy RL, Cingolani HE, Taylor RR, Graham TP Jr, Gilmore JP. Influence of sodium bicarbonate on myocardial performance. *Am J Physiol.* 1967;212:917-923.

37. Kette F, Weil MH, von Planta M, Gazmuri RJ, Rackow EC. Buffer agents do not reverse intramyocardial acidosis during cardiac resuscitation. *Circulation.* 1990;81:1660-1666.

38. Foster GT, Vaziri ND, Sassoon CSH. Respiratory alkalosis. *Respir Care.* 2001;46:384-391.

39. Mizock BA, Falk JL. Lactic acidosis in critical illness. *Crit Care Med.* 1992;20:80-93.

40. Dugas MA, Proulx F, de Jaeger A, Lacroix J, Lambert M. Markers of tissue hypoperfusion in pediatric septic shock. *Intensive Care Med.* 2000;26:75-83.

41. Hatherill M, Waggie Z, Purves L, Reynolds L, Argent A. Mortality and the nature of metabolic acidosis in children with shock. *Intensive Care Med.* 2003;29:286-291.

42. Siegel LB, Dalton HJ, Hertzog JH, Hopkins RA, Hannan RL, Hauser GJ. Initial postoperative serum lactate levels predict survival in children after open heart surgery. *Intensive Care Med.* 1996;22:1418-1423.

43. Munoz R, Laussen PC, Palacio G, Zienko L, Piercey G, Wessel DL. Changes in whole blood lactate levels during cardiopulmonary bypass for surgery for congenital cardiac disease: an early indicator of morbidity and mortality. *J Thorac Cardiovasc Surg.* 2000;119:155-162.

44. Hannan RL, Ybarra MA, White JA, Ojito JW, Rossi AF, Burke RP. Patterns of lactate values after congenital heart surgery and timing of cardiopulmonary support. *Ann Thorac Surg.* 2005;80:1468-1474.

45. Forsythe SM, Schmidt GA. Sodium bicarbonate for the treatment of lactic acidosis. *Chest.* 2000;117:260-267.

46. Levraut J, Grimaud D. Treatment of metabolic acidosis. *Curr Opin Crit Care.* 2003;9:260-265.

47. Glaser N, Barnett P, McCaslin I, et al. Risk factors for cerebral edema in children with diabetic ketoacidosis. The Pediatric Emergency Medicine Collaborative Research Committee of the American Academy of Pediatrics. *N Engl J Med.* 2001;344:264-269.

48. Stephens RC, Mythen MG. Saline-based fluids can cause a significant acidosis that may be clinically relevant. *Crit Care Med.* 2000;28:3375-3377.

49. Skellett S, Mater A, Durward A, Tibby SM, Murdoch IA. Chasing the base deficit: hyperchloraemic acidosis following 0.9% saline fluid resuscitation. *Arch Dis Child.* 2000;83:514-516.

50. Hatherill M, Salie S, Waggie Z, et al. Hyperchloaemic metabolic acidosis following open cardiac surgery. *Arch Dis Child.* 2005;90:1288-1292.

51. Khanna A, Kurtzman NA. Metabolic alkalosis. *Respir Care.* 2001;46:354-365.

52. Narins RG, Emmett M. Simple and mixed acid-base disorders: a practical approach. *Medicine.* 1980;59:161-187.

53. Brewer ED. Disorders of acid-base balance. *Pediatr Clin North Am.* 1990;37:429-447.

CHAPTER 6

Drug–Nutrient Interactions

Joy Lehman

- INTRODUCTION
- RESPIRATORY
- SEIZURES
- ANTI-INFECTIVES
- PARENTERAL NUTRITION
- GLUCOSE HOMEOSTASIS
- ELECTROLYTE METABOLISM
- CONCLUSION
- KEY POINTS
- References

INTRODUCTION

From the time a fetus is viable through adolescence, the body is undergoing exponential growth and development. However, the development of organ function and body composition does not occur in a linear fashion. How the body processes nutrients and medications from birth through age 2 changes rapidly. There is also a significant change as the body begins the growth spurt through adolescence.[1] Critical illness, whether in the setting of extreme prematurity, sepsis, or chronic illness, may significantly impact growth and development as well as organ function. Electrolyte abnormalities, glucose intolerance, and protein malnutrition are common in the pediatric intensive care unit (PICU) patient.[2] Medications may impact these changes, and likewise the organ function disruptions that occur in critical illness may affect how the body processes medications.[3] When considering drug–nutrient interactions within the PICU setting, the clinician should consider the physiologic state of the patient, as well as the pharmacokinetic, pharmacodynamic and therapeutic properties of both medications and nutrients. There is a delicate balance between maintaining nutritional and therapeutic goals in the PICU setting, but these should never be considered mutually exclusive.

Chan defines drug–nutrient interactions as "physical, chemical, physiologic, or pathophysiologic relationships between a drug and a nutrient."[4] Numerous conditions and disease states involve a countless number of medications that are used in the neonatal intensive care unit (NICU) and PICU. Various classifications of drug–nutrient interactions have been proposed, but one useful classification that is based on the drug's course through the body is as follows[4]:

1. Ex-vivo bioinactivation refers to the interaction between the drug and the nutritional formulation through biochemical or physical reactions. A classic example of this form of interaction is the creation of a precipitate in an enteral feeding tube by a drug that has been administered before all the enteral formula has been flushed through. This form of interaction occurs when the drug and the nutrient are in physical contact, and usually occurs in the feeding tube or the central venous catheter.
2. Interactions affecting absorption affect drugs and nutrients delivered orally or enterally. These interactions have the potential to cause either an increase or decrease in the bioavailability of the drug. A variety of medications, including carbamazepine, quinolones, phenytoin, and warfarin, have significantly

impaired absorption in the presence of enteral formulas.

3. Interactions affecting systemic disposition occur after the drug and the nutrient have entered the systemic circulation. The mechanisms may involve changing the tissue distribution and/or systemic metabolism or transport. In this case, the classic example is grapefruit juice causing inhibition of the cytochrome P450 3A4 system and increasing the bioavailability of drugs like cyclosporine.
4. The final type of drug–nutrient interaction affects the elimination of drugs or nutrients, which may involve the modulation of renal or enterohepatic elimination.

This chapter will focus on the most common conditions and medications and potential nutrient interactions. Unanticipated drug–nutrient interactions may result in an adverse outcome or effect of the medication and/or decrease the effectiveness of the nutrients needed for optimal growth and development.

■ RESPIRATORY

Respiratory distress is one of the most common reasons for admission to the PICU for a child. This can either be acute (respiratory distress syndrome, bronchiolitis, asthma exacerbation) or chronic (bronchopulmonary dysplasia, or BPD). Maintaining adequate hydration without compromising respiratory efficiency is particularly important. In addition, providing adequate nutrition while restricting fluids may be a challenge.[5]

Caffeine is a respiratory stimulant primarily used in the NICU to treat apnea of prematurity. Caffeine can increase the resting metabolic rate, which may result in a higher caloric requirement for the patient.[6] Theophylline, like caffeine, is a respiratory stimulant, but is used more commonly in older children. It has a narrow therapeutic window, and levels should be monitored to routinely to check for toxicity. The bioavailability of oral theophylline is greatly influenced by food intake. High-fat and high-protein meals increase gut transit time of theophylline and may cause the sustained-release product to release suddenly and result in a short-term toxic level of the medication. Increased protein intake and decreased carbohydrate intake both decrease the half-life of theophylline, which may result in decreased efficacy of the medication.[7-9]

Albuterol and other beta agonists used to treat bronchiolitis, asthma, or BPD can all cause hyperglycemia, particularly in those patients who are diabetic. Blood glucose should be monitored whenever a patient is started on a scheduled beta agonist. In addition, use of beta agonists may result in hypokalemia. Clinicians should carefully monitor electrolyte status and replace potassium as necessary to avoid potential cardiac dysrhythmias.[10,11]

Furosemide, a loop diuretic, may be used to optimize fluid balance in the setting of respiratory insufficiency by decreasing fluids in the interstitial space. Furosemide can cause acute depletion of magnesium, sodium, and potassium. Chronic use can result in calcium depletion and thiamine deficiency. Acute electrolyte changes can affect cardiac function, so electrolytes should be monitored regularly while the patient is receiving furosemide. Long-term electrolyte depletion (addressed later in this chapter) can affect metabolic efficiency and growth, particularly bone metabolism, which can result in nonstress-related fractures and osteopenia.[12,13] Thiamine deficiency can lead to poor cardiac function. If a patient is placed on chronic therapy with furosemide, electrolytes—particularly calcium, magnesium, and phosphorus—and thiamine should be monitored monthly and/or prophylactically replaced.[11,14,15]

Systemic corticosteroids are used for numerous indications within the PICU setting. In the management of respiratory distress, steroids can be used in the acute phase or for long-term management of chronic respiratory diseases. Steroids have a lengthy list of drug–nutrient interactions, most commonly hyperglycemia.[16]

Blood glucose should be monitored closely upon initiation and with dose adjustments.[17,18] Steroids may cause sodium retention, whether used acutely or chronically. This effect can subsequently lead to fluid imbalance; therefore, fluid intake and output and serum electrolytes should be monitored routinely and replaced or restricted as necessary. Long-term steroid use may also cause changes in fat metabolism. The patient can experience an increase in total cholesterol and triglycerides, with a decrease in high-density lipoprotein (HDL) levels. A lipid panel should be evaluated at baseline and every 6 months if the patient will require an extended course of steroids.[19] In addition, and particularly concerning in the growing child, is the effect on bone metabolism. Long-term steroids can lead to bone demineralization. Therefore, calcium, vitamin D, and phosphorus supplements should be given through a complete multivitamin and levels monitored on a quarterly basis.[20]

SEIZURES

Children with seizures are frequently managed in the PICU and the NICU. Many of the medications used to treat seizures, whether given orally or intravenously, can have nutrient interactions.

Both phenobarbital and phenytoin interfere with vitamin D metabolism. Vitamin D plays a role in bone development and maintains calcium homeostasis. It is crucial that 25 OH-vitamin D levels are monitored and replaced appropriately while patients are receiving either phenobarbital or phenytoin.[21] There are limited options to replace vitamin D if the patient is completely nil per os (NPO). Current parenteral multivitamin formulations do not meet the American Academy of Pediatrics or the Academy of Nutrition and Dietetics recommendations for vitamin D replacement. In addition, hypocalcemia may cause the patient to experience seizures even when drug levels are therapeutic.[22] Phenytoin, phenobarbital, and valproic acid can all decrease levels of folate. If not adequately replaced, folic acid deficiency may cause megaloblastic anemia. The dose of supplementation will depend on the age of the patient and if the patient is receiving a multivitamin.[23,24] Recommendations for vitamin D and folic acid by age are shown in Table 6-1.[25,26] Pyridoxine (vitamin B_6) may decrease the effectiveness of phenobarbital, and levels should be monitored if pyridoxine is administered outside of a daily multivitamin regimen.[21]

Valproic acid (VPA) may induce a deficiency in L-carnitine, which is considered a conditionally essential amino acid in neonates and infants. This deficiency usually presents as hyperammonemia that can lead to mental status changes and encephalopathy. In addition, L-carnitine plays a role in both glucose and lipid metabolisms. Patients may develop hypertriglyceridemia and in severe deficiency, may develop hypoglycemia. L-carnitine can be supplemented at 50 mg/kg per day to prevent or treat VPA-induced deficiency.[27]

Oral phenytoin absorption is greatly influenced by enteral feeds. Phenytoin should be taken on an empty stomach 1 hour before a meal or 2 hours after. If the patient is on continuous tube feeds, then the tube feeding should be held for 2 hours before and 2 hours after each dose.[28,29]

TABLE 6-1. Folate and Vitamin D Recommended Dietary Allowances (RDAs) by Age

Age	Folate	Vitamin D
Birth-6 months	65 mcg*	–
7-12 months	80 mcg*	–
1-3 years	150 mcg	600 IU
4-8 years	200 mcg	
9-13 years	300 mcg	
14-18 years	400 mcg	600IU

*These are adequate intakes (AIs).

ANTI-INFECTIVES

Sepsis can be a reason for admission or can occur after admission to the PICU. Anti-infectives are one of the most widely used classes of medications in the PICU and are the most prone to drug–nutrient interactions. These medications can affect nutrient absorption, as well as cause organ dysfunction that can lead to disruption in metabolism. Conversely, many oral forms of anti-infectives are affected by food administration. Enteral feeds can decrease or increase the absorption of many oral anti-infectives, as seen in Table 6-2.[12,30,31]

TABLE 6-2. Anti-infective and Food Interactions

Decreased absorption when given with food	Increased absorption when given with food
Ampicillin	Cefuroxime
Azithromycin	Erythromycin estolate or ethyl succinate
Cefaclor	Ganciclovir
Cefixime	Griseofulvin
Cephalexin	Itraconazole
Ciprofloxacin	Ketoconazole
Doxycycline	Nelfinavir
Famciclovir	Nitrofurantoin
Indinavir	Ritonavir
Isoniazid	Saquinavir
Nafcillin	
Penicillin G or V	
Rifampin	
Tetracycline	

PARENTERAL NUTRITION

Parenteral nutrition (PN) may be indicated for the PICU patient who is unable to tolerate adequate enteral nutrition. One of the challenges to delivering PN is appropriate central venous access. Often, the PICU patient will need several intravenous (IV) therapies but will have limited IV access. The clinician should be aware of the compatibility of medications with PN to avoid complications such as precipitation of PN, loss of central access from thrombophlebitis, and potential embolization in cases where an inline filter is not present. Table 6-3 shows common medications used in the PICU setting and their compatibility with PN.[32-34]

TABLE 6-3. Medication Compatibility with Parenteral Nutrition

	Admixture Type		
Medication	**2-in-1**	**3-in-1**	**Lipids**
Acyclovir	I	I	I
Amikacin	C	C	I
Aminophylline	C	C	I
Amphotericin	I	I	I
Ampicillin sodium	C	C	C
Ampicillin-sulbactam	C	C	
Bumetanide	C	C	
Calcium gluconate	C	C	
Cefazolin	C	C	C
Cefotaxime	C	C	
Cefotetan	C	C	
Ceftazidime	C	C	
Ceftriaxone	C	C	
Clindamycin	C	C	C
Cyclosporine	I	I	C
Dexamethasone	C	C	C
Digoxin	C	C	C
Dobutamine	C	C	
Dopamine	C	I	
Famotidine	C	C	C
Fentanyl	C	C	
Fluconazole	C	C	
Furosemide	C	C	C
Gentamicin	C	C	C
Haloperidol	C	I	

(Continued)

■ **TABLE 6-3.** ***(Continued)***

	Admixture Type		
Medication	**2-in-1**	**3-in-1**	**Lipids**
Heparin	C	I	I
Hydralazine	C		
Hydrocortisone	C	C	C
Hydromorphone	C	I	C
Insulin, regular	C	C	C
Lorazepam	C	I	I
Magnesium sulfate	C	I	I
Methotrexate	I	C	
Methylprednisolone	C	C	
Metronidazole	C	C	
Midazolam	C	I	
Morphine	C	C*	
Nafcillin	C	C	
Norepinephrine	I	I	
Octreotide	C	C	
Ondansetron	C	C	
Penicillin GK	I	C	C
Pentobarbital	C	I	
Phenobarbital	C	I	I
Phenytoin	I	I	I
Piperacillin sodium	C	C	
Piperacillin-tazobactam	C	C	C
Potassium chloride	C	C	
Potassium phosphate	I	I	
Promethazine	I	C	
Propofol	C		
Ranitidine	C	C	C
Sodium bicarbonate	I	C	
Sodium phosphate	I	I	
Sulfamethoxazole-trimethoprim	C	C	

(Continued)

TABLE 6-3. (Continued)

Medication	Admixture Type 2-in-1	3-in-1	Lipids
Tacrolimus	C	C	
Ticarcillin-clavulanate	C		
Tobramycin	C	C	
Vancomycin	C	C	
Zidovudine	C	C	

All compatibility information refers to terminal site ("Y-site" injection port or other access port) between the parenteral nutrition solution and the central venous catheter.
C, Compatible; I, Incompatible.
2-in-1: Dextrose and amino acids; 3-in-1: Dextrose, amino acids, and lipids.
*Morphine in a 1 mg/ml concentration is compatible.

Another consideration for the patient on PN is fluid status. Patients in the PICU may require multiple continuous IV infusions that can contribute to the total daily fluid intake. If a patient is fluid restricted and on numerous medications, it becomes difficult for the clinician to write a PN formula that will meet energy requirements but not cause fluid overload. In some cases, the pharmacist can concentrate the medications being delivered so there is more fluid available to compound the appropriate PN formula.[35, 36]

GLUCOSE HOMEOSTASIS

Blood glucose abnormalities are one of the most common adverse events that occur in the PICU setting. Both hyper- and hypoglycemia are associated with increased morbidity and mortality in the PICU setting. These conditions can result from the endogenous response to critical illness, such as increased levels of glucagon, cortisol, and catecholamines or increased levels of insulin. However, many medications used in the PICU setting can affect blood glucose levels (Table 6-4). Many IV medications are delivered in a dextrose-based solution, and this may also contribute to hyperglycemia. When evaluating blood glucose abnormalities, the clinician should consider the total glucose infusion rate (GIR) from all sources, including medications and maintenance IV fluids.[12,37]

TABLE 6-4. Medications That May Affect Glucose Response

Medication/Drug Class	Response
Corticosteroids	Hyperglycemia
Diuretics	Hyperglycemia
Epinephrine	Hyperglycemia
Fosphenytoin	Hypoglycemia
Glucagon	Hyperglycemia
Megestrol	Hyperglycemia
Nelfinavir	Hyperglycemia
Octreotide	Hyper/hypoglycemia
Penicillamine	Hypoglycemia
Phenytoin	Hyperglycemia
Sertraline	Hyperglycemia
Tacrolimus	Hyperglycemia

ELECTROLYTE METABOLISM

Maintaining appropriate electrolyte balance is crucial to vital organ function. Acute changes in electrolyte levels can cause severe consequences such as seizures, heart failure, respiratory failure, or death. Table 6-5 summarizes medications that can affect electrolyte balance.[4,10,16,38,39] As with blood glucose, the imbalance may be due to the disease state itself or can be a combination of factors. For example, decreased kidney function will decrease potassium elimination that subsequently leads to increased serum potassium levels. If a patient is also receiving a medication that increases potassium levels (e.g., spironolactone), then the patient could become dangerously hyperkalemic very

TABLE 6-5. Medication-Nutrient Interactions

Medication/Drug Class	Nutrient	Interaction
Aminoglycosides	Potassium, magnesium, sodium, calcium	Electrolyte wasting
Amphotericin	Magnesium, potassium, sodium	Electrolyte wasting
Digoxin	Calcium, magnesium, potassium	Hypomagnesemia or hypokalemia may increase digoxin toxicity, cardiac arrhythmias
Fluconazole	Potassium	Hypokalemia
Foscarnet	Calcium, magnesium, potassium, sodium	Electrolyte depletion
Furosemide	Calcium, magnesium, potassium, sodium, chloride	Electrolyte depletion
H_2 receptor antagonists (ranitidine, famotidine)	Vitamin B_{12}, zinc	Depletion of vitamin B_{12} and zinc
Methotrexate	Folic acid	Folate deficiency; folic acid replacement may decrease methotrexate efficacy
Nonsteroidal anti-inflammatory agents	Potassium	Hyperkalemia in renal deficiency or in patients receiving potassium supplements
Proton pump inhibitors	Iron, vitamin B_{12}	Decreased absorption
Spironolactone	Sodium, potassium	Hyponatremia, hyperkalemia
Warfarin	Vitamin K, vitamin E	Vitamin K may inhibit effectiveness of warfarin; vitamin E may enhance anticoagulation effect
Zidovudine	Carnitine, folic acid	May cause carnitine deficiency, megaloblastic anemia

quickly.[40] Therefore, it is crucial that electrolytes be monitored on a regular basis, especially when medications that can affect electrolyte balance are started or stopped.

CONCLUSION

The PICU patient undergoes a tremendous metabolic response to meet the hormonal and energy demands of critical illness. Every aspect of nutrient and medication management, from delivery to elimination, is affected by critical illness. Understanding the delicate balance and interactions between nutrients and medications can help the clinician deliver safe and effective care and thereby optimize outcomes for the critically ill child. A dedicated pharmacist in the PICU is an invaluable resource to facilitate safe therapeutic prescriptions, for monitoring and avoiding undesirable drug-nutrient interactions.

KEY POINTS

- A variety of potential drug-nutrient interactions occur frequently in the intensive care unit. Diuretics, beta agonists, steroids, antiepileptics, antimicrobials are drugs that require careful consideration of these interactions and close monitoring.
- Unanticipated drug–nutrient interactions may result in an adverse outcome or effect of the medication and/or decrease the effectiveness of the nutrients needed for optimal growth and development.
- Awareness of the compatibility of commonly used medications with parenteral nutrition (PN) is essential to avoid complications such as precipitation.
- A dedicated pharmacist is invaluable for delivering safe and effective therapies in the complex PICU environment.

REFERENCES

1. Kearns GI, Abdel-Rahman SM, Alander SW, et al. Developmental pharmacology-drug disposition, action and therapy in in infants and children. *N Engl J Med.* 2003;349:1157-1167.
2. Mehta NM, Jaksic T. The critically ill child. nutrition in pediatrics. In: Duggan C et al, eds. *Nutrition in Pediatrics,* 4th edition. Hamilton, ON: BC Decker, Inc; 2008:663-673.
3. Kearns GL, Abdel-Rahman SM, Alander SW, et al. Developmental pharmacology-drug disposition, action, and therapy in infants and children. *N Engl J Med.* 2003:349;1157-1167.
4. Chan LN. Drug-nutrient interactions. *J Parent Enteral Nutr.* 2013;37:450-459.
5. Kair LR, Leonard DT, Anderson JM. Bronchopulmonary dysplasia. *Pediatrics in Review.* 2012;33:255-264.
6. Schmidt B, Roberts RS, Davis P, et al. Caffeine therapy for apnea of prematurity. *N Engl J Med.* 2006;254:2112-2121.
7. Feldman CH, Hutchinson VE, Pigpenger CE, et al. Effect of dietary protein and carbohydrate on theophylline metabolism in children. *Pediatrics.* 1980;66:956-962.
8. Kappas A, Anderson KE, Conney AH, et al. Influence of diet and fluid on bioavailability of theophylline metabolism in man. *Clin Pharmacol Ther.* 1976;20:643-653.
9. Welling PG, Lyons LL, Craig, WA, Trochta GA. Influence of diet and fluid on bioavailability of theophylline. *Clin Pharmacol Ther.* 1976:17:475-480.
10. Gura KM, Chan LN, Drug therapy and role of nutrition. In: Duggan C. et al eds. *Nutrition in Pediatrics,* 4th ed. Hamilton, ON: BC Decker; 2005.
11. Albuterol. In: *Drug Information Handbook,* 22nd ed. Hudson, NY: Lexi-Comp Inc.41
12. Gura KM. Drug-nutrient interactions. In: Hendricks KM, Duggan C, eds. *Manual of Pediatric Nutrition,* 4th ed. Hamilton, ON: BC Decker; 2005;540-549.
13. Gura KM, Couris RR. Drug-induced bone disease. *US Pharmacist.* 2002;27:HS43-HS57.
14. Seligmann H, Halkin H, Rauchefleisch S, et al. Thiamine deficiency in patients with congestive heart failure receiving long-term furosemide therapy: a pilot study. *Am J Med.* 1991;91:151-155.
15. Brady JA, Rock CL, Horneffer MR. Thiamine status, diuretic medications and the management of congestive heart failure. *J Am Diet Assoc.* 1995;95:541-544.
16. Chan LN. Drug-nutrient interactions in transplant recipients. *J Parenter Enteral Nutr.* May 2001:25:132-141.
17. Dellinger RP, Levy MM, Rhodes A et al. Surviving Sepsis Campaign: international guidelines for management of severe sepsis and septic shock, 2012. *Intensive Care Med.* 2013;39:165-228.
18. Kinsella JP, Greenough A, Abman SH. Bronchopulmonary dysplasia. *Lancet.* 2006;267:1421-1431.
19. Henkin J, Como JA, Oberman A. Secondary dyslipidemia: inadvertent effects of drugs in clinical practice. *JAMA.* 1992;267:961-968.
20. LoCascio V, Bonucci E, Imbinbo B, et al. Bone loss in response to long term glucocorticoid therapy. *Bone Miner.* 1990;20:251-262.
21. Kotzer LM, Mascarenhas MR, Wallace E. Drug-nutrient interactions in infancy and childhood. In: *Handbook of Drug-Nutrient Interactions.* Boullata JI, Armenti VT, eds. Humana Press, Totowa, NJ: 2010;331-345.
22. Holick, MF. Vitamin D deficiency. *N Engl J Med.* 2007;357:266-281.
23. Lambie DG, Johnson RH. Drugs and folate metabolism. *Drugs.* 185;30:145-155.
24. Seligmann H, Potasman I, Weller B, et al. Phenytoin-folic acid interaction: a lesson to be learned. *Clin Neuropharmacol.* 1999;22:268-272.
25. Office of Dietary Supplements National Institutes of Health: Vitamin D Fact Sheet. 2011/2013. http://ods.od.nih.gov.factsheets/VitaminD-HealthProfessional.
26. Office of Dietary Supplements National Institutes of Health: Folate Fact Sheet. 2012/2013. http://ods.od.nig.gov.factsheets/folate-HealthProfessional.
27. Ohtani Y, Endo F, Mastuda I. Carnitine deficiency with hyperammonemia associated with valproic acid therapy. *J Pediatr.* 1982:101;782-785.
28. Marvel ME, Bertino JS. Comparative effects of an elemental and a complex enteral feeding formulation on the absorption of phenytoin suspension. *J Parenter Enteral Nutr.* 1991;15:316-318.
29. Doak KK, Haas CI, Dunnigan KJ, et al. Bioavailability of phenytoin acid and phenytoin sodium with enteral feedings. *Pharmacotherapy.* 1998;18:637-645.
30. Singh BN. Effects of food on clinical pharmacokinetics. *Clin Pharmacokinet.* 1999;37:3-231-255.
31. Welling PG. Effects of food on drug absorption. *Annu Rev Nutr.* 1996;16:383-415.
32. Trissel LA, Gilbert DL, Martinez JF, Baker MB, Walter WV, Mirtallo JM. Compatibility of parenteral nutrient solutions with selected drugs during simulated Y-sited administration. *Am J Health Syst Pharm.* 1997;54(11):1295-1300.
33. Trissel A. *Handbook on Injectable Drugs.* 17th ed. Bethesda, MD: American Society of Health-System Pharmacists; 2013.
34. NEOFAX® System [Internet database]. Greenwood Village, CO: Thomson Healthcare. 2013.

35. Langley G, Tajchman S. Fluids, electrolytes and acid-base disorders. In: *A.S.P.E.N Adult Nutrition Support Core Curriculum,* 2nd ed. Mueller CM, ed. Silver Spring, MD. :A.S.P.E.N;2012:98-121.

36. Moritz ML, Ayus JC. Intravenous fluid management for the acutely ill child. *Curr Opin Pediatr.* 2011;23:186-193.

37. Pandit MK, Burke J, Gustafson AB, et al. Drug-induced disorders of glucose tolerance. *Ann Intern Med.* 1993;118:529-539.

38. Shetty AK, Rogers NI, Mannick EE, Viles DH. Syndrome of hypokalemic metabolic alkalosis and hypomagnesemia associated with gentamicin therapy: case reports. *Clin Pediatr.* 2000;39:529-533.

39. Sonneblick M, Friedlander Y, Rosin AJ. Diuretic-induced severe hyponatremia. Review and analysis of 129 reported patients. *Chest.* 1993;103;601-606.

40. Tolstoi LG. Drug-induced hyperkalemia. *Hosp Pharm.* 1996;31:221-228.

SECTION 2

Delivery of Nutrition Support to the Critically ill Child

CHAPTER 7

Parenteral Nutrition Support in the Critically ill Child

Katelyn Ariagno and Christopher Duggan

- INTRODUCTION
- INDICATIONS FOR PARENTERAL NUTRITION
- PARENTERAL NUTRITION REQUIREMENTS
- FLUIDS AND ELECTROLYTES
- CARBOHYDRATE
- PROTEIN
- FAT
- MICRONUTRIENTS
- PARENTERAL NUTRITION COMPLICATIONS
- TRANSITION FROM PARENTERAL NUTRITION TO ENTERAL NUTRITION
- KEY POINTS
- References

INTRODUCTION

The prevalence of both acute and chronic malnutrition in the critically ill child continues to be documented.[1] Vigilant nutrition screening to assess for malnutrition and the development of an appropriate nutrition prescription are important goals for nutrition support in the critically ill child.[2] During critical illness, energy and macronutrient utilization is altered, resulting in glucose and lipid intolerance, as well as altered protein metabolism, making the design of appropriate nutrition support a challenge.[3] Other barriers to nutrition delivery also commonly exist during critical illness, including fluid restrictions, interruptions in the advancement of nutrition support due to procedures, and the inability to obtain dedicated venous or enteral access.[4]

Compared to adults, critically ill neonates and children are at increased risk of loss of lean body mass due to their decreased energy stores and increased basal energy requirements, which can ultimately place them at risk for increased morbidity and mortality.[5] A nutrition prescription consisting of a mixed substrate fuel system, including adequate protein, will not fully suppress the ensuing metabolic response, but can offset the catabolism and eventually lead to anabolism, ensuring continued growth and development.[6]

The field of parenteral nutrition (PN) dates only from the 1960s, when pioneering studies by Dudrick and others were described in patients with chronic gastrointestinal diseases, which set the stage in supporting the use of PN to address malnutrition in hospitalized patients.[7] In this chapter, we will discuss the role of both primary and supportive PN in terms of delivering adequate nutrition to critically ill children. We will also discuss the importance of delivering a PN solution that will reduce the risk of morbidity and mortality. PN has considerably improved the survival of previously fatal pediatric conditions. Specialized enteral and PN solutions have made significant advancements and play an essential role in the overall management of critically ill children.[8]

INDICATIONS FOR PARENTERAL NUTRITION

Although current research supports enteral nutrition (EN) as the preferred mode of nutrition support, PN can be a judicious choice in terms of delivering adequate nutrition prescriptions when the function of the gastrointestinal tract is altered. Table 7-1 lists common clinical conditions that result in altered gastrointestinal function wherein PN use should be considered.[8,9]

Determining the timing of PN initiation in the pediatric population is related to the age and underlying nutritional status of the patient. Premature, very-low-birth-weight (VLBW) infants have minimal nutritional reserves; therefore, early nutrition support is commonly initiated within the first 12 to 24 hours after birth to optimize energy and protein balance, as well as to prevent growth failure and delays in neurodevelopment. In comparison, it is common for full-term, appropriate-for-gestational-age (AGA) infants to be started on PN by day 3 to 4 if no EN support is planned, and in older children, PN is often initiated by day 5 to 7 of EN deprivation.[8] Children with preexisting malnutrition and an inability to be fed by the enteral route should be initiated on PN sooner.

Deciding whether a patient should be initiated on PN should involve a thoughtful discussion with a dedicated nutrition support service to weigh the benefits versus the known risks associated with PN. These risks include metabolic, mechanical, and infectious complications. A patient with significant fluid and electrolyte derangements associated with hemodynamic instability should not be initiated on PN. Parenteral nutrition is safe to start once a patient's fluid and electrolyte status is corrected. Other conditions in which PN may be contraindicated include if a patient has a severe egg or soy allergy, due to the presence of egg yolk phospholipids and soybean oil in the sterile fat emulsion.

Parenteral nutrition can serve as a primary therapy for some patients, and for others, a supportive therapy in combination with EN support. Examples of when PN is used in combination with EN include when a patient is unable to advance to the prescribed goal volume of enteral feeds over an extended period or when a patient is receiving only trophic enteral feeds for gastrointestinal benefit versus energy intake, such as in intestinal failure. (Please see chapter 8 in which EN is discussed in greater detail.)

It is important to ensure that patients for whom PN is considered have a dedicated venous catheter access. For central venous access, the distal tip of the catheter must be in the central venous circulation in order for a hypertonic PN solution to safely infuse into the circulation. Similar to adults, central venous access in pediatrics is defined by the distal tip of the catheter being located in the superior vena cava (SVC), the junction of the SVC and the right atrium (RA), or the inferior vena cava (IVC). These venous locations allow for maximum flow and distribution of hypertonic PN

TABLE 7-1. Indications for PN[8,9]

Clinical Condition	
Surgical gastrointestinal disorders	Gastroschisis, omphalocele, intestinal atresias, meconium ileus, Hirschsprung disease, diaphragmatic hernia, gastrointestinal fistula, postoperative ileus
Prematurity	
Short bowel syndrome	
Congenital heart disease	Compromised blood supply to the mesentery
Intestinal disease	Severe inflammatory bowel disease, chronic or secretory diarrhea, microvillus inclusion disease and tufting enteropathy
Motility disorders	Intestinal pseudo-obstruction, total colonic Hirschsprung disease, mitochondrial and metabolic disorders
Bone marrow transplant	Anorexia, mucositis, feeding intolerance related to side effects of therapy
Hypermetabolic states	Trauma, burns, sepsis

solutions: >900 mOsm/L. The determination of catheter tip location usually involves radiographic confirmation.[10,11]

In general, PN administered through a peripheral venous catheter provides inadequate energy for those completely unable to meet nutrient needs enterally, and is associated with increased infectious and mechanical risks compared with central PN.[10] In patients who are able to tolerate high intravenous fluid volumes, peripheral PN use can be a way to meet energy and nutrient goals, or as a bridge while awaiting the placement of central venous access. In some instances, a patient can continue on peripheral PN for 5 to 7 days if they have stable electrolytes and are not hypermetabolic.[12] Peripheral PN solutions are recommended to be limited to ≤900 mOsm/L to reduce the risk of venous thrombosis, phlebitis, or infiltration.

When deciding on the mode of nutrition support that best suits the patient, the route of administration of macro- and micronutrient prescriptions are often the first to be determined. However, current research in nutrition support is also focusing on the optimal timing in which nutrition support should be initiated, specifically with PN. Recent studies in adult critical care have evaluated the effects of early versus late initiation of PN, as well as using PN as a supplement, when energy goals are not being met with EN alone. In a large, randomized, multicenter adult trial, Casaer et al. compared early initiation of PN within 48 hours (2,312 patients) with late initiation after day 7 (2,328 patients) in the intensive care unit (ICU) to supplement insufficient EN. They found that late initiation of PN was associated with fewer infections, faster recovery from organ failure, and reduced hospital stay as compared to the group that received PN earlier.[13] In contrast, Doig and colleagues showed that early initiation of PN in adult patients that have short-term contraindications to EN led to fewer invasive ventilation days and less muscle and fat mass losses without any mortality difference.[14] The investigators enrolled 1,372 patients from 27 centers who were ineligible or unable to receive EN. They were randomized to receive either early PN (on day 1) or to receive standard care (as determined by the bedside team). No difference was reported in 60-day mortality between groups (22.8% vs. 21.5%). Although patients receiving early PN had lower duration of mechanical ventilation, their ICU or hospital stay was similar to the standard care group. There were no differences in infectious morbidity or PN-related adverse events between the groups. Due to the limited number of published studies available that are specific to the critically ill child, nutrition support practice continues to be based in part on interpretation of these adult data.

PARENTERAL NUTRITION REQUIREMENTS

Hospitalized pediatric patients may have reduced total energy requirements compared to healthy children. The components of total energy expenditure (TEE) are as follows:

$$TEE = BMR + SDA + E_{activity} + E_{growth} + E_{losses}$$

Where BMR = basal metabolic rate, which is the largest component of TEE (energy required by the body at rest while fasted, 60% to 70%),

SDA = specific dynamic action of food or thermic effect of food (energy produced as heat during digestion and metabolism of food, 8% to 10%),

$E_{activity}$ = energy required for physical activity,

E_{growth} = energy required for somatic growth, and

E_{losses} = obligatory energy lost in urine and stool due to inefficiencies of absorption and metabolism.

Of the 5 components of TEE, 4 are often significantly reduced in the critically ill hospitalized patient. Energy required for physical activity is minimal due to bed rest and use of sedative and paralytic agents. Energy required for growth is often reduced, since the catabolic response following severe injury or illness presumably results in a temporary halt to anabolism (accretion of lean body mass). The thermic effect of food is reduced in patients receiving PN support as opposed to patients receiving EN. Also, in patients receiving PN, obligatory gastrointestinal losses of nutrients are generally less.[15] A clinician who is not aware of these facts may end up prescribing an energy goal that exceeds a patient's actual energy expenditure, resulting in overfeeding.

Estimated energy prescriptions obtained from predicted energy equations continue to be used, despite studies demonstrating a high rate of inaccuracy. The most accurate clinical measure of resting energy expenditure is obtained through indirect calorimetry (IC). Mehta et al. developed criteria to select patients at increased risk of metabolic derangements in the pediatric intensive care unit (PICU) who would greatly benefit from IC.[16] (Please see chapter 3 for more details on energy and macronutrient requirements in the PICU.)

As discussed in earlier chapters in this book, under- and overfeeding a critically ill child can result in significant complications that affect both treatment and recovery. Under- and overfeeding not only apply to EN, but also to the nutrition prescription provided via PN. Concerns exist that by providing both PN and EN, patients may be at increased risk of overfeeding, which can result in a longer time on mechanical ventilator support, infection, hyperglycemia, and organ dysfunction.[16] The presumed altered metabolic response following critical illness cannot always be accurately predicted due to the dynamic changes that occur throughout the hospital course. This alteration in metabolism, specifically in children with less substrate reserves, can result in malnutrition. Appropriate provision and necessary modifications to both macro- and micronutrients during critical illness will help guide the composition of PN.[17]

FLUIDS AND ELECTROLYTES

Fluid management plays a significant role in a critically ill child's hospital course. A detailed account of fluid and electrolyte management during critical illness can be found in chapter 5 of this book. Following the resuscitation phase, which aims to increase cardiac output and optimize tissue blood flow and oxygen delivery to vital organs, fluid is often allotted to nutrition support.[18] A child's overall fluid status, as well as their age, size, and underlying disease condition, may influence the daily fluid balance goals.

If a patient has increased insensible losses related to fever or tachycardia, or increased sensible losses related to vomiting, diarrhea, urine, ostomy, or nasogastric output, they may require fluid intake greater than their maintenance needs. If only a small amount of fluid is available for nutrition support due to fluid overload or renal and kidney dysfunction, optimizing the PN solution can be a challenge.

TABLE 7-2. Holliday-Segar Method[19]

Body Weight	Fluid Requirements
0-10 kg	100 mL/kg
10-20 kg	1000 mL + 50 mL/kg over 10 kg
>20 kg	1500 mL + 20 mL/kg over 20 kg

Fluid available for the PN prescription should be reviewed daily with the critical care and nutrition support teams to ensure the patient does not become fluid overloaded or dehydrated. The PN infusion rate should not be rapidly titrated up and down to account for fluid shifts or used as replacement fluids to avoid wide variation in the delivery of glucose, electrolytes, and other components of PN. Maintenance fluid requirements in children can be assessed using the Holliday-Segar method (Table 7-2).[19] It is important to consider fluids from all sources, as many critically ill patients are receiving additional infusions such as medications and/or blood products.

Electrolyte contents in PN solutions will vary, depending on the patient's underlying condition and organ function. Table 7-3 lists electrolyte requirements of children. Of note, these are not specific to critical illness; electrolyte requirements in critically ill children are often altered by the effects of illness, medications (diuretic use), and other factors.[20] If a patient develops electrolyte derangements, it is important to understand all potential causes to

TABLE 7-3. Electrolyte Requirements in Children

	Standard Daily Requirements		
Nutrient	Preterm Neonate	Infants/Children	Adolescents
Sodium (mEq)	2-5/kg	2-5/kg	1-2/kg
Potassium (mEq)	2-4/kg	2-4/kg	1-2/kg
Phosphorus (mmol)	1-2/kg	0.5-2/kg	10-40/day
Calcium (mEq)	2-4/kg	0.5-4/kg	10-20/day
Magnesium (mEq)	0.3-0.5/kg	0.3-0.5/kg	10-30/day
Chloride	As needed to maintain acid–base balance		
Acetate	As needed to maintain acid–base balance		

Reproduced with permission from Mirtallo, J., Canada, T., Johnson, D., Task force for the revision of safe practices for parenteral nutrition. Safe practices for parenteral nutrition, *J Parenter Enteral Nutr* 2004;28(6):S39-S70

assist with properly adjusting the composition of the PN solution. When possible, PN should be modified to support therapeutic efforts intended to re-establish fluid and electrolyte balance.[21] Daily monitoring of a patient's hydration status, including daily intakes and outputs, as well as electrolyte trends, is crucial in any patient receiving PN.

CARBOHYDRATE

Carbohydrate (CHO) metabolism during critical illness is characterized by an increase in glucose production. Gluconeogenesis ensures a steady energy source for glucose-dependent organs, such as the brain, erythrocytes, and renal medulla.

In PN solutions, dextrose (D-glucose) provides the primary source of nonprotein energy, with an energy density of 3.4 kcal/gram. Dextrose infusions are often initiated at a glucose infusion rate (GIR) of 5 mg CHO/kg/minute, which is thought to be the endogenous glucose production of premature infants and neonates. Advancement of the GIR is done daily, pending tolerance, increasing by 2 to 5 mg/kg/min until goal energy needs are met. For infants, the recommended upper range of the GIR is 12 to 14 mg CHO/kg/min; however, other clinical reasons may require a patient to receive a GIR that exceeds this range.[22] It is important to be mindful of the possible risk of overfeeding with an excessive GIR, which some studies have shown can lead to the development of hyperglycemia, hepatic steatosis, and cholestasis.[23]

Tolerance of the GIR advancement often depends on the patient's age and size, as well as their underlying condition, such as sepsis. A critically ill child may also be receiving other dextrose-containing infusions that need to be taken into account, or medication requirements that are affecting adequate glycemic control despite their GIR seeming appropriate for their age. Blood glucose checks as well as checking the urine for glucose are two methods of assessing a patient's tolerance of dextrose provided via PN. Temporary adjustments can be made to the GIR if a patient demonstrates inadequate glycemic control with hyperglycemia and glucosuria. Insulin may also need to be considered to ensure a patient receives an adequate nutrition prescription and is utilizing CHO appropriately.

Many current studies are evaluating the relationship between elevated serum glucose levels and morbidity and mortality during critical illness.[24-26] This relationship has prompted studies examining the role of tight glucose control using insulin in the ICU. In a large, randomized trial of tight glycemic control in children after cardiac surgery, this approach was not associated with decrease in infections, rates of mortality, or length of hospital stay.[27]

PROTEIN

Provision of optimal protein delivery and intake during critical illness to prevent unintended loss of lean body mass is one of the primary goals of nutrition support in critically ill children. Critical illness is characterized by increased protein turnover, with ongoing protein degradation and synthesis.[28,29] This adaptive response allows amino acids to be available to the free amino acid pool, which are then redistributed away from skeletal muscle for tissue repair, wound healing, and participation in a variety of inflammatory response pathways. This contribution to the amino acid pool, as well as overall protein breakdown during critical illness, can exceed dietary protein intake, creating a net negative nitrogen balance. Recent studies have suggested that a minimum of 1.5 gram/kilogram of protein intake may be necessary to maintain a positive balance during critical illness.[30,31] This is consistent with the recommendation made by the American Society of Parenteral and Enteral Nutrition (A.S.P.E.N) pediatric critical care nutrition guidelines.[32]

Providing amino acids parenterally affects their utilization and recommended requirements, in comparison to when they are being provided enterally. Parenteral nutrition bypasses the splanchnic area, and amino acids arrive at the liver via the hepatic arterial circulation instead of the portal venous circulation. Amino acid needs are influenced by age, but specific amino acid needs are also thought to change during critical illness.[3]

With the variety of amino acid formulations available for use, studies have evaluated the composition of both essential and nonessential amino acids. A balance of these amino acids needs to exist in order to optimize protein synthesis.[3] If essential amino acids are limited, protein breakdown will continue to occur in order to maintain the synthesis of essential amino acids. This is also thought to be the case with conditionally essential amino acids, such as during a period of critical illness. Glutamine, a nonessential amino acid, has been considered conditionally essential during critical illness. In a recent study by Heyland et al., a randomized, blinded trial was conducted in which 1,223 critically ill adults in 40 ICUs with multiorgan failure on mechanical ventilation were assigned to receive glutamine, antioxidants, glutamine and antioxidants together, or a placebo. Both intravenous and enteral supplementation were initiated within 24 hours after admission. They concluded that early administration of glutamine in critically ill adults with multiorgan failure was harmful, reporting a nonsignificant increase in 28-day mortality and significant increases in in-hospital and 6-month mortality.[33] Additional parenteral glutamine supplementation in the pediatric critically ill population is not well supported at this time.[3]

Crystalline amino acids make up the protein source in PN solutions. In the United States (US), the common amino acid solutions used in the pediatric population include TrophAmine® (B. Braun Medical), Aminosyn PF® (Hospira), and Premasol® (Baxter). The compositions of the amino acid solutions vary, aiming to meet the specific needs of infants, children, and adults. Pediatric amino acid solutions contain more glutamic and aspartic acid and taurine, while having less glycine, methionine, and phenylalanine.[9] (9). Table 7-4 outlines the composition of the common amino acid solutions available in the United States. Premature infants, especially those weighing less than 1,000 grams at birth, are not able to efficiently metabolize methionine into cysteine and taurine; therefore, cysteine is considered a

TABLE 7-4. Brand-Specific Pediatric Parenteral Amino Acid Solutions

	Solutions Designed for Infants		Solutions Appropriate for >1+ year of age					
Product (Manufacturer)	Aminosyn PF (Hospira)	TrophAmine (B. Braun) Premasol (Baxter)	Aminosyn (Hospira)	Aminosyn II (Hospira)	FreAmine III (B. Braun)	Novamine (Hospira)	Travasol (Baxter)	Prosol (Baxter)
Nitrogen mg per 100 mL of 1% solution	152	155	157	153	153	158	165	161
Amino Acids (Essential) mg per 100 mL of a 1% solution								
Isoleucine	76	82	72	66	69	50	60	54
Leucine	120	140	94	100	91	69	73	54
Lysine	68	82	72	105	73	79	58	68
Methionine	18	34	40	17	53	50	40	38
Phenylalanine	43	48	44	30	56	69	56	50
Threonine	51	42	52	40	40	50	42	49
Tryptophan	18	20	16	20	15	17	18	16
Valine	67	78	80	50	66	64	58	72
Amino Acids (Nonessential) mg per 100 mL of a 1% solution								
Alanine	70	54	128	99	71	145	207	138
Arginine	123	120	98	102	95	98	115	98
Histidine	31	48	30	30	28	60	48	59
Proline	81	68	86	72	112	60	68	67
Serine	50	38	42	53	59	39	50	51
Taurine	7	2.5						
Tyrosine	4	4.4	4.4	27		2.6	4	2.5
Glycine	39	36	128	50	140	69	103	103
Glutamic Acid	62	50		74		50		51
Aspartic Acid	53	32		70		29		30
Cysteine		<1.6			<2.4			
N-ac-L-tyrosine	0	24	0		0	0	0	

Reproduced with permission from Sonneville K, Duggan C: Manual of Pediatric Nutrition, 5th edition, Shelton, CT: PMPH-USA; 2013

conditionally essential amino acid in this population. Amino acid solutions specific to the infant population are designed to maintain the plasma amino acid composition compared to healthy breastfed infants. Because of the added cysteine, it also has a reduced pH, which allows for a greater amount of calcium and phosphorus to be added to the PN solution, avoiding precipitation.[34] The small amount of taurine added to these solutions aids in solubilizing bile salts for adequate biliary secretion and reabsorption from the ileum.[35]

Recent studies examining early PN and amino acid provision in VLBW infants support initiation within hours after birth, with amino acid dosing at 2 to 2.5 grams of protein/kg/day and advancing daily by 1 gram/kg to an upper range of 3 to 4 grams/kg/day. Results demonstrated positive nitrogen retention with no noted increase in metabolic derangements.[36,37] For older children and adolescents, an upper range of 1.5 to 2 grams/kg/d is thought to be adequate. One study examined the relationship of protein and energy intake together and its response to nitrogen balance in PICU patients. Results of this systematic review suggest that administration of >1.5 grams protein/kg/day and >57 kcal/kg/day is associated with achievement of positive protein balance (see **Fig. 7-1**).[30]

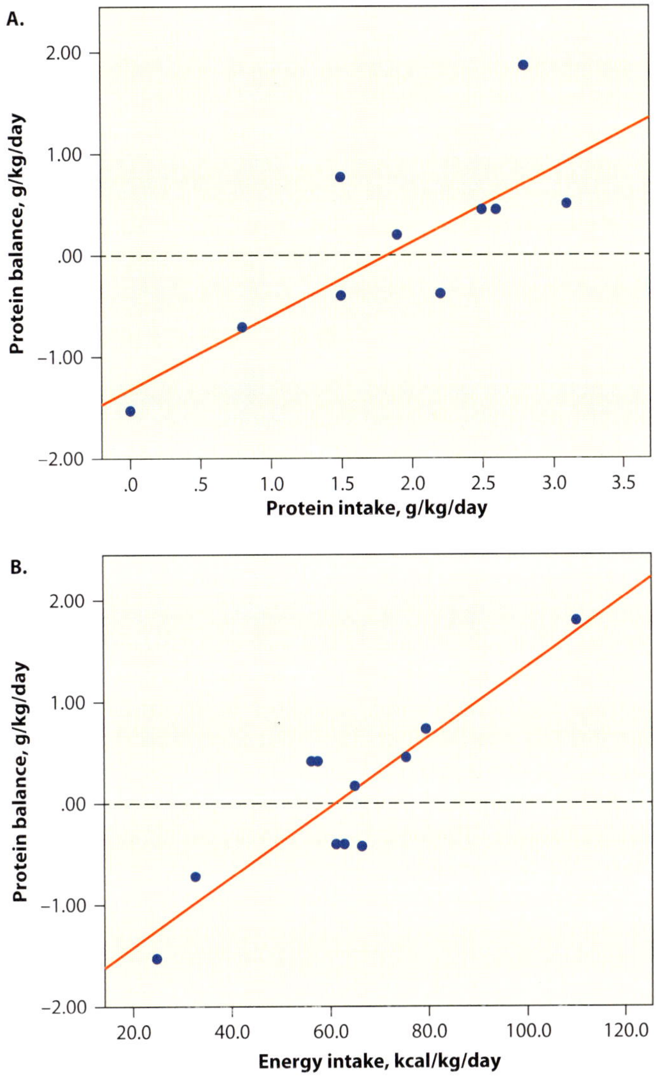

FIGURE 7-1. Protein balance associated with corresponding level of A, protein intake (Spearman r = 0.729; P = .011) and B, energy intake (r = 0.721; P = .012) in critically ill children.

Reproduced with permission from Bechard LJ, Parrott JS, Mehta NM: Systematic Review of Energy and Protein Intake on Protein Balance in Critically Ill Children, J Pediatr 2012;161(2):333-339

Due to the current research supporting the importance of providing adequate protein provision, it is often recommended that protein provided in the PN not be included in the calculation of energy intake to allow for efficient utilization and accretion of lean body mass. This ratio of nonprotein calories to protein is also a way to ensure that the macronutrient distribution provided is balanced. The recommended ratio of nonprotein (kcal) to nitrogen (g) is 150 to 200:1. Critically ill conditions that support increased protein needs, such as burn patients, may benefit from a ratio closer to 100:1.

Despite being aware of minimum protein goals during critical illness, delivering these recommendations is not always achieved, and in some studies, found to be much lower.[38] Current protein recommendations for injured children with the aim to achieve protein balance are based on limited data and consensus, which supports the need for further research.[30,31] In addition, upper intake limits of amino acids provided via long-term PN in children need to be further investigated.

FAT

Similar to protein and CHO, lipid turnover increases during critical illness, with free fatty acids acting as the primary source of energy for patients under inflammatory stress.[39] Adequate delivery of essential fatty acids is crucial during critical illness in order to prevent deficiency. This is usually achieved by providing 30% to 40% of the total calories from fat, which is the recommended upper limit to maintain a mixed fuel system of macronutrients while preventing associated complications. In the critically ill pediatric patient, most nutrition support teams initiate intravenous fat emulsion (IVFE) at 1 gram/kg/day and advance daily by 1 gram/kg to an upper limit of 2 to 3 grams/kg/day, depending on the age of the patient.[32] At our institution, we commonly restrict the IVFE dose to 1 gram/kg/day in infants who are anticipated to be dependent on PN for an extended period due to the perceived link between intravenous fat intake and a the risk of PN-associated liver disease.

Currently in the United States, the IVFE choice is limited to a soy-based 18-carbon omega-6 fatty acid preparation, which studies have demonstrated have proinflammatory characteristics in the ICU population.[40]

Carnitine plays a role in the transport and metabolism of long-chain fatty acids. It is not routinely included in PN solutions, but can be added if deficiency is suspected. In neonates receiving PN, carnitine has been shown to aid in mobilization of hepatic fat stores and prevention of steatosis.[41]

Assessing tolerance to IVFE is done by routine monitoring of serum triglyceride (TG) levels. It is not uncommon during periods of critical illness that IVFE are poorly tolerated, with serum TG levels >300 to 400 mg/dL. Medications can also cause hypertriglyceridemia.[42] Increasing the duration of time that lipid is infused, reducing the lipid dose, or infusing lipids on limited days during the week are examples of strategies that nutrition support teams will trial in attempts to improve serum TG levels. It is important to be aware of essential fatty acid deficiency (EFAD) if a reduced lipid dose is required. To prevent against EFAD, it is recommended that at least 3% to 5% of total calories be provided as fat. In infants, this often equates to 0.5 gram of IVFE/kg/day.[9]

The role of omega-3 fatty acids as an anti-inflammatory agent in critical illness is an area of current research. Studies have demonstrated that fish oil–based fat emulsions are effective in reducing serum bilirubin levels in infants with intestinal failure.[43] Further studies of omega-3 fatty acids in the critically ill population are needed.

MICRONUTRIENTS

Micronutrients include both vitamins and minerals and serve an important role in metabolism and critical illness. Critically ill pediatric patients are at risk of micronutrient deficiencies even at the onset of the injury/illness, due to the redistribution of micronutrients to certain tissues, losses from wounds, or third spacing of fluid, any of which can create an imbalance of micronutrients.[44,45] Micronutrients in critical illness are described in more detail in chapter 4. This section highlights standard micronutrients available in PN solutions, as well as specific vitamins and minerals that are at risk for abnormalities during periods of critical illness.

Minerals or trace elements serve an important role for many functions related to metabolism. The 4 trace elements commonly available in PN solutions include zinc, manganese, chromium, and copper. Iron, molybdenum, and iodine are other trace elements that can be supplemented in the PN solution, depending on patient needs. Copper and manganese should be reduced in the PN if a patient has chronic cholestasis, since they are excreted via the biliary system. Patients with renal dysfunction should avoid standard doses of selenium and chromium.[9]

Pediatric multivitamin solutions contain more vitamin D and K and less of the B vitamins in comparison to adult multivitamin solutions.[9] It is recommended that patients who are not able to receive the standard age-appropriate multivitamin solution at least receive parenteral thiamine to avoid thiamine deficiency.[46] Currently, parenteral multivitamin solutions specifically designed for premature infants do not exist.[47]

Depending on the center, selenium is not always initially included in the PN, but is often added once a patient has remained on PN for an extended period. Depressed selenium levels have been reported in patients who demonstrate systemic inflammatory response syndrome (SIRS). Further research is needed to evaluate the role of selenium supplementation for antioxidant benefits.[48,49]

Zinc acts as a cofactor in multiple metabolic processes, including immune function, with antioxidant properties and wound healing. During critical illness, depressed serum zinc levels have been reported, although evaluating zinc status via serum levels is not always reliable.[50]

Calcium and phosphate needs are greater in infants and children in comparison to adults due to the increased demands for bone growth. It is important to evaluate the dosing being provided via the PN to optimize bone mineralization and attempt to prevent metabolic bone disease when a patient is unable to receive any enteral supplementation.[51,52]

It is important to be aware of certain medications that can alter micronutrient blood concentrations due to side effects such as increased urinary losses while on loop diuretics. Water-soluble vitamins may be excreted at a higher rate during stress or illness, and certain medical conditions may require altered dosing of multivitamin solutions to account for increased losses.[8]

As with most nutrients, if a vitamin or mineral dose is adjusted outside of the standard, it is important to closely follow serum levels to make sure a patient does not become deficient or develops signs of toxicity. Pediatric parenteral vitamin and trace element formulations were designed to meet the rapidly changing nutrient needs of children. However, currently, there exist widespread shortages of vitamins and minerals, making it more challenging to consistently meet their needs. Most recently, the Centers for Disease Control and Prevention (CDC) reported zinc deficiency dermatitis in cholestatic, extremely premature infants following a nationwide shortage of injectable zinc. The infants all had severe cholestasis and had received PN for a prolonged period that included 1 month without any zinc due to shortages. Zinc deficiency was confirmed with serum levels and skin biopsy. Once enteral zinc supplementation was initiated, the infants' serum zinc levels improved, as well as their dermatitis.[53] This case supports the importance of practitioners being aware of the vitamin and mineral solutions available at their institution and the need for routine monitoring of both serum levels and correlation with physical exam findings. When feasible, enteral supplementation should be undertaken.

PARENTERAL NUTRITION COMPLICATIONS

Complications from PN are commonly categorized as being mechanical, infectious, or metabolic. Due to this wide variety of systemic complications, patients receiving PN, both short term and long term, require close monitoring by the nutrition support team. Experienced clinicians who are familiar with what to monitor may prevent complications from becoming severe.

Mechanical complications include catheter occlusions, thrombotic occlusions, cracking of the catheter, or malfunctioning of the intravenous fluid pump. Catheter occlusions are the most common noninfectious complication that can occur in which the clinician is unable to infuse parenteral solutions or aspirate blood without resistance. Thrombotic occlusions are related to vessel wall damage, changes in blood flow, or coagulation changes.[11]

Infectious complications are one of the most common complications associated with venous catheters, specifically catheter-related blood stream infections (CR-BSI). Patients with CR-BSI are at an increased risk of mortality.[54] Strict aseptic precautions during line placement, use of tunneled catheters, appropriate dressing techniques, avoidance of the femoral venous site, hand hygiene, sterilization of the catheter hub, and other infection-control practices at the time of accessing the catheter; use of ethanol locks in home PN-dependent patients; and prompt removal of the catheter when no longer needed or when infection is confirmed are some of the strategies often incorporated as a care bundle to minimize the incidence of CR-BSI. These practices need to be supported by adoption of uniform definitions, diligent monitoring for new cases, prompt and prudent antimicrobial therapy, and a multidisciplinary commitment to preventing CR-BSI in vulnerable patients.

Hyperglycemia is a metabolic complication that can occur frequently in patients receiving PN. As discussed earlier in this chapter, critically ill patients may be at increased risk of developing hyperglycemia due to stress or sepsis that is associated with insulin resistance, increased gluconeogenesis and glycogenolysis, and reduced insulin sensitivity.[55] Other metabolic complications seen with patients receiving PN include hypertriglyceridemia and fluid and electrolyte imbalances. Hyperglycemia and hypertriglyceridemia observed in critically ill children have been correlated with a greater length of time on mechanical ventilatory support, as well as an increased length of stay.[56,57]

In addition to laboratory abnormalities, patients receiving long-term PN can develop organ dysfunction specifically related to the liver. Exposure to high amounts of soybean oil lipid emulsions have been recently implicated as a causative factor, but in the setting of critical illness, other etiologies may apply, including hypoperfusion, sepsis, drug effects, and others.

TRANSITION FROM PARENTERAL NUTRITION TO ENTERAL NUTRITION

An important role of the nutrition support team is to continually assess the readiness of a patient to begin EN, as this is the preferred mode of nutrition support and has many noted benefits, which will be discussed in the following chapter (see chapter 8). Whether a patient is receiving PN, EN, or a combination of both, it is important to be aware of nutrition support goals in order for the patient to fully benefit from the nutrition prescription that includes both macro- and micronutrients. These goals include preserving lean body mass, preventing metabolic complications whenever possible, decreasing disease severity and organ dysfunction, decreasing hospital length of stay, and most importantly, improving a critically ill child's outcome.[39]

This chapter summarized the role of PN support in the critically ill hospitalized patient. Aiming to provide energy prescriptions to this population is a challenge in itself; however, this chapter also emphasizes the importance of macro- and micronutrient support during critical illness in improving patient outcomes and in optimizing their nutritional status. More research is needed in the area of pediatric nutrition support, specifically randomized control trials, in order to develop evidenced-based practices to better guide our recommendations.[58] Until then, a prudent approach, with careful selection of patients eligible for PN support, attention to macronutrient and micronutrient composition, diligent attention to infection control, monitoring for tolerance and complications while on PN, and assessing readiness to transition to EN will allow safe and effective nutrient delivery in critically ill children.

KEY POINTS

- Parenteral nutrition is associated with mechanical, infectious, and metabolic complications.
- Intravenous fat emulsion choice in the ICU population is an area of ongoing investigation. Soy-based lipid emulsion available in the United States is pro-inflammatory in nature.
- Parenteral nutrition must be used judiciously to achieve nutrition delivery goals in patients with altered gastrointestinal tract function.
- The optimal timing of PN in critically ill children needs further investigation.

REFERENCES

1. Joosten KF, Hulst JM. Prevalence of malnutrition in pediatric hospital patients. *Curr Opin Pediatr.* 2008;20: 590-596.
2. Mehta N M, Bechard LJ, Dolan M, et al. Energy imbalance and the risk of overfeeding in critically ill children. *Pediatr Crit Care Med.* 2011;12(4):398-405.
3. Verbruggen S, Sy J, Arrivillaga A. Parenteral amino acid intakes in critically ill children: a matter of convenience. *J Parenter Enteral Nutr.* 2010;34(3):329-340.
4. Mehta NM, McAleer D. Challenges to optimal enteral nutrition in a multidisciplinary pediatric intensive care unit. *J Parenter Enteral Nutr.* 2010;34(1):38-45.
5. Shew SB, Jaksic T. The metabolic needs of critically ill children and neonates. *Semin Pediatr Surg.* 1999;8(3): 131-139.
6. Agus MSD, Jaksic T. Nutritional support of the critically ill child. *Curr Opin Pediatr.* 2002;14:470-481.
7. Blackburn GL, Wollner S, Bistran BR. Nutrition support in the intensive care unit; an evolving science, *Arch Surg.* 2010;145(6)533-538.
8. Herman R, Btaiche I, Teitelbaum DH. Nutrition support in the pediatric surgical patient. *Surg Clin N Am.* 2011;91:511-541.
9. Collier S, Gura KM, et al. Parenteral nutrition. In: *Manual of Pediatric Nutrition*, 5th edition, Sonnevillek, Dugganc, eds, 2013. PMPH-USA: Shelton, CT.
10. Rocadio JM, Doellman DA, Johnson ND. Pediatric peripherally inserted central catheters: complication rates related to catheter tip location. *Pediatrics.* 2001;107.E28.
11. Krzywda EA, Andris DA, Edmistron CE. Parenteral access devices. In: *The A.S.P.E.N. Nutrition Support Core Curriculum*, Mueller CM, Editor-in-chief. 2012; A.S.P.E.N: Silver Spring, MD.
12. Gura KM. Is there still a role for peripheral parenteral nutrition? *Nutr Clin Pract.* 2009;24(6):709-717.
13. Casear MP, Dieter M, Hermans G, et al. Early versus late parenteral nutrition in critically ill adults. *N Engl J Med.* 2011;365:506-517.

14. Doig GS. Parenteral versus enteral nutrition in the critically ill patient: additional sensitivity analysis supports benefit of early parenteral compared to delayed enteral nutrition. *Intensive Care Med.* 2013. In press.

15. Ariagno K, Duggan C. Nutrition assessment in sick or hospitalized children. In: *Manual of Pediatric Nutrition*, 5th edition, Sonnevillek, Dugganc, eds. 2013. PMPH-USA: Shelton, CT.

16. Mehta N M, Bechard LJ, Leavitt K, et al. Cumulative energy imbalance in the pediatric intensive care unit: role of targeted indirect calorimetry. *J Parenter Enteral Nutr.* 2009;33(3):336-344.

17. Skillman H, Wischmeyer P. Nutrition therapy in critically ill infants and children. *J Parenter Enteral Nutr.* 2008;32(5):520-534.

18. Raman S, Peters MJ. Fluid management in the critically ill child, *Pediatr Nephrol.* 2013. In print.

19. Holliday MA, Segar WE. The maintenance need for water in parenteral fluid therapy. *Pediatrics.* 1957;19:823-832.

20. Mirtallo J, Canada T, Johnson D. Task force for the revision of safe practices for parenteral nutrition. Safe practices for parenteral nutrition. *J Parenter Enteral Nutr.* 2004;28:39-70.

21. Whitmire SJ. Nutrition-focused evaluation and management of dysnatremias. *Nutr Clin Practice.* 2008;23:108-121.

22. Sheridan R, Yu YM, Prelack K, et al. Maximal parenteral glucose oxidation in hypermetabolic young children: a stable isotope study. *J Parenter Enteral Nutr.* 1998;22:212-216.

23. Preissig CM, Rigby MR. Pediatric critical illness hyperglycemia: risk factors associated with development and severity of hyperglycemia in critically ill children. *J Ped.* 2009;155:734-739.

24. Branco R G, Garcia P C, Piva JP, et al. Glucose level and risk of mortality in pediatric septic shock. *Pediatr Crit Care Med.* 2005;6(4):470-472.

25. Krinsley JS. Association between hyperglycemia and increased hospital mortality in a heterogeneous population of critically ill patients. *Mayo Clin Proc.* 2003;78(12):1471-1478.

26. Laird AM, Miller PR, Kilgo PD, et al. Relationship of early hyperglycemia to mortality in trauma patients. *J Trauma.* 2004;56(5):1058-1062.

27. Agus MSD, Steil GM, Wypij D. Tight glycemic control versus standard care after pediatric cardiac surgery. *N Engl J Med.* 2012;367:1208-1219.

28. Hulst JM, Joosten KF, Tibboel D, et al. Causes and consequences of inadequate substrate supply to pediatric ICU patients. *Curr Opin Clin Nutr Metab Care.* 2006;9(3):297-303.

29. Mehta N, Jaksic T. The critically ill child. In: *Nutrition in Pediatrics*, Watkinsj, Dugganc, Walker, eds. 2008, B. C. Decker, Inc.: Hamilton, Ontario.

30. Bechard LJ, Parrott JS, Mehta NM. Systematic review of energy and protein intake on protein balance in critically ill children. *J Ped.* 2012;161(2):333-339.

31. Hoffer JL, Bistrian BR. Appropriate protein provision in critical illness: a systematic and narrative review. *Am J Clin Nutr.* 2012;96:591-600.

32. Mehta N, Compher C. A.S.P.E.N clinical guidelines: nutrition support of the critically ill child. *J Parenter Enteral Nutr.* 2009;33(3):260-276.

33. Heyland D, Muscedere J, Wischmeyer PE, et al. A randomized trial of glutamine and antioxidants in critically ill patients. *N Engl J Med.* 2013;368:1489-1497.

34. Fitzgerald KA, MacKay MW. Calcium and phosphate solubility in neonatal parenteral nutrient solutions containing TrophAmine. *Am J Hosp Pharm.* 1986;43:88.

35. Spencer AU, Sunkyung Y, Tracy TF, et al. Parenteral nutrition-associated cholestasis in neonates: multivariate analysis of the potential protective effect of taurine. *J Parenter Enteral Nutr.* 2005;29:337-344.

36. Valentine CJ, Fernandez S, et al. Early amino-acid administration improves preterm infant weight. *J Perinatology.* 2009;29:428-432.

37. Ibrahim HM, Jeroudi MA, Baier RJ, et al. Aggressive early total parenteral nutrition in low birth weight infants. *Perinatol.* 2004;24:482-486.

38. Mehta NM, Bechard LJ, Cahill N, et al. Nutritional practices and their relationship to clinical outcomes in critically ill children–an international multicenter cohort study. *Crit Care Med.* 2012;40(7):2204-2210.

39. Jaksic T. Effective and efficient nutritional support for the injured child. *Surg Clin N Am.* 2002;82:379-391.

40. McClave SA, Martindale RG, et al. Guidelines for the provision and assessment of nutrition support therapy in the adult critically ill patient: Society of Critical Care Medicine (SCCM) and American Society for Parenteral and Enteral Nutrition (A.S.P.E.N). *J Parenter Enteral Nutr.* 2009;33(3):277-316.

41. Btaiche IF, Khalidi N. Parenteral nutrition-associated liver complications in children. *Pharmacotherapy.* 2002;22:188-211.

42. Colomb V, Jobert-Giraud A, Lacaille F, et al. Role of lipid emulsion in cholestasis associated with long-term parenteral nutrition in children. *J Parenter Enteral Nutr.* 2000;24:345-350.

43. Gura KM, Lee S, Valim C, et al. Safety and efficacy of a fish-oil-based fat emulsion in the treatment of parenteral

nutrition associated liver disease. *Pediatrics*. 2008;121: 678-686.

44. Galloway P, McMillan DC, Sattar N. Effect of the inflammatory response on trace element and vitamin status. *Ann Clin Biochem*. 2000;37(Pt 3):289-297.
45. Maehira F, Luyo GA, Miyagi I, et al. Alterations of serum selenium concentrations in the acute phase of pathological conditions. *Clin Chim Acta*. 2002;316(1-2):137-146.
46. Green H, Hambridge KM, Schanler R., et al. Guidelines for the use of vitamins, trace elements, calcium, magnesium, and phosphorus in infants and children receiving total parenteral nutrition. Report of the subcommittee on Clinical Practice Issues of the American Society for Clinical Nutrition. *Am J Clin Nutr*. 1988;48:1324-1342.
47. Hurwitz M, Garcia MG, Poole RL, et al. Copper deficiency during parenteral nutrition: a report of four pediatric cases. *Nutr Clin Pract*. 2004;19:305-308.
48. Cherry-Bukowiec JR. Optimizing nutrition therapy to enhance mobility in critically ill patients. *Crit Care Nurs Q*. 2013;36(1):28-36.
49. Hardy G, Hardy I, Manzanares W. Selenium supplementation in the critically ill. *Nutr Clin Pract*. 2012;27(1):21-33.
50. Heyland DK, Jones N, Cvijanovich NZ. Zinc supplementation in critically ill patients: a key pharmaconutrient? *J Parenter Enteral Nutr*. 2008;32(5):509-519.
51. Karlen J, Aperia A, Zetterstorm R. Renal excretion of calcium and phosphate in preterm and term infants. *J Pediatr*. 1985;106:814-819.
52. Prestridge LL, Schanler RJ, Shulman R, et al. Effect of parenteral calcium and phosphorus on mineral retention and bone mineral content in very low birth weight infants. *J Pediatr*. 1993;122:761-768.
53. Control and Prevention (CDC). Notes from the field: Zinc deficiency dermatitis in cholestatic extremely premature infants after a nationwide shortage of injectable zinc. Washington, DC, December 2012. *Centers for Disease MMWR Morb Mortal Wkly Rep*. 2013;62(7):136-137.
54. Safdar N, Fine JP, Maki DG. Meta-analysis: methods for diagnosing intravascular device-related bloodstream infection. *Ann Intern Med*. 2005;142(6):451-466.
55. Lewis KS, Kane-Gill SL, Bobek MB, et al. Intensive insulin therapy for critically ill patients. *Ann Pharmacother*. 2004;38:1243-1251.
56. Alaedeen DI, Walsh MC, Chwals WJ. Total parenteral nutrition associated hyperglycemia correlates with prolonged mechanical ventilation and hospital stay in septic infants. *J Pediatr Surg*. 2006;41:239-244.
57. Hulst JM, van Goudoever JB, Zimmermann LJ. The role of initial monitoring of routine biochemical nutritional markers in critically ill children. *J Nutr Biochem*. 2006;17:57-62.
58. Joffe A, Anton N, Lequier L, et al. Nutritional support for critically ill children (Review). *Cochrane Database of Syst Rev*, 2009.

CHAPTER 8

Enteral Nutrition in the Critically ill Child

Heather E. Skillman

- INTRODUCTION
- EARLY ENTERAL NUTRITION
  - Benefits of Early Enteral Nutrition
  - Risks of Early Enteral Nutrition
- ENTERAL NUTRITION ROUTE
  - Gastric versus Postpyloric Feeding
  - Advantages and Disadvantages of Gastric Feeding
  - Advantages and Disadvantages of Postpyloric Feeding
- POSTPYLORIC FEEDING TUBE PLACEMENT
  - Blind Feeding Tube Placement
  - Fluoroscopic Feeding Tube Placement
  - Electromagnetic Feeding Tube Placement
- ENTERAL NUTRITION FORMULA SELECTION
  - Infant and Pediatric Enteral Formulas
  - High-Calorie and/or High-Protein Enteral Formulas
  - High-Carbohydrate Enteral Formulas
- EVALUATION AND MAINTENANCE OF ENTERAL NUTRITION
  - Enteral Nutrition Tolerance
  - Barriers to Optimal Enteral Nutrition
  - Strategies to Optimize Enteral Nutrition
- SUMMARY OF ENTERAL NUTRITION BEST PRACTICES
- KEY POINTS
  - References

INTRODUCTION

Enteral nutrition (EN) is the preferred method of nutrition support in critically ill children, as parenteral nutrition (PN) is associated with increased costs, infections, and other complications.[1] Enteral feeding is tolerated by most pediatric intensive care unit (PICU) patients and can effectively meet energy and protein goals. The time from admission to initiation, route, composition, and cumulative intake of EN have the potential to positively influence the course of critical illness. Multiple obstacles to enteral feeding are common to the PICU environment; these must be anticipated and minimized to achieve improved outcomes with EN therapy.

EARLY ENTERAL NUTRITION

Although there is enthusiasm for EN, the optimal timing for introducing enteral feeds in a critically ill child remains unclear. In an effort to maximize the benefits of EN and to achieve nutrient delivery goals, the concept of early EN is gaining traction. The benefits of this approach need to be balanced against the potential of EN intolerance in the early phase of illness or injury.

Benefits of Early Enteral Nutrition

Few randomized controlled studies have evaluated the effects of early versus delayed EN in pediatric critical illness, and those conducted in children with burn injuries have demonstrated multiple benefits. In a large study, 688 children with a mean of 20% total body surface area (TBSA) burns were randomized to early (fed within 6 hours) or delayed (no sooner than 48 hours from injury) EN.[2] Length of hospital stay (12.6 ± 1.3 days vs. 16.4 ± 3.7 days, $P < .05$) and mortality (8.5% vs. 12%, $P < .05$) were significantly lower in the group that received early EN.

In another study, 21 children with a median of 30% TBSA burns were randomized either to early enteral resuscitation and early EN or intravenous resuscitation with late EN.[3] All children were fed via nasojejunal tubes (NJT) placed under fluoroscopy or at the bedside. Enteral nutrition was initiated by a median of 10.7 hours and reached the target in 16 hours in the early group. In children randomized to late EN, feeding commenced at a median of 54 hours, with the goal rate achieved in the next 10 hours. Significantly higher serum insulin and lower growth hormone levels were demonstrated in the early compared to delayed group, suggesting an improved anabolic response with early enteral resuscitation and feeding. Recipients of early EN were reported to have decreased incidence of weight loss (3% vs. 7.75%), antibiotic treatment (11 days vs. 14 days), and diarrhea. In a similar study, 77 critically ill children with severe burns of approximately 50% TBSA were randomized to EN via postpyloric feeding tube within 24 hours or delayed after 48 hours.[4] Significantly reduced caloric deficits and protein breakdown were demonstrated in the early EN group. Serum insulin was also significantly higher in children receiving early EN. The definition of early EN in these studies was varied in terms of time to initiate EN, time required to reach goal, and the definition of daily goal. Nevertheless, these studies demonstrate that early EN can be safely delivered in children with burn injury, and may be associated with attenuation of the stress response. In a recent retrospective study of 5,105 critically ill children from 12 PICUs in North America, early EN was achieved with approximately a quarter of the cohort, with lower odds of mortality (odds ratio, 0.51; 95% confidence interval, 0.34-0.76; P = .001) compared to those who did not receive early EN.[5]

Risks of Early Enteral Nutrition

Although early compared to delayed EN can improve the postinjury anabolic response and reduce hospital stay and mortality, the potential risks and benefits must be carefully balanced (see Table 8-1). Increased incidence of bowel necrosis and mortality were reported in children with burn injury randomized to early EN.[4] Patients with bowel infarction had a mean 71% TBSA burns, and 4 (80%) also had inhalation injury. All children with bowel necrosis had preceding fever, tachycardia, hypotension requiring vasopressor support, leukocytosis, and increased abdominal pressure. Critically ill children with shock are at risk for gastrointestinal (GI) intolerance with early EN, which is likely associated with decreased gastric and intestinal perfusion and motility. To evaluate cytokines in septic shock, 38 children received an immune-enhanced or standard formula via nasogastric tube (NGT) within 12 hours of admission.[6] Enteral nutrition was gradually advanced to meet estimated caloric requirements in 4 days. Eight patients (21%) were excluded from the study for feeding intolerance, although the symptoms were not further described. Of the 30 children included, 16% receiving the immune-enhanced formula and 7% on standard formula experienced transient diarrhea. In a prospective investigation

TABLE 8-1. Benefits and Risks with Early Enteral Nutrition

Potential Benefits	Potential Risks
Improved gastrointestinal tolerance	Gastrointestinal intolerance
Decreased small-bowel permeability	Abnormal small-bowel permeability
Increased serum insulin	Bowel necrosis, necrotizing enterocolitis
Reduced protein breakdown	
Positive nitrogen balance	Bowel perforation
Reduced caloric deficits	
Improved weight retention	
Decreased length of hospital stay	
Reduced mortality	

of critically ill children who received postpyloric feeding, 44/65 (67.7%) of those with shock and 284/461 (61.6%) of patients without shock received EN within 48 hours.[7] Gastrointestinal complications were significantly higher in children admitted with shock. Abdominal distention (15.4% vs. 5%, $P = .004$), diarrhea (20% vs. 4.6%, $P = .0001$), necrotizing enterocolitis (1.5% vs. 0.4%, $P = .432$), and other complications were more prevalent in the children with shock versus other diagnoses. One death was related to duodenal perforation during feeding tube placement in a child with shock. In another retrospective study of 55 critically ill children receiving EN concomitant with cardiovascular medications, 16 (29.1%) experienced vomiting, abdominal distention, diarrhea, and constipation.[8] Significant GI bleeding occurred in 2 patients (3.6%), but was believed to be secondary to underlying disease.

These studies emphasize the importance of balancing the risks and benefits of early EN. Careful selection of patients with a low risk of serious GI complications and close monitoring for tolerance, especially in infants and children with vasopressor requirement or shock, will allow safe administration of early EN in the PICU.

ENTERAL NUTRITION ROUTE

Once the amount and timing for initiating EN are confirmed, the most appropriate route or site for delivering the nutrients needs to be determined. While feeding into the stomach is most physiologic, the risk of aspiration of gastric contents in the setting of altered GI motility has prompted the consideration for feeding into the small bowel.

Gastric versus Postpyloric Feeding

The selection of gastric or postpyloric feeding has the potential to affect timing of initiation, feeding tolerance, daily intake, and outcomes in pediatric critical illness (see Table 8-2). To compare the incidence of aspiration, 44 mechanically ventilated critically ill children were prospectively randomized to NGT or NJT feeding.[9] Two patients unable to achieve NJT placement within 24 hours of randomization were moved to the NGT group, resulting in 17 assigned to NJT feeding and 27 NGT. Endotracheal tube aspirates were analyzed every 8 hours for the presence of glucose, and spectrophotometry was used to detect methylene blue added to color the enteral formula. No patient developed aspiration pneumonia or had tracheal secretions positive for glucose. A significant delay (median 24 hours vs. 6 hours, $P = .0002$) in initiating EN and an increase in radiographs for feeding tube placement (median 4 vs. 1, $P = .0001$) occurred in the NJT compared to the NGT group. Authors of this study concluded that selection of the NGT versus NJT feeding route can result in faster initiation of EN without an increased risk of aspiration.

In another evaluation of critically ill children randomized to gastric or small-bowel feeding, aspiration was defined by the presence of pepsin in endotracheal tube aspirates.[10] Twelve of the 42 randomized to the small-bowel group were excluded from the study due to unsuccessful bedside feeding tube placement, and 32 were assigned to NGT feeding. Several children required feeding tube replacement during the study; 5 in the small-bowel group could not be repositioned beyond the stomach. These children received NGT feeding for the remainder of the

TABLE 8-2. Gastric versus Postpyloric Feeding

	Advantages	Disadvantages
Gastric Feeding	Faster initiation Easy tube placement Meets requirements Well tolerated Physiologic More options for administration	Risk of aspiration of gastric contents, especially in patients with history of delayed emptying, severe reflux, or unprotected airway
Postpyloric Feeding	Improved intake Shorter time to goal Reduced fasting Decreased PN use and cost Well tolerated May decrease pneumonia	Delayed initiation Increased radiographs May not prevent aspiration

study, but following an intent-to-treat design, were included for analysis in the small-bowel group. Pepsin was identified in 59% of tracheal aspirates in the NGT group and 67% of the small-bowel group ($P = 0.8$). No differences in time to initiate EN, abdominal distention, vomiting, diarrhea, number of feeding interruptions, duration of mechanical ventilation, length of stay, or mortality were demonstrated between feeding routes. Children randomized to small-bowel feeding received a higher proportion of the caloric goal versus those in the NGT group (47 ± 23% vs. 30 ± 23%, $P = .01$), possibly due to shorter feeding interruptions.

Neither of these 2 studies revealed a significant difference in aspiration risk between the 2 feeding strategies; however, the methods of detection and the incidence of tracheal aspiration varied. While 1 study showed earlier initiation of EN and fewer x-rays in the gastric group,[9] the other demonstrated increased caloric intake with small-bowel feeding.[10] When these 2 pediatric studies were combined with 13 adult trials in a meta-analysis including 966 critically ill patients, those randomized to postpyloric versus gastric feeding demonstrated a significant reduction in the incidence of pneumonia (risk reduction 0.63, 95% confidence interval 0.48-0.83, $P = .001$).[11] No difference in vomiting or aspiration was seen between groups. Differences in institutional practices may influence success with placement of enteral access[1] and the duration of fasting prior to procedures according to the route of feeding. Larger randomized trials are required to determine whether postpyloric versus gastric EN reduces the incidence of pneumonia in critically ill infants and children. Until then, individual centers must base their practice on resources available to place and maintain postpyloric tubes. Ultimately, the success of this strategy will be dependent on careful selection of patients that are most likely to benefit from postpyloric feeding.

Advantages and Disadvantages of Gastric Feeding

Compared to the postpyloric route, gastric feeding is more physiologic and easier to implement. The stomach provides a larger reservoir than does the small intestine, which helps regulate GI osmotic load and transit. The simplicity and lack of specialized procedures required for NGT placement may promote early initiation of EN.[9,12] Prospective investigations have demonstrated early gastric feeding is well tolerated and meets predicted energy requirements in acutely ill and injured children.[13,14] A majority (67/71, 94.4%) of critically ill children with sepsis, traumatic brain injury, respiratory failure, and burns received early EN via NGT and met 150% of predicted basal metabolic rate by the fifth day.[13] Furthermore, EN implemented via NGT within hours of admission met the energy target by an average of 18.5 ± 15.2 hours in 92 critically ill pediatric patients.[12] Early EN per NGT was also achieved in 30/38 children admitted with septic shock.[6] The gastric feeding route appears to offer many potential benefits for the majority of critically ill children, including the ease of early implementation and the ability to achieve energy and protein targets. However, those with delayed gastric emptying, severe gastroesophageal reflux, intractable vomiting, an unprotected airway, and others at high risk for aspiration may be inappropriate candidates for gastric feeding.

Advantages and Disadvantages of Postpyloric Feeding

In critically ill children unable to receive adequate EN via the gastric route, postpyloric feeding can successfully meet caloric goals, avoid use of PN, and reduce associated costs.[14,15] In a 12-month retrospective review, 110 patients received EN via postpyloric tubes placed at bedside, of whom 42 were too unstable to transport for fluoroscopic feeding tube placement.[14] All required mechanical ventilation, and most were on at least 1 vasoactive medication, and 50% were on neuromuscular blockade. A majority (31/42, 74%) achieved the estimated caloric goal within 24 hours from the initiation of feeding, and the remainder (11/42, 26%) within 48 hours. Postpyloric EN was reported to be well tolerated without incidence of reflux, aspiration, or necrotizing enterocolitis. With the charges for PN approximately 10 times that of EN, the cost savings from 42 patients utilizing EN instead of PN for a total of 256 days was considered clinically significant.

During the second year of a 4-year retrospective study, postpyloric EN was implemented to replace PN in PICU patients with intolerance or contraindication to gastric feeding.[15] Of 1,636 children admitted, 240 (14.6%) received PN or EN. Over the course of the study, exclusive PN use declined from 16% to 5.5%, $P = .01$, while utilization of postpyloric EN as the sole means of nutrition support increased from 3.2% to 10.5%, $P < .05$. Although there were no significant outcome differences between those who received exclusive EN versus PN, the total estimated costs for nutrition therapy per patient were reduced by approximately 55%.

Critically ill children fed via the postpyloric route may experience abbreviated periods of fasting for procedures and subsequently an improved caloric intake.[10,16] Fifty-nine

PICU patients receiving postpyloric EN and mechanical ventilation were randomized to continuous or interrupted feeding in which feeds were held 4 hours prior to and after tracheal extubation.[17] Adverse events, including abdominal distention, emesis, and diarrhea, were not different between the continuous and interrupted groups (4/29, 13.4% vs. 3/30, 10%), and aspiration did not occur. The percent of caloric goal achieved was significantly higher on the day prior to ($92 \pm 2.5\%$ vs. $76 \pm 4.2\%$, $P < .004$) and the day of tracheal extubation ($93 \pm 3.2\%$ vs. $43 \pm 4.3\%$, $P < .001$) in the continuous versus the interrupted feeding groups. Postpyloric EN may also reduce the time to achieve the energy target in some patients. In a multicenter trial of 102 infants and children with acute lung injury randomized to supine or prone positioning, those fed via NJT reached the caloric goal in a median of 4 days versus 7 days with NGT feeding, $P = .03$.[18]

While studies report that the majority of critically ill children tolerate postpyloric EN and achieve the energy goal within 48 hours of initiation,[3,4,14] this feeding route confers potential disadvantages. Delays in EN initiation, higher exposure to abdominal radiographs, and feeding interruptions have been demonstrated with postpyloric compared to gastric EN.[9,18] Additional research is needed to evaluate postpyloric feeding in critically ill children. Until more evidence is available, the American Society for Parenteral and Enteral Nutrition recommends consideration of postpyloric EN for critically ill children at high risk of aspiration, or for those intolerant to gastric feeding.[1]

POSTPYLORIC FEEDING TUBE PLACEMENT

A variety of techniques to facilitate bedside postpyloric feeding tube placement in children have been studied. Important considerations when evaluating methods of feeding tube placement include safety, risk of adverse events, efficacy, and resources required, such as time, expertise, technology, and cost.

Blind Feeding Tube Placement

Some critically ill children who are appropriate candidates for postpyloric feeding are too unstable to transport for feeding tube placement under fluoroscopy. In these patients, bedside insertion of a feeding tube into the small bowel may be the only option to achieve optimal EN.[14] Blind placement of postpyloric feeding tubes necessitates the least technology compared to other techniques, but may require more expertise and increase the risk of complications. A case series described feeding tube misplacement in the respiratory tract in 5 PICU patients; 2 were unharmed, 1 developed a pneumothorax requiring a chest tube and mechanical ventilation, and 2 died.[19] Early recognition of tube misplacement can be achieved by mandatory abdominal radiography prior to the usage of blindly placed NJTs.

The combination of metoclopramide administration, body positioning, and air insufflation led to small-bowel feeding tube placement in 84/90 (93%) of critically ill children by a mean of 15 minutes,[20] and in 63/71 (89%) in an average of 7 minutes.[21] In 2 randomized controlled trials of critically ill children, postpyloric feeding tube placement was significantly more successful with air insufflation in 33/38 (87%) of patients versus 18/40 (45%) without air insufflation.[22] Critically ill children were randomized to bedside small-bowel feeding tube placement using positioning with addition of air insufflation or erythromycin; all methods were equally effective, with success in 71/75 (95%) by the second attempt.[23] No major complications were related to feeding tube placement in any of the patients. Potential concerns regarding neurologic and cardiac side effects of prokinetics and gastric perforation from air insufflation may limit use of these adjuncts in some patients. Skilled providers have demonstrated a high achievement rate of successfully placing postpyloric feeding tubes without prokinetics or air insufflation.[23] In addition, a training and audit process can improve successful bedside NJT placement in pediatric patients.[24]

Fluoroscopic Feeding Tube Placement

Methods of bedside postpyloric tube insertion that can improve safety and accuracy are desired. Fluoroscopic feeding tube placement is highly accurate and can help prevent malposition, but radiation exposure is a concern, and it is not widely available for use at the bedside. After implementation of a training session, the mean time for postpyloric tube placement in pediatric burn patients using bedside fluoroscopy was reduced from 4.1 minutes to 2.3 minutes, $P < .0001$.[25]

Electromagnetic Feeding Tube Placement

Electromagnetic technology is similar to fluoroscopy, with use of three-dimensional, real-time imaging. Bedside small-bowel feeding tube placement was achieved in 41/50 (82%) of critically ill children randomized to an electromagnetic device, versus 22/57 (38%) assigned to standard institutional protocol of blind insertion using a tube without a stylette, $P < .0001$.[26] Median placement time was shorter (1.7 hours vs. 21 hours, $P < .0001$) and fewer mean abdominal radiographs were required ($1.3 \pm .06$ vs. 2.4 ± 1.4, $P < .0001$) with the electromagnetic device compared to the standard group, and no complications occurred during the investigation. In another randomized trial in critically ill children, the electromagnetic device was equally successful as the standard method of positioning, air insufflation, and metoclopramide for postpyloric tube placement (22/22, 100% vs. 24/26, 92%, $P = .49$).[27] Although feeding tubes were rapidly placed by skilled practitioners, more time was required with use of the electromagnetic technology versus standard method (median 9.5 minutes vs. 5 minutes, $P = .03$).

A multicenter prospective study was conducted to compare confirmation of bedside feeding tube placement by interpretation of electromagnetic device or by an abdominal radiograph.[28] Of 194 enrolled, 18 (9%) were children, with methods of feeding tube confirmation in agreement for all except 1 adult patient. A majority of tubes were successfully placed in the small bowel (191/194, 98%; 100% of children), with airway malposition prevented in 15/194 (8%), including 4/18 (22%) children. Feeding tube placement required a median of 12 minutes for the entire study group, and 20 minutes per child. To attain the benefits of EN therapy, feeding tube placement is usually necessary; therefore, the risks must be minimized. Electromagnetic technology appears to be accurate and may help prevent feeding tube malposition. In centers where specialized equipment is not available, a training program can improve successful feeding tube placement at the bedside. An abdominal radiograph is recommended following blind feeding tube insertion in children, as all other confirmation methods have been shown to be inaccurate.[29]

ENTERAL NUTRITION FORMULA SELECTION

Enteral formulas are available for specific age groups, and with specific nutrient content.

Infant and Pediatric Enteral Formulas

An increasing number of EN formulas are available for infants and children with a variety of conditions, but none have been specifically manufactured for critical illness or wound healing.[30] A majority of the formulas are based on cow milk protein and contain casein and/or whey, but some include soy protein, amino acids, or food ingredients (see Table 8-3). Compared to those with casein as the predominant protein source, whey-based formulas accelerate gastric emptying in infants with gastroesophageal reflux and in children with cerebral palsy.[31,32] Whey protein provides cysteine to synthesize glutathione, provides branched-chain amino acids to aid tissue repair, and may positively impact GI motility and absorption during critical illness.[33] These potential benefits of whey protein have not been studied in critically ill children. Some polymeric or intact protein pediatric formulas are available with whey as the predominant protein source, while semielemental formulas are manufactured with hydrolyzed whey and/or casein. In an observational study, variables significantly associated with the initial choice of a peptide-based formula in the PICU included malnutrition, use of vasoactive medications, and prior fasting >2 days.[34] Research is needed to determine if the increased costs of hydrolyzed formulas can be offset with improved nutrition and clinical outcomes.

High-Calorie and/or High-Protein Enteral Formulas

Modified enteral formulas may be required to meet increased protein requirements of critically ill infants and children.[35] Standard-term infant formulas can be reconstituted with less water to yield a proportionately higher concentration of energy, macronutrients, vitamins, minerals, and electrolytes. This method fails to supply the suggested 2 to 3 g/kg/d protein[1] to the acutely ill or injured infant unless intake provides ~100 to 140 kcal/kg/d. In a systematic review of 6 studies including 239 mechanically ventilated children, intake >1.5 g/kg/d protein and >57 kcal/kg/d was required to achieve positive protein balance.[36] Severe catabolism induced by burn injury or extracorporeal membrane oxygenation may necessitate higher protein intakes approaching 3 to 4 g/kg/d.[1,37] To achieve the increased protein requirements of critically ill pediatric patients, enteral protein supplements or higher-protein formulas are needed.

In some countries, a high-protein and high-energy formula is available for infants up to 18 months with growth faltering, increased nutrient requirements, or fluid restriction. In a randomized, controlled, double-blind design, 20 critically ill infants with respiratory syncytial virus requiring mechanical ventilation were assigned to high protein-energy (100 kcal, 2.6 g protein per 100 mL) or standard infant formula (67 kcal, 1.4 g protein

TABLE 8-3. Enteral Nutrition Formulas

Category	Types
Infant Formula	
• Most contain docosahexaenoic and arachidonic acids	Cow milk protein
• Some available with nucleotides, prebiotics, probiotics	Hydrolyzed casein and/or whey
	Soy protein
	Amino acids
	Lactose free
	Added rice starch
	Added fiber
	Carbohydrate free/reduced
	High medium-chain triglycerides
	High protein energy
	Reduced electrolytes and minerals
	For preterm infants
	For inborn errors of metabolism
Pediatric Formula	
• Most are lactose free, gluten free	Cow milk protein
• Some available with fiber, prebiotics, docosahexaenoic acid	Hydrolyzed casein and/or whey
	Soy protein
	Amino acids
	Food ingredients
	High calorie
	Reduced calorie
	Low fat
	High medium-chain triglycerides
	High fat, low carbohydrate (ketogenic)
	For inborn errors of metabolism

per 100 mL).[38] Enteral nutrition was started within 24 hours from admission and reached the target within 36 hours of initiation. Formulas were well tolerated without vomiting, diarrhea, or abdominal distention. As per the protocol, the intervention group demonstrated increased energy (112 ± 13 kcal/kg/d vs. 82 ± 4 kcal/kg/d) and protein intake (2.8 ± 0.3 g/kg/d vs. 1.5 ± 0.1 g/kg/d) on day 5 compared to the standard cohort. Nitrogen balance was significantly higher on study days 2 through 5 in the high protein-energy group. Mean resting energy expenditure measured by indirect calorimetry was similar (54 ± 3 kcal/kg/d vs. 50 ± 3 kcal/kg/d) during the 5-day investigation, but respiratory quotient (0.96 ± 0.02 vs. 0.91 ± 0.01, $P < .01$) was increased in the high protein-energy versus standard group on day 5. The durations of mechanical ventilation and PICU stay were not statistically different between groups. Using stable phenylalanine and tyrosine isotope tracers, whole-body protein synthesis and balance were significantly increased, despite higher breakdown, indicating positive anabolic function in the high protein-energy versus standard group.[39] High-energy density feeding improves caloric and protein balance in critically ill infants and appears to be well tolerated.

To meet increased protein requirements during critical illness or following severe traumatic injury, enteral protein supplements are often administered. To evaluate the safety and efficacy of this practice, 51 critically ill infants and children were randomized to receive standard feeding with or without a cow milk protein supplement.[40] Infants up to 12 months received human milk (70 kcal, 1.1 g protein per 100 mL) or infant formula (70 kcal, 1.6 g protein per 100 mL), while those >12 months received a standard pediatric formula (122 kcal, 2.6 g protein per 100 mL). The intervention group received 1.1 g of the protein supplement added to every 100 mL human milk or formula. Patients in both groups were a median 7 months of age, and 85% were postoperative from cardiac surgery. Enteral nutrition was initiated via NGT or postpyloric tube within 24 to 36 hours from admission and reached goal within the next 24 hours. From days 1 to 5, the range of median energy expenditure (46 to 52 kcal/kg vs. 44 to 53 kcal/kg) and caloric intake (65 to 77 kcal/kg vs. 62 to 68 kcal/kg) were similar, while protein intake was higher according to design (2.6 to 3.1 g/kg/d vs. 1.5 to 1.7 g/kg/d) between the protein-enriched and standard groups. Nitrogen balance became positive on day 5 only in the protein-enriched group. None of the patients developed feeding intolerance or abnormal biochemical parameters. Enteral protein supplementation is an important adjunct to optimize protein intake and achieve positive nitrogen balance in critically ill infants and children.

High-protein and high-energy feeding is also beneficial during recovery from critical illness, injury, or surgery. Infants with acute perinatal brain injury randomized to 120% versus 100% of usual energy and protein intake demonstrated improved weight, length, head circumference, and brain growth.[41] After surgery for congenital heart disease and transfer to the ward, 46 infants were randomized to rapid advancement to high-energy and high-protein formula (from 80 kcal/100 mL to 100 kcal/100 mL in 3 days) or usual care (from 67 kcal/100 mL to 90 kcal/100 mL in 6 days).[42] Energy intake 3 days prior to hospital discharge reached a higher percentage of estimated requirements (98% vs. 78%, $P = .01$) and weight gain improved in the rapid advancement versus usual care groups. One patient had emesis, likely related to the high-energy and high-protein formula.

High-Carbohydrate Enteral Formulas

A high-carbohydrate (CHO) diet may promote anabolism in children with severe burn injuries by stimulating endogenous insulin production. Fourteen children with a mean of 65% TBSA burns were randomized to a high CHO or high-fat formula for 1 week and crossed over to the other diet for 1 week.[43] Protein kinetics using cross-leg stable isotope infusions demonstrated no change in protein synthesis, but a significant reduction in protein breakdown with the high-CHO diet. In all patients, net protein balance significantly improved and plasma insulin levels were higher during the high-CHO diet.

In a retrospective cohort study, children with severe burns >40% TBSA were divided into groups according to type of diet.[44] A total of 944 children were evaluated; from 1985 to 1995, a high-fat diet was given to 426 patients, and from 1996 to 2004, 518 received a high-CHO formula. Demographics were not different between groups; however, the incidence of sepsis and length of ICU stay were significantly reduced in children who received the high-CHO diet. Autopsy results of 135 patients demonstrated significantly less hepatic steatosis in those fed the high-CHO formula. Although advancements in burn and ICU care were achieved during the period studied, the type of feeding also likely contributed to the observed outcomes.

Enteral formulas with arginine, glutamine, omega-3 fatty acids, and/or other ingredients designed to modulate immune function are reviewed in chapter 19.

EVALUATION AND MAINTENANCE OF ENTERAL NUTRITION

Despite early initiation of EN, a number of barriers impede ongoing EN delivery in the PICU. A multidisciplinary commitment to maintaining EN during critical illness is necessary.

Enteral Nutrition Tolerance

Effective management of feeding tolerance is essential to maximize the benefits of EN. Use of objective parameters or technology to assess GI function, perfusion, motility, absorption, and aspiration in critically ill children are highly desirable, but may not be readily available at the bedside. Feeding intolerance is not associated with severity of illness; therefore, regular monitoring of GI function is necessary for all patients receiving EN.[45] A variety of signs and symptoms are used as surrogate markers for EN intolerance in critically ill children, and there is lack of uniformity in defining intolerance.

Measurement of abdominal girth is a simple assessment tool to detect abdominal distention in children. Increased abdominal girth may be alleviated with treatment of constipation, venting air from the GI tract, or smaller volume, more concentrated feedings.[46] Severe abdominal distention can lead to altered GI motility and perfusion and impaired respiratory mechanics, requiring temporary cessation of EN.[47]

Opioid-related constipation is prevalent in critically ill children, but can be reduced with a step-wise approach using stool softeners, prokinetics, laxatives, and enemas.[11] Enteral naloxone effectively increased stool output compared to a randomly sampled matched control group, but caused opiate withdrawal in 2 out of 23 patients.[48] Diarrhea, more than 4 to 6 loose stools per 24 hours, is associated with altered GI flora or transit due to antibiotics, sorbitol-containing medications, opioid withdrawal, and underlying illness; less frequently, malabsorption, *Clostridium difficile*, or the type of formula.[49-51] Efforts should be taken to address the etiology of diarrhea and avoid cessation of EN while monitoring fluid and electrolyte status. If all other factors have been ruled out, a change to an isotonic, semielemental formula or the addition of soluble fiber may be considered.[51] Probiotics are not recommended for critically ill children due to inadequate safety and efficacy data.[52,53]

Vomiting may require short-term interruption of EN, but can be ameliorated with head of bed elevation, a change to postpyloric feeding, medications to reduce gastric acid and nausea, and decreasing the infusion rate. In 46 critically ill children randomly assigned to continuous or intermittent feeding every 2 hours via the gastric route, there was no difference in vomiting or diarrhea between groups.[54] In a secondary analysis of these patients, the proportion of patients with gastric residual volume >5 mL/kg was similar with continuous and intermittent feeding.[55] Gastric residuals are a poor predictor of vomiting and aspiration in adults,[56] and no uniform threshold has been identified for critically ill children. In addition, no safe and accurate bedside tool to detect aspiration is available.[57] Until more research clarifies the markers and predictors of EN intolerance in the PICU population, safe EN delivery requires careful monitoring of abdominal girth, stool pattern, clinical signs of perfusion and oxygenation, and symptoms of overt intolerance such as vomiting and aspiration. Appropriate patient selection, uniform definitions and approach to intolerance, and multidisciplinary commitment are key factors that will ensure safe and effective EN in critically ill children.

Barriers to Optimal Enteral Nutrition

Achieving and maintaining optimal EN requires that feeding interruptions are consistently minimized and prevented. Cessation of EN is appropriate in many circumstances, such as prior to endotracheal intubation, extubation, or general anesthesia, and in cases of pneumatosis intestinalis, hemodynamic instability, significant GI bleeding, vomiting, and aspiration. Use of arbitrary gastric residual volume cutoffs without other significant findings results in inappropriate EN deprivation and negatively effects nutrition status.[46] In 80 consecutive, prospectively evaluated critically ill children receiving EN, feeds were interrupted an average of 3.7 $\pm$ 3.1 times in 24 (30%) patients.[18] A majority (58%) of the episodes of EN cessation were deemed avoidable and were associated with an increased utilization of PN. Mechanically ventilated patients were at the highest risk for inadequate EN. Significantly, more avoidable and unavoidable feeding interruptions were observed in 20 children receiving postpyloric EN compared to 60 fed via the gastric route. In 55 critically ill children, failure to meet energy goal for >50% of EN days was associated with airway and other procedures, clinical instability, and feeding tube removal; however, vasoactive medications and GI complications were the only significant factors identified.[58] Requirement for vasoactive or neuromuscular blocking medications also correlated with inadequate EN in 84 mechanically ventilated children in another study.[59] Fluid restriction was a major barrier to adequate nutrition in 42 PICU patients, and the 22 who were postoperative from cardiac surgery suffered a significant decline in weight-for-age Z-scores.[60] Cumulative energy and protein deficits were also associated with decreased weight and arm circumference Z-scores in 261 critically ill children prospectively evaluated.[61]

Strategies to Optimize Enteral Nutrition

Several strategies can reduce the impact or duration of inadequate enteral intake (see Table 8-4). Interruptions can be minimized by adhering to objective definitions of intolerance and guidelines for withholding feeds before procedures, use of technology and expertise for postpyloric tube insertion, and prompt reinstatement of feeding as soon as feasible. When gastric residuals are not measured in critically ill mechanically ventilated adults, enteral formula intake is significantly higher without an increase in the incidence of ventilator-associated pneumonia.[62] Neuromuscular blocking agents paralyze skeletal muscles, not the smooth muscles of the GI tract, and therefore should not prevent optimal EN. In addition, low-volume enteral feeding may be initiated and cautiously advanced in hemodynamically stable patients requiring consistent or decreasing doses of vasoactive medications with adequate perfusion and oxygenation. Reduction or elimination of fasting prior to bedside, operative, and airway procedures has also been demonstrated to improve EN intake in critically ill children and adults.[16,63] When enteral feeding interruptions are unavoidable, the administration rate may be temporarily increased to achieve the 24-hour volume goal in a shorter period (catch-up).[64-66] In addition, concentrated enteral formulas can be provided to meet protein and energy requirements despite fluid restriction.[64] Implementation of dietitian recommendations has been shown to increase delivery of early EN, energy, and protein intake in critically ill adults.[67] Computerized information systems can track energy and protein intake versus requirements and help prompt initiation of early EN.[68] Ongoing audits and updates of nutrition

TABLE 8-4. Barriers and Strategies to Achieve Optimal Enteral Nutrition

Barrier	Strategy
Lack of enteral access	Use education and technology for rapid tube placement
Vasoactive medications	If hemodynamics, perfusion, oxygenation adequate: start low volume feeds, monitor, slowly increase to meet nutrition goals
Neuromuscular blocking medication	Initiate feeds, monitor, increase to meet nutrition goals
Fasting for procedure	Reduce period of fasting when appropriate Increase hourly formula administration rate
Fluid restriction	Use concentrated enteral formula
Elevated gastric residuals	Use objective measures of feeding tolerance Postpyloric feeding route
Vomiting	Elevate head of bed Medications to reduce gastric acid and nausea Postpyloric feeding route
Constipation	Medications: stool softeners, laxatives, enemas Increase enteral fluid intake To maintain stool output in hemodynamically stable patients, change to fiber-containing formula
Diarrhea	Discontinue or reduce laxatives Rule out enteric infection and malabsorption Eliminate sorbitol from medications Change to isotonic or semielemental formula Hemodynamically stable patients: add soluble fiber
Abdominal distention	Treat constipation Vent air from the gastrointestinal tract Use lower volume, more concentrated formula Postpyloric feeding route

practices and guidelines over several years in one PICU led to a continued reduction in the time to start EN and in the use of PN.[69] A protocolized, step-wise approach to EN in the PICU has been shown to improve nutritional outcomes and achievement of daily goals in single centers, and needs to be examined in larger studies.

SUMMARY OF ENTERAL NUTRITION BEST PRACTICES

Early EN within 24 hours of admission or injury not only reduces energy and protein deficits, but may also decrease length of hospital stay and mortality in critically ill children. Selection of the gastric feeding route promotes a faster implementation of EN, but for those intolerant or at high risk for aspiration, postpyloric feeding should be considered. Although the postpyloric versus gastric route has not been shown to reduce aspiration in critically ill children, it may help avoid the use of PN and the associated increased costs and complications. A high-protein enteral formula or protein supplementation is necessary to meet the increased requirements of critical illness and injury, and objective measures of feeding tolerance should be monitored. Cumulative feeding interruptions result in caloric deficits, deterioration of nutritional status in the hospital, and an increased reliance on PN; barriers must be expected and prevented to maximize the benefits of EN. A regular audit of enteral feeding practices can identify areas for improvement to promote positive outcomes in the PICU.

KEY POINTS

- Enteral nutrition is preferred during critical illness.
- Early EN within 24 hours of PICU admission should be considered in critically ill children with a functional gut.
- The gastric feeding route is preferred, as it promotes faster achievement of nutrient delivery goals. However, for those intolerant to gastric feeds or at high risk for aspiration, postpyloric feeding should be considered.
- A high-protein enteral formula or protein supplementation may be necessary to meet the increased requirements of critical illness.
- Cumulative feeding interruptions result in caloric deficits, deterioration of nutritional status, and an increased reliance on PN; barriers must be anticipated and prevented to maximize the benefits of EN.
- The role of protocols or guidelines to promote uniform EN practices has improved nutrient delivery in single centers.

REFERENCES

1. Mehta NM, Compher C. A.S.P.E.N Clinical Guidelines: nutrition support of the critically ill child. *J Parenter Enteral Nutr.* 2009;33(3):260-276.
2. Khorasani EN, Mansouri F. Effect of early enteral nutrition on morbidity and mortality in children with burns. *Burns.* 2010;36(7):1067-1071.
3. Venter M, Rode H, Sive A, Visser M. Enteral resuscitation and early enteral feeding in children with major burns—effect on McFarlane response to stress. *Burns.* 2007;33(4):464-471.
4. Gottschlich MM, Jenkins ME, Mayes T, et al. The 2002 Clinical Research Award. An evaluation of the safety of early vs. delayed enteral support and effects on clinical, nutritional, and endocrine outcomes after severe burns. *J Burn Care Rehabil.* 2002;23(6):401-415.
5. Mikhailov TA, Kuhn EM, Manzi J, et al. Early enteral nutrition is associated with lower mortality in critically ill children. *J Parenter Enteral Nutr.* 2014;38(4):459-66.
6. Briassoulis G, Filippou O, Kanariou M, Hatzis T. Comparative effects of early randomized immune or non-immune-enhancing enteral nutrition on cytokine production in children with septic shock. *Intensive Care Med.* 2005;31(6):851-858.
7. Lopez-Herce J, Mencia S, Sanchez C, Santiago MJ, Bustinza A, Vigil D. Postpyloric enteral nutrition in the critically ill child with shock: a prospective observational study. *Nutr.* 2008;7:6.
8. King W, Petrillo T, Pettignano R. Enteral nutrition and cardiovascular medications in the pediatric intensive care unit. *J Parenter Enteral Nutr.* 2004;28(5):334-338.
9. Kamat P, Favaloro-Sabatier J, Rogers K, Stockwell JA. Use of methylene blue spectrophotometry to detect subclinical aspiration in enterally fed intubated pediatric patients. *Pediatr Crit Care Med.* 2008;9(3):299-303.
10. Meert KL, Daphtary KM, Metheny NA. Gastric vs. small-bowel feeding in critically ill children receiving mechanical ventilation: a randomized controlled trial. *Chest.* 2004;126(3):872-878.
11. Jiyong J, Tiancha H, Huiqin W, Jingfen J. Effect of gastric versus post-pyloric feeding on the incidence of pneumonia in critically ill patients: observations from traditional and Bayesian random-effects meta-analysis. *Clin Nutr.* 2012.
12. Petrillo-Albarano T, Pettignano R, Asfaw M, Easley K. Use of a feeding protocol to improve nutritional support through early, aggressive, enteral nutrition in the pediatric intensive care unit. *Pediatr Crit Care Med.* 2006;7(4):340-344.
13. Briassoulis GC, Zavras NJ, Hatzis MT. Effectiveness and safety of a protocol for promotion of early intragastric feeding in critically ill children. *Pediatr Crit Care Med.* 2001;2(2):113-121.
14. Chellis MJ, Sanders SV, Webster H, Dean JM, Jackson D. Early enteral feeding in the pediatric intensive care unit. *J Parenter Enteral Nutr.* 1996;20(1):71-73.
15. de Lucas C, Moreno M, Lopez-Herce J, Ruiz F, Perez-Palencia M, Carrillo A. Transpyloric enteral nutrition reduces the complication rate and cost in the critically ill child. *J Pediatr Gastroenterol Nutr.* 2000;30(2):175-180.
16. Lyons KA, Brilli RJ, Wieman RA, Jacobs BR. Continuation of transpyloric feeding during weaning of mechanical ventilation and tracheal extubation in children: a randomized controlled trial. *J Parenter Enteral Nutr.* 2002;26(3):209-213.
17. Fineman LD, LaBrecque MA, Shih MC, Curley MA. Prone positioning can be safely performed in critically ill infants and children. *Pediatr Crit Care Med.* 2006;7(5):413-422.
18. Mehta NM, McAleer D, Hamilton S, et al. Challenges to optimal enteral nutrition in a multidisciplinary pediatric intensive care unit. *J Parenter Enteral Nutr.* 2010;34(1):38-45.
19. Creel AM, Winkler MK. Oral and nasal enteral tube placement errors and complications in a pediatric intensive care unit. *Pediatr Crit Care Med.* 2007;8(2):161-164.
20. Chellis MJ, Sanders SV, Dean JM, Jackson D. Bedside transpyloric tube placement in the pediatric intensive care unit. *J Parenter Enteral Nutr.* 1996;20(1):88-90.

21. Joffe AR, Grant M, Wong B, Gresiuk C. Validation of a blind transpyloric feeding tube placement technique in pediatric intensive care: rapid, simple, and highly successful. *Pediatr Crit Care Med.* 2000;1(2):151-155.

22. Da Silva PS, Paulo CS, de Oliveira Iglesias SB, de Carvalho WB, Santana e Meneses F. Bedside transpyloric tube placement in the pediatric intensive care unit: a modified insufflation air technique. *Intensive Care Med.* 2002;28(7):943-946.

23. Phipps LM, Weber MD, Ginder BR, Hulse MA, Thomas NJ. A randomized controlled trial comparing three different techniques of nasojejunal feeding tube placement in critically ill children. *J Parenter Enteral Nutr.* 2005;29(6):420-424.

24. Meyer R, Harrison S, Cooper M, Habibi P. Successful blind placement of nasojejunal tubes in paediatric intensive care: impact of training and audit. *Journal of Advanced Nursing.* 2007;60(4):402-408.

25. Cone LC, Gilligan MF, Kagan RJ, Mayes T, Gottschlich MM. Enhancing patient safety: the effect of process improvement on bedside fluoroscopy time related to nasoduodenal feeding tube placement in pediatric burn patients. *J Burn Care Res.* 2009;30(4):606-611.

26. October TW, Hardart GE. Successful placement of postpyloric enteral tubes using electromagnetic guidance in critically ill children. *Pediatr Crit Care Med.* 2009;10(2):196-200.

27. Kline AM, Sorce L, Sullivan C, Weishaar J, Steinhorn DM. Use of a noninvasive electromagnetic device to place transpyloric feeding tubes in critically ill children. *American Journal of Critical Care: An official Publication, American Association of Critical-Care Nurses.* 2011;20(6):453-459; quiz 460.

28. Powers J, Luebbehusen M, Spitzer T, et al. Verification of an electromagnetic placement device compared with abdominal radiograph to predict accuracy of feeding tube placement. *J Parenter Enteral Nutr.* 2011;35(4):535-539.

29. Bankhead R, Boullata J, Brantley S, et al. Enteral nutrition practice recommendations. *J Parenter Enteral Nutr.* 2009;33(2):122-167.

30. Joeckel RJ, Phillips SK. Overview of infant and pediatric formulas. *Nutr Clin Pract.* 2009;24(3):356-362.

31. Tolia V, Lin CH, Kuhns LR. Gastric emptying using three different formulas in infants with gastroesophageal reflux. *J Pediatr Gastroenterol Nutr.* 1992;15(3):297-301.

32. Savage K, Kritas S, Schwarzer A, Davidson G, Omari T. Whey- vs. casein-based enteral formula and gastrointestinal function in children with cerebral palsy. *J Parenter Enteral Nutr.* 2012;36(1 Suppl):118S-123S.

33. Abrahao V. Nourishing the dysfunctional gut and whey protein. *Curr Opin Clin Nutr Metab Care.* 2012; 15(5):480-484.

34. Vidigal MV, Leite HP, Nogueira PC. Factors associated with peptide-based formula prescription in a pediatric intensive care unit. *J Pediatr Gastroenterol Nutr.* 2012;54(5):620-623.

35. Skillman HE, Wischmeyer PE. Nutrition therapy in critically ill infants and children. *J Parenter Enteral Nutr.* 2008;32(5):520-534.

36. Bechard LJ, Parrott JS, Mehta NM. Systematic review of the influence of energy and protein intake on protein balance in critically ill children. *J Pediatr.* 2012;161(2): 333-339 e331.

37. Jaksic T, Hull MA, Modi BP, et al. A.S.P.E.N. Clinical Guidelines: nutrition support of neonates supported with extracorporeal membrane oxygenation. *J Parenter Enteral Nutr.* 2010;34(3):247-253.

38. van Waardenburg DA, de Betue CT, Goudoever JB, Zimmermann LJ, Joosten KF. Critically ill infants benefit from early administration of protein and energy-enriched formula: a randomized controlled trial. *Clin Nutr.* 2009;28(3):249-255.

39. de Betue CT, van Waardenburg DA, Deutz NE, et al. Increased protein-energy intake promotes anabolism in critically ill infants with viral bronchiolitis: a double-blind randomised controlled trial. *Arch Dis Child.* 2011;96(9):817-822.

40. Botran M, Lopez-Herce J, Mencia S, Urbano J, Solana MJ, Garcia A. Enteral nutrition in the critically ill child: comparison of standard and protein-enriched diets. *J Pediatr.* 2011;159(1):27-32 e21.

41. Dabydeen L, Thomas JE, Aston TJ, Hartley H, Sinha SK, Eyre JA. High-energy and -protein diet increases brain and corticospinal tract growth in term and preterm infants after perinatal brain injury. *Pediatrics.* 2008;121(1):148-156.

42. Pillo-Blocka F, Adatia I, Sharieff W, McCrindle BW, Zlotkin S. Rapid advancement to more concentrated formula in infants after surgery for congenital heart disease reduces duration of hospital stay: a randomized clinical trial. *J Pediatr.* 2004;145(6):761-766.

43. Hart DW, Wolf SE, Zhang XJ, et al. Efficacy of a high-carbohydrate diet in catabolic illness. *Crit Care Med.* 2001;29(7):1318-1324.

44. Lee JO, Gauglitz GG, Herndon DN, Hawkins HK, Halder SC, Jeschke MG. Association between dietary fat content and outcomes in pediatric burn patients. *J Surg Res.* 2011;166(1):e83-90.

45. Sanchez C, Lopez-Herce J, Mencia S, Urbano J, Carrillo A, Maria Bellon J. Clinical severity scores do not predict tolerance to enteral nutrition in critically ill children. *The British Journal of Nutrition.* 2009;102(2):191-194.

46. Weckwerth JA. Monitoring enteral nutrition support tolerance in infants and children. *Nutr Clin Pract.* 2004;19(5):496-503.

47. Bernard AC, Magnuson B, Tsuei BJ, Swintosky M, Barnes S, Kearney PA. Defining and assessing tolerance in enteral nutrition. *Nutr Clin Pract.* 2004;19(5):481-486.

48. Tofil NM, Benner KW, Faro SJ, Winkler MK. The use of enteral naloxone to treat opioid-induced constipation in a pediatric intensive care unit. *Pediatr Crit Care Med.* 2006;7(3):252-254.

49. Mehta NM. Approach to enteral feeding in the PICU. *Nutr Clin Pract.* 2009;24(3):377-387.

50. Thakkar K, Kien CL, Rosenblatt JI, Herndon DN. Diarrhea in severely burned children. *J Parenter Enteral Nutr.* 2005;29(1):8-11.

51. McClave SA, Martindale RG, Vanek VW, et al. Guidelines for the Provision and Assessment of Nutrition Support Therapy in the Adult Critically Ill Patient: Society of Critical Care Medicine (SCCM) and American Society for Parenteral and Enteral Nutrition (A.S.P.E.N). *J Parenter Enteral Nutr.* 2009;33(3):277-316.

52. Honeycutt TC, El Khashab M, Wardrop RM, 3rd, et al. Probiotic administration and the incidence of nosocomial infection in pediatric intensive care: a randomized placebo-controlled trial. *Pediatr Crit Care Med.* 2007;8(5):452-458; quiz 464.

53. Simakachorn N, Bibiloni R, Yimyaem P, et al. Tolerance, safety, and effect on the faecal microbiota of an enteral formula supplemented with pre- and probiotics in critically ill children. *J Pediatr Gastroenterol Nutr.* 2011;53(2):174-181.

54. Horn D, Chaboyer W. Gastric feeding in critically ill children: a randomized controlled trial. *Am J Crit Care.* 2003;12(5):461-468.

55. Horn D, Chaboyer W, Schluter PJ. Gastric residual volumes in critically ill paediatric patients: a comparison of feeding regimens. *Aust Crit Care.* 2004;17(3):98-100, 102-103.

56. McClave SA, Lukan JK, Stefater JA, et al. Poor validity of residual volumes as a marker for risk of aspiration in critically ill patients. *Crit Care Med.* 2005;33(2): 324-330.

57. Maloney JP, Ryan TA. Detection of aspiration in enterally fed patients: a requiem for bedside monitors of aspiration. *J Parenter Enteral Nutr.* 2002;26 (6 Suppl):S34-41; discussion S41-32.

58. de Oliveira Iglesias SB, Leite HP, Santana e Meneses JF, de Carvalho WB. Enteral nutrition in critically ill children: are prescription and delivery according to their energy requirements? *Nutr Clin Pract.* 2007;22(2):233-239.

59. de Neef M, Geukers VG, Dral A, Lindeboom R, Sauerwein HP, Bos AP. Nutritional goals, prescription and delivery in a pediatric intensive care unit. *Clin Nutr.* 2008;27(1):65-71.

60. Rogers EJ, Gilbertson HR, Heine RG, Henning R. Barriers to adequate nutrition in critically ill children. *Nutrition.* 2003;19(10):865-868.

61. Hulst JM, van Goudoever JB, Zimmermann LJ, et al. The effect of cumulative energy and protein deficiency on anthropometric parameters in a pediatric ICU population. *Clin Nutr.* 2004;23(6):1381-1389.

62. Reignier J, Mercier E, Le Gouge A, et al. Effect of not monitoring residual gastric volume on risk of ventilator-associated pneumonia in adults receiving mechanical ventilation and early enteral feeding: a randomized controlled trial. *JAMA.* 16 2013;309(3):249-256.

63. Pousman RM, Pepper C, Pandharipande P, et al. Feasibility of implementing a reduced fasting protocol for critically ill trauma patients undergoing operative and nonoperative procedures. *J Parenter Enteral Nutr.* 2009;33(2): 176-180.

64. Hulst JM, Joosten KF, Tibboel D, van Goudoever JB. Causes and consequences of inadequate substrate supply to pediatric ICU patients. *Curr Opin Clin Nutr Metab Care.* 2006;9(3):297-303.

65. Heyland DK, Cahill NE, Dhaliwal R, et al. Enhanced protein-energy provision via the enteral route in critically ill patients: a single center feasibility trial of the PEP uP protocol. *Crit Care.* 2010;14(2):R78.

66. Lichtenberg K, Guay-Berry P, Pipitone A, Bondy A, Rotello L. Compensatory increased enteral feeding goal rates: a way to achieve optimal nutrition. *Nutr Clin Pract.* 2010;25(6):653-657.

67. Soguel L, Revelly JP, Schaller MD, Longchamp C, Berger MM. Energy deficit and length of hospital stay can be reduced by a two-step quality improvement of nutrition therapy: the intensive care unit dietitian can make the difference. *Crit Care Med.* 2012;40(2):412-419.

68. van Schijndel RJ, de Groot SD, Driessen RH, et al. Computer-aided support improves early and adequate delivery of nutrients in the ICU. *Neth J Med.* 2009;67(11):388-393.

69. Meyer R, Harrison S, Sargent S, Ramnarayan P, Habibi P, Labadarios D. The impact of enteral feeding protocols on nutritional support in critically ill children. *J Hum Nutr Diet.* 2009;22(5):428-436.

CHAPTER 9

Guidelines and Algorithms for Feeding the Critically ill

Enid E Martinez

Lauren Sorce

Susan Hamilton

■ INTRODUCTION

■ COMMON GUIDELINE AND ALGORITHM COMPONENTS

Preinitiation

Initiation and Advancement of Enteral Nutrition

Enteral Nutrition Intolerance

Enteral Nutrition Maintenance and Adjuncts

■ DEVELOPMENT AND IMPLEMENTATION OF AN ENTERAL NUTRITION GUIDELINE/ALGORITHM

Key Stakeholders

Guideline Development Process

Implementation of an EN Guideline

Barriers to Successful Implementation

Auditing Practice Change

■ CONCLUSIONS

■ KEY POINTS

References

■ INTRODUCTION

Optimal nutrition therapy of critically ill children has emerged as an important goal. Studies indicate up to 64% of children admitted to pediatric intensive care units (PICUs) are malnourished,[1-4] and these children are at a greater risk for prolonged mechanical ventilation and hospital stay, compared to their well-nourished counterparts.[4,5] The degree of malnutrition depends on the disease type, duration, and comorbidities. The provision of adequate nutrition to the critically ill child is paramount to reducing further nutritional deterioration in an already compromised host. Malnutrition evolves during critical illness and most prominently affects newborns and infants.[2] The American Society for Parenteral and Enteral Nutrition (A.S.P.E.N) guidelines (Please see Table 9.1) recommend early enteral nutrition (EN) in critically ill children with a functional gastrointestinal (GI) tract.[6]

There are emerging data supporting the role of enteral feeds in critically ill children. Enteral nutrition in this population is well tolerated,[7-11] is associated with reduced complications compared with parenteral nutrition (PN),[4,7] and can be delivered via the gastric or transpyloric route.[12,13] Enteral nutrition is also associated with reduced mortality and length of stay in this population.[4,14] Despite its perceived benefits, EN delivery in the PICU remains challenging. When enteral feeding is

TABLE 9-1. A.S.P.E.N Pediatric Nutrition Support Guideline Recommendations

Nutrition Support Guideline Recommendations in the Critically ill Child		
#	Guideline Recommendations	Grade
1	1A) Children admitted with critical illnesses should undergo nutrition screening to identify those with existing malnutrition and those who are nutritionally-at-risk.	D
	1B) A formal nutrition assessment with the development of a nutrition care plan should be required, especially in those children with premorbid malnutrition.	E
2	2A) Energy expenditure should be assessed throughout the course of illness to determine the energy needs of critically ill children. Estimates of energy expenditure using available standard equations are often unreliable.	D
	2B) In a subgroup of patients with suspected metabolic alterations or malnutrition, accurate measurement of energy expenditure using indirect calorimetry (IC) is desirable. If IC is not feasible or available, initial energy provision may be based on published formulas or nomograms. Attention to imbalance between energy intake and expenditure will help to prevent overfeeding and underfeeding in this population.	E
3	There are insufficient data to make evidence-based recommendations for macronutrient intake in critically ill children. After determination of energy needs for the critically ill child, the rational partitioning of the major substrates should be based upon understanding of protein metabolism and carbohydrate- and lipid-handling during critical illness.	E
4	4A) In critically ill children with a functioning gastrointestinal tract, enteral nutrition (EN) should be the preferred made of nutrient provision, if tolerated.	C
	4B) A variety of barriers to EN exist in the pediatric intensive care unit (PICU) Clinicians must identify and prevent avoidable interruptions to EN in critically ill children.	D
	4C) There are insufficient data to recommend the appropriate site (gastric vs postpyloric/transpyloric) for enteral feeding in critically ill children. Post-pyloric or transpyloric feeding may improve caloric intake when compared to gastric feeds. Post-pyloric feeding may be considered in children at high risk of aspiration or those who have failed a trial of gastric feeding.	C
5	Based on the available pediatric data, the routine use of immunonutrition or immune-enhancing diets/nutrients in critically ill children is not recommended.	D
6	A specialized nutrition support team in the PICU and aggressive feeding protocols may enhance the overall delivery of nutrition, with shorter time to goal nutrition, increased delivery of EN, and decreased use of parenteral nutrition. The affect of these strategies on patient outcomes has not been demonstrated.	E

Reproduced with permission from Mehta NM, Compher C, A.S.P.E.N. Board of Directors: A.S.P.E.N. Clinical Guidelines: nutrition support of the critically ill child, J Parenter Enteral Nutr 2009;33(3):260-276.

protocolized or supported through a nutrition support team, time to feeding and tolerance improve.[15,16-20] Children who are in intensive care units (ICUs) for whom a feeding protocol is implemented experience fewer infections[4] are more likely to meet energy needs[19] and achieve positive protein and energy balance[21] sooner than do those who do not received protocolized enteral feeding. However, a majority of critically ill children do not meet recommended daily allowance of energy and protein intake,[3] and even with feeding protocols, children may be under- or overfed when using respiratory quotient (RQ) as a measurement.[22]

Determining algorithmic approaches to the provision of enteral feeds will enable standardization of processes, which may ultimately facilitate the development of clinical trials.

COMMON GUIDELINE AND ALGORITHM COMPONENTS

Nutrient delivery guidelines or protocols provide recommendations related to screening for malnutrition, determination of macronutrient goals, selection of the best route (enteral or parenteral), site (gastric or postpyloric) and rate of nutrient administration, detection and management of feeding intolerance, and the use of adjuncts for enteral nutrition. Please see Figure 9-1 for an example of an EN algorithm from a North American PICU.

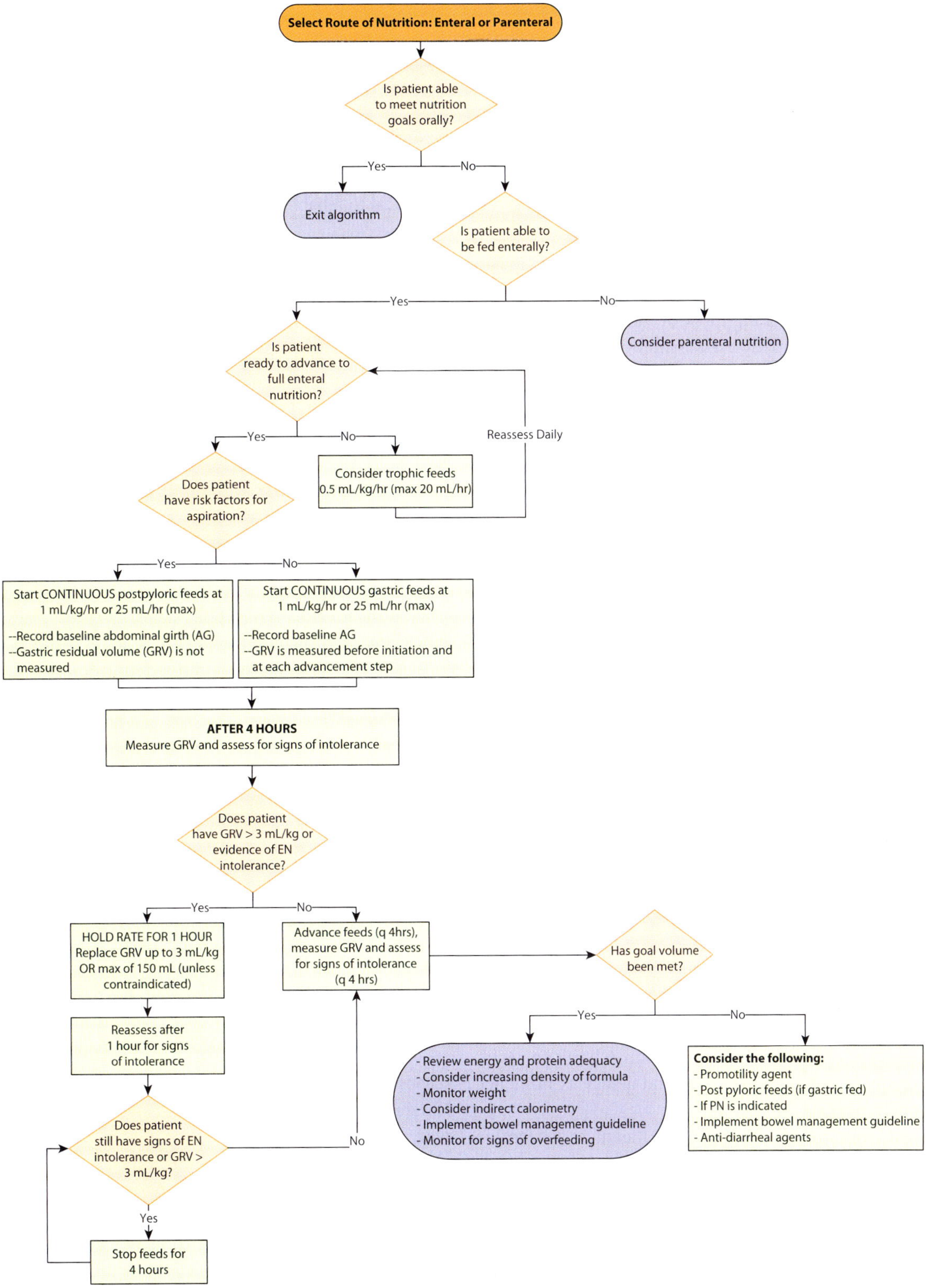

FIGURE 9-1. Components of the PICU Enteral Nutrition Algorithm at Boston Children's Hospital.

Preinitiation

Nutrition assessment is among the few evidence-based recommendations in the 2009 A.S.P.E.N. Clinical Guidelines on nutrition support of the critically ill child.[6] Performing a nutrition assessment prior to implementing a nutrition plan is critical, given the high prevalence of both acute and chronic malnutrition in the pediatric critically ill population. The aim of a nutrition screen is to identify patients who would require a more in-depth nutrition assessment, targeting those who are already malnourished or at a high risk of nutritional deterioration. Objective nutrition assessment includes anthropometric measurements and biochemical assessment. Anthropometric measurements should at least include height or length and weight, which are then normalized to classify the nutritional state based on Z-scores for weight-for-age, height/length-for-age, weight-for-length or body mass index (BMI)-for-age.[23] Skinfold measurements and mid-upper-arm circumference measurements are used to assess body composition, particularly fat content. All values should be evaluated in the context of challenges to obtaining measurements in critically ill patients (e.g., recumbent lengths or the use of bed scales) and the patient's fluid balance. Algorithms should include recommendations for the type and frequency of measurements and describe standard techniques and the personnel assigned to anthropometry on admission and during the course of PICU stay.

Biochemical testing has been suggested to assess duration and severity of malnutrition and inflammation. Albumin and prealbumin are most commonly tested to assess nutritional status; however, these are not reliable in the critically ill patient due to alterations in fluid balance and inflammation resulting in decreased levels of both. Inflammation in particular alters prealbumin levels due to a shift in the liver toward increased production of acute-phase reactants such as C-reactive protein.[6] Consequently, some have suggested obtaining C-reactive protein, procalcitonin, and interleukin-6 levels to assess the patient's inflammatory state and assess its influence on nutritional status.

Nutrition assessment tools as a means to determine nutritional status exist, but are not widely implemented or recommended by national nutrition guidelines. Subjective global nutritional assessment (SGNA) is a pediatric modification of a nutrition assessment tool developed for adults that has been evaluated in children. Two separate studies, one in critically ill children and another in children undergoing thoracic or abdominal surgery, showed the SGNA nutrition classification to correlate fairly to moderately with nutritional assessments based on anthropometric measurements.[24,25] Ultimately, whether assessment is performed by a validated tool or traditional anthropometric measurements, a skilled provider, likely a dietitian, is critical to reliable assessments.

Defining Energy Intake Goal

The metabolic demands of critically ill patients vary depending on pre-illness nutritional status, disease severity, and stages of that disease. Consequently, the most accurate and gold standard measure of energy requirement is indirect calorimetry (IC). IC is not widely implemented, however, given that it requires trained personnel and resources.[26] The current A.S.P.E.N. guidelines recommend the consideration of IC, and studies have shown that up to 71% of pediatric critically ill patients meet indications for IC.[27]

Alternatively, the most common practice is the use of population-based equations to estimate the energy requirements, with the possible inclusion of stress factors accounting for altered metabolic states. The most common equations used include the WHO, Schofield, and White equations.[28-30] Estimated energy requirements (EER) have been shown to be inaccurate when compared to measured resting energy expenditure by IC in critically ill patients; this could result in the risk of overestimating or underestimating energy requirements.[28-31] Use of EER for determining energy needs should include accurate anthropometric measurements, close follow-up for possible energy imbalance, and consideration of IC in special populations, such as those at higher risk of energy imbalance as recommended by A.S.P.E.N.[6] Algorithms should include guidance on the best available method for assessing energy requirements for individual institutions. Energy prescriptions must be based on this assessment and must be regularly revisited during the course of illness as the clinical condition changes.

Considerations for Route of Nutrient Delivery

Enteral nutrition is recommended over PN in patients with a functional GI tract. Adult studies have consistently shown decreased infection morbidity associated with EN over PN.[32] Individual studies have shown decreased mortality, shorter length of stay, and decreased nutrition costs as well.[33,34] Parenteral nutrition may be used in cases where delays in initiating EN could result in prolonged suboptimal nutrition intake in a vulnerable host.

For EN delivery, the gastric or postpyloric route may be considered. In adults, systematic reviews have not revealed a significant difference in total energy intake, risk of aspiration pneumonia, and length of stay between gastric or postpyloric EN delivery.[35,36] Some studies have suggested that feeds are initiated earlier when using the gastric route, likely due to delays in initiating feeds when choosing the postpyloric route, which in turn are due to difficulties in bedside postpyloric tube placement.[37,38] Notwithstanding the limited evidence, the postpyloric feeding route should be considered in patients receiving gastric feeds with feeding intolerance and subsequent poor advancement of feeds, or patients with known high risk or history of aspiration.[6,39] Algorithms for EN in the PICU may include the indications for postpyloric feeding based on the available local expertise and resources for placing postpyloric feeding tubes.

Contraindications for Enteral Nutrition

Most contraindications for EN are relative and based on clinical judgment. Abdominal surgery or pathology (e.g., GI bleeding) and active ongoing resuscitation with escalation of vasopressor support are the most commonly stated contraindications for EN.[39] In well-nourished older patients, if it is projected that nutrition goals will not be met enterally by 5 to 7 days due to a contraindication or as a result of feeding intolerance and failure to advance calories, initiation of PN may be considered. Parenteral nutrition is usually initiated earlier in newborns and in malnourished children.

Initiation and Advancement of Enteral Nutrition

This section of the algorithms is probably the most important. Bedside teams benefit from stepwise guidance on starting and advancing EN. In particular, specific starting rate and frequency of rate increase are desirable. Most institutions recommend early EN initiation—within 24 to 48 hours after admission. If the goal of nutrition is to provide trophic feeds, initiation of feeding volumes with isotonic formula or human milk range from 0.5 mL/kg/hr to 2 mL/kg/hr, depending on the condition and size of the patient.[40] In children for whom the plan is to provide full nutrition via enteral feeds, feedings may start at this volume and be advanced by 1 to 5 mL/hr every 4 hours in infants[40] and 5 to 20 mL/hr every 2 to 4 hours in children.[7,40] While initiating trophic feeds with electrolyte solution for infants with hypoplastic left heart syndrome has been described, the real utility of this approach instead of using human milk or formula as the first step is questionable.[15]

Evidence is lacking on the benefits of bolus versus continuous feeds in critically ill children. Using tolerance and risk for aspiration as a guide, critically ill children may progress from continuous to bolus feeds as their clinical condition directs.[41]

The overall limiting factors related to the volume of enteral feeds are intolerance (diarrhea, high gastric residual volume, abdominal distention, constipation) and fluid restriction. For children who develop feeding intolerance, reducing the feed volume may improve tolerance. For children whose enteral feeds are limited by fluid restriction, maximizing energy density may improve nutritional intake; however, monitoring the child for feeding intolerance is critical with hyperosmolar feeds.

Enteral Nutrition Intolerance

Enteral feeding intolerance is described in the critically ill population with prevalence rates of approximately 60% in both adult and pediatric populations.[42-44] Critical illnesses such as sepsis, increased intracranial pressure,[45] certain medications, and poor systemic perfusion can result in abnormal GI motility.[46] Diagnostic tests of poor GI motility such as the paracetamol absorption test[47] are not practical for routine use. Bedside clinical signs, such as gastric residual volume measurement, abdominal distension, emesis, diarrhea, and lack of bowel sounds, are commonly used as markers of feeding intolerance in the PICU.[48,49] Perceived intolerance to EN is one of the principal factors resulting in failure to reach EN goals. A uniform definition and approach to managing EN intolerance in the algorithm is highly desirable.

Gastric Residual Volume

Increased gastric residual volume (GRV) is the most cited cause for stopping feeds and subsequently the most common definition of enteral feeding intolerance reported. Adult studies report increased GRV in 35% to 45% of enterally fed critically ill patients.[32,50,51] However, the threshold for defining increased GRV is highly variable. Stopping feeds for GRVs <500 mL is not recommended in adult nutrition guidelines.[51] In the pediatric population, GRV thresholds for defining feeding intolerance have not been studied. They vary greatly between institutions, and hence their use as a lone marker of intolerance is not recommended in pediatric guidelines.[6] In the pediatric population, aspiration by small enteric tubes might make GRV measurements inaccurate. After measurement, the residual volume may be wasted or refed. Though no definitive data are available, refeeding GRVs, and possibly holding ongoing feeds if needed, is a common practice in PICUs. In the absence of pediatric data, it may be reasonable to consider GRVs in association with other symptoms of feeding intolerance, particularly abdominal distention and emesis. While a high GRV by itself is probably not an indication of feeding intolerance, the additional presence of other GI symptoms may indicate a true feeding intolerance.

Diarrhea, Constipation, and Emesis

The second most commonly cited clinical sign of possible feeding intolerance is diarrhea. Diarrhea has been reported in one-third to one-half of the critically ill population, including pediatric subsets.[48,52] The most common definition of diarrhea is more than 3 loose stools a day, though broader definitions such as sudden increase in frequency, volume, and fluidity of stool have also been used.[7,42,44] Constipation, lack of bowel movements, or infrequent bowel movements are also poorly defined, with prevalence ranging between 33% and 79%.[46,47,53] Slowed GI motility, though multifactorial in etiology, is highly influenced by commonly administered medications in ICUs, such as narcotics, and is treated with stimulants and softeners. Algorithms may include a uniform institutional approach to diarrhea and constipation.

Emesis and reflux of gastric contents are concerning possible symptoms of GI intolerance due to the risk of aspiration in the critically ill patient. Both may be common, gastroesophageal reflux (GER) more so, as critical illness and many medications used in the PICU cause relaxation of the lower esophageal sphincter, facilitating the retrograde flow of gastric contents into the esophagus and potentially the upper airway.[7] Increased gastric contents possibly due to delayed gastric emptying can potentiate these symptoms, and medications can also lead to nausea and emesis. Emesis is reported in in 10% to 45.2% of the PICU population.[7,44]

Abdominal Distension and Bowel Sounds

Abdominal distension is a potential sign of feed intolerance, as poor GI motility results in accumulation of contents and subsequently GI distension. However, it is unclear what degree of change in abdominal girth is an indication of poor feeding tolerance. More importantly, abdominal distention has not been correlated with other signs of feeding intolerance such as increased GRV.[54,55] The reported prevalence of abdominal distension is between 6%[56] and 9.5%[34] in the pediatric population, though higher in the adult population, 12% to 28%.[57,58]

Presence or absence of bowel sounds is an imprecise clinical sign of feeding tolerance or altered GI motility. Auscultation of bowel sounds does not correlate accurately with feed tolerance, as even in the setting of an ileus, bowel sounds may be appreciated.

Management of Intolerance

Many strategies are employed to overcome feeding intolerance despite minimal to no scientific evidence to support any one of them. Most interventions address slow GI motility and its associated clinical signs: abdominal distension and high GRVs. The simplest of these is reducing the volume or slowing the rate of advancement of feeds. Feeding tolerance may improve when changing the rate of advancement, but it may delay the achievement of energy goals or result in failure to meet energy goals. Prokinetics can improve GI motility—mostly delayed gastric emptying and partially small-bowel dysmotility. Prokinetic use is limited by the associated adverse drug reactions, medication interactions, and loss of effect with prolonged use or tachyphylaxis.[59] The postpyloric feeding route is a commonly adopted strategy to overcome the intolerance to gastric feeds. However, it does require a skilled provider for placement, may be challenging to place at the bedside, and there is no convincing evidence to favor the postpyloric route to the gastric route in critically ill children.[6] A stepwise escalating bowel regimen helps promote regular bowel movements, prevents constipation, and might improve feeding tolerance in critically ill children. Hence, it is incorporated into the enteral feeding guidelines in the PICU.

Enteral Nutrition Maintenance and Adjuncts

The benefits of early initiation of EN have been well described and hence adopted at most centers. The ongoing challenge lies in maintaining optimal EN over time for critically ill patients that have a longer ICU length of stay. Ongoing intolerance, fasting for procedures, tube malfunction, and changes in patient condition, as well as rotating practitioners caring for these patients, have all been implicated as reasons why a patient may not be able to maintain goal EN.[41,60] Enteral nutrition algorithms may include some of the following guidelines to help maintain EN delivery.

Fasting Guidelines

Critically ill children undergo a variety of procedures and tests that may require fasting. As such, adhering to fasting guidelines is required. The American Society of Anesthesiologists published an updated guideline in 2011[61] that addresses fasting recommendations for the healthy child (see Table 9-2).

Ongoing Nutrition Surveillance

Ongoing nutritional surveillance is important to evaluate the success of a patient's EN regimen. Monitoring for weight gain may serve as an indicator of meeting the EER and energy goals. However, obtaining accurate weight data can be challenging in the PICU. In a recent survey of nutrition practices in the UK, less than one-third of the units had a specific policy for frequency of weighing patients on the unit.[60] The actual act of obtaining a weight may place some critically ill patients at risk for extubation or hemodynamic instability, and the risk/benefit ratio must be considered prior to obtaining a weight in such cases. Weight data can sometimes be difficult to interpret due to fluid shifts. New and innovative strategies for accurately weighing patients are greatly needed.

Other anthropometric measures may also be relevant, particularly in the setting of patients with prolonged admissions and chronic illnesses. In newborns and infants, who have faster growth rates, frequent measurement of head circumference and length is vital to confirm matching of energy expenditure to energy intake and provision. Protein malnutrition due to protein loss and inadequate intake is common in critically ill patients, resulting in risk of morbidity, including delayed wean from mechanical ventilation, poor wound healing, and loss of skin integrity. Monitoring lean body mass via anthropometric variables such as the mid-upper arm circumference can gauge loss or gain in lean body mass as protein intake is maximized. Finally, routine biochemical and micronutrient testing, including vitamin levels, may be necessary in prolonged illness and must be included as part of the institutional algorithm.

TABLE 9-2. ASA Recommended Fasting Times

Ingested Material	Minimum Fasting Time
Clear liquids	2 hours
Human milk	4 hours
Infant formula	6 hours
Nonhuman milk	6 hours
Light meal (toast and clear liquid)	6 hours
Fried or fatty food meal	8 hours or more

Reproduced with permission from American Society of Anesthesiologists Committee: Practice guidelines for preoperative fasting and the use of pharmacologic agents to reduce the risk of pulmonary aspiration: application to healthy patients undergoing elective procedures: an updated report by the American Society of Anesthesiologists Committee on Standards and Practice Parameters, Anesthesiology 2011;114(3):495-511.

Feeding Tube Management

In PICUs that use nasally or orally inserted feeding tubes, there is the risk of tube dislodgement or obstruction. Gastric feeding tubes are easily replaced, but specialized skills are necessary for replacing postpyloric feeding tubes. In a study by Mehta et al., 43% of patients with postpyloric feeding tubes experienced prolonged EN deprivation due to tube-related complications.[41] Development of strategies that expedite tube replacement and limit the amount of time of EN deprivation are worthwhile as part of an EN guideline.

Other Enteral Nutrition Adjuncts

Providing guidelines for the use of adjunctive therapies such as a bowel management, motility agents, and antacids are pivotal to the success of preventing and treating EN intolerance.

Bowel regimen Underlying severity of disease, prolonged nil per os (NPO) status, abdominal surgery, negative fluid balance, and medications, particularly narcotics, sedation, and muscle relaxants, are all reasons why critically ill patients may have changes in their bowel movements, including constipation. Constipation can result in abdominal distension and subsequent concern for feeding intolerance and interruption of feeds, as well as possible small intestinal bacterial overgrowth and, in some studies, has been associated with prolonged ICU stay.[62,63] Application of a bowel regimen has been shown to reduce constipation,[64] and some studies have suggested that early defecation is associated with shorter hospital length of stay.[65] Insufficient evidence is available to guide the use of specific stool softeners and laxatives. In the setting of multifactorial etiology for constipation, preventive agents against constipation, such as stool softeners and fiber, and active agents against constipation, such as enemas and laxatives, should be considered. One special consideration is the use of peripherally acting mu-opioid receptor antagonists (PAMORAs), such as methylnaltrexone, which reverses the effect of narcotics primarily on the GI tract and the bladder, or oral naloxone in patients where narcotic use is thought to be a primary cause of constipation.[66] Peripherally acting mu-opioid receptor antagonists have been studied primarily in adults and most prominently in the chronically ill patient population, though recent published case reports of a pediatric patient and a neonate proved methylnaltrexone to be effective in promoting bowel movements with no major side effects.[67-69]

Prokinetics Prokinetics, drugs that increase motility of the GI tract, are considered first-line treatment for feeding intolerance.[50] The most commonly studied and approved prokinetics are erythromycin and metoclopramide. Erythromycin, a macrolide antibiotic, improves contractility of the stomach and duodenum.[59,70] Metoclopramide, a selective dopamine and serotonin receptor antagonist, improves contractility not only of the stomach and the duodenum, but also the esophagus and jejunum, and is hence used to facilitate nasojejunal tube placement.[64,66] Both agents, as monotherapy or combined therapy, have been shown to improve motility, and in some studies result in faster attainment of feeding goal volume.[71,72] However, not all studies have reached a similar conclusion, and both agents result in decreased effect with time due to tachyphylaxis and have significant side effects.[73,74] Erythromycin most importantly can cause QT prolongation, an important side effect given that ICU patients are often on multiple QT-prolonging medications. Metoclopramide has a black box warning for its risk of permanent tardive dyskinesia, a disorder of involuntary movements, when used long term. The risk from short-term use in the ICU is smaller, but not zero.

Antacids Gastric stress ulcers are thought to develop commonly in ICU patients, but the incidence of actual significant bleeding is quite low. Cook et al. place the risk of clinically significant bleeding at 1.5% for adult ICU patients.[75] Most published studies to date have focused on adult ICU patients. There is a paucity of evidence in the PICU population. To date, there are no evidence-based data to confirm the need for stress ulcer prophylaxis while receiving EN in the ICU or whether EN in and of itself can constitute prophylaxis in a critically ill child. In their review of the literature on this topic, Quenot et al. found that routine use of antacid medications for stress ulcer prophylaxis could not be justified in an adult population.[76] The authors recommend that patients should be screened for risk for stress ulcer bleeding and those patients found to be at risk should receive prophylaxis. The most commonly cited risk factors are mechanical ventilation for >48 hours, coagulopathy, splanchnic hypoperfusion, history of GI bleeding within 1 year, sepsis, ICU admission >1 week, and glucocorticoid therapy.[76,77] The practice of prescribing antacid therapy varies widely from ICU to ICU, and standardized risk assessment is not commonly undertaken. The most common agents currently used for ICU stress ulcer prophylaxis are proton pump inhibitors, which block acid secretion, and histamine 2 receptor antagonists, which decrease acid secretion. The American Society of Health System Pharmacists suggest that both agents are safe for acid suppression in critically ill patients, but the proton pump inhibitors offer the advantage of fewer drug interactions and decreased need to adjust the dosing for renal insufficiency.[78]

DEVELOPMENT AND IMPLEMENTATION OF AN ENTERAL NUTRITION GUIDELINE/ALGORITHM

This section describes some of the key steps and strategies involved in the successful implementation of a uniform feeding guideline or algorithm in the PICU.

Key Stakeholders

Prior to developing EN guidelines, it is necessary to identify key stakeholders to participate in the development process, as well as who the end users will be. While it is the physician, nurse practitioner, or physician's assistant who prescribes EN, the bedside nursing staff implements any guidelines. The more specific and self-directed the guideline is, the greater the likelihood that it will be adhered to. It is necessary to have full cooperation from all levels of staff.

Minimum recommendations of disciplines to be involved in guideline development include:

- Pediatric critical care physicians with an interest in critical care nutrition and an understanding of institutional hierarchy

- Intensive care unit staff nurses
- Clinical registered dietician
- Clinical pharmacist
- Gastrointestinal/nutrition specialist
- Pediatric surgeon

Others may include:

- Administrative support
- Nurse educator/leader

If special patient populations are involved, it is critical to have input from those specialists that have a vested interest in the population. Examples of special populations may include neonates, children with congenital heart disease, solid organ transplant patients, and stem cell transplant patients.

Guideline Development Process

In the first half of this chapter, we discussed key components of an EN guideline that are important to implementing a successful protocol. Each unit is unique, however, with its own distinct challenges. Developing guidelines without surveying current practices in the PICU may result in missing local practice challenges. Mehta et al.[41] found in a presurvey of EN practices that avoidable interruptions accounted for 58% of all EN interruptions. These interruptions were mostly related to excessive fasting times around intubation/extubation and subjective symptoms of intolerance. These interruptions led to higher PN use in these patients with associated higher costs.

Components of a presurvey may include collecting data of daily EN usage over a specified period, including time to goal feeds, feed interruptions, feeding route, staff perceptions of feed intolerance, fasting times, and the use of adjunctive therapies.

Recommended steps to developing an EN guideline include:

- Develop a multidisciplinary team.
- Establish a timeline for each phase of guideline development.
- Conduct a presurvey of current EN practices.
- Analyze predata and utilize to identify priorities for guideline development.
- Develop evidence-based questions for each area of concern.

Example: Preferred route for feeding in the PICU. Questions may include the following: What are indications for bolus versus continuous gastric feeds? What are the indications for postpyloric feeds? What patient populations are at risk for pulmonary aspiration of gastrointestinal contents?

- Assign team members to answer specific directed questions.
- Convene as a group to review evidence.
- Create a guideline based on a review of literature, expert consensus, and the specific needs or challenges of the PICU.
- Create a document in a form that is user friendly, easy to follow, explicit, and self-directed whenever possible.

The entire process is time consuming and cannot be expected to be completed quickly. Disseminating the results of presurvey data during the development process may be helpful to maintain focus on EN issues during this time.

Implementation of an EN Guideline

The implementation of a nutrition guideline requires a stepwise effort to educate, using multiple avenues to disseminate the information to the entire group. Nutrition champions play an important role in providing bedside support to nursing and physician groups as the new guidelines are being adopted.

Education

Prior to implementing the new guideline, support/approval should be garnered from the appropriate overseeing bodies, such as an ICU governance committee or a nutrition oversight committee. An assessment of the multidisciplinary team's knowledge of critical care nutrition may be helpful in identifying areas of concentration for education at the time of guideline implementation. A pretest or survey can be implemented online, with questions focused on each component of the guideline. Results of the pretest can be objectively shared with members of the multidisciplinary team to highlight areas for growth/improvement. It can also be used to highlight areas of needed education.

Implementing any type of comprehensive practice change takes a multipronged approach to ensure success. Enrolling the assistance of a nurse educator to help plan a sequential rollout that meets the needs of all disciplines may be prudent. Widespread introduction to the guideline by all disciplines is necessary. Education can be personalized to fit the needs of each discipline.

A learning module may be created to highlight important aspects of the guideline. Visual reminders, such as posting the guideline on the front page of a unit's website or at the bedside, are helpful. Developing a plan to include discussion of nutritional goals in multidisciplinary rounds is paramount in creating a culture that values nutritional care. Weekly rounds by members of the guideline development team for the first 1 to 2 months after implementation to maintain a focus on the guidelines may also be helpful.

Barriers to Successful Implementation

Any time a new practice is introduced, there is the potential for resistance. Some components of a new EN guideline may call for a re-evaluation of long-held clinical practices and caregiver beliefs. Status quo can be difficult to affect. A study of nutritional practices in the UK and Ireland found that among the reasons that clinicians did not start feeds in the PICU, some were highly subjective, such as nurses did not start feeds in a timely manner or the patient was "too ill" to be fed.[60] In a survey of adult ICUs in the UK that had either a local or national EN guideline, Judges et al.[79] found that the more experienced a clinician was, the more their EN practice was influenced by experience over a written guideline. A lack of definitive evidence for some nutritional practices may be put forward as an argument to not adhere to newly established guidelines. Overcoming an ingrained culture can be difficult, but it has been shown that the more comprehensive a guideline is, the more likely it will be followed with good outcomes.[7]

Auditing Practice Change

Any comprehensive practice change that is implemented will take a minimum of 3 to 6 months to become ingrained in daily practice. The timing for collecting postimplementation data will be contingent on the size of the unit, the numbers of staff that require training, how homogeneous or heterogeneous the patient population is, and other competing initiatives.

The postimplementation survey should closely mimic the preimplementation survey. When feasible, the survey should be implemented by the same data collectors as the presurvey to maintain reliability. Demographic variables can be compared for similarities in the 2 patient populations. Time to EN initiation; time to goal volume feeds; PN usage; and the number, duration, and reasons for feed interruptions can be compared. Challenges not met after implementation can then be identified and prioritized for ongoing education. Deficiencies in the guidelines may also become evident from the results of the postimplementation survey. Ongoing refinements to the actual guideline document based on new evidence and feedback from the institutional implementation are an expected and necessary part of the process.

CONCLUSIONS

The development of guidelines and algorithms to support the initiation and management of enteral feedings can be done successfully when the right multiprofessional team is gathered. These guidelines should include steps to assess the nutritional needs, selection of the appropriate route of nutrient delivery, emphasis on enteral feeding in eligible patients, uniform guidelines to address intolerance, and the use of adjuncts to maintain the nutrient delivery during the PICU course. The guidelines should be based on institutional challenges and barriers. Once implemented, outcomes should be monitored and guidelines should be modified as patient outcomes, institutional feedback and new evidence emerge.

The A.S.P.E.N. guidelines recommend providing EN to critically ill children. While the existing data overall support the use of enteral feeds to improve outcomes in critically ill children, challenges continue, given the lack of definitive randomized controlled trials evaluating this practice. It remains unclear whether the unfounded concerns about feeding critically ill children enterally will be supported or refuted. For now, given our best evidence, enteral feeding is known to reduce mortality, reduce infection risk, and reduce hospital length of stay.

KEY POINTS

- Nutrition algorithms facilitate uniform stepwise nutrient delivery and are associated with higher likelihood of achieving nutrition goals in the PICU.
- Nutrition algorithms must include recommendations for screening, assessment of nutritional status, route of feeding, EN initiation, and EN maintenance.
- Definition and management of EN intolerance are important considerations in an algorithm.
- A multidisciplinary approach, involvement of key stakeholders, assessment of local barriers, and review of best available evidence are important when developing an institutional feeding algorithm. Implementation of an algorithm requires education, phased implementation, and regular audits to examine problems with adherence.

REFERENCES

1. Pollack MM, Wiley JS, Kanter R, Holbrook PR. Malnutrition in critically ill infants and children. *J Parenter Enteral Nutr.* 1982;6(1):20-24.
2. Leite HP, Isatugo MK, Sawaki L, Fisberg M. Anthropometric nutritional assessment of critically ill hospitalized children. *Rev Paul Med.* 1993;111:309-13.
3. Hulst J, Joosten K, Zimmermann L, et al. Malnutrition in critically ill children: from admission to 6 months after discharge. *Clin Nutr.* 2004;23(2):223-232.
4. Mehta N, Bechard L, Cahill N, et al. Nutritional practices and their relationship to clinical outcomes in critically ill children—An international multicenter cohort study. *Crit Care Med.* 2012;40:2204-2211.
5. Menezes FS, Leite HP, Nogueira PC. Malnutrition as an independent predictor of clinical outcomes in critically ill children. *Nutrition.* 2012;28:267-270.
6. Mehta NM, Compher C, A.S.P.E.N. Board of Directors. A.S.P.E.N. clinical guidelines: nutrition support of the critically ill child. *J Parenter Enteral Nutr.* 2009;33(3):260-276.
7. Pettignano R, Davis R, Labuz M, Hart M. Total enteral nutition versus total parenteral nutrition duringpediatric extracorporeal membrane oxygenation. *Crit Care Med.* 1998; 26(2):358-363.
8. Briassoulis G, Zavras N, Hatzis T. Malnutrition nutritional indices, and early enteral feeding in critically ill children. *Nutrition.* 2001;*17*:548-557.
9. Briassoulis G, Filippou O, Hatzi E, Papassotiriou I, Hatzis T. Early enteral administration of immunonutrition in critically ill children: results of a blinded randomized controlled clinical trial. *Nutrition.* 2005;21:799-807.
10. Sánchez C, López-Herce J, Carillo A, Bustinza A, Sancho L, Vigil D. Transpyloric enteral feeding in the postoperative of cardiac surgery in children. *J Pediatr Surg.* 2006; 41:1096-1102.
11. Sánchez C, López-Herce J, Carrillo A, Mencía S, Vigil D. Early transpyloric enteral nutrition in critically ill children. *Nutrition.* 2007; 23:16-22.
12. Chellis MJ, Sanders SV, Webster H, et al. Early enteral feeding in the pediatric intensive care unit. *J Parenter Enteral Nutr.* 1996; 20:71-73.
13. Meert KL, Daphtary KM, Metheny NA. Gastric vs small-bowel feeding in critically ill children receiving mechanical ventilation: a randomized controlled trial. *Chest.* 2004; 126:872-878.
14. Khorasani EN, Mansouri F. Effect of early enteral nutrition on morbidity and mortality in children with burns. *Burns.* 2010;36:1067-1071.
15. Braudis NJ, Curley MAQ, Beaupre K, et al. Enteral feeding algorithm for infants with hypoplastic left heart syndrome post stage I palliation. *Pediatr Crit Care Med.* 2009;10: 460-466.
16. López-Herce J, Mencía S, Sánchez C, et al. Postpyloric enteral nutrition in the critically ill child with shock: a prospective observational study. *Nutr J.* 2008;7:6.
17. Gurgueira GL; Leite HP; de Aguiar Carrazedo Taddei JA, de Carvalho WB. *J Parenter Enteral Nutr.* 2005;29:176-185.
18. Petrillo-Albarano T, Pettignano R, MD, Asfaw M, et al. Use of a feeding protocol to improve nutritional support through early, aggressive, enteral nutrition in the pediatric intensive care unit. *Pediatr Crit Care Med.* 2006;7(4):340-344.
19. Meyer R, Harrison S, Sargent S, Ramnarayan P, Habibi P, Labadarios D. The impact of enteral feeding protocols on nutritional support in critically ill children. *J Hum Nutr Diet.* 2009;22:428-436.
20. Tume L, Latten L, Darbyshire A. An evaluation of enteral feeding practices in critically ill children. *Nurs Crit Care.* 2010;15(6):291-299.
21. Briassoulis G, Tsorva A, Zavras N, Hatzis T. Influence of an aggressive early enteral nutrition protocol on nitrogen balance in critically ill children. *J Nutr Biochem* 2002;13:560-569.
22. Hulst JM, van Goudoever JB, Zimmermann LJ, et al. Adequate feeding and the usefulness of the respiratory quotient in critically ill children. *Nutrition.* 2005;21: 192-198.
23. WHO Multicentre Growth Reference Study Group. "WHO Child Growth Standards: Length/Height-for-Age, Weight-for-Age, Weight-for-Length, Weight-for-Height and Body Mass Index-for-Age:Methods and Development," Geneva, Switzerland: World Health Organization 2006 (n.d.):1-312.
24. Secker DJ & Jeejeebhoy KN. Subjective global nutritional assessment for children. *Am J Clin Nutr.* 2007; 85(4): 1083-1089.
25. Vermilyea S, Slicker J, El-Chammas K, et al. Subjective global nutritional assessment in critically ill children. *J Parenter Enteral Nutr.* June 2012 (epub).
26. McClave S, Snider H. Use of indirect calorimetry in clinical nutrition. *Nutr Clin Prac.* 1992; 7(5):207-221.
27. Kyle UG, Arriaza A, Esposito M, Coss-Bu JA. Is indirect calorimetry a necessity or a luxury in the pediatric intensive care unit? *J Parenter Enteral Nutr.* 2012;36(2): 177-182.
28. Mehta NM, Bechard LJ, Leavitt K, Duggan C. Cumulative energy imbalance in the pediatric intensive care unit: role of targeted indirect calorimetry. *J Parenter Enteral Nutr.* 2009;33(3):336-344.

29. Hardy Framson CM, LeLeiko NS, Dallal GE, Roubenoff R, Snelling LK, Dwyer JT. Energy expenditure in critically ill children. *Pediatr Crit Care Med.* 2007;8(3):264-267.

30. White MS, Sheperd RW, McEniery JA. Energy expenditure in 100 ventilated, critically ill children: improving the accuracy of predictive equations. *Crit Care Med.* 2000;28(7):2307-2312.

31. Meyer R, Kulinskaya E, Briassoulis G, et al. The challenge of developing a new predictive formula to estimate energy requirements in ventilated critically ill children. *Nutr Clin Prac.* 2012;27(5):669-676.

32. Gramlich L, Kichian K, Pinilla J, Rodych NJ, Dhaliwal R, Heyland DK. Does enteral nutrition compared to parenteral nutrition result in better outcomes in critically ill adult patients? A systematic review of the literature. *Nutrition.* 2004;20(10):843-848.

33. Simpson F and Doig GS. Parenteral vs. enteral nutrition in the critically ill patient: a meta-analysis of trials using the intention to treat principle. *Intensive Care Med.* 2005;31(1):12-23.

34. Heyland DK, Dhaliwal R, Drover JW, Gramlich L, Dodek P. Canadian clinical practice guidelines for nutrition support in mechanically ventilated, critically ill adult patients. *J Parenter Enteral Nutr.* 2003;27(5):355-373.

35. Marik PE, Zaloga GP. Gastric versus post-pyloric feeding: a systematic review. *Crit Care.* 2003;7(3):46-51.

36. Ho KM, Dobb GJ, Webb SAR. A comparison of early gastric and post-pyloric feeding in critically ill patients: a meta-analysis. *Intensive Care Med.* 2006;32:639-649.

37. White H, Sosnowski K, Tran K, Reeves A, Jones M. A randomised controlled comparison of early post-pyloric versus early gastric feeding to meet nutritional targets in ventilated intensive care patients. *Crit Care.* 2009;13(6):187-195.

38. Meert KL, Daphtary KM, Metheny NA. Gastric vs small-bowel feeding in critically ill children receiving mechanical ventilation. A randomized controlled trial. *Chest.* 2004;126:872-878.

39. McClave SA, Martindale RG, Vanek VW, et al. Guidelines for the provision and assessment of nutrition support therapy in the adult critically ill patient: Society of Critical Care Medicine (SCCM) and American Society for Parenteral and Enteral Nutrition (A.S.P.E.N.). *J Parenter Enteral Nutr.* 2009;33(3):277-316.

40. Mehta NM. Approach to enteral feeding in the PICU. *Nutr Clin Pract.* 2009;24:377 .

41. Mehta N, McAleer D, Hamilton S, et al. Challenges to optimal enteral nutrition in a multidisciplinary pediatric intensive care unit. *J Parenter Enteral Nutr.* 2010; 34(1):38-45.

42. McClave SA, Sexton LK, Spain DA, et al. Enteral tube feeding in the intensive care unit: factors impeding adequate delivery. *Crit Care Med.* 1999;27(7):1252-1256.

43. Mentec H, Dupont H, Bocchetti M, Cani P, Ponche F, Bleichner Gl. Upper digestive intolerance during enteral nutrition in critically ill patients: frequency, risk factors, and complications. *Crit Care Med.* 2001;29(10):1955-1961.

44. Rogers EJ, Gilbertson HR, Heine RG, Henning R. Barriers to adequate nutrition in critically ill children. *Nutr.* 2003;19(10):865-868.

45. Kao CH, ChangLai SP, Chieng PU, Yen TC. Gastric emptying in head-injured patients. *Am J Gastro.* 1998; 3(7):1108-1112.

46. Ukleja A. Altered GI motility in critically ill patients: current understanding of pathophysiology, clinical impact, and diagnostic approach. *Nutr Clin Prac.* 2010;25(1):16-25.

47. Tarling MM, Toner CC, Withington PS, Baxter MK, Whelpton R, Goldhill DR. A model of gastric emptying using paracetamol absorption in intensive care patients. *Intensive Care Med.* 1997;23(3):256-260.

48. Taylor RM, Preedy VR, Baker AJ, Grimble G. Nutritional support in critically ill children. *Clin Nutr.* 2003;22(4):365-369.

49. Hulst JM, Joosten KF, Tibboel D, van Goudoever JB. Causes and consequences of inadequate substrate supply to pediatric ICU patients. *Curr Opin Clin Nutr Metab Care.* 2006;9(3):297-303.

50. Petros S, Engelmann L. Enteral nutrition delivery and energy expenditure in medical intensive care patients. *Clin Nutr.* 2006;25(1):51-59.

51. O'Leary-Kelley CM, Puntillo KA, Barr J, Stotts N, Douglas M. Nutritional adequacy in patients receiving mechanical ventilation who are fed enterally. *Am J Crit Care.* 2005;14(3):222-231.

52. Roberts SR, Kennerly DA, Keane D, George C. Nutrition support in the intensive care unit. Adequacy, timeliness, and outcomes. *Crit Care Nurs.* 2003;23(6):49-57.

53. Montejo JC. Enteral nutrition-related gastrointestinal complications in critically ill patients: a multicenter study. The Nutritional and Metabolic Working Group of the Spanish Society of Intensive Care Medicine and Coronary Units. *Crit Care Med.* 1999;27(8):1447-1453.

54. Metheny NA, Mills AC, Stewart BJ. Monitoring for intolerance to gastric tube feedings: a national survey. *Am J Crit Care.* 2012;21(2):e33-40.

55. McClave SA, Snider HL, Lowen CC, et al. Use of residual volume as a marker for enteral feeding intolerance: prospective blinded comparison with physical examination

and radiographic findings. *J Parenter Enteral Nutr.* 1992;16(2):99-105.

56. Sánchez C, Lopez-Herce J, Carrillo A, Mencia, Vigil D. Early transpyloric enteral nutrition in critically ill children. *Nutr.* 2007;23(1):16-22.
57. Montejo González JC, Culebras-Fernandez JM, Garcia de Lorenzo y Mateos A. Recommendations for the nutritional assessment of critically ill patients. *Rev Méd Chile.* 2006;134(8):1049-1056.
58. Adam S and Batson S. A study of problems associated with the delivery of enteral feed in critically ill patients in five ICUs in the UK. *Intensive Care Med.* 1997;23(3): 261-266.
59. Fraser RBL and Bryant L. Current and future therapeutic prokinetic therapy to improve enteral feed intolerance in the ICU patient. *Nutr Clin Pract.* 2010;25(1):26-31.
60. Tume L, Carter B, Latten L. A UK and Irish survey of enteral nutrition practices in paediatric intensive care units. *Br J Nutr*, 2012;Firstview (2):1-19.
61. American Society of Anesthesiologists (2011), Practice Guidelines for preoperative fasting and the use of pharmacologic agents to reduce the risk of pulmonary aspiration: application to healthy patients undergoing elective procedures. An updated report by the American Society of Anesthesiologists Committee on Standards and Practice Parameters. *Anesthesiology.* 2011;114:495-511.
62. Asai T. Constipation: does it increase morbidity and mortality in critically ill patients? *Crit Care Med.* 2007;35(12):2861-2862.
63. van der Spoel JI, Schultz MJ, van der Voort PHJ and de Jonge E. Influence of severity of illness, medication and selective decontamination on defecation. *Intensive Care Med.* 2006;32(6):875-880.
64. McPeake J, Glimour H, MacIntosh G. The implementation of a bowel management protocol in an adult intensive care unit. *Nurs Crit Care.* 2011;16(5):235-242.
65. van der Spoel JI, Straaten A, Kuiper MA, van Roon EN, Zandstra DF, van der Voort PHJ. Laxation of critically ill patients with lactulose or polyethylene glycol: a two-center randomized, double-blind, placebo-controlled trial. *Crit Care Med.* 2007;35(12):2726-2731.
66. Tofil NM, Benner KW, Faro SJ and Winkler MK. The use of enteral naloxone to treat opioid-induced constipation in a pediatric intensive care unit. *Pediatr Crit Care Med.* 2006;7(3):252-254.
67. Yuan CS, Foss JF, O'Connor M, Toledano A, Roizen MF d, Moss J. Methylnaltrexone prevents morphine-induced delay in oral-cecal transit time without affecting analgesia: a double-blind randomized placebo-controlled trial. *Clin Pharmacol Ther.* 1996;59:469-475.
68. Garten L, Degenhardt P, Buhrer C. Resolution of opioid-induced postoperative newborn infant after methylnaltrexone. *J Ped Surg.* 2011;46:E13-E15.
69. Lee JM, Mooney J. Methylnaltrexone in treatment of opioid-induced constipation in a pediatric patient. *Clin J Pain.* 2012;28:338-341.
70. Herbert MK, Holzer P. Standardized concept for the treatment of gastrointestinal dysmotility in critically ill patients: current status and future options. *Clin Nutri.* 2008;27(1):25-41.
71. Chapman MJ, Fraser RJ, Kluger MT, Buist MD, Nichilo DJ. Erythromycin improves gastric emptying in critically ill patients intolerant of nasogastric feeding. *Crit Care Med.* 2000;28(7):2334-2337.
72. Nguyen NQ, Chapman MJ, Fraser RJ, Bryant LK, Holloway RH. Erythromycin is more effective than metoclopramide in the treatment of feed intolerance in critical illness. *Crit Care Med.* 2007;35(2):483-489.
73. Nguyen NQ, Chapman M, Fraser RJ, Bryant LK, Burhstad C, Holloway RH. Prokinetic therapy for feed intolerance in critical illness: one drug or two? *Crit Care Med.* 2007;35(11):2561-2567.
74. Ng E, Shah VS. Erythromycin for the prevention and treatment of feeding intolerance in preterm infants. *Cochrane Database of Systematic Reviews (Online)* no. 3 (2008).
75. Cook DJ, Fuller HD, Guyutt GH, et al. Risk factors for gastrointestinal bleeding in critically ill patients. *New Eng J Med.* 1994;330:377-381.
76. Quenot JP, Thiery N, Barbar S. When should stress ulcer prophylaxis be used in the ICU? *Curr Opin Crit Care.* 2009,15:129-143.
77. Martindale R. Contemporary strategies for the prevention of stress-related mucosal bleeding. *American Journal of Health-System Pharmacy.* 2005; 62(10):Suppl 2 S11-17.
78. Welage L. Overview of pharmacologic agents for acid suppression in critically ill patients. *Am J Health Syst Pharm* 2005;62(10):Suppl 2 S4-10.
79. Judges D, Beverly S, Rio A, Goff LM. Clinical guidelines and enteral nutrition support: a survey of dietetic practice in the United Kingdom. *Eur J Clin Nutr.* 2012; 66:130-135.

SECTION 3

Disease-related Nutrition Considerations

CHAPTER 10

Nutritional Support of the Critically ill Neonate

Melissa S. Rice
Carrie Smith
Christina J. Valentine

- INTRODUCTION
- GOALS FOR GROWTH AND NUTRITION ASSESSMENT
  - Assessment of Neonatal Nutritional Status
  - Clinical Assessment Tools
  - Energy
  - Special Disease Considerations
  - Protein
  - Lipids
- MICRONUTRIENTS
  - Vitamins
  - Trace Elements
- PARENTERAL NUTRITION
  - Vitamins/Minerals
- ENTERAL NUTRITION
  - Human Milk
  - Pasteurized Donor Human Milk
  - Formulas
  - Intermittent Bolus Feedings
  - Continuous Feedings
- KEY POINTS
  - References

INTRODUCTION

Over the last 30 years, survival rates have improved among preterm infants of all gestational ages.[1] With increasing survival rates, it has become evident that neonatal nutrition is important to prevent postnatal growth restriction, achieve appropriate body composition, and prevent neurodevelopmental impairment.[2] Nutrition previously provided by the placenta can now be provided as parenteral or enteral support in an effort to allow these infants to mimic intrauterine growth as closely as possible. Studies have shown growth velocity alone to be associated with developmental outcomes, emphasizing the importance of appropriate nutrition for the neonatal population.[2,3] Providing the best nutrition for any high-risk, critically ill neonate is an evolving field, and determining how to deliver the best nutrition for gut maturation as well as effective nutrient absorption is still debated. Previous nutritional strategies emphasized catch-up growth through increased calories, with an emphasis on carbohydrate and lipid intake. This nutritional plan led to late catch-up growth, with infants that were shorter and fatter than term infants at the same corrected gestational age.[4] In addition to providing higher calories, new data have shown protein to be an important component for lean muscle mass synthesis and linear growth.[5] Appropriate nutrition is also important to prevent anemia of prematurity and osteopenia of prematurity, and appears to play an important role in prevention of necrotizing enterocolitis (NEC).[6]

GOALS FOR GROWTH AND NUTRITION ASSESSMENT

The goal set forth by the American Academy of Pediatrics is to provide neonatal nutrition to best mimic fetal accretion rates for the appropriate gestational age of each infant.[7] These intrauterine growth rates are estimated to be 20 to 30 grams per day, increasing with gestational age nearing a full-term fetus. Postnatal growth rate goals for preterm infants range from 16 to 18 g/kg per day.[8] Goal increase for length is 1.1 cm per week, while goal increase for head circumference is 0.7 to 1 cm per week. Once infants near term-corrected gestational age, a goal of 20 to 30 grams per day is appropriate, and infants should follow the trajectory of growth in the World Health Organization charts.[7]

Intrauterine growth rates are often not achieved until near the time of discharge from the neonatal intensive care unit (NICU), while needed catch-up growth does not occur until after discharge.[1] When growth mimicking fetal rates are achieved, infants are often found to be shorter than their term counterparts.[9] Achievement of appropriate postnatal growth will reduce the risks of developing morbidities such as cardiovascular disease and neurodevelopment impairment.[10]

Assessment of Neonatal Nutritional Status

Assessment of nutritional status can be difficult in the preterm infant where normative standardized data are limited, especially among the extremely low birth weight (ELBW) (<1500 gm) and very low birth weight (VLBW) (<1000 gm) populations. Anthropometric analysis remains the standard of care (head circumference, length, and weight), but can vary widely from infant to infant. These data are also difficult to obtain in a consistent manner on smaller, critically ill infants with endotracheal tubes, umbilical catheters, and large fluid fluctuations. Monitoring growth with at least weekly measurements plotted on the Fenton premature infant growth curves[8] not only shows whether adequate growth is being achieved at that time, but also displays trends of growth over time. Protein adequacy can be evaluated acutely by using the blood urea nitrogen (BUN), which has been established as an important tool to assess protein accretion, with levels less than 9 often a sign of suboptimal protein intake.[11] If the neonate is on parenteral nutrition (PN) for 2 weeks or longer, obtaining direct bilirubin is important to evaluate for cholestasis (direct bilirubin ≥2 mg/dL (≥34.2 mmol/L)).Electrolytes such as potassium, sodium, calcium, and phosphorus are important to evaluate 1 to 2 times in the first week of nutrition support and then can be spaced to biweekly or as needed. Bone health screening should also include alkaline phosphatase in the first week and then biweekly to evaluate for osteopenia.

Clinical Assessment Tools

New tools are currently being investigated for better assessment of neonatal nutrition, since the current standard use of anthropometrics has limits. Head circumference varies based on placement of the measuring tape. Length requires at least 2 individuals to measure accurately and can be difficult to obtain in neonates that cannot be moved easily. Weight is more standardized, but can vary based on fluid/hydration status. Air displacement plethysmography is a new technology that is noninvasive and can measure fat and fat-free mass.[12,13] Other methods of measurement, such stable isotope measurement and dual-energy x-ray absorptiometry (DEXA) scan to asses bone mineral density have been utilized for research purposes, but are not feasible in the clinical setting.

Energy

The resting energy expenditure (REE) in a growing fetus is estimated to be a minimum of 35 kcal/kg per day, which is provided by maternal glucose, placental lactate, and maternal amino acids.[9] The growing neonate, however, has a higher metabolic demand due to added demand of cold stress, nutritional processing, activity, and growth. The neonate has an REE of 45 kcal/kg per day.[14] Each gram of new tissue requires 4.5 to 5 kcal/g for synthesis. In order to achieve fetal accretion rates of 16 g/kg per day requires 72 to 80 kcal/kg above REE.[15,16] To provide adequate calories for REE and growth, a minimum of 80 to 90 parenteral kcal[17] or 120 enteral kcal/kg per day should be provided to the preterm infant,[18] or 100 to 110 kcal/kg per day for the full-term critically ill neonate.[19] The amount of nutrition provided should create a positive energy balance to prevent further nutritional deficits in a population with an already increased metabolic demand. Caloric deficits can result in the use of amino acids for anabolism, creating a possible protein deficit.[20] Younger gestational age and low birth weight can increase this baseline requirement.[15,21] See Table 10-1 for the estimated energy and protein intake recommendations for VLBW infants.

TABLE 10-1. Estimated Energy and Protein Needs of the Very Low Birth Weight Infant

	ESPGHAN (2009)	AAPCON (2009)	LSRO (2002)	CPS (1995)
Energy (kcal/kg per day)	130-150	105-130	110-135	105-135
Protein (g/kg per day)	3.8-4.4	3.4-4.2	3.4-4.3	3.0-3.6

Special Disease Considerations

During times of stress, the REE may not necessarily increase in the critically ill neonate. For example, neonates on extracorporeal membrane oxygenation may have highly variable changes in REE, but require 20% more protein due to high metabolic turnover. As a whole, infants immediately postprocedure may transiently need double the protein support to promote tissue healing.[22] The REE did not change in infants pre- and postpatent ductus arteriosus (PDA) ligation on PN.[23]

Protein

Protein accretion is dependent on protein intake, whether enteral or parental. A minimum of 1 to 1.5 g/kg per day of protein is required to prevent catabolism of protein or cumulative deficits.[18] Protein deficits occur quickly in neonates for many reasons. Although early enteral feeding within 24 hours of life is encouraged, infants are often not fed due to cardiorespiratory instability at the time of delivery.[24] Feedings are often slowly increased over time due to concern for the development of NEC, decreased perfusion to the intestinal vascular bed, and/or hypoxic injury in cases of traumatic birth. This is especially true in the ELBW and VLBW populations, where many centers currently follow protocols with gradual increases in feeding. This leaves the amino acid composition of PN as the primary source of protein, which may be less effective at preventing proteolysis.[25] Even if protein is provided parenterally within 24 hours of life, infants often begin life with an overall protein deficit,[26] which affects growth velocity in the short term and mental and motor developmental outcomes later.[3]

Providing ill neonates with the appropriate protein-to-calorie ratio is paramount, as this promotes skeletal muscle synthesis, prevents proteolysis, and allows for protein accretion. Estimated protein requirements for fetal growth and accretion range from 4.3 g/kg per day for the 700- to 1000-g fetus, 4.0 g/kg per day for the 1000- to 1500-g fetus, and 3.6 g/kg per day for the 1500- to 2000-g fetus.[27] Protein requirements for growth and accretion increase as gestation age decreases.[28] Whey and casein are the major protein sources in human milk and formula for the neonate. Whey has increased solubility, provides more rapid gastric emptying, and an increased amount of branched-chain amino acids (BCAA). The content of BCAA in whey protein has also been found to be associated with increased skeletal muscle protein synthesis and transient rise in leucine oxidation.[29] Protein content has been shown to decrease as breast milk matures. Whey-to-casein ratio in colostrum is 80:20, which later changes to 55:45 in mature milk.[30] Preterm formulas are higher in protein content than standard-term formulas, providing a 60:40 composition of protein, more closely mimicking that found in breast milk, but only providing 3 to 3.6 g/kg per day without fortification.[31] Current formulas and fortifiers require volumes of 165 to 180 mL/kg per day in order to achieve protein goal intakes of 4 g/kg per day.[27] Often, pasteurized donor milk is provided to ill infants for its vital biological value when mother's milk is not available, but nutritionally, the protein content averages only 0.4 to 0.7 g/dL of protein. Donor milk is also significantly lower in glycine, aspartate, valine, phenylalanine, proline, lysine, arginine, and serine.[32] Unfortified human milk would need to be provided in volumes of 180 to 200 mL/kg per day to achieve appropriate protein accretion rates.[33] Higher-protein formulas are now available, providing up to 4.6 g/kg per day. Studies have shown that initial concerns of acidosis and elevated BUN do not occur with the use of these formulas,[20] and adequate growth parameters are achieved when infants fed human milk are supported with these products.

Prevention of proteolysis and promotion of skeletal muscle synthesis in the preterm infant require an adequate protein-to-energy ratio. Studies comparing early amino acid intake 1 g/kg per day vs. 3 g/kg per day showed a 35% higher protein synthesis rate when infants were given 3 g/kg per day.[16] A linear relationship has been observed with increased amino acid intake and accretion when infants were provided with at least 3 g/kg per day of protein.[25]

Skeletal muscle synthesis has been shown to increase with the postprandial rise in insulin and amino acids in the neonate. Both insulin and essential amino acids appear to promote synthesis independently.[29] Providing nutrition with an increased protein-to-energy ratio has been shown to increase lean muscle mass weight gain in neonates.[34] The protein-to-calorie ratio should be maintained close to 4.3 g:120 kcal. Excessive calories provided by a nonprotein source will be stored as fat, which can lead to detrimental side effects later in life based on the theory of "programming." Following this theory, former preterm infants with increased fat mass are at greater at risk for development of hypertension, diabetes mellitus, and renal disease as they age.[2]

Lipids

Preterm infants miss a large portion of the accretion of the longer-chain fatty acid docosahexaenoic acid (DHA) that occurs over the last trimester of pregnancy,[35,36] making it essential that they receive this nutrient in their dietary management in the NICU.

All mammals require the fatty acids linoleic (C18:2n-6) and alpha-linolenic acid (C18:3n-3) in the diet because they are incapable of inserting the cis double bond at the n-6 and n-3 position from the carboxyl terminus.[35] The liver is the predominant organ that receives the triglyceride form of the fat in the diet and, using a series of lipases, extracts the nonesterified fatty acid[37] and in the endoplasmic reticulum desaturates (adds a double bond) and elongates the acyl chain of the parent fatty acid to its longer chain and more unsaturated compounds arachidonic acid (ARA) (C20:4n-6) and docosahexaenoic acid (DHA) (C22:6n-3)[38] (see **Fig. 10-1**). These long-chain polyunsaturated fatty acids (LCPUFA) not only produce different prostaglandins, but DHA has related products called resolvins that can promote the resolution of inflammation.[39] Docosahexaenoic acid is also the predominant fatty acid in the cerebral cortex, retinal rods, and cones and significantly influences function.[40] Historically, there was a balance of the n-6 and n-3 fatty acids to provide a homeostasis between the two, but as dietary habits have changed over the 20th century,[41] there has been a dramatic increase in n-6 fatty acid consumption, thus altering the balance between pro- and anti-inflammatory events.[42]

In addition, the biosynthesis dependent on the desaturase and elongase enzyme activities may not be able to

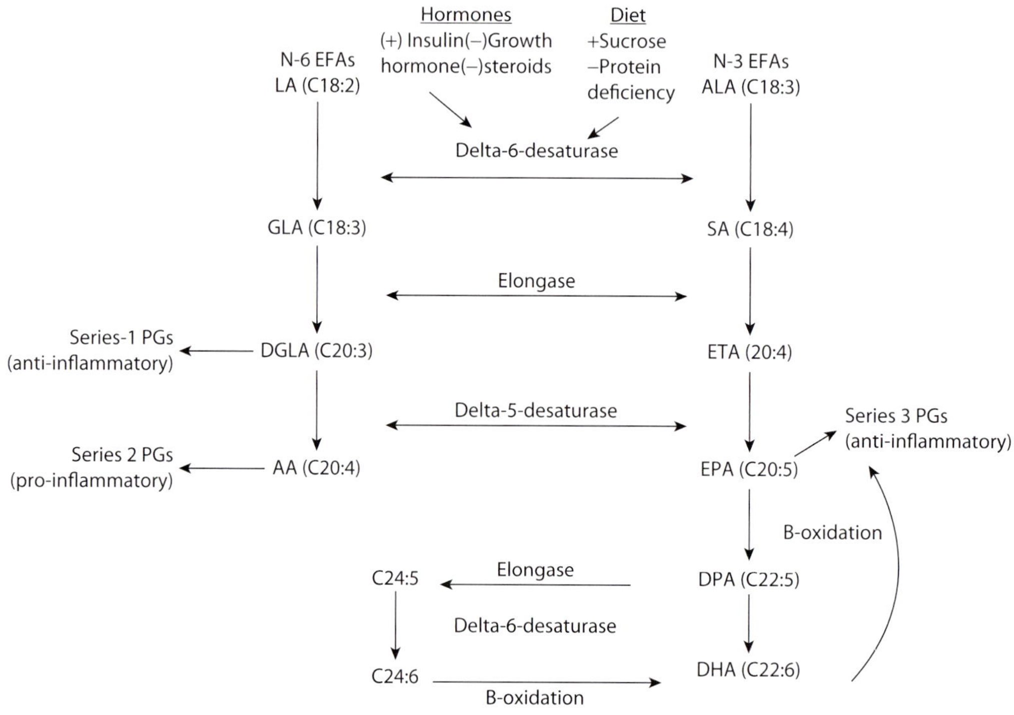

FIGURE 10-1. Lipid metabolism in the newborn infant.

produce enough DHA because of the competition the fatty acids have for the same enzymes.[43] Maternal dietary sources for linoleic and alpha-linolenic acid are found primarily in plant oils such as corn, olive, poppy seed, palm, soybean, rapeseed, safflower, sunflower, and wheat germ.[39] Dietary sources of preformed ARA are in animal products; DHA can be found in oily marine sources such as salmon, mackerel, tuna, and herring. Eggs that are the product of hens fed omega-3s are also good sources of DHA for the nursing mother.[44] The advisable intakes (AIs) for a nursing mother are 13 grams per day of linoleic acid and 1.3 grams of alpha-linolenic acid per day.[45] The recommendation for the infant is to ingest 4.4 grams per day of linoleic acid and 0.5 grams per day of alpha-linolenic acid to prevent essential fatty acid deficiency.[46] Recommendations have not been officially made for DHA, but based on randomized controlled trials, it is suggested that women who are pregnant or nursing receive a minimum of 200 mg/day of DHA in the diet.[47] For the preterm infant, an enteral intake of 12 to 30 mg/kg per day of DHA is recommended by the European Society for Pediatric Gastroenterology, Hepatology, and Nutrition Committee on Nutrition.[48]

Term infants fed human milk receive 750 mL/day of milk, and that dietary fat provides 55% of the total calories and 4 grams per deciliter, which provides ample essential fatty acids.[40] Commercial term and preterm formulas are designed to provide a minimum of a 5:1 ratio of linoleic to alpha-linolenic acids to reach a minimum standard when compared to human milk samples. Formulas with a lower 4:1 ratio resulted in a fatty acid erythrocyte composition of the formula-fed infants to be lower than in the reference breastfed group.[41]

Dietary fatty acid intake is reflected in the plasma or erythrocyte fatty acid measurements.[49] A significant correlation can also be measured in red blood cell phospholipids, which increase with corresponding increases in dietary DHA intake.[43,49] Laboratory documentation of essential fatty acid deficiency is determined by an increased concentration of either the nonessential fatty acid eicosatrienoic ("triene") or mead acid of the n-9 family compared to the ARA concentration from the n-6 family ("tetraene"), or the triene-to-tetraene ratio measured in the plasma >0.4 mg/dL.[42] Preterm neonates exhibit laboratory evidence of fatty acid deficiency by 5 days of life when they are not fed essential fatty acids.[50] Clinical deficiency signs for the essential fatty acids include a scaly dermatitis and platelet dysfunction.[51] Deficiency symptoms have not been described for DHA, but preterm infants have demonstrated slow growth when ratio of their intake with ARA was altered in earlier fish oil supplement studies.[52]

The preterm infant, unlike the term infant, is not ingesting 750 mL per day of human milk or formula for months, and is often on small amounts of enteral milk at 20 mL/kg for days and is supplemented with intravenous nutrition as feedings are advanced. Current intravenous sources of lipid emulsions in the United States provide adequate essential fatty acids but only trace amounts of ARA and DHA. Compassionate therapy with an intravenous emulsion that contains fish oil that has DHA in the product has been prescribed in the NICU, but has primarily been reserved for the infant with hepatic cholestasis.[53] Reliance on enteral sources of DHA is, therefore, vital. The biosynthesis of LCPUFA from the dietary ingestion of the precursor fatty acids can be of concern, however, for the preterm infant, unlike the term infant, because of additional confounders. Preterm infants have enzymes available for conversion, but total quantity of DHA produced may be small.[50] In preterm infants, the effects of DHA on developmental indices is even more striking, particularly in the most premature infants.[54] Henriksen et al. directly supplemented preterm infants with 32 mg of DHA and 31 mg ARA to their human milk feedings in the NICU and found that the supplemented group had higher problem-solving scores at 6 months of age.[55] Most recently, increased whole-blood concentrations of DHA have been retrospectively found to correlate with decreased bronchopulmonary dysplasia.[56]

Based on the clinical evidence, milk sources with 1% to 1.5% fatty acid as DHA have been suggested for the premature infant.[57] Preterm formulas contain both DHA and ARA but not at these suggested concentrations. The practice of direct supplementation of the neonate's milk with an exogenous supplement is compelling, but can be difficult in the intensive care unit (ICU). Most practical is the direct supplementation of the mother ensuring her optimal health, preventing premature deliveries, and improving the quality of her milk to ensure an adequate balance of fatty acids. It appears an intake of DHA of 1 gram per day in the maternal diet would meet the dietary needs of the high-risk infant that is receiving human milk.[58]

MICRONUTRIENTS

In utero, infants have a high accretion rate of micronutrients during the third trimester, while neonates born prematurely have an increased demand for micronutrients due to their targeted catch-up growth and ineffective metabolism. They are, therefore, at high risk for micronutrient deficiency if they are not provided with the appropriate vitamins and minerals through enteral or parenteral nutrition during this period. Neonates are also at risk for vitamin toxicity due to their altered urinary excretion rates.

Vitamins

Water-soluble vitamins, such as the B and C vitamins, do not accumulate in the body (with the exception of vitamin B_{12}), and therefore need to be provided on a daily basis to prevent neonatal deficiency from developing.[59,60] The human milk fortifiers and commercial preterm formulations are adequate to meet the needs of the high-risk infant. Infants on PN require special dosing based on term compared to preterm standards.[61] Fat-soluble vitamins such as A, D, E, and K are produced by precursors and are stored in the body. They do not need to be provided in addition to the diet on a daily basis, with the exception of a few disease states such as cystic fibrosis. Vitamin D is now recommended for all infants on human milk or <500 mL of formula.[7] Because these vitamins are stored, potential for toxicity exists.

Vitamin A (retinol) is important for pulmonary epithelial growth and cellular differentiation. Deficiency may play a role in chronic lung disease, and a randomized control trial of 5000 IU administered intramuscularly 3 times per week in a preterm cohort was associated with 55% incidence of chronic lung disease when compared to 62% in control patients.[62] However, an oral dose of vitamin A did not demonstrate similar effects.[63]

Vitamin D is necessary to prevent rickets and hypocalcemia.[64] Free vitamin D is not increased in the infant until the third trimester, leaving preterm infants at greater risk for rickets or osteopenia. Vitamin D plays an active role in the absorption of calcium and phosphorus in the neonatal gut, as well as metabolism of bone.[65] In the face of vitamin D deficiency in the neonate, calcium is not adequately absorbed from the intestine, minerals are reabsorbed from the bone, and new bone is not adequately mineralized, creating a rachitic and weak skeleton.[64] Breast milk is naturally low in vitamin D, and therefore infants require supplementation. Neonates being fed human milk are at high risk for vitamin D deficiency and should receive supplementation of at least 400 IU per day to prevent the development of rickets and hypocalcemia.[66]

Vitamin E (tocopherol) provides antioxidant properties. Deficiency leads to increased hemolysis, especially in the face of peroxide or other reactive oxygen species, anemia, thrombocytosis, and neurological deficits.[67]

Vitamin K is required for carboxylation of prothrombin into active form in the coagulation cascade.[68] The dietary recommended intake (DRI) is easily achieved by a standard intake of formula, but maternal milk is deficient in vitamin K. Deficiency can lead to hemorrhagic disease of the newborn,[69] which is now prevented with recommended intramuscular injections of vitamin K after birth in the United States.[7,68] Vitamin K does require optimal factors in the intestinal tract for absorption enterally, and thus innate deficiency, maternal medications (anticonvulsants and warfarin), malabsorptive or intestinal injury, the immature preterm liver, or lack of intestinal microorganisms that synthesize vitamin K could each lead to deficiency.[68,70] While most infants do not need further supplementation of vitamin K beyond the recommended injection provided to the newborn, infants with cholestatic liver disease and other conditions that interfere with vitamin K absorption will need additional supplements.

Trace Elements

Trace elements play an important role in regulation of metabolic pathways and cofactor function, but there is a paucity of research in the neonatal field. Chromium is important for insulin metabolism and can affect glucose regulation. Copper is integral for red blood cell production and iron absorption.[71] Iron is a component of hemoglobin, critical for oxygen and carbon dioxide transport, as well as neurodevelopment.[72] Manganese plays a role in activation of superoxide dismutase and is a component of normal bone structure and carbohydrate metabolism. Zinc plays a role in several enzymes and is important for growth.[73] Derangement of these pathways can lead to detrimental effects such as anemia, osteopenia of prematurity, failure to thrive, neutropenia, dermatitis, and malabsorption.[72,73]

PARENTERAL NUTRITION

In order to achieve adequate intake of nutrients for REE and growth, PN is initiated due to a preterm or critically ill infant's inability to tolerate large volumes of enteral nutrition immediately after birth.[28,74,75] It is used as a bridge to full enteral nutrition, as well as the sole source of nutrition for those conditions where enteral nutrition is contraindicated. Parenteral nutrition should be initiated within hours after delivery to help prevent starvation, normalize glucose levels, and improve nitrogen balance.[28,76]

The provision of carbohydrate is an immediate priority because of the fetal abruption of glucose delivery and the brain's requirements.[9] The exact glucose infusion rate (GIR) (usually expressed in mg/kg of body weight per minute) has yet to be determined; however, for euglycemia, it may be beneficial to begin with a GIR that is similar to the fetus, such as of 4 to 8 mg/kg per minute (with a tighter range of 4 to 6 mg/kg per minute for ELBW infants and infants that are critically ill).[77,78] Factors to consider when initiating and advancing GIRs are gestational age, enteral nutrition advancement, glucose concentration levels, and laboratory values.[78] Glucose infusion rates should be increased as tolerated to reach a goal of 10 to 13 mg/kg per minute.[77] Insulin is necessary if a normal GIR is not obtainable.[79] The operational threshold for blood glucose goals is >40 mg/dL.[80]

Along with glucose, a parenteral source of amino acids for protein should be initiated. Early administration of intravenous amino acids has been shown to be beneficial for preterm infants with no known harm.[81-85] Early amino acid administration is essential to prevent catabolism, improve nitrogen balance, decrease growth failure, and improve neurodevelopmental outcomes.[76,81,85,86] Hyperglycemic episodes in neonates can be reduced by administering amino acids, and the reduction in episodes can be maximized with early administration of amino acids.[82] This is possibly due to the promotion of insulin secretion by amino acids.[78] Full enteral nutrition can be achieved sooner and PN duration shortened with the administration of amino acids.[85] It is suggested that early amino acid administration of 3 gm/kg per day be initiated to match in utero accretion rates.[28,87]

Next, lipids are important for overall nutrition and allow for increased energy intake early in life, as well as prevention of essential fatty acid deficiency.[76,88] An intravenous lipid dose of 0.5 to 1 gm/kg per day is needed to prevent essential fatty acid deficiency.[76,81] Lipids also influence oxidative stress, immune responses, and inflammation.[57] Early lipid administration amounts are still controversial; however, lipid administration should occur as soon as possible, ideally on the day of birth or by the day after birth.[28] A review of intravenous lipids suggests that lipids not be started any greater than 0.5 to 1 gm/kg per day for the preterm infant and specifically for those with birth weights <800 gm.[77,88] Hypertriglyceridemia (defined as >201 mg/dL) is more likely to occur when lipids are initiated at 2 gm/kg per day.[86]

Electrolytes in PN should include sodium and potassium. Early administration, however, should be restricted to allow for appropriate diuresis.[89] Once diuresis has occurred, a goal of 2 to 5 mEq/kg/day of sodium and 2 to 4 mEq/kg/day of potassium should be provided to achieve optimal fluid and electrolyte balance.[77] These amounts should be adjusted based on clinical findings such as edema and laboratory values.

Vitamins/Minerals

Calcium and phosphorus are vital during PN to help prevent/minimize osteopenia of prematurity.[76] A Ca:P ratio of 1.7:1 by weight is recommended for mineral retention.[76] Magnesium should be provided at 0.3 to 0.5 mEq/kg per day, as magnesium is important in calcium and potassium homeostasis, as well as activation for coenzymes needed for metabolism of carbohydrates and protein.[76] Zinc, involved in tissue building and skin integrity, is important for a neonate due to the loss of in utero accretion during the third trimester, and therefore must be included in PN solutions at 400 mcg/kg per day.[76,89,90] Copper deficiency, although rare, can occur in neonates if supplementation does not occur. It is recommended that PN solutions contain 20 mcg/kg per day, with a reduction if cholestasis occurs.[76,91] However, if copper provision is decreased due to cholestasis, regular monitoring is recommended to prevent deficiency. Manganese should be avoided for those infants receiving short-term PN due to the potential for toxicity, as trace element mixtures often contain manganese as a contaminant.[92] Selenium, an important antioxidant, should be included in PN solutions at 2 mcg/kg per day.[93] Neonates receiving long-term PN may benefit from carnitine administration of 2 to 5 mg/kg per day due to carnitine's involvement in transporting fatty acids to mitochondria for oxidation. Carnitine may also help prevent cholestasis as well as hypertriglyceridemia.[77,94]

Parenteral nutrition support is maximized when provided via a central catheter. However, central catheters are often a cause of bloodstream infections, which are responsible for nosocomial infections and account for approximately three-quarters of all health care–associated infections.[95] The use of PN should be minimized, if possible, with the goal to advance to full enteral nutrition support as quickly as possible after birth based on the infant's stability.

ENTERAL NUTRITION

Trophic enteral nutrition, or minimal enteral nutrition, is initiated to promote gut maturity as well as to prevent gut atrophy and should begin as soon as the infant is medically stable.[28,75,76,96-98] This is usually initiated at 10 to

20 mL/kg per day, with advancement in increments of 20 to 35 mL/kg per day thereafter.[99] Preterm infants with early enteral nutrition administration reach full enteral nutrition quicker and achieve better growth than those with delayed initiation.[74,96-98] Early enteral nutrition has also been associated with faster maturation of motor patterns and less feeding intolerance with no increases in the incidence of NEC.[98] It is beneficial to create feeding protocols in NICUs to establish when to initiate trophic feedings and how and when to advance them.[28,96,100] Once enteral nutrition is at volumes that can provide adequate nutrients, PN should be discontinued. In addition to human milk, many milk products and choices are available in the United States to feed a neonate. Deciding on the most appropriate feeding product can be crucial to survival, growth, and neurodevelopmental outcomes.

Human Milk

Human milk contains immunoprotective properties such as immunogloblulins, lactoferrin, lymphocytes, oligosaccharides, and lysozyme that inhibit bacterial growth and minimize inflammation[74,98,101] and is therefore considered the best feeding choice for all infants, regardless of gestational age.[81,102] The use of human milk has been shown to decrease the risk for such conditions as late-onset sepsis and NEC compared to the use of formula in preterm infants.[74,81,96,103-105] Human milk is also associated with improved neurodevelopmental outcomes[104,106] and improved gastric emptying.[74] There is evidence to suggest that the benefit of human milk increases as the amount of human milk provided to the infant in the first weeks of life increases.[96,100,104,107] When breast milk is pumped and stored for later use, it should be provided to the infant in chronological order of pumping to maximize these benefits.[101] Colostrum, which can only be provided by an infant's own mother, has been shown to stimulate growth in the intestinal mucosa and stimulate digestive enzymes when provided as the first feed.[107]

Pasteurized Donor Human Milk

Human milk has been shown to have such beneficial qualities that the American Academy of Pediatrics states all infants less than 1500 grams at birth receive human milk, and if the mother's own milk is not available, then donor milk should be utilized.[104] It is often difficult for mothers of preterm infants to provide an adequate initial supply of breast milk. Early and frequent pumping is necessary to establish and maintain a milk supply.[106] Skin-to-skin contact has also been shown to increase/maintain maternal milk supply.[106] Pasteurized donor milk from milk banks such as the Human Milk Banking Association of North America (HMBANA)[101] has become a more widely accepted and utilized alternative to mother's own milk. Donor milk has been associated with lower rates of NEC than in formula-fed infants.[96,105] Donor milk has also been shown to provide many of the immunoprotective qualities of mother's own milk, as well as protection from cardiovascular risks.[108] Breast milk pumped by mothers of preterm infants is higher in protein, calcium, sodium, and calories for several weeks.[101,105,109] One downside to the use of donor milk is the decreased amounts of protein and other nutrients such as DHA, which may affect neurodevelopment and retinal maturation.[105,108] This is likely due to the donor milk being a product that is produced during later lactation.

Human milk has been shown to be low in nutrients (calories, protein, calcium, phosphorus, vitamin D, and sodium) necessary for a preterm infant or high-risk critically ill infant on volume restriction and, therefore, fortification of human milk is necessary for appropriate growth and to minimize osteopenia risk, late hyponatremia, and negative nitrogen balance.[57,81,87,99,109] The previously available human milk fortifiers have been inadequate in terms of protein concentration to meet the increased protein needs of the preterm infant.[102] Often, fortified human milk feedings need to be further fortified with additional protein to meet these increased protein needs.[28,99] Increased protein administration via a human milk fortifier has been shown to improve weight gain and result in fewer length measurements plotted less than the tenth percentile on preterm growth charts without adverse side effects.[102] A higher-protein human milk fortifier and a liquid protein fortifier are currently available in the United States.

Previously, only powder forms of human milk fortifiers were available. Two liquid versions of human milk fortifiers are now available: a bovine-based fortifier and a human milk-based fortifier. These liquid versions provide for a more sterile method of fortifying human milk. Another method for increasing the caloric content of breast milk is the use of hindmilk, which is higher in calories and fat than foremilk[101] and therefore may be beneficial in terms of weight gain. Fortification, however, is still required for essential nutrient provision[110] and to increase protein content.

Formulas

Preterm infant formulas are designed to meet the nutritional needs of a preterm infant in the absence of maternal breast milk. Preterm infant formulas contain ~50% of calories as fat, ~10% of calories as protein (cow's milk), and ~40% of calories as carbohydrates (glucose polymers to aid in digestion).[110] They were also designed to provide increased calories and protein for improved growth, as well as additional calcium and phosphorus to aid in the prevention of osteopenia of prematurity; furthermore, they are iron fortified.[110-111] With the knowledge of the role that DHA and ARA play in a preterm infant's cognitive and visual development, preterm infant formulas now contain DHA and ARA.[48,104] Protein hydrolysate formulas (where protein is in the form of di- and tripeptides) can be helpful in cow milk allergy, and elemental formulas (where protein is in the form of free amino acids) can be helpful in intestinal injury, where they have been shown to reduce the time to get off PN when human milk is not available.[112] Soy formulations should not be used for the preterm infant because of concerns that they may adversely affect bone mineralization.[7]

See **Fig. 10-2** for an algorithm suggested to choose a formulation based on physiology.

Intermittent Bolus Feedings

An intermittent bolus feeding is a set volume of milk provided over a short period, usually over 10 to 20 minutes every 2 to 3 hours by gravity.[113] This administration of enteral nutrition is more physiologic for an infant; however, there may be an increase in energy expenditure, reflux, and abdominal distention.[76,113]

Continuous Feedings

A continuous feeding consists of a set volume of milk infused continuously on a pump.[113] If there are any issues with tolerance to bolus enteral nutrition and/or reflux or respiratory distress, then continuous feedings may be warranted.[76] It has been noted that there are more significant nutrient losses (calcium, phosphorus, and fat) of fortified human milk in continuous feeding administration as opposed to bolus feedings.[114] It has also been noted that a decrease in fat content of human milk occurs when enteral nutrition is given via continuous feeding administration and that the decrease in fat content could be minimized if the syringe is in a vertical position.[115]

The critically ill neonate requires nutrients for growth and development. A systematic approach to providing early parenteral and enteral nutrition can improve these outcomes.

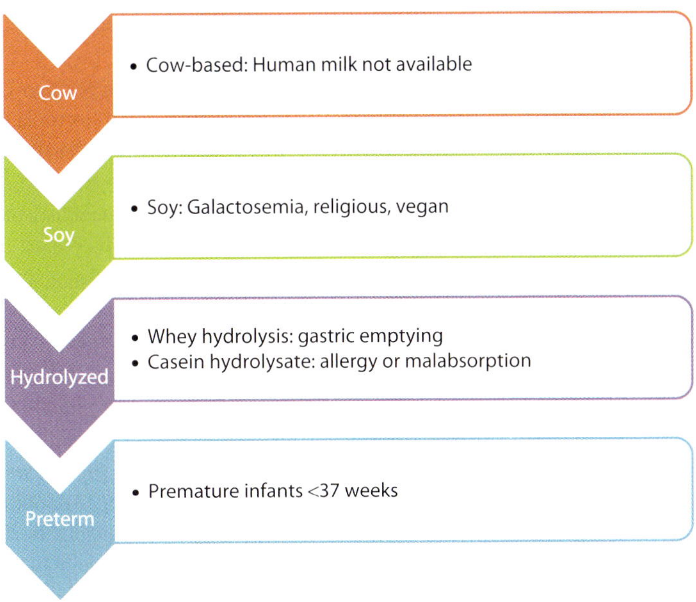

FIGURE 10-2. Choosing the appropriate nutritional formulation.

KEY POINTS

- Growth velocity is closely related to neurodevelopment.
- Nutrient requirements of the preterm infant in critical care are unique and should be tailored to the individual infant.
- Preterm infants require early amino acids with dextrose immediately after delivery.
- A high protein:energy ratio and DHA are particularly important for the preterm infant that missed intrauterine nutrition.
- Human milk is recommended for all neonates except for those with galactosemia or HIV-positive mothers.

REFERENCES

1. Clark RH, Wagner CL, Merritt RJ, Bloom BT, et al. Nutrition in the neonatal intensive care unit: how do we reduce the incidence of extrauterine growth restriction? *J Perinatol.* 2003;23:337-344.
2. Ehrenkranz RA, Dusick AM, Vohr BR, et al. Growth in the neonatal intensive care unit influences neurodevelopmental and growth outcomes of extremely low birth weight infants. *Pediatrics.* 2006;117:1253-1261.
3. Isaacs EB, Morley R, Lucas A. Early diet and general cognitive outcome at adolescence in children born at or below 30 weeks gestation. *J Pediatr.* 2009;155:229-234.
4. Cooke RJ, Griffin IJ, McCormick K, et al. Feeding preterm infants after hospital discharge: effect of dietary manipulation on nutrient intake and growth. *Pediatr Res.* 1998; 43:355-360.
5. Adamkin DH. Late preterm infants: severe hyperbilirubinemia and postnatal glucose homeostasis. *J Perinatol.* 29 Suppl. 2009;2:S12-17.
6. Weiler HA, Yuen CK, Seshia MM. Growth and bone mineralization of young adults weighing less than 1500 g at birth. *Early Hum Dev.* 2002;67:101-112.
7. AAP. *Pediatric Nutrition Handbook*; Kleinman RE, editor. Elk Grove Village, IL: American Academy of Pediatrics. 2009;1470 p.
8. Fenton TR. A new growth chart for preterm babies: Babson and Benda's chart updated with recent data and a new format. *BMC Pediatr.* 2003;3:13.
9. Hay WW, Jr. Strategies for feeding the preterm infant. *Neonatology.* 2008;94:245-254.
10. Lucas A. Long-term programming effects of early nutrition — implications for the preterm infant. *J Perinatol.* 2005;25 Suppl 2:S2-6.
11. Arslanoglu S, Moro GE, Ziegler EE. Adjustable fortification of human milk fed to preterm infants: does it make a difference? *J Perinatol.* 2006;26:614-621.
12. Butte NF, Hopkinson JM, Wong WW, Smith EO, Ellis KJ. Body composition during the first 2 years of life: an updated reference. *Pediatr Res.* 2000;47:578-585.
13. Ellis KJ, Yao M, Shypailo RJ, et al. Body-composition assessment in infancy: air-displacement plethysmography compared with a reference 4-compartment model. *Am J Clin Nutr.* 2007;85:90-95.
14. Pencharz PB, Azcue MP. Measuring resting energy expenditure in clinical practice. *J Pediatr.* 1995;127:269-271.
15. Rigo J. Body composition during the first year of life. *Nestle Nutr Workshop Ser Pediatr Program.* 2006. 58: 65-76; discussion 76-68.
16. Thureen PJ, Melara D, Fennessey PV, Hay WW, Jr. Effect of low versus high intravenous amino acid intake on very low birth weight infants in the early neonatal period. *Pediatr Res.* 2003;53:24-32.
17. Zlotkin SH. TrophAmine. *Pediatrics.* 1998;82:388-390.
18. Embleton ND. Optimal protein and energy intakes in preterm infants. *Early Hum Dev.* 2007;83:831-837.
19. de Betue CT, van Waardenburg DA, Deutz NE, van Eijk HM, et al. Increased protein-energy intake promotes anabolism in critically ill infants with viral bronchiolitis: a double-blind randomised controlled trial. *Arch Dis Child.* 2001;96:817-822.
20. Cooke R, Embleton N, Rigo J, Carrie A, et al. High protein pre-term infant formula: effect on nutrient balance, metabolic status and growth. *Pediatr Res.* 2006;59:265-270.
21. Rivera A, Jr., Bell EF, Bier DM. Effect of intravenous amino acids on protein metabolism of preterm infants during the first three days of life. *Pediatr Res.* 1993;33:106-111.
22. Jaksic T, Shew SB, Keshen TH, Dzakovic A, Do critically ill surgical neonates have increased energy expenditure? *J Pediatr Surg.* 2001;36:63-67.
23. Garza JJ, Shew SB, Keshen TH, Dzakovic A, et al. Energy expenditure in ill premature neonates. *J Pediatr Surg.* 2002;37:289-293.
24. Adamkin D. *Nutritional Strategies for the Very Low Birth Weight Infant*; Adamkin D, ed. Cambridge, UK: Cambridge University Press, 2009.
25. Denne SC. Regulation of proteolysis and optimal protein accretion in extremely premature newborns. *Am J Clin Nutr.* 2007;85:621S-624S.

26. Poindexter BB, Langer JC, Dusick AM, Ehrenkranz RA. Early provision of parenteral amino acids in extremely low birth weight infants: relation to growth and neurodevelopmental outcome. *J Pediatr*. 2006;148:300-305.

27. Kashyap S. Enteral intake for very low birth weight infants: what should the composition be? *Semin Perinatol.* 2007;31:74-82.

28. Ziegler EE. Meeting the nutritional needs of the low-birth-weight infant. *Ann Nutr Metab*. 58 Suppl. 2011;1:8-18.

29. Suryawan A, Orellana RA, Nguyen HV, Jeyapalan AS, et al. Activation by insulin and amino acids of signaling components leading to translation initiation in skeletal muscle of neonatal pigs is developmentally regulated. *Am J Physiol Endocrinol Metab*. 2007;293:E1597-1605.

30. Valentine CJ. Maternal dietary DHA supplementation to improve inflammatory outcomes in the preterm infant. *Adv Nutr*. 2012;3:370-376.

31. Florendo KN, Bellflower B, van Zwol A, Cooke RJ. Growth in preterm infants fed either a partially hydrolyzed whey or an intact casein/whey preterm infant formula. *J Perinatol.* 2009;29:106-111.

32. Valentine CJ. *Maternal Supplementation of DHA and Donor Milk Composition*; 2010; Washington, D.C.

33. Cohen RS, McCallie KR. Feeding premature infants: why, when, and what to add to human milk. *J Parenter Enteral Nutr*. 2012;36:20S-24S.

34. Amesz EM, Schaafsma A, Cranendonk A, Lafeber HN. Optimal growth and lower fat mass in preterm infants fed a protein-enriched postdischarge formula. *J Pediatr Gastroenterol Nutr*. 2010;50:200-207.

35. Innis SM. Essential fatty acid transfer and fetal development. *Placenta*. 2005;26 Suppl A:S70-75.

36. Montgomery C, Speake BK, Cameron A, Sattar N, Weaver LT. Maternal docosahexaenoic acid supplementation and fetal accretion. *Br J Nutr*. 2003;90:135-145.

37. Engelmann B, Wiedmann MK. Cellular phospholipid uptake: Flexible paths to coregulate the functions of intracellular lipids. *Biochim Biophys Acta*. 2010;1801:609-616.

38. Brenna JT, Lapillonne A. Background paper on fat and fatty acid requirements during pregnancy and lactation. *Ann Nutr Metab.* 2009;55:97-122.

39. Hong S, Lu Y, Yang R, Gotlinger KH, et al. Resolvin D1, protectin D1, and related docosahexaenoic acid-derived products: Analysis via electrospray/low energy tandem mass spectrometry based on spectra and fragmentation mechanisms. *J Am Soc Mass Spectrom*. 2007;18:128-144.

40. Jeffrey BG, Weisinger HS, Neuringer M, Mitchell DC. The role of docosahexaenoic acid in retinal function. *Lipids*. 2001;36:859-871.

41. Blasbalg TL, Hibbeln JR, Ramsden CE, Majchrzak SF, Rawlings RR. Changes in consumption of omega-3 and omega-6 fatty acids in the United States during the 20th century. *Am J Clin Nutr.* 2011;93:950-962.

42. German JB. Dietary lipids from an evolutionary perspective: sources, structures and functions. *Matern Child Nutr.* 2011;7 Suppl 2:2-16.

43. German JB, Dillard CJ. Composition, structure and absorption of milk lipids: a source of energy, fat-soluble nutrients and bioactive molecules. *Crit Rev Food Sci Nutr.* 2006;46:57-92.

44. Jensen CL, Maude M, Anderson RE, Heird WC. Effect of docosahexaenoic acid supplementation of lactating women on the fatty acid composition of breast milk lipids and maternal and infant plasma phospholipids. *Am J Clin Nutr*. 2000;71:292S-299S.

45. Institute of Medicine of the National Academies. *Dietary Reference Intakes (DRIs): For Energy, Carbohydrate, Fiber, Fat, Fatty Acids, Cholesterol, Protein and Amino Acids*. Washington, D.C.: The National Academies Press. 2005;1331.

46. Querques G, Forte R, Souied EH. Retina and omega-3. *J Nutr Metab.* 2011;2011:748361.

47. Koletzko B, Cetin I, Brenna JT. Dietary fat intakes for pregnant and lactating women. *Br J Nutr.* 2007;98:873-877.

48. Agostoni C, Buonocore G, Carnielli VP, De Curtis M, et al. Enteral nutrient supply for preterm infants: commentary from the European Society of Paediatric Gastroenterology, Hepatology and Nutrition Committee on Nutrition. *J Pediatr Gastroenterol Nutr.* 2010;50:85-91.

49. Kuratko CN, Salem N, Jr. Biomarkers of DHA status. *Prostaglandins Leukot Essent Fatty Acids*. 2009;81:111-118.

50. Clandinin MT, Chappell JE, Heim T, Swyer PR, Chance GW. Fatty acid utilization in perinatal de novo synthesis of tissues. *Early Hum Dev*. 1981;5:355-366.

51. Hansen AE, Wiese HF, Boelsche AN, Haggard ME, et al. Role of linoleic acid in infant nutrition. *Pediatrics*. 1963;31:171-192.

52. Carnielli VP, Simonato M, Verlato G, Luijendijk I, et al. Synthesis of long-chain polyunsaturated fatty acids in preterm newborns fed formula with long-chain polyunsaturated fatty acids. *Am J Clin Nutr*. 2007;86:1323-1330.

53. Innis SM, Elias SL. Intakes of essential n-6 and n-3 polyunsaturated fatty acids among pregnant Canadian women. *Am J Clin Nutr*. 2003;77:473-478.

54. Makrides M, Gibson RA, McPhee AJ, Yelland L, et al. Effect of DHA supplementation during pregnancy on maternal depression and neurodevelopment of young children: a randomized controlled trial. *JAMA*. 2010;304: 1675-1683.

55. Schanler RJ, Lau C, Hurst NM, Smith EO. Randomized trial of donor human milk versus preterm formula as substitutes for mothers' own milk in the feeding of extremely premature infants. *Pediatrics.* 2005;116: 400-406.

56. Martin CR, Dasilva DA, Cluette-Brown JE, Dimonda C, et al. Decreased postnatal docosahexaenoic and arachidonic acid blood levels in premature infants are associated with neonatal morbidities. *J Pediatr.* 2011;159:743-749;e 741-742.

57. Lapillonne A, Jensen CL. Reevaluation of the DHA requirement for the premature infant. *Prostaglandins Leukot Essent Fatty Acids.* 2009;81:143-150.

58. Valentine CJ, Morrow G, Pennell M, Morrow AL, et al. Randomized controlled trial of docosahexaenoic acid supplementation in midwestern U.S. human milk donors. *Breastfeed Med.* 2013;8(1):86-91.

59. Friel JK, Bessie JC, Belkhode SL, Edgecombe C, et al. Thiamine, riboflavin, pyridoxine, and vitamin C status in premature infants receiving parenteral and enteral nutrition. *J Pediatr Gastroenterol Nutr.* 2001;33:64-69.

60. Moore MC, Greene HL, Phillips B, Franck L, et al. Evaluation of a pediatric multiple vitamin preparation for total parenteral nutrition in infants and children. I. Blood levels of water-soluble vitamins. *Pediatrics.* 1986;77:530-538.

61. Greene HL, Phillips BL. Vitamin dosages for premature infants. *Pediatrics.* 1988;81:173-174.

62. Tyson JE, Wright LL, Oh W, Kennedy KA, et al. Vitamin A supplementation for extremely-low-birth-weight infants. National Institute of Child Health and Human Development Neonatal Research Network. *N Engl J Med.* 1999;340:1962-1968.

63. Wardle SP, Hughes A, Chen S, Shaw NJ. Randomised controlled trial of oral vitamin A supplementation in preterm infants to prevent chronic lung disease. *Arch Dis Child Fetal Neonatal Ed.* 2001;84:F9-F13.

64. Kovacs CS. Maternal vitamin D deficiency: Fetal and neonatal implications. *Semin Fetal Neonatal Med.* 2013;doi: 10.1016/j.siny.2013.01.005.

65. Czech-Kowalska J, Pludowski P, Dobrzanska A, Kryskiewicz E, et al. Impact of vitamin D supplementation on markers of bone mineral metabolism in term infants. *Bone.* 2012;51:781-786.

66. Cranney A, Horsley T, O'Donnell S, Weiler H, et al. Effectiveness and safety of vitamin D in relation to bone health. *Evid Rep Technol Assess* (Full Rep). 2007;158:1-235.

67. Lee JW, Davis JM. Future applications of antioxidants in premature infants. *Curr Opin Pediatr.* 2011;23:161-166.

68. Greer FR. Vitamins A, E and K. In: Tsang RC, Uauy R, Koletzle B, Zlotkin SH, eds. *Nutrition of the Preterm Infant: Scientific Basis and Practical Guidelines*, 2nd ed. Cincinnati, Ohio: Digital Educational Publishing. 2005;141-172.

69. Greer FR. Are breast-fed infants vitamin K deficient? *Adv Exp Med Biol.* 2001;501:391-395.

70. Litwack G. Vitamin K. Preface. *Vitam Horm.* 2008; 78:XIX-XX.

71. AAP. *Pediatric Nutrition Handbook*, Kleinman RE, ed. Elk Grove Village, IL: Committee on Nutrition, American Academy of Pediatrics, 1998.

72. Georgieff MK, Innis SM. Controversial nutrients that potentially affect preterm neurodevelopment: essential fatty acids and iron. *Pediatr Res.* 2005;57:99R-103R.

73. Taneja S, Bhandari N, Rongsen-Chandola T, Mahalanabis D, et al. Effect of zinc supplementation on morbidity and growth in hospital-born, low-birth-weight infants. *Am J Clin Nutr.* 2009;90:385-391.

74. Gregory KE, Connolly TC. Enteral feeding practices in the NICU: results from a 2009 Neonatal Enteral Feeding Survey. *Adv Neonatal Care.* 2012;12:46-55.

75. Lucchini R, Bizzarri B, Giampietro S, De Curtis M. Feeding intolerance in preterm infants. How to understand the warning signs. *J Matern Fetal Neonatal Med.* 2011;24 Suppl 1:72-74.

76. Mayhew SL, Gonzalez ER. Neonatal nutrition: a focus on parenteral nutrition and early enteral nutrition. *Nutr Clin Pract.* 2003;18:406-413.

77. Wanten GJ, Calder PC. Immune modulation by parenteral lipid emulsions. *Am J Clin Nutr.* 2007;85:1171-1184.

78. Hay WW. Early postnatal nutritional requirements of the very preterm infant based on a presentation at the NICHD-AAP workshop on research in neonatology. *J Perinatol.* 2006;26 Suppl 2:S13-18.

79. Meetze W, Bowsher R, Compton J, Moorehead H. Hyperglycemia in extremely- low-birth-weight infants. *Biol Neonate.* 1998;74:214-221.

80. Committee on F, Newborn, Adamkin DH. Postnatal glucose homeostasis in late-preterm and term infants. *Pediatrics.* 2011;127:575-579.

81. Ellard D. Optimizing nutritional management for the very low-birth-weight infant. *Nutr Clin Pract.* 2001;16:243-245.

82. Mahaveer A, Grime C, Morgan C. Increasing early protein intake is associated with a reduction in insulin-treated hyperglycemia in very preterm infants. *Nutr Clin Pract.* 2012;27:399-405.

83. Senterre T, Rigo J. Reduction in postnatal cumulative nutritional deficit and improvement of growth in extremely preterm infants. *Acta Paediatr.* 2012;101:e64-70.

84. Stephens BE, Walden RV, Gargus RA, Tucker R, et al. First-week protein and energy intakes are associated with

18-month developmental outcomes in extremely low birth weight infants. *Pediatrics*. 2009;123:1337-1343.

85. Valentine CJ, Fernandez S, Rogers LK, Gulati P, et al. Early amino-acid administration improves preterm infant weight. *J Perinatol*. 2009;29:428-432.
86. Drenckpohl D, Niehaus M, Schneider C, McConnell C, et al. A randomized trial of micropreemies receiving higher amounts of intravenous fat emulsion during the first week of life. *ICAN: Infant, Child, & Adolescent Nutrition*. 2012;4:58-66.
87. Civardi E, Tzialla C, Garofoli F, Mazzucchelli I, et al. Nutritional needs of premature infants. *J Matern Fetal Neonatal Med*. 24 Suppl. 2011;1:27-29.
88. Kerner JA, Jr., Poole RL. The use of IV fat in neonates. *Nutr Clin Pract*. 2006;21:374-380.
89. Adamkin DH. *Nutritional Strategies for the Very Low Birthweight Infant*. New York: Cambridge University Press. 2009;p. 191.
90. Jeejeebhoy K. Zinc: an essential trace element for parenteral nutrition. *Gastroenterology*. 2009;137:S7-12.
91. Shike M. Copper in parenteral nutrition. *Gastroenterology*. 2009;137:S13-17.
92. Hardy G. Manganese in parenteral nutrition: who, when, and why should we supplement? *Gastroenterology*. 2009;137:S29-35.
93. Shenkin A. Selenium in intravenous nutrition. *Gastroenterology*. 2009;137:S61-69.
94. Calder PC, Jensen GL, Koletzko BV, Singer P, Wanten GJ. Lipid emulsions in parenteral nutrition of intensive care patients: current thinking and future directions. *Intensive Care Med*. 2010;36:735-749.
95. Zingg W, Tomaske M, Martin M. Risk of parenteral nutrition in neonates–an overview. *Nutrients*. 2012;4:1490-1503.
96. Adamkin DH. Mother's milk, feeding strategies, and lactoferrin to prevent necrotizing enterocolitis. *J Parenter Enteral Nutr*. 2012;36:25S-29S.
97. Donovan R, Puppala B, Angst D, Coyle BW. Outcomes of early nutrition support in extremely low-birth-weight infants. *Nutr Clin Pract*. 2006;21:395-400.
98. Neu J. Gastrointestinal maturation and implications for infant feeding. *Early Hum Dev*. 2007;83:767-775.
99. Groh-Wargo S, Sapsford A. Enteral nutrition support of the preterm infant in the neonatal intensive care unit. *Nutr Clin Pract*. 2009;24:363-376.
100. Parish A, Bhatia J. Feeding strategies in the ELBW infant. *J Perinatol*. 2008;28 Suppl 1:S18-20.
101. Lawrence RM, Lawrence RA. Breastfeeding: more than just good nutrition. *Pediatr Rev*. 2011;32:267-280.
102. Miller J, Makrides M, Gibson RA, McPhee AJ, et al. Effect of increasing protein content of human milk fortifier on growth in preterm infants born at <31 wk gestation: a randomized controlled trial. *Am J Clin Nutr*. 2012;95:648-655.
103. Ganapathy V, Hay JW, Kim JH. Costs of necrotizing enterocolitis and cost-effectiveness of exclusively human milk-based products in feeding extremely premature infants. *Breastfeed Med*. 2012;7:29-37.
104. Section on Breastfeeding. Breastfeeding and the use of human milk. *Pediatrics*. 2012;129:e827-841.
105. Valentine CJ, Morrow G, Fernandez S, Gulati P, et al. Docosahexaenoic acid and amino acid contents in pasteurized donor milk are low for preterm infants. *J Pediatr*. 2010;157:906-910.
106. Dougherty D, Luther M. Birth to breast–a feeding care map for the NICU: helping the extremely low birth weight infant navigate the course. *Neonatal Netw*. 2008;27:371-377.
107. Meier PP, Engstrom JL, Patel AL, Jegier BJ, Bruns NE. Improving the use of human milk during and after the NICU stay. *Clin Perinatol*. 2010;37:217-245.
108. Arslanoglu S, Ziegler EE, Moro GE, World Association of Perinatal Medicine Working Group on Nutrition. Donor human milk in preterm infant feeding: evidence and recommendations. *J Perinat Med*. 2010;38:347-351.
109. Di Natale C, Coclite E, Di Ventura L, Di Fabio S. Fortification of maternal milk for preterm infants. *J Matern Fetal Neonatal Med*. 2011;24 Suppl 1:41-43.
110. Joeckel RJ, Phillips SK. Overview of infant and pediatric formulas. *Nutr Clin Pract*. 2009;24:356-362.
111. O'Connor NR. Infant formula. *Am Fam Physician*. 2009;79:565-570.
112. Andorsky DJ, Lund DP, Lillehei CW, Jaksic T, et al. Nutritional and other postoperative management of neonates with short bowel syndrome correlates with clinical outcomes. *J Pediatr*. 2001;139:27-33.
113. Maggio L, Costa S, Zecca C, Giordano L. Methods of enteral feeding in preterm infants. *Early Hum Dev*. 2012;88 Suppl 2:S31-33.
114. Rogers SP, Hicks PD, Hamzo M, Veit LE, Abrams SA. Continuous feedings of fortified human milk lead to nutrient losses of fat, calcium and phosphorous. *Nutrients*. 2010;2:230-240.
115. Greer FR, McCormick A, Loker J. Changes in fat concentration of human milk during delivery by intermittent bolus and continuous mechanical pump infusion. *J Pediatr*. 1984;105:745-749.

CHAPTER 11

Trauma and Traumatic Brain Injury

Sabina Siddiqui
Keith Thatch
Samir K. Gadepalli

■ INTRODUCTION
■ METABOLIC RESPONSE TO TRAUMA
Measurement Of Energy Expenditure
Hormones, Hyperglycemia, and Protein Catabolism
■ PARENTERAL NUTRITION AND SUPPLEMENTS
Merits of Parenteral Nutrition
Complications of Parenteral Nutrition
■ ENTERAL NUTRITION AND FEEDING STRATEGIES
Indications and Contraindications
Benefits
Timing and Amount
Enteral Access
■ APPROACH TO SPECIFIC INJURIES
Traumatic Brain Injury
Obese Trauma Patient
The Open Abdomen
Duodenal Hematoma
Enterocutaneous Fistula
■ KEY POINTS
References

INTRODUCTION

Metabolic alterations following injury in children significantly affect survival. Though the response occurs in a predictable manner, much controversy exists in the medical literature on the mode, timing, and amount of feeding. With better understanding of the various approaches to providing nutrition support, additional opportunities for decreasing mortality after trauma can be identified.

Improving nutrition support of the pediatric trauma patient can not only affect survival, but also shorten the time needed for rehabilitation. Caloric support can ameliorate the protein catabolism that occurs following trauma. Wound healing and immune response are also reliant on adequate protein stores. Muscle breakdown can be ameliorated using nutrition support with parenteral and enteral approaches.

Enteral nutrition (EN) should be an early priority soon after achieving hemodynamic stability using adequate resuscitation. Parenteral nutrition (PN) can be an adequate substitute until injuries have been addressed and enteral access has been obtained. Both underfeeding and overfeeding can lead to unintended consequences.

Specific injuries after trauma require additional nutrition support and careful monitoring of nutritional needs. Burns, traumatic head injury, multiorgan system injury, and concomitant abdominal compartment syndrome all have unique characteristics that need to be addressed. In this chapter, we will focus on the metabolic response after injury, followed by parenteral and enteral approaches to providing nutrition, and finally, specific traumatic injuries that require distinct practices.

METABOLIC RESPONSE TO TRAUMA

As originally outlined by Cuthbertson in 1932, injury leads to a series of metabolic events that in turn lead to a loss of nitrogen in the urine from protein breakdown.[1] The response follows an "ebb and flow" pattern where there is an initial decrease in blood pressure, cardiac output, and temperature, with a subsequent increase in temperature, heart rate, and release of catabolic enzymes. Though the normal state of health prior to injury differs among individuals, the response involves release of catabolic enzymes promoting glycolysis, lipolysis, gluconeogenesis,[2] and an increase in the basal metabolic rate, which correlates with the severity of the injury.[3] Details of the metabolic stress response can be found in chapter 1.

In children, the metabolic response can be more challenging to predict than in adults. Children have a higher per weight baseline energy expenditure, which does not increase with injury. Instead, calories are shunted away from growth, as exhibited by the high rates of protein turnover.[4] Children are also more vulnerable to protein loss and more readily demonstrate complications secondary to this loss. Misinterpreting the metabolic response can lead to either underfeeding or overfeeding, and each may produce unintended consequences.

Adverse effects of the response also include insulin resistance and hyperglycemia; sarcopenia, osteopenia, and growth restriction; and deficient immune response and sepsis. Long-term metabolic effects of injury from a prolonged response or severe injury have been reported, including cardiovascular events, type 2 diabetes mellitus, and early-onset obesity.[2] Mucosal ischemia can also occur, since children require higher intestinal perfusion to absorb nutrients.[4] The metabolic response and potential for complications highlight the importance of precise measurements of the energy expenditure.

Measurement of Energy Expenditure

While body weight is considered the easiest and most convenient way of measuring baseline nutritional status,[5] indirect calorimetry (IC) is considered the gold standard for measuring caloric expenditure.[6] When IC is unavailable, traditionally equations include those by including Harris-Benedict, World Health Organization, Schofield, and White[4] have been used despite their limitations.

In addition to type and location of injuries, sedation and paralysis, pain, fever, and infection all play a role on the basal energy expenditure and calorie needs. Burns increase calorie needs and metabolic demand, while spinal cord injury resulting in paralysis may decrease the caloric requirement. The number of wounds and broken bones increase calorie needs, while sedation and paralysis result in decreased demand. Pain, fever, and infection all increase metabolism and concomitant calorie needs; therefore, frequent measurement and monitoring are required for precise estimation of baseline metabolism and targeting of calorie needs.

Overfeeding leads to adverse effects such as increased production of carbon dioxide and fat deposition in the liver.[4,7] Overfeeding can be detrimental to weaning from ventilator support and can create long-term changes in other systems.[8] Furthermore, giving excess protein has not been shown to stifle the posttraumatic catabolic response.[9] In some adult studies, underfeeding actually improved survival and lengths of hospital and intensive care unit (ICU) stays, but it is unclear if the same is true for children.[10]

Hormones, Hyperglycemia, and Protein Catabolism

Glucagon release causes gluconeogenesis and glycolysis, increasing glucose in the bloodstream. Children have decreased stores of hepatic glycogen,[4] and this supply is quickly exhausted, increasing the importance of gluconeogenesis in the maintenance of serum glucose. Certain organs, such as the brain, which incidentally is proportionately larger per kilogram in children, rely on a steady supply of glucose for nutrition. Hyperglycemia and protein loss can result from excess glucagon production.[4]

Another hormone causing hyperglycemia and protein loss is cortisol, released secondary to increases in adrenocorticotropic hormone production in the anterior pituitary. Through stimulation of cytokine release, cortisol promotes protein breakdown and gluconeogenesis.[4] Breakdown of protein releases alanine from muscle and glutamine from the gut. These amino acids are converted to glucose in the liver.[4] Loss of glutamine, the primary nutrient for enterocytes and lymphocytes, creates additional intestinal and immune dysfunction.[4] Similar to glucagon, cortisol also acts on the liver and stimulates glycolysis, promoting further hyperglycemia.

Hyperglycemia is further augmented by catecholamines (epinephrine, norepinephrine, and dopamine) released from the adrenal medulla after stimulation by the sympathetic nervous system. Through suppression of insulin release by the pancreas and promoting glycogenolysis (breakdown of glycogen) in the skeletal muscle, catecholamines worsen hyperglycemia.[4] Lipolysis (breakdown of fat into free fatty acids and glycerol) is also increased by catecholamines.

The effect of protein loss is intensified in children because they have a smaller lean body mass. Loss of diaphragmatic and intercostal muscle mass can lead to respiratory compromise, while loss of cardiac muscle can lead to hemodynamic compromise and fatal arrhythmias.[4] Though significant protein loss can have catastrophic effects, protein catabolism more commonly leads to gastrointestinal dysfunction (feeding intolerance, mucosal bleeding, and bacterial translocation), immune deficiency (infections, poor or delayed wound healing, wound breakdown), and need for prolonged rehabilitation.[11]

PARENTERAL NUTRITION AND SUPPLEMENTS

The ability to reach calorie and protein needs in such a hypermetabolic state as described earlier remains a significant challenge in the management of trauma patients. Enteral nutrition remains the preferred route for nutrition support over PN in trauma patients because it is safer, more physiologic, promotes better gastrointestinal function, prevents bacterial translocation, and improves outcome. Parenteral nutrition should be reserved for patients in whom the intestinal tract will remain unavailable and nonfunctional for a prolonged period, resulting in eventual malnutrition. Patients with questionable gastrointestinal function should be fed using a combination of EN and PN when possible. The enteral feeding should be increased or decreased according to tolerance, with PN adjusted accordingly. If the patient requires frequent procedures with inability to advance enteral feeds to caloric goals, then PN could be used preferentially.

Merits of Parenteral Nutrition

Parenteral nutrition provides intravenous administration of macronutrients and micronutrients to meet the nutritional requirements in patients when adequate EN is not feasible. In a study of patients with closed head injury, only a quarter of patients were able to spontaneously eat enough to meet their nutritional needs by discharge.[12] In another study of patients with traumatic brain injury (TBI), nutritional deficiencies and weight loss at 14 days were common, partially ameliorated by starting nutrition early (before 72 hours) and the presence of a dietitian.[13] The European Society for Clinical Nutrition and Metabolism (ESPEN) recommends that PN be considered in patients when enteral feeds cannot be started by 24 hours after ICU admission or injury.[14]

When compared head to head in the setting of a controlled study, short-term outcomes have been similar for PN and enteral feeds. In one study of patients with moderate-to-severe TBI, the PN group had increased protein intake, improved nitrogen balance, and improved outcome at 3 months over the enteral group without negatively affecting intracranial pressure.[15] Another study randomizing patients to early PN versus jejunal feeding found that both approaches were equally effective at achieving nutritional goals based on measured energy expenditure with equivalent hospital costs and infection rates.[12] A third prospective randomized study also demonstrated that PN use resulted in a more positive nitrogen balance, higher serum albumin and lymphocyte levels, and less mortality than standard EN in patients with TBI.[16] These patients also achieved higher calorie intake and reached full nutritional replacement by 7 days postinjury (compared with 14 days for those fed enterally). Finally, in a review of prospective studies examining the comparative efficacy of EN and PN on gut-barrier function and other clinical outcomes, no advantage was demonstrated between the two routes, aside from the fact that in patients with acute abdominal trauma, enteral feeding was associated with a reduction of sepsis.[17] More recently, in a retrospective cohort study of patients with blunt trauma across 8 centers, use of early PN was associated with increased infectious complications.[18] The literature commonly discusses the failures of achieving appropriate nutritional goals in a timely manner. The amount of nutrition provided during the first 5 days after a TBI is an independent risk factor for mortality.[19] Every 10 kcal/kg decrement was associated with a 30% to 40% increase in mortality rate.[19] Discrepancies between prescribed and delivered nutrients are mainly attributable to interruptions due to digestive intolerance and procedures such as surgery, diagnostic tests, and extubation attempts.[20] This phenomenon has led to measures to minimize the effects of such nutrition interruptions by (1) increased use of postpyloric feeding in children; (2)

reduced length of fasting for procedures when postpyloric feeds are used; (3) resumption of enteral feeds at the preinterruption rate when stopped; (4) anticipating and compensating for predicted caloric deficits by increasing rates periprocedurally; and (5) considering the combination of EN and PN early in patients with increased injury severity scores and anticipated procedures.[13]

Complications of Parenteral Nutrition

Although widespread in its application, PN is associated with mechanical, infectious, and metabolic complications and hence, should only be used in carefully selected patients. Parenteral nutrition in critical illness is discussed in more detail in chapter 7 of this book. Parenteral nutrition requires central venous access, which by itself can lead to complications. In a Cochrane review of central venous access, infectious complications included line sepsis, bacteremia, and colonization with gram-negative bacteria, while mechanical complications ranged from inadvertent arterial puncture, minor bleeding and hematoma to a displaced or broken catheter or thrombotic events.[21] Analysis of septic states in blunt trauma demonstrated that patients who received at least 40% of their nutrition by the enteral route developed less sepsis.[22]

There is considerable concern that the lipid component of PN is the primary factor in the metabolic complications associated with it. Battistella et al. suggest lipids be withheld from the PN of trauma patients able to tolerate at least 10% of their nutrition enterally. In their study, this group received fewer calories, but no intravenous lipids. They had fewer infections, shorter lengths of stay, and fewer days on a ventilator.[23]

ENTERAL NUTRITION AND FEEDING STRATEGIES

Enteral nutrition should be considered whenever possible because it is safer, more physiologic, promotes better gastrointestinal function, prevents bacterial translocation, and improves outcome.

Indications and Contraindications

Enteral nutrition remains the preferred method of providing nutritional support for the acutely injured child. In fact, even in the early postoperative abdominal trauma and open abdomen scenarios, enteral feeding may be of benefit.[24] Only a handful of situations exist where enteral support cannot be initiated in the postinjury state, including the child with a (1) mechanical bowel obstruction—either due to mass effect (e.g., duodenal hematoma) or due to surgically created discontinuity as part of a staged, damage-control laparotomy; (2) prolonged ileus; (3) distal or high output enterocutaneous or enteroenteric fistula where distal feeding access cannot be obtained; (4) severe feeding intolerance with refractory vomiting or osmotic diarrhea; and (5) need for high-dose or escalating vasoactive agent support due to hemodynamic instability. Further discussion on these scenarios is outlined later in this chapter. In these situations, the use of PN would be the preferred method of nutritional support.

Benefits

Enteral nutrition has been shown to have a number of metabolic and clinical benefits in addition to being a much more cost-effective strategy for nutrition support in the ICU. Numerous studies show that early EN blunts the systemic inflammatory response and attenuates the metabolic response, including attenuating the body's breakdown of glycogen, fat, and protein stores.[25] Over the last 20 years, use of EN in the postinjury patient has been shown to promote immune competence by maintaining gut mucosal integrity, decreasing bacterial translocation, and improving nitrogen retention and thus providing a significant decrease in infectious complications and enhanced wound healing.[25-28] Three separate small, randomized control trials in adult trauma have shown significant reductions in mortality in patients fed enterally within the first 48 hours of injury.[28-31]

Timing and Amount

In complex multitrauma, initiation of nutrition often takes a back seat to multiple other acute issues and needs. While this may be clinically appropriate postinjury day 1, expert opinion encourages initiation of a nutritional support plan by the third postinjury day.[13] Early initiation of nutritional support has consistently been associated with improved recovery in trauma patients.[12,32] This has been proven to be true even in the postoperative trauma patient after laparotomy, with early feeding initiated 12 to 18 hours after surgery in one study,[31] and some small retrospective reviews indicating that enteral feeding in patients with an open abdomen may actually decrease the time required to fascial closure.[33] In the case of complex abdominal trauma, it is important that the intensivist and the trauma surgeon formulate plans for enteral access during the initial or return trips to the operating room.

Trophic feeds are the amount of EN needed to supply the minimum support needed by enterocytes to maintain villous structures, mucosal barrier, and immunologic function. In situations where full goal calories cannot be achieved through the enteral route, a combination effort with trophic volume of enteral feeds and provision of the remaining calories through the parenteral route may be indicated. While there is evidence to support the use of trophic feeding strategies, determining this ideal amount can be difficult. Cook et al. make the argument that energy needs can be calculated based on oxygen delivery of the splanchnic system, estimated at 25% of the cardiac output.[4] Because approximately half of the splanchnic blood flow is received by the gut, they make a logical argument that 12% of per kilogram daily calories should provide adequate substrate support for enterocytes.[4] As recovery proceeds, the feeds can be slowly advanced to achieve goal caloric needs enterally.

Enteral Access

Short-term enteral access can be obtained by nasogastric or nasoenteric routes. Each route has a unique set of associated risks and benefits. The most common and easiest method of access is the orogastric or nasogastric route. Children receiving gastric feeds tolerate a higher osmolarity and volume than those being fed into the small bowel. Gastric acid may also benefit digestion and have a bactericidal effect; gastric feeds are associated with less frequent gastrointestinal complications such as diarrhea.[34] Complications of gastric feeding include some evidence of an increase in ventilator-associated pneumonia (VAP), feeding intolerance, and an inability to reach feeding goals. Small-bowel feeds have been used with the aim of decreasing aspiration, the rate of VAP, and the time to achieve caloric goals. However, the putative benefits of jejunal feeding have not been demonstrated in adult studies.[35,36] In a randomized controlled study of gastric versus jejunal feeding in critically ill mechanically ventilated children, children receiving jejunal feeds achieved higher percentage of goal calories delivered compared to those fed via the gastric route.[37] There was no significant difference in the rates of aspiration of gastric contents between the 2 groups. Despite the lack of evidence of benefit, nasoduodenal/nasojejunal access is often the standard in many ICUs. Jejunal feeds must be run at a continuous rate, as bolus feeds are contraindicated by this route. Placement and maintenance of placement in the small bowel can be time consuming and expensive: There is also a 40% incidence of dislodgement of nasoenteral tubes in ICUs.[38] There is also a reported increase in the rate of *Clostridium*-associated diarrhea with small-bowel feeding.[39]

For patients requiring more than 4 weeks of feeding access or in those undergoing abdominal surgery, surgical enteral feeding access should be considered and obtained. There are several methods by which a gastric feeding tube can be placed, the most common of which is the percutaneous endoscopic gastrostomy (PEG).[40] While the actual incidence of complications from gastrostomy tubes is low, several complications are known to occur, including improper placement of PEG, inadvertent placement of tube through or into other portions of the bowel, necrosis of tube tract, technical failure requiring laparotomy, and leak into the abdomen with subsequent peritonitis.[41] Interestingly enough, the PEG tube has been shown to confer the same decrease in VAP rates as nasojejunal feeds; therefore, a trial of gastric feeding to confirm intolerance is indicated prior to proceeding to the operating room for a jejunal feeding tube. Surgical jejunostomy tubes can be placed in patients who have undergone extensive foregut surgery and need for distal feeding is anticipated, or in patients in whom gastric feeding is contraindicated due to reflux and aspiration. Complications associated with jejunostomy tubes include intra-abdominal abscess, volvulus with bowel infarction, intestinal obstruction, and more commonly, diarrhea and other symptoms of dumping and catheter obstruction by inspissated feedings/medications.[42]

Our recommendations are to attempt to feed the child into the stomach with aspiration precautions, such as keeping the head of the bed elevated >30 degrees. Only if the child does not tolerate gastric feeds do we advance the feeding tube to the postpyloric position. If the child appears to require long-term feeding tube access, we prefer to place a PEG tube. In the child who has been receiving jejunal feeds, we will either attempt to trial gastric feeds again or obtain contrast studies prior to proceeding to surgical enteral access.

■ APPROACH TO SPECIFIC INJURIES

Certain traumatic injuries require distinct nutrition practices, and these include traumatic brain injury, the open abdomen, enterocutaneous fistula, duodenal hematoma, and the obese patient with trauma.

Traumatic Brain Injury

Traumatic brain injury is followed by a hypermetabolic, severely catabolic response. The subsequent need for sedation, paralytics, and muscle relaxants will further modulate this response. Energy requirements in the paralyzed or comatose patient are quite difficult to interpret and estimate. Indirect calorimetry for measured energy expenditure (MEE) has been found to be useful in these patients. In the first 48 hours, energy expenditure ranged from 75% to 200% predicted.[43] The average respiratory quotient was 0.68, indicating consumption of lipids as a predominant fuel. Borzotta and colleagues demonstrated that this hypermetabolic state not only occurs immediately after injury, but persists for 4 weeks as the MEE remains between 135% and 146% of predicted.[12] They also noted that both PN and EN were equally effective at meeting these needs.

The ability to reach nutritional needs and goals in within a timely matter has significant effect on morbidity and mortality. Taylor and colleagues demonstrated that an accelerated feeding regimen to meet nutritional goals within 7 days demonstrated improved outcomes at 3 months and decreased numbers of infections.[25] Other studies have shown that continuously fed TBI patients and/or those that receive nasojejunal feedings have increased caloric delivery, less feeding intolerance, and reach goals more quickly.[16,44] Our focus (**Fig. 11-1**) is to start feeds within a couple of days and reach nutritional goals by 7 days postinjury. The use of a dietitian and frequent measurements of caloric needs are pivotal to attempting to meet the TBI patient's needs and ameliorating the catabolic state.

Early nutrition support can be achieved, but special attention must be paid to prevent hyperglycemia, which has been shown to exacerbate ischemic brain injury. Hyperglycemia early after TBI has been shown to be associated with poor outcomes on bivariate analysis. These outcomes remained significant in multivariate analysis, adjusting for Glasgow coma score, type of trauma, hypoxia, hypotension, disseminated intravascular coagulation, and early posttraumatic seizures.[45] Furthermore, the level and severity of hyperglycemia at admission had direct correlation with mortality associated with moderate and severe TBI.[46]

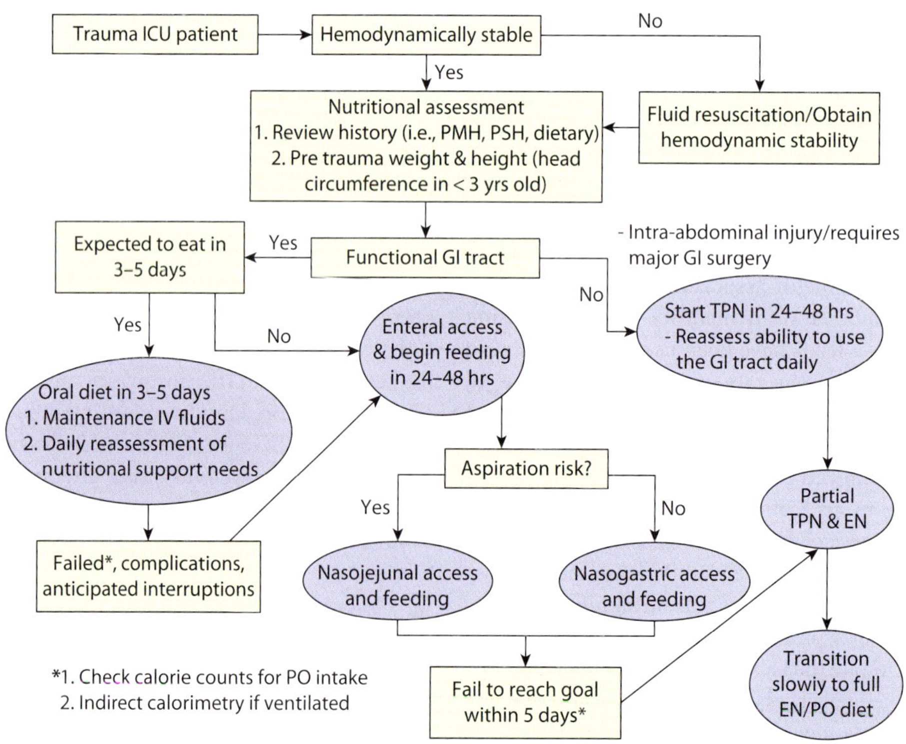

FIGURE 11-1. Algorithm for the management of nutrition in the pediatric trauma patient.

Obese Trauma Patient

Nutritional support for injured obese pediatric patients can pose unique problems for critical care physicians. (Please see chapter 21 for a detailed account on nutritional aspects of the obese child.) These patients often suffer from chronic diseases secondary to their obesity, including diabetes, hyperlipidemia, hypertension, sleep apnea, respiratory difficulties, and biliary disease. They also are more likely to develop complications from their injuries, such as nosocomial infections, wound dehiscence, and cardiorespiratory complications.[47] The MEE of obese pediatric patients is difficult to predict accurately, as many dietitians and physicians will attempt to find nutritional goals somewhere along the spectrum of a calculated ideal body weight and the patient's actual body weight. Thus, overfeeding and underfeeding can easily result.

The idea of a hypocaloric, high-protein feeding regimen has become increasingly attractive in the critically injured obese patient. Dickerson et al. examined outcomes of adult obese patients who received eucaloric or hypocaloric enteral feeds.[48] While obtaining an equivalent nitrogen balance, the hypocaloric group required significantly fewer ventilator days, fewer antibiotic days, and fewer ICU days. Working closely with our dietitian, we attempt to match MEE needs by utilizing a high-protein regimen to meet ideal body weight goals.

The Open Abdomen

In the context of trauma, the open abdomen is usually the result of surgery abbreviated due to a patient's unstable clinical condition or failure to achieve fascial closure due to large fluid shifts and edema of the bowel wall. First described in the 1980s, the principles of damage-control laparotomy are to stop acute hemorrhage, control enteric spillage into the abdominal cavity, and transfer to the ICU for continued resuscitation prior to performing any type of definitive repair.[49,50] The patient then returns to the operating room a number of times after resuscitation for eventual fascial closure over a period of days thereafter. The principles employed in damage-control laparotomy with the open abdomen have also been used in accessory trauma diagnoses of abdominal compartment syndrome and intra-abdominal sepsis.[51,52] Regardless of the underlying diagnosis, the burden of ongoing resuscitation then transfers from the operating room to the ICU.

While leaving the abdomen open has been shown to improve survival in the face of catastrophic abdominal injuries or abdominal compartment syndrome,[50] this strategy also places patients at risk for complications. Patients who are too sick to tolerate definitive surgical repair can be considered as being in a constant inflammatory and catabolic state, with ongoing protein and fluid loss from a large surgical wound with exposed viscera until the abdomen is closed.[53] Miller et al. described their experience with 344 adults and children with open abdomen, with a 25% complication rate, including wound infection, abscess, fistula, VAP, abdominal hernia, and fluid and protein losses.[54]

While there is minimal literature describing feeding limitations in management of the open abdomen, there is a body of evidence to support that EN can significantly dampen the inflammatory response to the catabolic state.[25-28] A handful of retrospective studies have shown the safety of early EN in the open abdomen,[24,55-57] with few complications associated with feeding, no difference in the ability to close the abdomen, and earlier achievement of goal feeds. Additional retrospective studies actually indicate that early feeding may allow for faster time to abdominal wall closure and fewer associated complications such as fistula formation and VAP.[33,58]

Given the known benefits of EN and the additional support to the safety of its use in the patients with an open abdomen, it is our recommendation that enteral feeds be initiated once the patient is fully resuscitated and hemodynamically stable. Parenteral nutrition should be reserved for the catastrophic abdomen where enteral feeds would not be anatomically feasible for prolonged periods (greater than 7 days).

Duodenal Hematoma

The duodenum is the fourth most commonly injured organ after blunt abdominal trauma, with an incidence of 2% to 10% in the pediatric population.[59] The duodenal hematoma can be a consequence of child neglect or abuse and is classically considered a nonoperative condition.[60] In the vein of all hollow-viscous injuries, the duodenal injuries are difficult to diagnose, and up to a third present with obstructive symptoms up to 72 hours after the injury.

The treatment algorithm for the isolated duodenal hematoma is conservative therapy with bowel rest, nasogastric decompression, and PN for up to 3 weeks of therapy, though the average length is 9 days.[59,61] Clinical symptoms of obstruction and repeat imaging with contrast studies (upper gastrointestinal series or computed tomography scan) are used to monitor for resolution of the hematoma and introduction of enteral feeds. If the symptoms do not resolve, operative exploration is recommended to evaluate for strictures, duodenal perforation, or injury to the head of the pancreas or some other factor contributing to the nonresolution of the obstruction.[59,61] It is important to realize that while the initial treatment of duodenal hematoma is nonoperative, there is a high rate of associated pancreatic injury, which may require some form of intervention and complicate the feeding plan.[59,60]

If the hematoma is encountered during trauma laparotomy, it is usually evacuated with mobilization and evaluation of the hematoma, and the child is treated like any other postoperative patient. If evaluation of the hematoma identifies a full-thickness duodenal wall injury, the operative management of this injury is complex and usually involves creating a proximal fistula, some form of diversion (pyloric exclusion and/or gastrojejunostomy), and a distal feeding plan (gastrojejunostomy or jejunostomy). The operative approach is similar for a duodenal hematoma treated nonoperatively for several weeks without resolution.

Enterocutaneous Fistula

The enterocutaneous fistula (ECF) and entero-entero fistula (EEF) are devastating complications of the trauma laparotomy associated with significant morbidity and mortality.[62] Enterocutaneous fistula develops in 1% to 2% of patients who have undergone a trauma laparotomy.[62] Risk factors of ECF development include penetrating trauma, multiple hollow viscous injuries, and the open abdomen. The open abdomen is a major risk factor for fistula development. Technically speaking, a fistula formed in this setting does not have a second epithelialized surface to which it opens, and is often referred to as an enteroatmospheric fistula.[54,62] The EEF is a fistulous tract between two areas of bowel, such as the small and large intestine. Any child with a history of abdominal trauma and feeding intolerance in the form of diarrhea refractory to medical management should be evaluated with a contrast study. Once the diagnosis is confirmed, the patient will require PN for nutrition until operative repair.

The initial management of the ECF is to manage fistula output, correcting associated fluid and electrolyte imbalances, protecting the skin and associated wound. The ECF is initially managed by bowel rest and PN. The management plan diverges depending on the location and volume of the fistula. Once the output is quantified, contrast studies are obtained to define the anatomy and location of the fistula. Approximately 60% of ECF will spontaneously heal with conservative management.[63] Most will heal within 2 weeks; if the fistula does not heal by 4 to 6 weeks of therapy, the fistulous portion will require surgical resection. The child is not limited to PN for nutrition at this time, as enteric feeds may be initiated with close monitoring and management of output. For the proximal, high-output fistula (e.g., duodenal perforation), a distal feeding access can be obtained and enteral feeds initiated similarly.

KEY POINTS

- Traumatic brain injury elicits a variable metabolic response. Resting energy expenditure measured by IC must guide energy prescriptions where available.
- When the gut is functional, enteral access available and the patient is hemodynamically stable, early EN is preferred. Where enteral feeding is not feasible, PN may be considered.
- Hyperglycemia should be anticipated in children with TBI and managed appropriately to improve outcomes.

REFERENCES

1. Cuthbertson DP. Observations on the disturbance of metabolism produced by injury to the limbs. *Q J Med.* 1932;1(2):233-246.
2. Pervanidou P, Chrousos GP. Metabolic consequences of stress during childhood and adolescence. *Metabolism.* 2012;61(5):611-619.
3. Winthrop AL, Wesson DE, Pencharz PB, Jacobs DG, Heim T, Filler RM. Injury severity, whole body protein turnover, and energy expenditure in pediatric trauma. *J Pediatr Surg.* 1987;22(6):534-537.
4. Cook RC, Blinman TA. Nutritional support of the pediatric trauma patient. *Semin Pediatr Surg.* 2010;19(4):242-251.
5. Chan MM, Chan GM. Nutritional therapy for burns in children and adults. *Nutrition.* 2009;25(3):261-269.
6. Suman OE, Mlcak RP, Chinkes DL, Herndon DN. Resting energy expenditure in severely burned children: analysis of agreement between indirect calorimetry and prediction equations using the Bland-Altman method. *Burns.* 2006;32(3):335-342.
7. Mizock B. Septic shock. A metabolic perspective. *Arch Intern Med.* 1984;144(3):579-585.
8. Shew SB, Keshen TH, Jahoor F, Jaksic T. The determinants of protein catabolism in neonates on extracorporeal membrane oxygenation. *J Pediatr Surg.* 1999;34(7):1086-1090.

9. Chwals WJ. Overfeeding the critically ill child: fact or fantasy? *New Horiz.* 1994;2(2):147-155.
10. Krishnan JA, Parce PB, Martinez A, Diette GB, Brower RG. Caloric intake in medical ICU patients: consistency of care with guidelines and relationship to clinical outcomes. *Chest.* 2003;124(1):297-305.
11. Mendonca Machado N, Gragnani A, Masako Ferreira L. Burns, metabolism and nutritional requirements. *Nutr Hosp.* 2011;26(4):692-700.
12. Borzotta AP, Pennings J, Papasadero B, et al. Enteral versus parenteral nutrition after severe closed head injury. *J Trauma.* 1994;37(3):459-468.
13. Malakouti A, Sookplung P, Siriussawakul A, et al. Nutrition support and deficiencies in children with severe traumatic brain injury. *Pediatr Crit Care Med.* 2012;13(1):e18-e24.
14. Kreymann KG, Berger MM, Deutz NE, et al. ESPEN Guidelines on Enteral Nutrition: Intensive care. *Clin Nutr.* 2006;25(2):210-223.
15. Young B, Ott L, Haack D, et al. Effect of total parenteral nutrition upon intracranial pressure in severe head injury. *J Neurosurg.* 1987;67(1):76-80.
16. Rapp RP, Young B, Twyman D, et al. The favorable effect of early parenteral feeding on survival in head-injured patients. *J Neurosurg.* 1983;58(6):906-912.
17. Lipman TO. Grains or veins: is enteral nutrition really better than parenteral nutrition? A look at the evidence. *J Parenter Enteral Nutr.* 1998;22(3):167-182.
18. Sena MJ, Utter GH, Cuschieri J, Maier RV, Tompkins RG, Harbrecht BG, Moore EE, O'Keefe GE. Early supplemental parenteral nutrition is associated with increased infectious complications in critically ill trauma patients. *J Am Coll Surg.* 2008;207(4):459-467.
19. Hartl R, Gerber LM, Ni Q, Ghajar J. Effect of early nutrition on deaths due to severe traumatic brain injury. *J Neurosurg.* 2008;109(1):50-56.
20. Bockenkamp B, Jouvet P, Arsenault V, Beauséjour M, Pelletier V-A. Assessment of calories prescribed and delivered to critically ill children. *E Spen Eur E J Clin Nutr Metab.* 2009;4(4):e172-e175.
21. Ge X, Cavallazzi R, Li C, Pan SM, Wang YW, Wang FL. Central venous access sites for the prevention of venous thrombosis, stenosis and infection. *Cochrane Database Syst Rev.* 2012;3:CD004084.
22. Border JR, Hassett J, LaDuca J, et al. The gut origin septic states in blunt multiple trauma (ISS = 40) in the ICU. *Ann Surg.* 1987;206(4):427-448.
23. Battistella FD, Widergren JT, Anderson JT, Siepler JK, Weber JC, MacColl K. A prospective, randomized trial of intravenous fat emulsion administration in trauma victims requiring total parenteral nutrition. *J Trauma.* 1997;43(1):52-58; discussion 58-60.
24. Dissanaike S, Pham T, Shalhub S, et al. Effect of immediate enteral feeding on trauma patients with an open abdomen: protection from nosocomial infections. *J Am Coll Surg.* 2008;207(5):690-697.
25. Taylor SJ, Fettes SB, Jewkes C, Nelson RJ. Prospective, randomized, controlled trial to determine the effect of early enhanced enteral nutrition on clinical outcome in mechanically ventilated patients suffering head injury. *Crit Care Med.* 1999;27(11):2525-2531.
26. Perel P, Yanagawa T, Bunn F, Roberts I, Wentz R, Pierro A. Nutritional support for head-injured patients. *Cochrane Database Syst Rev.* 2006(4):CD001530.
27. Marik PE, Zaloga GP. Early enteral nutrition in acutely ill patients: a systematic review. *Crit Care Med.* 2001; 29(12):2264-2270.
28. Kompan L, Kremzar B, Gadzijev E, Prosek M. Effects of early enteral nutrition on intestinal permeability and the development of multiple organ failure after multiple injury. *Intensive Care Med.* 1999;25(2):157-161.
29. Chuntrasakul C, Siltharm S, Chinswangwatanakul V, Pongprasobchai T, Chockvivatanavanit S, Bunnak A. Early nutritional support in severe traumatic patients. *J Med Assoc Thai.* 1996;79(1):21-26.
30. Kompan L, Vidmar G, Spindler-Vesel A, Pecar J. Is early enteral nutrition a risk factor for gastric intolerance and pneumonia? *Clin Nutr.* 2004;23(4):527-532.
31. Moore EE, Jones TN. Benefits of immediate jejunostomy feeding after major abdominal trauma--a prospective, randomized study. *J Trauma.* 1986;26(10):874-881.
32. Redmond C, Lipp J. Traumatic brain injury in the pediatric population. *Nutr Clin Pract.* 2006;21(5):450-461.
33. Collier B, Guillamondegui O, Cotton B, et al. Feeding the open abdomen. *J Parenter Enteral Nutr.* 2007;31(5):410-415.
34. Marian M. Pediatric nutrition support. *Nutr Clin Pract.* 1993;8(5):199-209.
35. Strong RM, Condon SC, Solinger MR, Namihas BN, Ito-Wong LA, Leuty JE. Equal aspiration rates from postpylorus and intragastric-placed small-bore nasoenteric feeding tubes: a randomized, prospective study. *J Parenter Enteral Nutr.* 1992;16(1):59-63.
36. White H, Sosnowski K, Tran K, Reeves A, Jones M. A randomised controlled comparison of early post-pyloric versus early gastric feeding to meet nutritional targets in ventilated intensive care patients. *Crit Care.* 2009;13(6):R187.

37. Meert KL, Daphtary KM, Metheny NA. Gastric vs small-bowel feeding in critically ill children receiving mechanical ventilation: a randomized controlled trial. *Chest.* 2004; 126(3):872-878.

38. Meer JA. Inadvertent dislodgement of nasoenteral feeding tubes: incidence and prevention. *J Parenter Enteral Nutr.* 1987;11(2):187-189.

39. Munshi IA, Steingrub JS, Wolpert L. Small bowel necrosis associated with early postoperative jejunal tube feeding in a trauma patient. *J Trauma.* 2000;49(1):163-165.

40. Gauderer MW, Ponsky JL, Izant RJ, Jr. Gastrostomy without laparotomy: a percutaneous endoscopic technique. *J Pediatr Surg.* 1980;15(6):872-875.

41. Beasley SW, Catto-Smith AG, Davidson PM. How to avoid complications during percutaneous endoscopic gastrostomy. *J Pediatr Surg.* 1995;30(5):671-673.

42. Holmes JH, Brundage SI, Yuen P, Hall RA, Maier RV, Jurkovich GJ. Complications of surgical feeding jejunostomy in trauma patients. *J Trauma.* 1999;47(6):1009-1012.

43. Foley N, Marshall S, Pikul J, Salter K, Teasell R. Hypermetabolism following moderate to severe traumatic acute brain injury: a systematic review. *J Neurotrauma.* 2008;25(12):1415-1431.

44. Pepe JL, Barba CA. The metabolic response to acute traumatic brain injury and implications for nutritional support. *J Head Trauma Rehabil.* 1999;14(5):462-474.

45. Chiaretti A, De Benedictis R, Langer A, et al. Prognostic implications of hyperglycaemia in paediatric head injury. *Childs Nerv Syst.* 1998;14(9):455-459.

46. Cochran A, Scaife ER, Hansen KW, Downey EC. Hyperglycemia and Outcomes from Pediatric Traumatic Brain Injury. *J Trauma.* 2003;55(6):1035-1038.

47. Slone DS. Nutritional support of the critically ill and injured patient. *Crit Care Clin.* 2004;20(1):135-157.

48. Dickerson RN, Boschert KJ, Kudsk KA, Brown RO. Hypocaloric enteral tube feeding in critically ill obese patients. *Nutrition.* 2002;18(3):241-246.

49. Stone HH, Strom PR, Mullins RJ. Management of the major coagulopathy with onset during laparotomy. *Ann Surg.* 1983;197(5):532-535.

50. Rotondo MF, Schwab CW, McGonigal MD, et al. 'Damage control': an approach for improved survival in exsanguinating penetrating abdominal injury. *J Trauma.* 1993;35(3):375-382; discussion 382-373.

51. Kritayakirana K, Maggio PM, Brundage S, Purtill MA, Staudenmayer K, Spain DA. Outcomes and complications of open abdomen technique for managing non-trauma patients. *J Emerg Trauma Shock.* 2010;3(2):118-122.

52. Ozguc H, Yilmazlar T, Gurluler E, Ozen Y, Korun N, Zorluoglu A. Staged abdominal repair in the treatment of intra-abdominal infection: analysis of 102 patients. *J Gastrointest Surg.* 2003;7(5):646-651.

53. Cheatham ML, Safcsak K, Brzezinski SJ, Lube MW. Nitrogen balance, protein loss, and the open abdomen. *Crit Care Med.* 2007;35(1):127-131.

54. Miller RS, Morris JA, Jr., Diaz JJ, Jr., Herring MB, May AK. Complications after 344 damage-control open celiotomies. *J Trauma.* 2005;59(6):1365-1371; discussion 1371-1364.

55. Tsuei BJ, Magnuson B, Swintosky M, et al. Enteral nutrition in patients with an open peritoneal cavity. *Nutr Clin Pract.* 2003;18(3):253-258.

56. Byrnes MC, Reicks P, Irwin E. Early enteral nutrition can be successfully implemented in trauma patients with an "open abdomen". *Am J Surg.* 2010;199(3):359-362; discussion 363.

57. Cothren CC, Moore EE, Ciesla DJ, et al. Postinjury abdominal compartment syndrome does not preclude early enteral feeding after definitive closure. *Am J Surg.* 2004;188(6):653-658.

58. Yuan Y, Ren J, Gu G, Chen J, Li J. Early enteral nutrition improves outcomes of open abdomen in gastrointestinal fistula patients complicated with severe sepsis. *Nutr Clin Pract.* 2011;26(6):688-694.

59. Desai KM, Dorward IG, Minkes RK, Dillon PA. Blunt duodenal injuries in children. *J Trauma.* 2003;54(4): 640-645; discussion 645-646.

60. Jewett TC, Jr., Caldarola V, Karp MP, Allen JE, Cooney DR. Intramural hematoma of the duodenum. *Arch Surg.* 1988;123(1):54-58.

61. Czyrko C, Weltz CR, Markowitz RI, O'Neill JA. Blunt abdominal trauma resulting in intestinal obstruction: when to operate? *J Trauma.* 1990;30(12):1567-1571.

62. Teixeira PG, Inaba K, Dubose J, et al. Enterocutaneous fistula complicating trauma laparotomy: a major resource burden. *Am Surg.* 2009;75(1):30-32.

63. Kaushal M, Carlson GL. Management of enterocutaneous fistulas. *Clin Colon Rectal Surg.* 2004;17(2):79-88.

CHAPTER 12

Burns and Wound Healing

Maggie L. Dylewski

Kathy Prelack

Robert L. Sheridan

- METABOLIC RESPONSE TO BURN INJURY
- NUTRITION ASSESSMENT
  - Determining Nutritional Status and Risk
  - Nutrition Assessment Tools
  - Monitoring Nutritional Status
  - Determining Energy Requirements
  - Estimating Protein Requirements
  - Vitamins and Minerals
- NUTRITION SUPPORT
  - Enteral Nutrition
  - Enteral Formula Selection
- PHARMACOLOGY
  - Glutamine
  - Oxandrolone
  - Propranolol
  - Insulin
- KEY POINTS
  - References

METABOLIC RESPONSE TO BURN INJURY

Adequate nutrition is required to support the metabolic alterations associated with burn injury. Although a surge in protein, carbohydrate, and fat catabolism occurs in all critically ill patients, the duration and intensity of the response are exaggerated in patients with large burn injuries.[1,2]

The basic etiology of the hypermetabolic response following a burn injury remains poorly understood despite years of well-funded investigation. Presumably, it is driven by the intensity of catecholamine, glucocorticoid, glucagon, and dopamine secretion, which activate several complex mediator cascades.[1,3-6] Endotoxin, tumor necrosis factor, interleukins 1 and 6, platelet-activating factor, arachidonic acid metabolites through the cyclooxygenase and lipooxygenase pathways, reactive oxygen species, neutrophil-adherence complexes, nitric oxide, and the complement and coagulation cascades are hypothesized to all play a major role in the regulation of the hypermetabolic response.[5]

The clinical consequences of these biochemical changes in burn victims can be profound and include elevated resting energy expenditure (REE), muscle and bone catabolism, and insulin resistance.[1] Despite aggressive treatment, a loss of up to 25% of total body mass is commonplace after large burn injuries.[7] Untreated burn injuries will result in severe wasting of lean body mass (**Fig. 12-1**).[8] Extensive lean body mass depletion is associated with morbidity and mortality.[9-12]

Strategies to blunt or counter the postinjury response include 2 general themes: (1) supportive care and (2) surgical intervention (Table 12-1). Supportive efforts focus on adequate nutrient intake; pharmacological interventions, including analgesia and infection

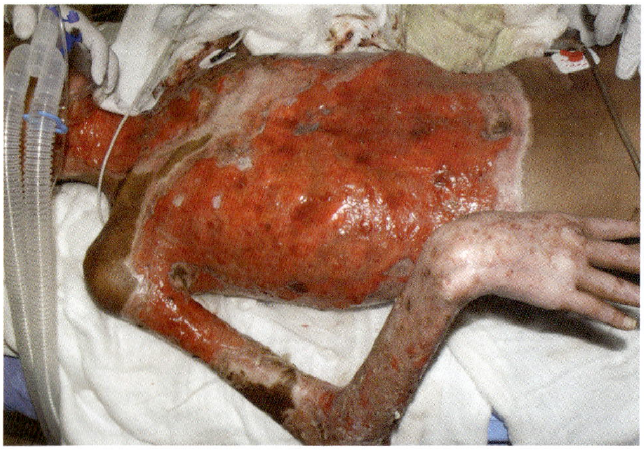

FIGURE 12-1. Severe wasting of lean body mass following an untreated burn injury.

control; and environmental manipulation. Continuous nutrition support, which focuses on optimal protein intake, is expected to offset muscle catabolism and preserve lean body mass. Optimal aseptic techniques help to minimize infectious complications. Sepsis increases protein catabolism and metabolic rate by approximately 40% in burn patients.[1] Evaporative losses and accompanying heat loss also increase the metabolic rate. Bacteria-controlled nursing units (BCNUs) (**Fig. 12-2**) provide a warm, isolated environment for patients with >30% total body surface area (TBSA) burn injuries. Inside the plastic walls of the BCNU, temperatures range from 84°F to 88°F with 80% humidity, and a laminar airflow unit reduces bacterial cross-colonization.[13] Overall, surgical interventions are the most successful approach to reducing the hyperdynamic effects of burn injury. Early excision and grafting of large full-thickness burn wounds significantly reduce metabolic rate.[1]

NUTRITION ASSESSMENT

The nutritional assessment of burn patients is an ongoing dynamic process that is directly related to the stage of injury. Upon admission, important demographic, anthropometric, laboratory, and dietary data must be collected in order to perform a complete nutritional assessment (Table 12-2). Subsequently, nutritional status and nutritional risk must be determined in tandem.

Determining Nutritional Status and Risk

Obesity and malnutrition should be identified on admission, since these factors will affect nutrition support strategies. Nutritional risk factors include all elements that can influence nutrient absorption and utilization, such as the severity of burn injury, age, and the presence of inhalation injury and organ dysfunction. In addition, it should be expected that, due to the physiologic response to trauma, nutritional status will decline over time, independent of the baseline status.[14]

Nutrition Assessment Tools

Anthropometric and laboratory data should be mindfully interpreted, as the physiological features of metabolic stress often confound these values. Body weight may be unreliable due to the influence of extracellular water expansion following acute burn injury.[15] Despite this limitation,

TABLE 12-1. Strategies to Blunt the Metabolic Response to Burn Injury

Nutrition Support	Pharmacologic	Environmental	Surgical
• Early initiation of nutrition support with minimal interruption • High nitrogen:calorie ratio	• Adequate sedation and pain control • Anabolic steroids • Beta-andrenergic blockade	• Infection control • Warm environment	• Early excision and wound closure • Drainage of septic foci

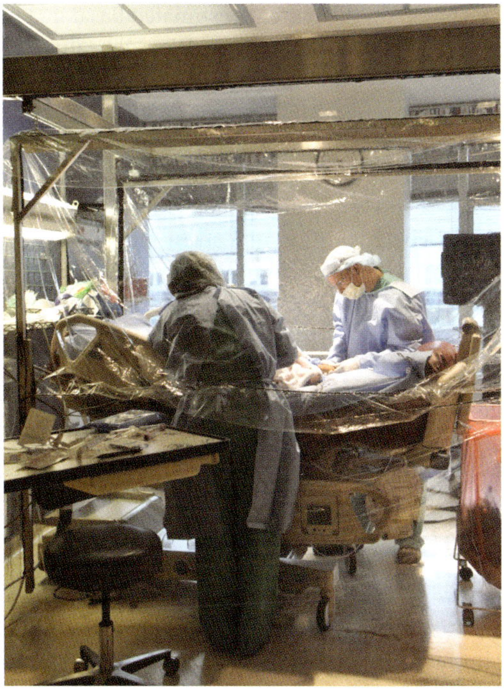

FIGURE 12-2. Bacteria-controlled nursing unit.

■ **TABLE 12-2. Elements of Nutrition Assessment**

Measurement	Monitoring Frequency
Weight	Twice a week
Prealbumin	Weekly
C-reactive protein	Weekly
Calorie and protein intake	Daily
Electrolytes, phosphorus, ionized calcium, magnesium	Every 6 hours for the first 48 hours, then twice daily
Glucose	Every 6 hours for the first 48 hours, then twice daily
Liver function tests	Weekly
Triglycerides	Every 2 weeks
Serum lipase, amylase	Weekly
BUN	Daily
Creatinine	Daily

longitudinal weight data, when judiciously evaluated, can be useful.

Similarly, obtaining accurate measurements of visceral proteins is nearly impossible, as most reasonable measures of nutritional status are down-regulated by the acute-phase response. Trending prealbumin measurements with the C-reactive protein, an acute-phase protein, is a common practice among burn units. There is evidence that prealbumin and C-reactive protein are related to morbidity and mortality among burn patients, but it is unclear that the prealbumin is truly related to nutrition status in these patients.[16,17]

Monitoring Nutritional Status

Nutritional parameters should be monitored regularly (Table 12-2). During the acute phase, weight should be obtained twice a week so that trends can be easily monitored. It is important to recognize that fluctuations in weight during the early acute phase of care are influenced by fluid shifts and may not indicate changes in dry weight. Once wound closure is achieved and the patient enters the rehabilitative phase, weekly weight checks may be sufficient.

The reliability of visceral protein levels also improves with wound closure. If nutritional intake is optimal throughout the course of injury, a gradual increase in prealbumin should occur as the acute phase subsides, evidenced by a decrease in C-reactive protein. Failure of prealbumin to rise despite declining C-reactive protein levels may indicate protein or calorie malnutrition.[14]

Evaluation of energy and protein intake is an important part of nutritional monitoring. Daily energy intake should be compared preferably to measured requirements, or when that option is unavailable, to estimated requirements by standard equations. If energy and protein intake are less than optimal, nutrition support strategies should be reevaluated.

Routine monitoring of biochemical parameters (Table 12-2) is necessary for assessing fluid and electrolyte balance, metabolic acidosis, organ function, and hyperglycemia. A decline in electrolytes, phosphorus, calcium, and magnesium levels is expected during the acute-phase response and may also occur during the initiation of aggressive nutrition support. Sodium levels are also influenced by silver-based dressing solutions. Hyperglycemia is common during burn injuries due to increased rates of glucose production and utilization accompanied by insulin resistance.[18] Other prominent burn-related changes in physiology and organ function include pancreatitis, renal failure, and liver dysfunction.

Determining Energy Requirements

Elevated energy expenditure is a well-recognized consequence of the inflammatory response. However, rates of energy expenditure following burn injury have gradually declined over the years, from historic measures of up to 200% of REE to a more manageable 120% to 130%.[19,20] Advances in burn care, including medical, surgical, environmental, and pharmacological strategies, can significantly reduce energy expenditure.[14] Early excision and grafting,[21] utilization of occlusive bandages,[22] and the provision of a bacteria-controlled, heated environment all reduce metabolic rate, regardless of open wound area. Similarly, vigilant management of pain and use of appropriate sedation lower energy requirements significantly.[2]

The American Society for Parenteral and Enteral Nutrition (A.S.P.E.N.) recommends that indirect calorimetry be used for measuring energy expenditure in critically ill patients.[23] This tool may be particularly useful among burn patients, as indirect calorimetry will capture the stress of disease as well as the various clinical factors that may be unique to each patient. An activity factor of 20% to 30% is added to the measured energy expenditure to account for daily activities (repositioning, dressing changes, physical therapy) that may contribute to the total energy expenditure.[24]

Serial indirect calorimetry measurements can provide early warning of over- and underfeeding,[25] which may occur when standard equations for energy expenditure estimation are utilized to prescribe the energy delivery goal. If indirect calorimetry is unavailable, energy goals may be based on the patient's estimated basal metabolic rate (BMR) with a stress factor.[14] Wound healing can be achieved if energy intake equals BMR with a stress factor of 1.3 to 1.4 and optimal dietary protein is provided.[23] For convalescent children, the stress factor of 1.2 is recommended.[23] In today's pediatric intensive care units (PICUs), severely burned patients are one of the few instances where addition of a stress factor to REE may be appropriate. When calories were delivered at 1.5 × REE, the patients accrued fat instead of muscle.[26]

Estimating Protein Requirements

Skeletal muscle catabolism after severe burn injury accommodates amino acid needs for wound healing, immune function, synthesis of acute-phase proteins, and gluconeogenesis.[1] Inadequate protein intake compromises these critical functions. It is now well known that exogenous protein will not completely abate protein breakdown during burn injury.[27,28] The goal of protein therapy after burn injury is to support wound healing and immune function by fostering protein synthesis. A positive protein balance can be achieved by supplying 3 to 4.5 g/kg of protein for children 0 to 6 years of age and 2.5 to 3 g/kg of protein to children older than 6 years.[29,30]

Vitamins and Minerals

Evidence-based practice guidelines for vitamin and mineral supplementation in burn patients are not available. Vitamins and minerals play an essential role in wound healing and immune function, and data are available to show that several of them are depleted following burn injury (Table 12-3). Regrettably, describing true micronutrient deficiencies following a burn injury can be a challenge, as

TABLE 12-3. Micronutrients Depleted During Burn Injuries

Micronutrient	Adults	Children	Reference
Vitamin C	x		70
Vitamin D		x	71
Vitamin E	x	x	70,72
Copper	x	x	73-77
Selenium	x	x	78-80
Zinc	x	x	73, 75-77

plasma levels are complicated by the acute-phase response. Many micronutrients rely on a protein carrier, which is often down-regulated during the inflammatory response.

Studies that focus on micronutrient supplementation for patients with burn injuries are scarce. Multitrace-mineral supplement cocktails receive the most attention in the burn literature, compared to specific vitamin or mineral supplements. Several randomized controlled trials among adults report that an intravenous trace-mineral cocktail, including selenium, copper, and zinc, resulted in reduced infection rates and graft loss among adult burn patients.[31-34] Corresponding pediatric data are not available. One small randomized control trial among pediatric burn patients did show improved rates of wound healing with a vitamin C, vitamin E, and zinc enteral cocktail.[35] Unfortunately, specific nutrient requirements cannot be elucidated from this data. It is also not clear as to what route—intravenous or enteral—is the most effective vehicle for micronutrient administration.

More data are needed to create evidence-based guidelines for micronutrient supplementation following burn injury. Of note, burn patients often receive 100% or more of the recommended dietary allowance for each micronutrient with their enteral feeding regimen. In fact, adult enteral nutrition (EN) products most likely provide pediatric patients with an ample supply of all required micronutrients. Unless a preexisting deficiency is suspected, additional supplementation is not warranted.

NUTRITION SUPPORT

Once the optimal nutrient delivery goals are determined, the best route for administration needs to be determined. As in other critical illnesses, there are many challenges to nutrient delivery in the child with burn injury.

Enteral Nutrition

When practical, EN is the ideal mode of nutrition support, as it may help to protect immune function, preserve gastrointestinal integrity, mitigate whole-body inflammation and stress, and provide the appropriate macro- and micronutrients the body requires.[36] Early initiation of EN (within 24 hours) among adult burn patients is associated with decreased length of ICU stay and wound infections.[37] The European Society for Clinical Nutrition and Metabolism (ESPEN) recommends that nutritional therapy be initiated early (within 12 hours) and by the enteral route.[38] Early enteral feeding, which is started within the first 12 hours after injury by the gastric route, is associated with numerous advantages, such as amelioration of the hypermetabolic response,[39] and also causes increased immunoglobulin production[40] while reducing the risk of malnutrition and of energy deficit.[41,42]

Most pediatric burn patients are capable of tolerating early EN. Of concern is the higher rate of adverse events, including bowel necrosis, reported with provision of early EN in pediatric burn patients. In one study, bowel necrosis seemed to be associated with burn size, resuscitation volumes, and inotropic requirements.[43] Exclusion criteria for aggressive early EN support include hemodynamic instability, high-dose vasopressor requirement, or significant abdominal distention. This practice is consistent with the A.S.P.E.N. guidelines, which state that EN should be held or delayed in patients with severe hemodynamic compromise until the patient is fully resuscitated or more stable.[44]

Since these children require frequent operative procedures, achieving nutritional requirements via the enteral route alone may not be practical.[36,45] Energy and protein deficits quickly accumulate when EN cannot be advanced to goal rate. In these situations, an alternative method of nutrition support that includes a combination of enteral and parenteral nutrition (PN) may be necessary to prevent consequences of suboptimal nutritional intake.

Historically, PN was associated with morbidity and mortality among burn patients.[46] However, we now know that when PN is used prudently, particularly when glucose infusions are capped at rates consistent with carbohydrate oxidation, PN is a safe alternative to suboptimal nutritional intake by the enteral route alone.[47]

When a patient is expected to receive inadequate EN support for longer than 12 hours, a high-nitrogen, hypocaloric PN formula (Table 12-4) should be started in conjunction with the abbreviated supply of EN.[48] The high amino acid content of this formula includes a nonprotein energy-to-protein ratio (85:1) that allows protein needs to be met without excessive volume infusion rates. To minimize the risk of overfeeding and hyperglycemia, it is imperative to limit glucose infusion to 5 mg/kg/min.[49] Unfortunately, with this limitation, PN can only approximate basal energy requirements. Supplemental EN may be needed to reduce the energy deficit associated with PN.

Two studies have shown that restricting lipid provision to patients with significant burns may be of benefit.[50,51] It has been recommended that lipid be kept <35% of total calorie intake while accounting for extraneous sources of lipid such as propofol.

TABLE 12-4. Parenteral Nutrition Composition and Administration Guidelines in Burned Children

Nutrient	Recommended Intake	Key Points
Total solution Dextrose 20%/7.4% amino acids	1.75 mL/kg/hr for infants and children <20 kg 1.5 mL/kg/hour for children >20 kg	Can be initiated at goal rate.
Carbohydrate	5 mg/kg/min	This is consistent with the maximum rate of glucose oxidation in burned children.
Protein	Goals of 2.5 to 4.0 g/kg ideal body weight	The high amino acid content enables protein goal to be met without excessive volume.
Fat (20% intravenous lipids)	Initiate at 0.5 g/kg for 12 hours Goal volume: 1.0 to 1.5 g/kg/day fat Ensure that fat is not >35% of total calories	Propofol contains a 10% soybean oil solution.
Sodium/potassium	100/50 mEq/L	Enhanced electrolytes to provide higher baseline needed for increased losses.
Calcium/magnesium	9/18 mEq/L	
Phosphorus	15 mmol	
Acetate/chloride	120/71 mEq/L	Acetate maximized to avoid acidosis with high amino acid content.
Intravenous multivitamin with trace minerals	5 mL/L, 0.5 mL/L	Vitamin K is added to PN weekly as 1 weight-based dose: 10 kg = 1 mg; 10 to 50 kg = 2 mg; >50 kg = 4 mg Trace mineral amounts: Zinc = 2,500 mcg; Copper = 500 mcg; Selenium = 30 mcg

Enteral Formula Selection

Standard high-protein EN formulas are sufficient to meet the heightened nutrient requirements of burn patients. A useful strategy in the pediatric burn unit is to utilize adult formulas, which typically contain more protein (~40 to 60 g/L) compared to pediatric versions (~30 g/L) with children >1 year of age. Adult formulas also supply higher amounts of electrolytes and micronutrients, which may reduce or eliminate the need for supplementation. Fiber-containing formulas may reduce the constipation seen almost invariably in these children.[38]

Many specialty EN formulas are also available on the market today, although their availability may exceed scientific support. Popular products contain key nutrients, such as glutamine, arginine, and omega-3 fatty acids, all believed to improve wound healing and/or immune function. Currently, there is no consistent evidence to suggest that immune-enhancing formulas reduce morbidity or mortality in critically ill patients[52] or burn patients.[53,54]

The gastric route is recommended for most patients; however, postpyloric placement has some distinct advantages in burn patients. Since these patients undergo frequent procedures in the operating room, use of postpyloric feeds leads to less nil per os (NPO) time, and some centers feed patients throughout their procedures. Postburn ileus typically involves the stomach and colon, and a postpyloric tube bypasses the stomach.

PHARMACOLOGY

The use of micronutrients or drugs that modify and alleviate the postburn catabolic response has been an area of great interest. A variety of interventions have been studied in this population with the intention of blunting the hypermetabolic response, promoting muscle mass accrual and wound healing, preventing infections, or controlling hyperglycemia.

Glutamine

Glutamine has several attractive features for adult burn patients, including improved wound healing[55,56] and fewer infections.[55,57] It is reasonable to assume that the benefits of glutamine supplementation in pediatric burn patients may be similar to those found in adults; however, no data exist to support this assumption. In fact, the only published study available among pediatric burn patients reported that enteral glutamine was not associated with improved protein turnover.[58] Therefore, no glutamine recommendation for pediatric burn patients can be proposed at this time.

Oxandrolone

Oxandrolone is an anabolic steroid used among burn patients to counteract the hypermetabolic response by promoting protein synthesis.[59-61] Data from one study showed that oxandrolone therapy (0.2 mg/kg/day) increased total body mass and lean body mass, and reduced length of stay among pediatric burn patients.[60] Treatment was also associated with increased liver function tests, but no hepatic failure was reported. Careful utilization of oxandrolone is necessary, as this drug comes with a black box warning from the Food and Drug Administration about lipid abnormalities, peliosis hepatitis, and hepatic tumors. Symptoms of peliosis hepatitis and hepatic tumors may be silent until they become life threatening. Withdrawal of oxandrolone often results in regression or cessation of symptoms. Pediatric patients can have a successful recovery following burn injury without the use of anabolic steroids. Due to the potential serious complications associated with oxandrolone, the decision to administer this drug to children should be carefully considered.

Propranolol

Propranolol is a nonselective, beta-adrenergic receptor antagonist. The rationale behind propranolol treatment is to blunt the catecholamine surge associated with the hypermetabolic response to burn injury. Doses of propranolol titrated to reduce heart rates by 20% significantly lessen cardiac work[62] and REE.[63] It is not possible to generalize this data to all critically ill children with burns, but side effects seem to be few and costs are low.[5] Although the impact of pain and anxiety control on postburn metabolism has not been well studied, propranolol may have a similar mechanism of action by reducing the intensity of catecholamine secretion.

Insulin

The inflammatory response associated with burn injuries is characterized by stress-induced hyperglycemia instigated by increased hepatic glucose production and cellular insulin resistance. Hyperglycemia is associated with increased incidence of infection, sepsis, and mortality among pediatric burn patients.[64,65] Correction of hyperglycemia may ameliorate these complications; however, the target range for serum glucose levels that is both safe and optimal remains ambiguous. Aggressive insulin therapy designed to maintain serum glucose levels between 80 and 121 mg/dL was reported to be associated with decreased infection and sepsis among pediatric burn patients.[66] However, strict glucose control was also related to mild hypoglycemia events (blood glucose <60 mg/dL) in 43% of the patients and severe hypoglycemic events (blood glucose <40 mg/dL) in 26% of the patients.

Given the hypoglycemic risks of intensive insulin therapy, a more liberal approach to glucose control is recommended. A blood glucose target of less than 140 mg/dL for critically ill patients appears effective and reasonable.[64,66-68] Recent Society of Critical Care Medicine guidelines on glucose control were developed for adult patients, but their relevance in children is unclear.[69] To optimize safety, some centers use a sliding-scale insulin protocol as the first line of therapy for hyperglycemia (serum glucose >140 mg/dL). If this approach is not effective, an insulin drip may be initiated.

KEY POINTS

- Enteral nutrition should be initiated within 12 hours of injury, if at all possible.
- Indirect calorimetry is a gold standard to assess energy requirements.
- Children with significant burns require large amounts of protein.

- Carbohydrate delivery should not exceed 5 mg/kg per minute in children.
- Energy from fat should not exceed 35% of total energy intake.

REFERENCES

1. Hart DW, Wolf SE, Chinkes DL, et al. Determinants of skeletal muscle catabolism after severe burn. *Ann Surg.* 2000;232:455-465.
2. Herndon DN, Tompkins RG. Support of the metabolic response to burn injury. *Lancet.* 2004;363:1895-1902.
3. Jeffries MK, Vance ML. Growth hormone and cortisol secretion in patients with burn injury. *J Burn Care Rehabil.* 1992;13:391-395.
4. Klein GL, Bi LX, Sherrard DJ, et al. Evidence supporting a role of glucocorticoids in short-term bone loss in burned children. *Osteoporos Int.* 2004;15:468-474.
5. Sheridan RL. A great constitutional disturbance. *N Engl J Med.* 2001;345:1271-12572.
6. Wilmore DW, Long JM, Mason AD, Jr, Skreen RW, Pruitt BA, Jr. Catecholamines: mediator of the hypermetabolic response to thermal injury. *Ann Surg.* 1974;180:653-669.
7. Newsome TW, Mason AD, Jr, Pruitt BA, Jr. Weight loss following thermal injury. *Ann Surg.* 1973;178:215-217.
8. Dylewski ML, Prelack K, Weber JM, et al. Malnutrition among pediatric burn patients: a consequence of delayed admissions. *Burns.* 2010;36:1185-1189.
9. Studley HO. Percentage of weight loss: a basic indicator of surgical risk in patients with chronic peptic ulcer. 1936. *Nutr Hosp.* 2001;16:141,3; discussion 140-141.
10. Windsor JA, Hill GL. Weight loss with physiologic impairment. A basic indicator of surgical risk. *Ann Surg.* 1988;207:290-296.
11. Kotler DP, Tierney AR, Wang J, Pierson RN,Jr. Magnitude of body-cell-mass depletion and the timing of death from wasting in AIDS. *Am J Clin Nutr.* 1989;50:444-447.
12. Hill GL, Blackett RL, Pickford I, et al. Malnutrition in surgical patients. An unrecognised problem. *Lancet.* 1977;1:689-692.
13. Weber JM, Sheridan RL, Schulz JT, Tompkins RG, Ryan CM. Effectiveness of bacteria-controlled nursing units in preventing cross-colonization with resistant bacteria in severely burned children. *Infect Control Hosp Epidemiol.* 2002;23:549-551.
14. Prelack K, Dylewski M, Sheridan RL. Practical guidelines for nutritional management of burn injury and recovery. *Burns.* 2007;33:14-24.
15. Prelack K, Sheridan R, Yu YM, et al. Sodium bromide by instrumental neutron activation analysis quantifies change in extracellular water space with wound closure in severely burned children. *Surgery.* 2003;133:396-403.
16. Gottschlich MM, Baumer T, Jenkins M, Khoury J, Warden GD. The prognostic value of nutritional and inflammatory indices in patients with burns. *J Burn Care Rehabil.* 1992;13:105-113.
17. Cynober L, Prugnaud O, Lioret N, Duchemin C, Saizy R, Giboudeau J. Serum transthyretin levels in patients with burn injury. *Surgery.* 1991;109:640-644.
18. Wolfe RR. Burn injury and increased glucose production. *J Trauma.* 1979;19:898-899.
19. Long CL, Schaffel N, Geiger JW, Schiller WR, Blakemore WS. Metabolic response to injury and illness: estimation of energy and protein needs from indirect calorimetry and nitrogen balance. *J Parenter Enteral Nutr.* 1979;3:452-456.
20. Gore DC, Rutan RL, Hildreth M, Desai MH, Herndon DN. Comparison of resting energy expenditures and caloric intake in children with severe burns. *J Burn Care Rehabil.* 1990;11:400-404.
21. Cone JB, Wallace BH, Caldwell FT, Jr. The effect of staged burn wound closure on the rates of heat production and heat loss of burned children and young adults. *J Trauma.* 1988;28:968-972.
22. Caldwell FT, Jr, Bowser BH, Crabtree JH. The effect of occlusive dressings on the energy metabolism of severely burned children. *Ann Surg.* 1981;193:579-591.
23. A.S.P.E.N Board of Directors and the Clinical Guidelines Task Force. Guidelines for the use of parenteral and enteral nutrition in adult and pediatric patients. *J Parenter Enteral Nutr.* 2002;26:1SA-138SA.
24. Goran MI, Peters EJ, Herndon DN, Wolfe RR. Total energy expenditure in burned children using the doubly labeled water technique. *Am J Physiol.* 1990;259: E576-585.
25. Saffle JR, Medina E, Raymond J, Westenskow D, Kravitz M, Warden GD. Use of indirect calorimetry in the nutritional management of burned patients. *J Trauma.* 1985;25:32-39.
26. Hart DW, Wolf SE, Herndon DN, et al. Energy expenditure and caloric balance after burn: increased feedings lead to fat rather than lean mass accretion. *Ann Surg.* 2002;235:152-161.
27. Wolfe RR, Goodenough RD, Wolfe MH. Isotopic approaches to the estimation of protein requirements in burn patients. *Adv Shock Res.* 1983;9:81-98.
28. Patterson BW, Nguyen T, Pierre E, Herndon DN, Wolfe RR. Urea and protein metabolism in burned children: effect of dietary protein intake. *Metabolism.* 1997;46:573-578.

29. Prelack K, Cunningham JJ, Sheridan RL, Tompkins RG. Energy and protein provisions for thermally injured children revisited: an outcome-based approach for determining requirements. *J Burn Care Rehabil.* 1997;18:177,81; discussion 176.

30. Prelack K, Yu YM, Dylewski M, Lydon M, Sheridan RL, Tompkins RG. The contribution of muscle to whole-body protein turnover throughout the course of burn injury in children. *J Burn Care Res.* 2010;31:942-948.

31. Berger MM, Spertini F, Shenkin A, et al. Trace element supplementation modulates pulmonary infection rates after major burns: a double-blind, placebo-controlled trial. *Am J Clin Nutr.* 1998;68:365-371.

32. Berger MM, Eggimann P, Heyland DK, et al. Reduction of nosocomial pneumonia after major burns by trace element supplementation: aggregation of two randomised trials. *Crit Care.* 2006;10:R153.

33. Berger MM, Chiolero RL. Antioxidant supplementation in sepsis and systemic inflammatory response syndrome. *Crit Care Med.* 2007;35:S584-590.

34. Berger MM, Shenkin A. Trace element requirements in critically ill burned patients. *J Trace Elem Med Biol.* 2007;21 Suppl 1:44-48.

35. Barbosa E, Faintuch J, Machado Moreira EA, et al. Supplementation of vitamin E, vitamin C, and zinc attenuates oxidative stress in burned children: a randomized, double-blind, placebo-controlled pilot study. *J Burn Care Res.* 2009;30:859-866.

36. Altintas ND, Aydin K, Turkoglu MA, Abbasoglu O, Topeli A. Effect of enteral versus parenteral nutrition on outcome of medical patients requiring mechanical ventilation. *Nutr Clin Pract.* 2011;26:322-329.

37. Mosier MJ, Pham TN, Klein MB, et al. Early enteral nutrition in burns: compliance with guidelines and associated outcomes in a multicenter study. *J Burn Care Res.* 2011;32:104-109.

38. Rousseau AF, Losser MR, Ichai C, Berger MM. ESPEN endorsed recommendations: nutritional therapy in major burns. *Clin Nutr.* 2013;32:497-502.

39. Mochizuki et al. Mechanism of prevention of postburn hypermetabolism and catabolism by early enteral feeding. *Ann Surg.* 1984; 200 :297-310.

40. Lam NN, Tien NG, Khoa CM. Early enteral feeding for burned patients: an effective method, which should be encouraged in developing countries. *Burns.* 2008; 34: 192-196.

41. Chiarelli A, et al. Very early nutrition supplementation in burned patients. *Am J Clin Nutr.* 1990; 51:1035-1039; 9.

42. Venter M, Rode H, Sive A, Visser M. Enteral resuscitation and early enteral feeding in children with major burns effect on McFarlane response to stress. *Burns.* 2007; 33:464-471.

43. Gottschlich MM, Jenkins ME, Mayes T, Khoury J, Kagan RJ, Warden GD. The 2002 Clinical Research Award. An evaluation of the safety of early vs delayed enteral support and effects on clinical, nutritional, and endocrine outcomes after severe burns. *J Burn Care Rehabil.* 2002;23:401-415.

44. McClave SA, Martindale RG, Vanek VW, et al. Guidelines for the Provision and Assessment of Nutrition Support Therapy in the Adult Critically Ill Patient: Society of Critical Care Medicine (SCCM) and American Society for Parenteral and Enteral Nutrition (A.S.P.E.N). *J Parenter Enteral Nutr.* 2009;33:277-316.

45. Woodcock NP, Zeigler D, Palmer MD, Buckley P, Mitchell CJ, MacFie J. Enteral versus parenteral nutrition: a pragmatic study. *Nutrition.* 2001;17:1-12.

46. Herndon DN, Barrow RE, Stein M, et al. Increased mortality with intravenous supplemental feeding in severely burned patients. *J Burn Care Rehabil.* 1989;10:309-313.

47. Dylewski ML, Baker M, Prelack K, et al. The safety and efficacy of parenteral nutrition among pediatric patients with burn injuries. *Ped Crit Care Med.* 2013 (in press).

48. Sheridan RL, Yu YM, Prelack K, Young VR, Burke JF, Tompkins RG. Maximal parenteral glucose oxidation in hypermetabolic young children: a stable isotope study. *J Parenter Enteral Nutr.* 1998;22:212-216.

49. Gottschlich MM, Alexander JW. Fat kinetics and recommended dietary intake in burns. *J Parenter Enteral Nutr.* 1987;11:80-85.

50. Bernier J, Jobin N, Emptoz-Bonneton A, Pugeat MM, Garrel DR. Decreased corticosteroid-binding globulin in burn patients: relationship with interleukin-6 and fat in nutritional support. *Crit Care Med.* 1998;26:452-60.

51. Garrel DR, Razi M, Larivière F, Jobin N, Naman N, Emptoz-Bonneton A, et al. Improved clinical status and length of care with low-fat nutrition support in burn patients. *J Parenter Enteral Nutr.* 1995; 19:482-489.

52. Montejo JC, Zarazaga A, Lopez-Martinez J, et al. Immunonutrition in the intensive care unit. A systematic review and consensus statement. *Clin Nutr.* 2003;22:221-233.

53. Martindale RG, Cresci GA. The use of immune enhancing diet in head injury. *J Parenter Enteral Nutr.* 2001;25:S27,8; discussion S28-29.

54. Marik PE, Zaloga GP. Immunonutrition in critically ill patients: a systematic review and analysis of the literature. *Intensive Care Med.* 2008;34:1980-1990.

55. Zhou YP, Jiang ZM, Sun YH, Wang XR, Ma EL, Wilmore D. The effect of supplemental enteral glutamine on plasma levels, gut function, and outcome in severe burns: a randomized, double-blind, controlled clinical trial. *J Parenter Enteral Nutr.* 2003;27:241-245.

56. Peng X, Yan H, You Z, Wang P, Wang S. Clinical and protein metabolic efficacy of glutamine granules-supplemented enteral nutrition in severely burned patients. *Burns.* 2005;31:342-346.

57. Garrel D, Patenaude J, Nedelec B, et al. Decreased mortality and infectious morbidity in adult burn patients given enteral glutamine supplements: a prospective, controlled, randomized clinical trial. *Crit Care Med.* 2003;31:2444-2449.

58. Sheridan RL, Prelack K, Yu YM, et al. Short-term enteral glutamine does not enhance protein accretion in burned children: a stable isotope study. *Surgery.* 2004;135:671-8.

59. Hart DW, Wolf SE, Ramzy PI, et al. Anabolic effects of oxandrolone after severe burn. *Ann Surg.* 2001;233:556-564.

60. Jeschke MG, Finnerty CC, Suman OE, Kulp G, Mlcak RP, Herndon DN. The effect of oxandrolone on the endocrinologic, inflammatory, and hypermetabolic responses during the acute phase postburn. *Ann Surg.* 2007;246:351,60; discussion 360-362.

61. Wolf SE, Thomas SJ, Dasu MR, et al. Improved net protein balance, lean mass, and gene expression changes with oxandrolone treatment in the severely burned. *Ann Surg.* 2003;237:801,10.

62. Williams FN, Branski LK, Jeschke MG, Herndon DN. What, how, and how much should patients with burns be fed? *Surg Clin North Am.* 2011;91:609-629.

63. Herndon DN, Hart DW, Wolf SE, Chinkes DL, Wolfe RR. Reversal of catabolism by beta-blockade after severe burns. *N Engl J Med.* 2001;345:1223-1229.

64. Jeschke MG, Kraft R, Emdad F, Kulp GA, Williams FN, Herndon DN. Glucose control in severely thermally injured pediatric patients: what glucose range should be the target? *Ann Surg.* 2010;252:521,7; discussion 527-528.

65. Pham TN, Warren AJ, Phan HH, Molitor F, Greenhalgh DG, Palmieri TL. Impact of tight glycemic control in severely burned children. *J Trauma.* 2005;59:1148-1154.

66. Brunkhorst FM, Engel C, Bloos F, et al. Intensive insulin therapy and pentastarch resuscitation in severe sepsis. *N Engl J Med.* 2008;358:125-139.

67. Finney SJ, Zekveld C, Elia A, Evans TW. Glucose control and mortality in critically ill patients. *JAMA.* 2003;290:2041-2047.

68. Preiser JC, Devos P. Clinical experience with tight glucose control by intensive insulin therapy. *Crit Care Med.* 2007;35:S503-507.

69. Jacobi J, Bircher N, Krinsley J, et al. Guidelines for the use of an insulin infusion for the management of hyperglycemia in critically ill patients. *Crit Care Med.* 2012;40:3251-3276.

70. Rock CL, Dechert RE, Khilnani R, Parker RS, Rodriguez JL. Carotenoids and antioxidant vitamins in patients after burn injury. *J Burn Care Rehabil.* 1997;18:269,78; discussion 268.

71. Klein GL, Langman CB, Herndon DN. Vitamin D depletion following burn injury in children: a possible factor in post-burn osteopenia. *J Trauma.* 2002;52:346-350.

72. Traber MG, Leonard SW, Traber DL, et al. Alpha-Tocopherol adipose tissue stores are depleted after burn injury in pediatric patients. *Am J Clin Nutr.* 2010;92:1378-1384.

73. Berger MM, Cavadini C, Bart A, et al. Cutaneous copper and zinc losses in burns. *Burns.* 1992;18:373-380.

74. Cunningham JJ, Leffell M, Harmatz P. Burn severity, copper dose, and plasma ceruloplasmin in burned children during total parenteral nutrition. *Nutrition.* 1993;9:329-332.

75. Gosling P, Rothe HM, Sheehan TM, Hubbard LD. Serum copper and zinc concentrations in patients with burns in relation to burn surface area. *J Burn Care Rehabil.* 1995;16:481-486.

76. Voruganti VS, Klein GL, Lu HX, Thomas S, Freeland-Graves JH, Herndon DN. Impaired zinc and copper status in children with burn injuries: need to reassess nutritional requirements. *Burns.* 2005;31:711-716.

77. Khorasani G, Hosseinimehr SJ, Kaghazi Z. The alteration of plasma's zinc and copper levels in patients with burn injuries and the relationship to the time after burn injuries. *Singapore Med J.* 2008;49:627-630.

78. Hunt DR, Lane HW, Beesinger D, et al. Selenium depletion in burn patients. *J Parenter Enteral Nutr.* 1984;8:695-699.

79. Berger MM, Cavadini C, Bart A, et al. Selenium losses in 10 burned patients. *Clin Nutr.* 1992;11:75-82.

80. Dylewski ML, Bender JC, Smith AM, et al. The selenium status of pediatric patients with burn injuries. *J Trauma.* 2010;69:584,8; discussion 588.

CHAPTER 13

Nutrition Management of Pediatric Patients Undergoing Liver Transplantation or Intestinal Transplantation

Renee Wieman

Samuel A. Kocoshis

NUTRITION AFTER LIVER TRANSPLANTATION
NUTRITION AFTER SMALL INTESTINAL TRANSPLANTATION
Pretransplant Nutritional Care
Nutritional Care During the Immediate Posttransplant Period
Nutrient Requirements within the Intensive Care Unit
Nutrition Care During the Late Posttransplant Period (and Long-Term Care)
KEY POINTS
References

NUTRITION AFTER LIVER TRANSPLANTATION

The rates of morbidity and mortality following liver transplantation are directly related to the degree of malnutrition at the time of transplantation. Pediatric patients, like adults, are predisposed to all of the consequences of end-stage liver disease, such as ascites, pruritus, encephalopathy, and portal hypertension, but the impact on growth and development is unique to the pediatric population.[1] Protein-energy malnutrition and growth failure are an inevitable consequence observed in 60% of infants and children with chronic liver disease.[2] Although the exact pathophysiology of this process is not fully understood, many different mechanisms within the disease process can contribute to the early onset of malnutrition. The nutritional care of infants and children with end-stage liver disease requires diligent monitoring and aggressive support by the entire health care team to ensure optimal transplant outcomes.

The rapid deterioration of nutritional status and the profound complications of end-stage liver disease have made early liver transplant evaluation imperative. Malnutrition is one of the major factors adversely affecting the survival of infants and children on transplant waiting lists, and the one in which we can have the greatest impact on outcome.[3] Therefore, the goals of nutritional support prior to transplant should be focused on the prevention of any further liver injury, the minimization of nutritional depletion, conservation of growth, maintenance of lean body mass (LBM), and control of disease-related complications. One valuable recommendation is that children with mid-upper arm muscle circumference (MUAC) falling below the fifth percentile be initiated on aggressive nutrition support regimens prior to transplantation.[4]

Liver transplantation has become a standard and effective life-saving intervention for infants and children with acute and chronic liver failure. With significant advances in surgical techniques, the development of variant technical procedures involving allograft reduction, and the improvement of long-term immunosuppressant medications, liver transplantation has now become a valid therapy for pediatric patients.[5] In the past, the need to size-match cadaveric livers had severely restricted pediatric transplantation and led to inflated rates of death among patients on transplant waiting lists. With the ability to use reduced-sized cadaveric grafts or living-related donation, more donor organs are now available. Survival rates in most experienced pediatric liver transplant centers approach 90% at 1 year, and the quality of life for most patients after transplant has significantly improved.[6] These advances have now shifted our principal focus from purely supportive disease management to treatment measures for improving the patient's clinical status before transplantation. The one metric that can make the most impact upon outcome is nutritional status. A child who is experiencing growth failure due to progressive liver disease is more likely to succumb prior to transplantation.[7]

Patients who have advanced liver disease are unable to maintain nutritional status, even with intakes above normal, because of increased energy requirements, the interference of the metabolism of nutrients, and vitamin/mineral deficiencies.[8] Infant formulas containing medium-chain triglyceride (MCT) oil, preferably those highest in MCT oil, are progressively calorie concentrated, up to a goal of 30 calories/oz (1 calorie/mL) with a balance of concentrated infant formula bases and modular additives of glucose polymers and/or MCT oil. (See chapter 16.) Children greater than 1 year of age should be trialed on oral MCT oil-containing pediatric formulas and modular nutrients added to food items in order to further boost calorie intake. These formulas generally contain at least 60% MCT oil and will enhance fat absorption. When patients are unable to consume adequate calories to maintain LBM measurements of MUAC and triceps skinfolds (TSF) in the normal range, supplemental enteral tube feeding should be initiated. Nasogastric tubes are the preferred route of administration if patients can tolerate adequate formula volume to achieve growth. However, in some instances, nasojejunal placement must be utilized because of reflux from gastric distension caused by ascites and organomegaly. Gastrostomy tubes are generally not placed because of this reason, as well as the predilection for developing peristomal varices due to portal hypertension.[9] These varices are particularly difficult to treat locally. Nocturnal drip feedings are commonly used so that preservation of oral feeding skills during the day can be maintained. This allows for supplementation during the normal hours of fasting, which may also prove beneficial in end-stage liver disease patients, particularly infants, who are unable to maintain fasting glucose levels overnight. Quite often, these patients will progress to require 24-hour continuous tube feeding infusions to achieve the increased nutrient intakes required to maintain nutritional status, as well as blood sugar control from a continuously delivered glucose infusion rate. Attempting to maintain oral motor function is essential during pretransplant care to ensure appropriate and opportune transition to normal feedings posttransplantation. In many instances, enteral tube feeding supplementation may be required for a short duration posttransplant until adequate oral intakes can be achieved. As posttransplant patients are able to normalize their daily schedules, pain subsides, and the added effect of appetite stimulation from higher-dose steroids is seen, oral intakes can quickly achieve and sometimes surpass goals.

Parenteral nutrition (PN) is employed pretransplant when complications such as severe varices, gastrointestinal (GI) bleeding, or excessive emesis make it difficult to safely provide the required nutrients enterally, or it can be employed as an adjunctive nutritional therapy in patients who are severely malnourished and in whom the goal enteral nutrient delivery is unattainable.[10] Parenteral nutrition solutions should be composed of a balance of standard amino acids, dextrose, lipids, electrolytes, and minerals designed to meet nutritional needs while minimizing metabolic complications. Amino acid mixtures enriched in branched-chain amino acids (BCAA), which are designed specifically for patients with liver disease have not been beneficial for pediatric patients with liver disease.[11,12] Whatever the modality of nutritional support is utilized pretransplant, serial anthropometric measurements are recommended to follow the effects and adequacy of nutritional interventions once deficiencies have been identified.[13]

The goals of nutritional therapy during the immediate posttransplant period are to manage the catabolic effect of the surgery, facilitate weaning from the ventilator, minimize infection risk, improve wound repair, and anticipate metabolic/electrolyte issues associated with liver regeneration, medications, and malnutrition, such as those seen in refeeding syndrome. Refeeding syndrome is a serious complication associated with aggressive nutritional rehabilitation of malnourished patients and is characterized by metabolic disturbances in potassium, magnesium, and phosphate levels; glucose and fluid intolerance; and potential cardiac and pulmonary dysfunction.[14]

Parenteral nutrition via a central venous catheter is generally initiated within 24 to 48 hours posttransplant after hemostasis is achieved with intravenous (IV) electrolyte and mineral replacement. In most instances, substantial potassium, phosphorus, and magnesium replacements are required. Parenteral nutrition is maintained until the patient is able to take 50% to 75% of his or her total caloric requirements enterally.[15] The intermittent shortages of some PN constituents in the United States have made parenteral replacement challenging and have led to the earlier use of enteral mineral replacements.

Oral or specialized enteral feeding should be reinstituted as soon as gut function is restored. If patients are unable to achieve nutrition goals with an oral diet and the use of high-calorie oral supplements or fortified infant formula, supplemental tube feeding support should be initiated to facilitate weaning from PN. Post-liver transplant, patients can be given standard infant or pediatric formulas or supplements, as liver function has been restored and long-chain fats can again be absorbed. As oral intake improves, tube feedings can be weaned and ultimately discontinued. Most children will resume a normal diet before discharge from the hospital after transplantation, although some may require additional oral supplements to achieve catch-up goals. A small portion of children and infants, particularly those with behavioral feeding issues secondary to pretransplant reliance on tube feeding, may require supplemental nocturnal enteral feedings for several months posttransplant. Some infants and younger children who have received enteral tube feeding supplementation pretransplant may have never developed normal feeding practices because they missed their normal developmental milestones for chewing and swallowing. These feeding problems can contribute to persistent growth failure during this posttransplant period through lack of adequate caloric intake. Data have shown that behavioral feeding problems are fairly common in children who were tube fed pretransplant, and are a major cause of growth failure in 10% of children.[16] Persistent inadequate caloric intake can sometimes be a factor in patients who experience posttransplant complications and necessitate longer term nutritional supplementation with tube feedings post-hospital discharge. Other iatrogenic factors such as the immunosuppressive drugs used posttransplant carry significant side effects that may affect nutrition (Table 13-1). However, with adequate support, 80% of children who survive liver transplantation will achieve normal growth patterns, body habitus, weight, MUAC, and TSF within 1 year posttransplant.[16,17]

Catch-up growth is defined as linear growth velocity that exceeds the limits of normal for age after a transient period of growth inhibition. Initial catch-up linear growth is slow during the first posttransplant year in most patients (possibly related to the effects of corticosteroids administered in the first 3 to 6 months posttransplant), but 80% achieve their ideal height by the twelfth posttransplant month. Virtually all children have satisfactory height standard deviation scores by 4 years posttransplant.[16,17]

Posttransplant maintenance goals ultimately revolve around quality of life issues. Long-term goals are focused on maximizing linear growth potential, as well as the development of optimal cognitive, physical, and emotional states.[6,19] Optimal nutrition support can improve these long-term quality of life issues in pediatric patients by reducing or avoiding linear growth failure, rickets from osteomalacia with related pathologic fractures, and neurodevelopmental delay.[20] Clearly, reaching a normal height is an important aspect of quality of life for these children because it affects social reintegration and self-esteem. The causes of poor growth after liver transplantation can be summarized as those caused from pretransplant growth failure, poor graft function, and the long-term use of glucocorticoid treatment. The efficacy and safety of recombinant growth hormone (rhGH) as a treatment of linear growth failure in liver transplant patients is presently under investigation. It has been used successfully to treat children after renal transplantation.[21] One of the primary goals posttransplantation is to decrease the complications associated with the chronic use of immunosuppressive drugs while optimizing graft survival. Reduced drug doses are the key to minimizing the potential for long-term complications. Target blood

TABLE 13-1. Most Commonly Employed Posttransplant Medications and Nutrition Related Side Effects[18]

Primary Immunosuppressants:

Cyclosporine: Immunosuppressant used in the prophylaxis of graft rejection.

Adverse reactions: Nephrotoxicity, hepatotoxicity, increased susceptibility to infection and lymphoma, hypertension, hirsutism, and gum hyperplasia.

Methylprednisolone: Immunosuppressive adjunct for the prevention and treatment of solid organ rejection.

Adverse reactions: Increased calcium excretion leading to osteoporosis,* sodium and fluid retention leading to cushingoid state,* hypertension, suppression of linear growth in children,* secondary decreased carbohydrate tolerance,* impaired wound healing, peptic ulcers, pancreatitis, muscle weakness, steroid myopathy, subcapsular cataracts, and glaucoma.

Tacrolimus: Immunosuppressant. Prophylaxis of graft rejection in liver and kidney transplants. Adverse reactions: Increased incidence of posttransplant diabetes mellitus,* neurotoxicity, acute nephrotoxicity characterized by non-anion gap metabolic acidosis, hypomagnesemia and hyperkalemia* due to type IV renal tubular acidosis, chronic nephrotoxicity characterized by glomerulosclerosis and chronic renal failure, increased risk of infection and lymphomas, hypertension that may require treatment with antihypertensive agents, and headaches.

Antithymocyte globulin (thymoglobulin)**:** Immunosuppressant sometimes used for induction of immunosuppression or to treat severe rejection refractory to corticosteroids.

Adverse reactions: Anaphylaxis, cytokine-release syndrome (cytokine storm characterized by tachycardia, pulmonary edema, adult respiratory distress syndrome, myocardial infarction), thrombocytopenia, neutropenia, fever, chills, flulike symptoms.

Immunosuppressants Used to Treat Acute Rejection:

Mycophenolate mofetil: Prophylaxis of graft rejection.

Adverse reactions: Increased susceptibility to infection and lymphoma, neutropenia, and gastrointestinal hemorrhage may occur.

Rapamycin Prevention and treatment of allograft rejection.

Adverse reactions: Thrombocytopenia and hyperlipidemia.

Key: *Adverse reactions with nutrition support implications

levels of cyclosporine or tacrolimus can usually be reduced within the first 1 to 2 years posttransplant pending no episodes of acute rejection. Aggressive prednisone wean is attempted over the first 3 to 6 months posttransplant.

Complications for younger children are generally related primarily to growth impairment and osteopenia from steroid use and are more serious than those observed in older children. These children frequently have metabolic bone disease from their chronic liver disease, as well as the secondary osteoporosis seen with chronic glucocorticoid use.[22] Multiple factors contribute to the development of osteopenia in patients with chronic liver disease awaiting liver transplantation, including immobility, malnutrition, poor muscle mass, poor renal function, and chronic cholestasis. In the posttransplant period, high-dose corticosteroids have long been implicated as the main cause of bone loss. In a retrospective study of children with end-stage liver disease who underwent orthotopic liver transplantation, 16% had bone fractures in the postoperative period. Irrespective of the postoperative bone density, most liver transplant recipients lose bone mass for 3 to 6 months after transplantation, but by 6 months, the bone loss typically ceases in patients with normal allograft function and then stabilizes or increases.[23,24] Adequate calcium and vitamin D supplementation during the pre- and posttransplant phases, as well as the promotion of physical activity and minimizing the use of osteopenia-producing medications, are keys in the preservation of bone mass during the early posttransplant phase.

Nephrotoxicity and abnormal renal function characterized by decreased glomerular filtration rate (GFR) have been associated with the long-term use of immunosuppressive drugs such as cyclosporine and tacrolimus, other nephrotoxic drugs, rejection episodes, and hypertension. Hypertension occurs in approximately one-third of all children at any given time posttransplant,[25] and remains a serious posttransplant complication, with 10% to 28% of children requiring long-term antihypertensive treatment.[26] Blood pressures should be routinely monitored during postoperative medical follow-ups.

Hyperlipidemia following liver transplantation is primarily associated with the use of cyclosporine, rapamycin, high-dose corticosteroids, obesity, and diabetes mellitus, and is seen more in prepuberty and adolescence. Familial predisposition to hyperlipidemia can also be a contributing factor. Using tacrolimus as the primary immunosuppressive drug has a relatively minor effect on serum lipid levels as compared to rapamycin.[27] One major focus of treatment for hyperlipidemia remains dietary intervention. Patient and family education on proper food-purchasing selections and low-fat substitutions, preparation techniques, and menu planning, as well as lifestyle modifications that include an exercise regimen, are essential.

Posttransplant diabetes mellitus (PTDM) is a complication sometimes seen in children post-liver transplantation. The most significant factor that influences the development of PTDM is the use of diabetogenic immunosuppressive medications.[28] Hyperglycemia may occur in some children on tacrolimus alone or in combination with high-dose corticosteroids used to treat rejection episodes. In most instances, hyperglycemia resolves when corticosteroid doses are weaned. In those instances when hyperglycemia is sustained, treatment with insulin injections will be required. Detailed diabetes education on dietary modifications (carbohydrate counting), monitoring, and insulin therapy should be implemented upon diagnosis. Patients with a family history of diabetes mellitus or a diagnosis of an autoimmune liver disease appear to have a greater risk of developing diabetes mellitus in this postoperative period.[29]

Obesity after liver transplantation is seen more frequently in adult patients than in children, but can affect adolescent patients and children who are transplanted during their prepubertal years. The goal of treatment should focus on lifestyle changes and behavior modification rather than calorie-restricted diets, as the tendency for weight gain will be present throughout their life.

In summary, the provision of nutrition therapy to pediatric patients with liver disease who are listed for liver transplantation is a concerted multidisciplinary team effort. Pretransplant goals are to preserve LBM and to medically manage the innate complications associated with the disease process. Posttransplant goals should focus primarily on quality of life issues: the development of cognitive, physical, and emotional states and minimizing the side effects inherent to the use of posttransplant medications. Rigorous attention to metabolic management and aggressive nutritional support during all phases of the disease are essential in maximizing outcomes for transplantation. Liver transplantation offers patients a therapeutic option for an otherwise fatal disease and the ultimate goal of offering a new beginning with a better quality of life.

NUTRITION AFTER SMALL INTESTINAL TRANSPLANTATION

With the development of PN in the early 1970s, those with irreversible intestinal failure are now capable of surviving much longer on waiting lists before intestinal transplantation is completed. Another factor that has been essential to the survival of these patients is the care provided by multidisciplinary teams within intestinal rehabilitation programs.[30] The outcomes and cost effectiveness of intestinal transplantation are directly related to the quality of care delivered by these intestinal rehabilitation programs. These teams should be composed of gastroenterologists, general surgeons, transplant surgeons, dietitians, social workers, pharmacists, and nurse clinicians, as well as many outside consultants such as intensivists, neonatologists, pulmonologists, nephrologists, and speech/occupational therapists, depending on the comorbidities of these infants and children with intestinal failure.[31] The spectacular improvements in liver protection by either reducing the parenteral soybean oil–based lipid load[32] or using fish oil–based lipid[33] have reduced the need for combined liver/bowel transplantation. Furthermore, the utilization of ethanol locks[34] and improved central line care have increased the average age of patients undergoing transplantation. Hence, according to the Scientific Registry of Transplant Recipients (SRTR), the annual number of transplants performed in 2011 is less than half the annual number performed during the earlier part of the millennium.[35]

Several variants of intestinal transplantation are utilized today. In patients with surgical short-bowel syndrome but without liver disease, an isolated intestinal transplantation may be performed. Patients with diffuse motility disorders involving stomach and duodenum who have not developed significant liver dysfunction may undergo a modified multivisceral transplant, which implies that the patient is completely eviscerated of native organs, which are then replaced by the stomach and small intestine en bloc. If severe intestinal failure–associated liver disease has developed, the patient may undergo a liver/intestine transplant or a multivisceral transplant including the liver. The details of the surgery and immunosuppressive regimens are too complex for this chapter, but are covered extensively by several excellent review articles.[36,37] Most patients emerge from surgery with a gastrostomy and an ileostomy. The gastrostomy is for feeding and venting of the stomach, and the ileostomy is to facilitate frequent ileoscopic monitoring of graft appearance and histopathology in order to rule in or rule out rejection or allograft enteritis. Generally, the immunosuppressive regimens are similar to, but more rigorous than, those utilized for liver transplantation, but the characteristics of typical immunosuppressive agents are identical to those utilized for liver transplantation and are cited in Table 13-1.

There are three chief periods of concentrated nutritional care management of these patients to assure the best achievable outcomes throughout their continuum of care, which the following sections describe.

Pretransplant Nutritional Care

Optimal pretransplant care depends heavily on minimizing/delaying intestinal failure–associated liver disease (IFALD) and maximizing the patient's chance for survival with a successful outcome.

Keys in this pursuit include diligent PN delivery and monitoring of nutritional substrates, vitamins, minerals, and fluids to ensure appropriate hydration to replace losses, yet avoid overfeeding. Attempts to cycle PN and initiate trophic enteral feeding if possible have been shown to impede IFALD. This strategy is, in many instances, very difficult to accomplish in small infants with liver insufficiency or injury. These infants may experience hypoglycemia due to impaired glycogenolysis or hyperinsulinism if PN delivery is compressed into too few hours. The deleterious effect of excessive phytosterols on the liver can be attenuated by the delivery of either a reduced lipid load or a reduced lipid load with fish oil–based lipid.[32,33] However, the calories not provided by lipid must be replaced by glucose calories, and many infants may then receive glucose infusion rates beyond their maximum oxidative capacity.[38]

Monitoring and maintaining proper vitamin and mineral levels are definite challenges. It is important to provide appropriate, yet not excessive, intakes of zinc and copper. Copper, in particular, is difficult to dose because too little may result in copper deficiency manifested by pancytopenia that mimics the hypersplenism of portal hypertension, and too much may produce oxidative hepatic damage. Ultimately, frequent measurements of serum copper and ceruloplasmin are crucial for guiding therapy.

Maintaining some form of oral stimulation is fundamental for infants and children pretransplant, as it will facilitate the transitioning from enteral tube feedings to oral feedings during the posttransplant period. Infants and children who have not received adequate oral stimulation during this early phase of care can require years of intensive therapy posttransplant to achieve adequate oral feeding to eliminate the need for enteral tube feeding supplementation.[39]

The choice of gastrostomy versus gastrojejunostomy as the route for enteral feeding must be evaluated individually for each patient based upon whether the patient is prone to vomit and based upon how much functioning residual bowel is present.

Nutritional Care During the Immediate Posttransplant Period

Parenteral nutrition support is generally initiated within the first 24 to 48 hours postoperatively when the patient is hemodynamically stable. Parenteral nutrition is run over 24 hours and, in many instances, is maintained with less than maintenance volumes to accommodate the additional IV fluid requirements of replacement fluids and IV medications. Fluid restriction during this early postoperative period may be essential for weaning from assisted ventilator support. Concentrating PN ensures adequate caloric and protein intake during this metabolically erratic period of support.

Indirect calorimetry can be used to obtain a more accurate assessment of resting energy expenditure.[40] Many clinicians will utilize baseline caloric assessment formulas, but these could over- or underpredict actual needs.[41]

Intensive laboratory monitoring during the early postoperative period is critical, as numerous metabolic complications can develop, such as steroid-induced hyperglycemia, renal insufficiency, refeeding syndrome, and medication-induced electrolyte and mineral losses. Biochemical markers need to be monitored carefully by the transplant team and appropriate adjustment must be made in PN fluids.[42]

The electrolyte and mineral components of PN solutions need to be adjusted regularly based on metabolic requirements; titrating drug effects; and losses from urine, enterostomy, and vacuum dressings. It is customary to deliver large quantities of potassium, phosphorus, and magnesium during the immediate postoperative period because the allograft organs, having suffered ischemia/reperfusion, become profoundly depleted of these elements. Furthermore, tacrolimus-induced renal tubular magnesium wasting is greatest when the tacrolimus level is highest in the first days posttransplantation. Sometimes, supplemental albumin is added to total parenteral nutrition (TPN) for Jackson Pratt drain replacements.

Nutrient Requirements within the Intensive Care Unit

Caloric requirements are determined based on age, weight, preoperative caloric requirements, and current level of respiratory and medical support, as well as postoperative complications such as infection and surgical problems. The dietitian needs to take into account these frequent changes in a patient's early postoperative course and adjust nutritional intakes accordingly. Consider the potential for increased energy needs in the setting of infection, spontaneous respiration with increased work of breathing, steroid-induced catabolism, and wound healing. There is a potential for decreased energy requirements in the setting of ventilator-assisted respiration, sedation/paralysis, and decreased activity. Hence, measurement of resting energy expenditure can be helpful during this assessment period.[43]

Protein requirements are normally estimated at 150% to 200% of the age-related recommended dietary allowances (RDAs) for protein, but vary greatly based on wound losses or protein losses in urine and enterostomy. Nitrogen balance studies may be performed to determine actual losses, but in many instances, are not practical clinically in children, and the factor used for stool output must be estimated and based on current enterostomy output.[44]

During the immediate postoperative period, patients do not need high quantities of fat, but essential fatty acid deficiency should be prevented or treated. A fat intake of only 4% of the total calorie requirement is enough to prevent essential fatty acid deficiencies. However, it is important to be aware that some patients may be deficient in essential fatty acid prior to their transplant. Many of these patients have been managed on lipid-sparing PN regimens (0.5 to 1 gram of fat/kg per day) preoperatively, and essential fatty acid levels should be measured before and after transplantation. Lipids can be an excellent source of calories in patients with drug- or stress-induced hyper-glycemia, but need to be monitored closely to prevent hypertriglyceridemia.

The initiation of continuous enteral feeding generally occurs after bowel viability is assured by a screening ileoscopy 4 to 7 days after the transplant. The graft is evaluated by both gross observation and histology before feedings are initiated. At our institution, initial feedings are started with a very-low-fat elemental formula at half-strength (isotonic at 1.0 kcal/mL) and advanced every 12 hours by 0.2 mL/kg to a goal rate. Once two-thirds of the goal rate is achieved, the strength is advanced by 25% and TPN weaning is initiated. Parenteral nutrition is weaned gradually as enteral tube feedings are advanced. Advancement to full-strength formula is attempted once goal rate is achieved, but if the high osmolality is not tolerated, the formula is maintained at three-quarters strength and the rate is increased further to achieve estimated goals. The rationale for the use of a very low-fat enteral formula is that the surgical division of all of the mesenteric lymphatics prevents significant long-chain triglyceride absorption for several weeks. Eventually, lymphatics regenerate, but until that time, long-chain triglyceride absorption is severely perturbed.[45]

At our institution, nasojejunal tubes are placed at the time of transplant proximal to the transplanted jejunum and maintained until the patient is able to tolerate full gastric feeding through the gastrostomy. Most patients have indwelling gastrostomy tubes at the time of transplant for trophic feedings or drainage. Jejunal feedings are converted to gastric feedings as soon as tolerated to take advantage of increased emptying time from the stomach to the duodenum. This sometimes decreases enterostomy output and increases intestinal transit time.

After 4 to 6 weeks, patients are transitioned to an elemental hypoallergenic MCT-containing formula. Hypoallergenic formulas are utilized post-small-bowel transplant because these patients are predisposed to develop eosinophilic bowel disease and food allergies. Posttransplant eosinophilic enteritis is increasingly recognized after solid organ transplants, presumably due to immune dysregulation induced by calcineurin inhibitors and the loss of optimal antigen processing because of increased macromolecular penetration after transplant. Many patients have clear-cut symptoms when challenged with specific foods such as cow's milk, soy, eggs, nuts, or other highly allergenic foods. Therefore, the use of hypoallergenic enteral formulas and avoiding foods with high allergenicity for the first 6 posttransplant months are recommended.[46]

Supplemental fluid and electrolyte replacements are based on enterostomy losses and urine sodium levels. In many instances, these patients require magnesium supplementation in their supplemental IV fluids during the early postoperative period to replace the prodigious losses incurred in urine (due to high tacrolimus levels) and in the ileostomy effluent. Enteral magnesium supplementation is generally poorly tolerated by these patients, as it has a strong laxative effect. After the immediate posttransplant period, as lower tacrolimus levels are accepted and the renal tubular wasting diminishes, parenteral magnesium needs are reduced. Because serum magnesium levels poorly reflect total body magnesium stores,[47] serum levels of <1.5 mEq/L (<0.75 mmol/L) but >1.0 mEq/L (>0.5 mmol/L) are customarily acceptable.

Oral feeding rehabilitation usually starts with a speech therapy assessment of swallowing and incorporation of oral desensitizing techniques. For infants, significant use of oral foods is usually not begun until the patient's tube feedings can be held for a few hours and the patient shows some interest in the tastes and textures of foods. Older children may begin eating solids within a few days of the time that enteral tolerance is established. Depending upon age at transplant, patients are offered by mouth small amounts of hypotonic fluids (formulas or Pedialyte for infants or electrolyte sport drinks low in sugar for older children) and small tastes of pureed or mechanically soft foods. Dietary advancement is customarily according to patient tolerance. Large quantities of water or ice chips are to be avoided insofar as water is not a contributor of significant nutrition or electrolytes.

Careful monitoring of intake and output is essential for maintaining appropriate fluid balance between oral, enteral tube, and parenteral fluid intakes and enterostomy and urine losses. Intravenous fluids are weaned as appropriate free-water-containing fluids can be administered enterally without causing a significant increase in enterostomy losses.[48]

Nutrition Care During the Late Posttransplant Period (and Long-Term Care)

In general, infants and children who have undergone small-bowel, liver/intestine, or multivisceral transplant can be weaned from PN support and onto all enteral tube feedings or a combination of tube feedings and oral intake within 2 to 4 weeks. Until their ileostomies are closed (approximately 6 to 12 months after transplant), they may require additional IV fluids administered overnight to maintain fluid balance and to compensate for enterostomy losses. As the new bowel adapts and enteral fluid volumes are tolerated, IV administration of supplemental fluids can sometimes be eliminated (even prior to ileostomy closure) during uncomplicated periods of recovery.

Again, multidisciplinary teams with an intestinal rehabilitation/transplant focus are essential in maximizing appropriate and rapid transition to normal feeding patterns, as well as minimizing long-term complications of infections, rejection, growth stunting, and food allergies. Any of these complications can lead to impaired absorption and weight loss requiring periods of PN support. An overriding principle that should inform nutrition therapy is that allograft intestines, which are impeccable in most aspects of function, display nutrient-absorptive deficits. Fat and energy balances are rarely better than 75% and 85%, respectively.[49,50]

Before small-bowel transplant, patients are severely nutritionally challenged, with height/length affected more than weight. Posttransplant patients show linear growth improvement over a 1- to 2-year period.[51-53] Periods of rejection and high-dose steroid cycles are primary reasons for these delays in catch-up growth.[53] Despite assiduous monitoring, many macro- and micronutrient deficiencies may occur. More than 90% of patients will experience one or multiple micronutrient deficiencies after weaning onto full oral or enteral feedings.[51,54] The most commonly deficient elements are magnesium, iron, and zinc, respectively. While most water-soluble vitamins are expected to be normally absorbed following transplantation, a curious deficiency in pyridoxine levels has been reported following intestinal transplantation.[55] The mechanism is unknown, but it is possible that calcineurin inhibitors such as tacrolimus accelerate catabolism of this vitamin.

After patients' ileostomies are taken down and continuity with colon is established, a new set of nutritional and developmental issues arises. Most younger children undergoing transplantation have never undergone toilet training and now must learn and experience the elimination of stool and urine into a toilet. Their buttocks are prone to a great deal of skin breakdown during the early transition period, and liberal use of skin protection ointments and sealants is encouraged. Fiber supplementation in formulas and/or foods or fluids can sometimes prove helpful in bulking the stool.

The number of long-term survivors with functioning intestinal grafts is growing yearly. These patients are faced with a lifetime of immunological and nutritional challenges. These patients have to learn for the first time how to sustain themselves through oral feeding, and their nutritional status must be closely monitored for life. Hence, they are best followed chronically by a multidisciplinary intestinal rehabilitation and transplant center long term in order to prevent late adverse nutritional events. If they are followed assiduously, restoration of nutritional independence to these patients is an achievable goal, and many children having undergone intestinal transplantation can be fully integrated with their family, their peers, and the community at large.

KEY POINTS

- Protein-energy malnutrition is an inevitable consequence of chronic liver disease and affects posttransplant survival in children.
- Infant formulas containing MCTs are preferably used pretransplant; PN is used pretransplant when complications make it difficult to safely provide the required nutrients enterally, or as an adjunctive therapy.
- Parenteral nutrition is generally initiated within 24 to 48 hours posttransplant and continued until the child is able to tolerate 50% to 75% of total caloric requirements enterally; standard formulas can be used posttransplantation.
- In intestinal failure, cycling of PN, maximizing enteral feeding, and limiting phytosterols (by the delivery of either a reduced soy-based lipid load or use of a fish oil–based lipid) can prevent IFALD.
- Patients post-liver and small-bowel transplantation require large quantities of potassium, phosphorus, and magnesium during the immediate postoperative period because the allograft organs, having suffered ischemia/reperfusion, become profoundly depleted of these elements.

REFERENCES

1. Squires RH. End-stage liver disease in children. *Curr Treat Options Gastroenterol.* 2001;4(5):409-421.
2. Heubi JE, Heyman MB, Shulman RJ. The impact of liver disease on growth and nutrition. *J Ped Gastro Nutr.* 2002;35(Suppl 1):S55-59.
3. Shepherd RW, Chin SE, Cleghorn GJ, et al. Malnutrition in children with chronic liver disease accepted for liver transplantation: clinical profile and effects on outcome. *J Paediatr Child Health.* 1991;27(5):295.
4. Goulet OJ, de Ville de Goyet, Otte JB, Ricour C. Preoperative nutritional evaluation and support of liver transplantation in children. *Transplant Proc.* 1987;19(4):3249-3255.
5. National Institute of Health Consensus Development Conference statement: liver transplantation-June 20-23, 1982. *Hepatology.* 1984;4(Suppl 1):107S.
6. Ryckman FC, Bucuvalas JC, Nathan J, Alonso M, Tiao G, Balistreri WF. Outcomes following liver transplantation. *Semin in Pediatr Surg.* 2008;17(2):123-130.
7. Whitington PF, Balistreri WF. Liver transplantation in pediatrics: indications, contraindications, and pretransplant management. *J Pediatr.* 1991;118:169-177.
8. Kleinman R, Warnman KY. Nutrition in liver disease. In: *Pediatric Enteral Nutrition.* Baker SB, Baker RD, Davis A, Eds. New York, NY: Chapman and Hall;1994:261-279.
9. Wolfsen HC, Kozarek RA, Bredfeldt JE, Fenster LF, Brubacher LL. The role of endoscopic injection sclerotherapy in the management of bleeding peristomal varices. *Gastroint Endosc.* 1990;36(5):472-474.
10. Sullivan JS, Sundaram SS, Pan Z, Sokol RJ. Parenteral nutrition supplementation in biliary atresia patients listed for liver transplant. *Liver Transpl.* 2012;18(1):120-128.
11. Novy MA, Schwartz KB. Nutritional considerations and management of the child with liver disease. *Nutrition.* 1997;13(3);177-184.
12. Setty AK, Schmidt-Sommerfeld E, Undall JN Jr. Nutritional aspects of liver disease in children. *Nutrition.* 1999;15(9);727-729.
13. Goulet OJ, de Ville de Goyet, Otte JB, Ricour C. Preoperative nutritional evaluation and support of liver transplantation in children. *Transplant Proc.* 1987;19(4):3249-3255.
14. Dunn RL, Stettler N, Mascarenhas MR. Refeeding Syndrome in hospitalized pediatric patients. *Nutr Clin Pract.* 2003;18(4):327-332.
15. Becht MB, Pedersen SH, Ryckman FC, Balistreri WF. Growth and nutrition management of pediatric patients after orthotopic liver transplantation. *Gastroenterol Clin North Am.* 1993;22(2):367-380.

16. Kelly DA. Nutritional factors affecting growth before and after liver transplantation. *Pediatr Transplant.* 1997;1(1):80-84.

17. Codoner-Franch P, Bernard O, Alvarez F. Long-term follow-up growth in height after successful liver transplantation. *J Pediatr.* 1994;124(3):368-373.

18. Pirsch J, Simmons W, Sollinger H, *Transplant Drug Manual,* 3rd edition, Landes Bioscience, Austin, Texas, 1999.

19. Kleinman R, Warnman KY. Nutrition in liver disease. In: *Pediatric Enteral Nutrition.* Baker SB, Baker RD, Davis A, Eds. New York, NY: Chapman and Hall; 1994:261-279.

20. Molleston JP. Acute and chronic liver disease. In *Nutrition in Pediatrics.* 2nd ed. Walker WA, Watkins JB, Eds. Hamilton, Ontario: BC Decker, Inc.; 1996:565.

21. Santiago, JM. Nutritional therapies in liver disease. *Semin Liver Dis.* 1991;11(4):278-291.

22. Sanchez AJ, Aranda-Michel J. Liver disease and osteoporosis. *Nutr Clin Pract.* 2006;21:(3)273-278.

23. Guthery SL, Pohl JF, Bucuvalas JC, et al. Bone mineral density in long-term survivors following pediatric liver transplantation. *Liver Transplant.* 2003;9(4):365-370.

24. Argao EA, Balistreri WF, Hollis BW, Ryckman FC, Heubi JE. Effects of orthotopic liver transplantation on bone mineral content and serum vitamin D metabolites in infants and children with chronic cholestasis. *Hepatology.* 1994;20(3):598-603.

25. Bartosh SM, Alonso EM, Whitington PF. Renal outcome in pediatric liver transplantation. *Clin Transplant.* 1997;11 (5 pt 1):354-360.

26. Whitington PF, Alonso EM, Piper JB. Pediatric liver transplantation. *Sem Liver Dis.* 1994;14(3):303-317.

27. Munoz SJ. Hyperlipidemia and other coronary risk factors after orthotopic liver transplantation: pathogenesis, diagnosis, and management. *Liver Transplant Surg.* 1995; 1(Suppl):29-38.

28. Obayashi PA. Post-transplant diabetes mellitus: cause, impact, and treatment options. *Nutr Clin Pract.* 2004; 19(2):165-171.

29. Lohmann T, List C, Lamesch P, et al. Diabetes mellitus and inlet cell specific autoimmunity as adverse effects of immunosuppression therapy with FK506/Tacrolimus. *Exp Clin Endocrinol* Diabetes. 2000;108(5):347-352.

30. Koehler AN, Yaworski JA, Gardner M, Kocoshis S, Reyes J, Barksdale EM Jr. Coordinated interdisciplinary management of pediatric intestinal failure: a 2-year review. *J Pediatr Surg.* 2000;35(2):380-385.

31. Venick RS, Wozniak LJ, Colangelo J, et al. Long-term nutrition and predictors of growth and weight gain following pediatric intestinal transplantation. *Transplantation.* 2011;92(9):1058-1062.

32. Cober MP, Killu G, Brattain A, Welch KB, Kunisaki SM, Teitelbaum DH. Intravenous fat emulsions reduction for patients with parenteral nutrition-associated liver disease. *J Pediatr.* 2012;160(3):421-427.

33. Gura KM, Lee S, Valim C, et al. Safety and efficacy of a fish-oil-based fat emulsion in the treatment of parenteral nutrition-associated liver disease. *Pediatrics.* 2008;121(3):e678-686.

34. Jones BA, Hull MA, Richardson DS, et al. Efficacy of ethanol locks in reducing central venous catheter infections in pediatric patients with intestinal failure. *J Pediatr Surg.* 2010;45(6):1287-1293.

35. http://www.srtr.org/csr/current/Centers/TransplantCenters.aspx?organcode=IN.

36. Mazariegos GV, Squires RH, Sindhi RK. Current perspectives in pediatric intestinal transplantation. *Curr. Gastroenterol Reports.* 2009;11(3):226-233.

37. Nayyer NS, McGhee W, Martin D, et al. Intestinal transplantation in children: a review of immunotherapy regimens. *Paediatr Drugs.* 2011;13(3):149-159.

38. Jones MO, Pierro A, Hammond P, Nunn A, Lloyd DA. Glucose utilization in the surgical newborn infant receiving total parenteral nutrition. *J Pediatr Surg.* 1993;28(9): 1221-1225.

39. Krawinkel MB, Scholz D, Busch A, Kohl M, Wessel LM, Zimmer, K-P. Chronic intestinal failure in children. *Dtsch Arztebl Int.* 2012;109(22-23):409-415.

40. Matarese LE. Indirect calorimetry: technical aspects. *J Am Diet Assoc.* 1997;97(Suppl.):154S-160S.

41. Seashore JH. Nutritional support of children in the intensive care unit. *Yale J Biol Med.* 1984;57:111-134.

42. Hauser GJ, Kaufman SS, Matsumoto CS, Fishbein TM. Pediatric intestinal and multivisceral transplantation: a new challenge for the pediatric intensivist. *Intensive Care Med.* 2008;34:1570-1579.

43. Strohm S, Reyes J, Koehler A. Pediatric small bowel transplantation. In: *Comprehensive Guide to Transplant Nutrition.* JM Hasse, LS Blue, Eds. Chicago, IL. American Dietetic Association. 2002:216-225.

44. Weseman R, Gilroy R. Nutrition management of small bowel transplant patients. *Nutr Clin Pract.* 2005;20(5): 509-516.

45. Olivier C, Rettori R, Camilleri J P. Interruption of the lymphatic vessels and its consequences in total homotransplantations of the small intestine and right side of the colon in man. *Lymphology.* 1972;5(1):24-31.

46. Saeed SA, Integlia MJ, Pleskow RG, et al. Tacrolimus-associated eosinophilic gastroenteritis in pediatric liver transplant recipients: Role of potential food allergies in pathogenesis. *Pediatr Transplant.* 2006;10(6):730-735.

47. Martin KJ, Gonzalez EA, Slatopolsky E. Clinical consequences and management of hypmagnesemia. *J Am Soc Nephrol.* 2009;20(11):2291-2295.

48. Gupte GL, Beath SV. Update on intestinal rehabilitation after intestinal transplantation. *Curr Opin Organ Transplant.* 2009;14(3):267-273.

49. Kaufman SS, Lyden ER, Brown CR, Iverson AK, et al. Disaccharidase activities and fat assimilation in pediatric patients after intestinal transplantation. *Transplantation.* 2000;69(3):362-365.

50. Ordonez F, Barbot-Trystram L, Lacaille F, et al. Intestinal absorption rate in children after small intestinal transplantation. *Am J Clin Nutr.* 2013;97(4):741-749.

51. Venick RS, Farmer DG, Saikali D, et al. Nutritional outcomes following pediatric intestinal transplantation. *Transplant Proc.* 2006;38(6):1718-1719.

52. Rovera GM, Strohm S, Bueno J, et al. Nutritional monitoring of pediatric intestinal transplant recipients. *Transplant Proc.* 1998;30(6):2519-2520.

53. Nucci AM, Strohm S, Squires RH, Mazariegos GV, Sun Q, Sindhi R. Growth pre and post implementation of a steroid free induction protocol in a large pediatric intestinal transplant population. *J Pediatr Gastroenterol Nutr.* 2011;52(5):601-606.

54. Ubesie AC, Cole CR, Nathan JD, et al. Micronutrient deficiencies in pediatric and young adult intestinal transplant patients. *Pediatr Transplant.* 2013;17(7):638-645.

55. Matarese LE, Dvorchik I, Costa G, et al. Pyridoxal-5'-phosphate deficiency after intestinal and multivisceral transplantation. *Am J Clin Nutr.* 2009;89(1):204-209.

CHAPTER 14

Renal Failure

Poyyapakkam R. Srivaths

■ ACUTE RENAL FAILURE
Etiology
Outcome
Metabolic Consequences of Acute Renal Failure
Energy Requirements
Glucose Metabolism and the Kidney
Protein Metabolism
Lipid Metabolism
Fluid and Electrolyte Management
Impact of Renal Replacement Therapy
Nutrition Route
■ SUMMARY
■ KEY POINTS
References

■ ACUTE RENAL FAILURE

The term "acute renal failure" (ARF) for alteration in kidney function in an acute setting was first introduced by Smith[1] to define changes in kidney function due to traumatic injuries. Since the kidney's physiological role is the excretion of water-soluble solutes and urine production, changes in these parameters are often included in the definition of ARF. However, since the magnitude of changes is not uniformly defined, there is a large ascertainment bias when epidemiology of ARF is examined. For example, in a pediatric intensive care unit (PICU) study that defined ARF as doubling of serum creatinine (Cr), the incidence of ARF in all children admitted to the PICU was reported as 4.5%. However, in another PICU study that defined ARF as elevation of serum Cr to 1.5 times the normal value, the incidence of ARF was 82% in children with severe illness.[2,3] This discrepancy led to the adoption of a consensus definition of ARF by the Acute Dialysis Quality Initiative. The objective was to arrive at a definition of ARF that uses standardized terminology and includes a broad range of acute impairment of renal function. This definition is referred by the acronym RIFLE,[4] which stands for risk, injury, failure, loss of function, and end-stage renal disease (ESRD). These criteria have been modified in children to account for normal variations in serum Cr with somatic growth, referred to as pRIFLE (Table 14-1).[3]

Etiology

In the past, the etiologies of ARF in the pediatric hospital setting were limited to primary renal diseases such as hemolytic uremic syndrome and acute glomerulonephritis. However, ARF is now more likely secondary to systemic illness or its treatment, such as sepsis, nephrotoxic medications, and ischemia due to other organ involvement.[3,5] Acute renal failure in the current intensive care setting is due to multiple organ dysfunction syndrome (MODS) following cardiopulmonary bypass surgery for congenital heart disease, liver failure, or stem

TABLE 14-1. Pediatric RIFLE (pRIFLE) Criteria[3]

Category	Estimated Creatinine Clearance (eCCl) Using Schwartz Formula	Urine Output
Risk	eCCl decrease by 25%	Less than 0.5 mL/kg per hr for 8 hours
Injury	eCCl decrease by 50%	Less than 0.5 mL/kg per hr for 16 hours
Failure	eCCl decrease by 75% or eCCl <35 mL/min/1.73 m^2	Less than 0.5 mL/kg per hr for 24 hours or anuric for >12 hours
Loss of function	Persistent failure for >4 weeks	
End-stage renal disease	Persistent renal failure >3 months	

cell transplantation. This poses difficult challenges in prescribing fluid and meeting nutrition needs, since each of these conditions has unique requirements.

Outcome

Pediatric ARF has a definite and serious impact on both short-term and long-term outcomes. Previous thinking was that children in the PICU would die with ARF and not necessarily due to ARF. However, recent studies have reported mortality rates between 15% and 50% in children with ARF.[6,7] Even small changes in serum Cr are now recognized to contribute to adverse patient outcomes.[7] Long-term outcome data from pediatric ARF have not been studied in detail. Recent small studies indicate that about 30% of children with hospital-acquired ARF either had reduced renal function or were dialysis dependent at the time of discharge.[8] On follow-up of this cohort for 3 to 5 years, 60% of patients had some evidence of kidney damage as evidenced by hypertension, hyperfiltration, or microalbuminuria.[9] So similar to adults, pediatric ARF can have profound consequences.

Metabolic Consequences of Acute Renal Failure

Acute renal failure is considered a pro-inflammatory state,[10] with even a mild degree of acute kidney injury eliciting systemic immune responses, which can at times lead to a catabolic state. This can lead to lean body mass wasting and fat mass depletion.[11] Protein-energy wasting is thought to be a prognostic indicator of outcomes in ARF. However, whether addressing this state would improve outcomes has not been tested in any intervention trial in pediatric ARF. Moreover, available evidence regarding nutrient requirements during ARF and the effect of meeting these requirements on both organ recovery and overall recovery has not been tested rigorously in children.

Energy Requirements

Energy requirements in ARF seem to be determined by the underlying disease and its complication rather than by ARF itself. Overfeeding should be avoided, since it can cause hyperglycemia, excess lipid deposition, and worsening azotemia. In hypermetabolic situations such as sepsis or MODS, energy requirements should be 100% to 130% of basal energy expenditure, which can be derived from the Caldwell-Kennedy equation.[12] Resting energy expenditure (REE) should be measured in patients with renal insufficiency when possible. The effect of renal replacement therapy (RRT) on indirect calorimetric testing remains unclear. Indirect calorimetry (IC) may be performed when the child is not receiving RRT. In the absence of IC, when relying on basal energy expenditure estimations using standard equations, it is prudent to use an ideal body weight or previous known weight, since actual body weight can be influenced by fluid overload.

Glucose Metabolism and the Kidney

Plasma glucose is freely filtered across the glomerulus, and if the efficient reabsorptive capacity of the tubules is compromised, it may result in enormous losses in the urine. Glucose is primarily reabsorbed in proximal tubules. The transfer of glucose from the tubular lumen to the interstitial space is executed by an active process via sodium-dependent glucose transporters (SGLTs) on the apical membrane that take glucose from the lumen to the cell and facilitate diffusion of glucose on the basolateral membrane to release it into the interstitium. Best characterized among the apical transporters are SGLT1 and SGLT2. Once glucose has been concentrated in epithelial cells to a level above interstitial glucose levels, it diffuses out to the interstitium across specific facilitative glucose transporters (GLUTs), which are localized to the basolateral membrane. The arrangement of the transporters in series enables the kidney to reabsorb glucose in an energy-efficient manner. In experimental models of sepsis, differential expression of both the apical and basolateral transporters causing altered glucose metabolism have been shown.[13] Also, the kidney is an important organ for gluconeogenesis, with defective mechanisms in ARF further increasing risk for hypoglycemia. Exogenous insulin is metabolized mainly in the kidneys, further complicating glucose metabolism in critically ill patients. All these changes can often lead to hypoglycemia; however, the most common abnormality seen in critical illness seems to be hyperglycemia due to insulin resistance observed in "stress states." The results of 2 large-scale studies in critically ill adults[14,15] suggest that intensive glycemic control (maintaining blood glucose 80 to 110 mg/dL) results in fewer episodes of ARF. However, a recent large randomized control trial has shown increased mortality with intensive glucose control when compared to a less intensive regimen in critically ill adult.[16] Thus, the kidney disease–improving global outcomes (KDIGO) recommendations do not support intensive glycemic control and recommend less rigorous control of blood sugar between 110 and 150 mg/dL.[12]

Protein Metabolism

As alluded to before, ARF is a pro-inflammatory state characterized by release of several cytokines such as tumor necrosis factor-α causing protein breakdown. Acute renal failure is a catabolic state with excessive protein breakdown, mainly from skeletal muscle, resulting in a negative nitrogen balance.[17] This protein breakdown seems to result from insulin resistance.[18] However, acidosis can also result in protein breakdown, as often seen in chronic kidney disease.[19] Hyperparathyroidism occasionally seen in ARF can worsen this protein breakdown. Provision of inadequate nutrition and protein losses seen in renal replacement therapy can further worsen the protein balance.[17]

The optimal requirement of protein is not known; however, in hypercatabolic states and in patients on continuous renal replacement therapy (CRRT), higher protein intake is needed to offset the catabolic losses and maintain a positive nitrogen balance. Adult studies have indicated nearly twice the dietary recommended intake (DRI) protein delivery goals for hypercatabolic states and CRRT. Since children have a higher DRI to begin with, it is reasonable to provide ~2 to 2.5 gm/kg of protein per day in younger children. A recent survey of daily protein intake in pediatric patients receiving CRRT revealed 2.4 gm/kg provided for infants, 1.9 gm/kg for children ages 1 to 13, and 1.3 gm/kg for children older than 13 years.[20] These are good starting points for protein provision in children receiving CRRT.

Lipid Metabolism

Though it is customary to observe lipolysis in critical illness, acute kidney injury is associated with an impairment of lipolysis, which causes hypertriglyceridemia.[21] The impaired lipolysis can decrease the elimination of enteral or parenterally delivered lipids in ARF, complicating critical illness.[22] It is reasonable to provide 0.8 to 1.2 gm/kg of lipids for patients with ARF, with close monitoring of triglyceride levels in these patients.

Fluid and Electrolyte Management

Careful attention to fluid and electrolyte balance is critical in preventing or reducing morbidities associated with ARF. Fluid-responsive or otherwise prerenal ARF requires fluid resuscitation, while acute tubular necrosis, which is often seen in the critical care setting, may require fluid restriction. Some causes of ARF, such as nephrotoxic medications or acute interstitial nephritis, may not have oliguria and may have increased fluid needs. It is important to realize that "maintenance fluids" are not appropriate in ARF, since two-thirds of maintenance fluids are determined by adequate urine output. A safe method to start fluid calculation would be to provide insensible fluid losses and replace urine output as well as any other ongoing losses. Insensible losses are generally calculated as 400 mL/m^2 per day; however, this fluid requirement may be reduced in children receiving mechanical ventilation through a humidified circuit. Urine output is generally replaced as 0.45% normal saline, but may require measurement of urine sodium to tailor therapy. In oliguric ARF, it is reasonable not to provide potassium or phosphorus unless one encounters hypokalemia or hypophosphatemia. Sodium should be restricted to avoid fluid overload and hypertension in oliguric ARF. In the setting of fluid restriction, as in cases of oliguric ARF, the provision of adequate energy and protein may be challenging due to fluid restriction, A concentrated parenteral solution or caloric-dense enteral formula may be required. Fluid overload has been demonstrated to be independently associated with increased mortality in children receiving RRT.[23-25] There is reluctance to provide adequate nutrition in children with ARF because of fear of fluid overload and worsening azotemia.[26] However, meeting nutritional needs in an ARF patient should be the goal and may often be an important consideration to start RRT in critically ill children.

Impact of Renal Replacement Therapy

The choice of RRT has to be tailored to the individual patient and clinical situation causing renal failure. Peritoneal dialysis (PD) is a reasonable modality to provide renal replacement in ARF in children and often is the preferred modality in neonates and infants. Peritoneal dialysis can cause 100 to 300 mg/kg of protein losses per day, which often need to be replaced.[27] Since PD dialysate has dextrose, its absorption can contribute to energy intake and result in hyperglycemia. The amount of dextrose absorbed during PD depends on the volume infused, the dwell time, the dialysate dextrose concentration, and the condition of the patient's peritoneal membrane. The energy derived from this dextrose absorbed from the dialysate must be taken into account when planning a child's nutrition.[28] Peritoneal dialysis in ARF, particularly in infants, is prescribed as a continuous therapy, resulting in some relaxation of fluid restriction. Intermittent hemodialysis (HD) can result in loss of water-soluble vitamins and some trace elements, which need to be provided while prescribing enteral or parenteral nutrition.[29] Vitamins A and D and the water-soluble vitamins—cyanocobalamin (B_{12}), vitamin C, folic acid, thiamin (B_1), and pyridoxine (B_6)—are removed with HD. Vitamin requirements with CRRT tend to mirror those needed in HD.[30,31] However, the disadvantage of HD is that the very nature of intermittent therapy is not well tolerated by critically ill and hemodynamically unstable children. Continuous renal replacement therapy is often the modality prescribed in critically ill and hemodynamically unstable children, but requires specialized equipment and personnel. The major advantage of CRRT over other modalities is precise control of fluid balance and adjustment of ultrafiltrate to meet the demands posed by ARF and critical illness. Continuous renal replacement therapy can cause profound electrolyte losses, resulting in hypokalemia and hypophosphatemia, which requires frequent monitoring and provision of these electrolytes and minerals in dialysate fluids. Continuous renal replacement therapy can also cause 10% to 20% of the amino acid provided to be lost in the dialysate,[32,33] which needs to be taken into account while prescribing nutrition needs. Some of the citrate mixed with dextrose (anticoagulant dextrose citrate solution), which is employed in some centers for regional anticoagulation, can enter systemic circulation and provide additional energy supplementation[11] as well as cause dyelectrolytemia, especially hypocalcemia.

Nutrition Route

The enteral route of nutrition is preferred over the parenteral route, as it keeps the intestinal mucosa active and reduces bacterial translocation.[33,34] Moreover, in adult studies, enteral nutrition was associated with improved outcomes in critically ill patients with ARF.[35] Gastrointestinal motility is often impaired in critically ill patients and in patients with ARF, so parenteral nutrition may be needed to supplement nutrition needs. Enteral formulas that provide less potassium, sodium, and phosphorus are available for different age groups and are the preferred method to start nutrition in children with ARF. In children receiving CRRT, regular age-appropriate enteral formula is often well tolerated, as excellent metabolic control is often achieved by this method.

A reasonable starting point of fluid and electrolyte therapy is provided in the following table (Table 14-2), which can serve as an initial guide to providing nutrition in children with ARF.

TABLE 14-2. Fluid and Electrolyte Therapy for Children with Acute Renal Failure in the Critical Care Unit

Nutrient	Conservative	Continuous Renal Replacement Therapy
Fluid	Insensible (400 mL/m^2 per day) + ongoing losses, including urine/stool/ostomy	Near normal fluid requirement
Electrolyte	Close attention to potassium and phosphorus	Often, additional potassium and phosphorus supplements
Energy	100% to 130% of basal energy expenditure	100% to 130% of basal energy
Protein	At least meet RDA; in hypercatabolic state, may require twice RDA	Twice RDA (~2 to 2.5 gm/kg per day)
Vitamins	At least meet RDA	Twice RDA
Trace elements	At least meet RDA	Meet RDA

RDA, recommended daily allowance.

SUMMARY

Nutrition therapy in ARF patients is often complicated by the fluid and electrolyte changes accompanying renal dysfunction. In addition, the pro-inflammatory state of ARF poses additional demands on the nutritional needs of the critically ill child. There are challenges to delivering adequate nutrition, such as fluid restriction and dysmotility, when ARF complicates critical illness. However, it is essential that optimal nutrient delivery be achieved, since it has profound consequences on outcomes and recovery in this population.

KEY POINTS

- The Pediatric RIFLE criteria should be used to describe impairment in renal function.
- Provision of inadequate calories and protein in renal failure can worsen muscle breakdown; however, optimal requirements have not been clearly defined.
- Careful attention to fluid and electrolyte balance is critical in preventing or reducing morbidities associated with ARF.
- Peritoneal dialysis results in absorption of dextrose from the dialysate, which provides additional energy.
- Hemodialysis results in loss of vitamins and minerals in the dialysate.

REFERENCES

1. Smith HW, ed. *The Kidney: Structure and Function in Health and Disease.* Oxford University Press, Cary; 1951.
2. Bailey D, Phan V, Litalien C, et al. Risk factors of acute renal failure in critically ill children: a prospective descriptive epidemiological study. *Pediatr Crit Care Med.* 2007;8(1):29-35.
3. Akcan-Arikan A, Zappitelli M, Loftis LL, Washburn KK, Jefferson LS, Goldstein SL. Modified RIFLE criteria in critically ill children with acute kidney injury. *Kidney Int.* 2007;71(10):1028-1035.
4. Bellomo R, Ronco C, Kellum JA, Mehta RL, Palevsky P. Acute renal failure - definition, outcome measures, animal models, fluid therapy and information technology needs: the Second International Consensus Conference of the Acute Dialysis Quality Initiative (ADQI) Group. *Crit Care.* 2004;8(4):R204-212.
5. Hui-Stickle S, Brewer ED, Goldstein SL. Pediatric ARF epidemiology at a tertiary care center from 1999 to 2001. *Am J Kidney Dis.* 2005;45(1):96-101.
6. Schwilk B, Wiedeck H, Stein B, Reinelt H, Treiber H, Bothner U. Epidemiology of acute renal failure and outcome of haemodiafiltration in intensive care. *Intensive Care Med.* 1997;23(12):1204-1211.
7. Zappitelli M, Bernier PL, Saczkowski RS, et al. A small post-operative rise in serum creatinine predicts acute kidney injury in children undergoing cardiac surgery. *Kidney Int.* 2009;76(8):885-892.

8. Symons JM, Chua AN, Somers MJ, et al. Demographic characteristics of pediatric continuous renal replacement therapy: a report of the prospective pediatric continuous renal replacement therapy registry. *Clin J Am Soc Nephrol.* 2007;2(4):732-738.
9. Askenazi DJ, Feig DI, Graham NM, Hui-Stickle S, Goldstein SL. 3-5 year longitudinal follow-up of pediatric patients after acute renal failure. *Kidney Int.* 2006;69(1):184-189.
10. Ratliff BB, Rabadi MM, Vasko R, Yasuda K, Goligorsky MS. Messengers without borders: mediators of systemic inflammatory response in AKI. *J Am Soc Nephrol.* 2013;24(4):529-536.
11. Fiaccadori E, Maggiore U, Cabassi A, Morabito S, Castellano G, Regolisti G. Nutritional evaluation and management of AKI Patients. *J Ren Nutr.* 2013;12.
12. Kellum JA. KDIGO clinical practice guideline for acute kidney injury. *Kidney Inter.* 2012;2(1):1-137.
13. Schmidt C, Hocherl K, Bucher M. Regulation of renal glucose transporters during severe inflammation. *Am J Physiol Renal Physiol.* 2007;292(2):F804-811.
14. Van den Berghe G, Wilmer A, Milants I, et al. Intensive insulin therapy in mixed medical/surgical intensive care units: benefit versus harm. *Diabetes.* 2006;55(11):3151-3159.
15. van den Berghe G, Wouters P, Weekers F, et al. Intensive insulin therapy in critically ill patients. *N Engl J Med.* 2001;8;345(19):1359-1367.
16. Finfer S, Chittock DR, Su SY, et al. Intensive versus conventional glucose control in critically ill patients. *N Engl J Med.* 2009:26;360(13):1283-1297.
17. Leblanc M, Garred LJ, Cardinal J, et al. Catabolism in critical illness: estimation from urea nitrogen appearance and creatinine production during continuous renal replacement therapy. *Am J Kidney Dis.* 1998;32(3):444-453.
18. Basi S, Pupim LB, Simmons EM, et al. Insulin resistance in critically ill patients with acute renal failure. *Am J Physiol Renal Physiol.* 2005;289(2):F259-264.
19. Mehrotra R, Kopple JD, Wolfson M. Metabolic acidosis in maintenance dialysis patients: clinical considerations. *Kidney Int Suppl.* 2003;(88):S13-25.
20. Zappitelli M, Goldstein SL, Symons JM, et al. Protein and calorie prescription for children and young adults receiving continuous renal replacement therapy: a report from the Prospective Pediatric Continuous Renal Replacement Therapy Registry Group. *Crit Care Med.* 2008;36(12):3239-3245.
21. Druml W, Zechner R, Magometschnigg D, et al. Post-heparin lipolytic activity in acute renal failure. *Clin Nephrol.* 1985;23(6):289-293.
22. Druml W, Fischer M, Sertl S, Schneeweiss B, Lenz K, Widhalm K. Fat elimination in acute renal failure: long-chain vs medium-chain triglycerides. *Am J Clin Nutr.* 1992;55(2):468-472.
23. Goldstein SL. Pediatric acute kidney injury: it's time for real progress. *Pediatr Nephrol.* 2006;21(7):891-895.
24. Goldstein SL, Currier H, Graf C, Cosio CC, Brewer ED, Sachdeva R. Outcome in children receiving continuous veno-venous hemofiltration. *Pediatrics.* 2001;107(6):1309-1312.
25. Sutherland SM, Zappitelli M, Alexander SR, et al. Fluid overload and mortality in children receiving continuous renal replacement therapy: the prospective pediatric continuous renal replacement therapy registry. *Am J Kidney Dis.* 2010;55(2):316-325.
26. Kyle UG, Akcan-Arikan A, Orellana RA, Coss-Bu JA. Nutrition support among critically ill children with AKI. *Clin J Am Soc Nephrol.* 2013;8(4):568-574.
27. Quan A, Baum M. Protein losses in children on continuous cycler peritoneal dialysis. *Pediatr Nephrol.* 1996;10(6):728-731.
28. Mactier R, Khanna R. Peritoneal cavity lymphatics. In: *Peritoneal Dialysis*, 3rd ed. Nolph, K, Ed. Boston, MA: Kluwer Academic Publishing; 1989:48-66.
29. Ikizler TA, Flakoll PJ, Parker RA, Hakim RM. Amino acid and albumin losses during hemodialysis. *Kidney Int.* 1994;46(3):830-837.
30. Blumberg A, Hanck A, Sander G. Vitamin nutrition in patients on continuous ambulatory peritoneal dialysis (CAPD). *Clin Nephrol.* 1983;20; 244-250.
31. Makoff R, Gonick H. Renal failure and the concomitant derangement of micronutrient metabolism. *Nutr Clin Pract.* 1999;14:238-246.
32. Fiaccadori E, Maggiore U, Giacosa R, et al. Enteral nutrition in patients with acute renal failure. *Kidney Int.* 2004;65(3):999-1008.
33. Maxvold NJ, Smoyer WE, Custer JR, Bunchman TE. Amino acid loss and nitrogen balance in critically ill children with acute renal failure: a prospective comparison between classic hemofiltration and hemofiltration with dialysis. *Crit Care Med.* 2000;28(4):1161-1165.
34. Heyland DK, Dhaliwal R, Drover JW, Gramlich L, Dodek P. Canadian clinical practice guidelines for nutrition support in mechanically ventilated, critically ill adult patients. *J Parenter Enteral Nutr.* 2003;27(5):355-373.
35. Kreymann KG, Berger MM, Deutz NE, et al. ESPEN Guidelines on Enteral Nutrition: intensive care. *Clin Nutr.* 2006;25(2):210-223.
36. Metnitz PG, Krenn CG, Steltzer H, et al. Effect of acute renal failure requiring renal replacement therapy on outcome in critically ill patients. *Crit Care Med.* 2002;30(9):2051-2058.

CHAPTER 15

Respiratory Failure

Jennifer N. Manzi
Jennifer A. McArthur
Theresa A. Mikhailov

■ OVERVIEW OF PEDIATRIC RESPIRATORY FAILURE
Upper Airway Obstruction
Parenchymal Lung Disease
Acute Lung Injury and Acute Respiratory Distress Syndrome
■ TYPES OF MECHANICAL VENTILATORY SUPPORT
Noninvasive Ventilation
Mechanical Ventilation Through an Endotracheal Tube
Conventional Mechanical Ventilation
Neurally Adjusted Ventilatory Assist
High-Frequency Oscillatory Ventilation
■ IMPORTANCE OF PROVIDING NUTRITION TO CRITICALLY ILL CHILDREN WITH RESPIRATORY FAILURE
Nutrition Goal
Nutritional Strategies in Mechanically Ventilated Patients
Underfeeding and Overfeeding Mechanically Ventilated Patients
■ OXIDATIVE STRESS, RESPIRATORY FAILURE, AND SPECIAL NUTRITIONAL CONSIDERATIONS
Omega Fatty Acids
Vitamins and Trace Elements
Future Complementary Nutritional Therapies
■ CONCLUSIONS
■ KEY POINTS
References

■ OVERVIEW OF PEDIATRIC RESPIRATORY FAILURE

The etiology of respiratory failure in children requiring mechanical ventilation is diverse. Children may develop respiratory failure due to primary lung disease, upper airway disease, central nervous system disease, or neuromuscular disorders.

Upper Airway Obstruction

Children may require endotracheal intubation and mechanical ventilation due to upper airway obstruction. Most commonly in children this is due to (1) infections such as croup, bacterial tracheitis, epiglottitis, neck abscesses, or laryngeal papillomatosis; (2) congenital or acquired malformations such as vascular rings, laryngeal webs, subglottic stenosis, soft tissue masses, bronchomalacia, tracheomalacia, or laryngomalacia; or (3) airway trauma from previous intubations, foreign body aspiration, burn injury, or traumatic injury.[1] Some of these upper airway diseases, such as the congenital malformations, are chronic. As such, infants may present with an acute exacerbation of their chronic upper airway obstruction causing respiratory failure and may be malnourished at the time of presentation. Chronic upper airway obstruction in infants can adversely affect their ability to coördinate sucking and swallowing and impede their ability to gain weight appropriately.[2] Once a stable airway is established, these infants should have a comprehensive feeding plan established to help them attain catch-up growth.

Parenchymal Lung Disease

The focus of this chapter will be on nutritional considerations in infants and children with respiratory failure from parenchymal lung disease. The most common cause of parenchymal lung disease requiring intubation in children is infectious pneumonitis caused by a variety of viruses and bacteria.

In a recent international epidemiologic study by the Pediatric Acute Lung Injury and Sepsis Investigators (PALISI) group, 94% of children receiving mechanical ventilation had a pulmonary illness. The most common pulmonary pathology in this population was pneumonia.[3] Other causes of pulmonary illnesses seen in decreasing frequency were pulmonary edema or effusion, pulmonary dysfunction after surgery or trauma, apnea or respiratory distress, pulmonary aspiration, bronchiolitis, asthma, upper airway obstruction, and chest trauma. In this study, most (75%) of the children received conventional mechanical ventilation, while 16% received high-frequency oscillatory ventilation (HFOV) and 8.5% received noninvasive mechanical ventilation. Each mode of ventilation is characterized by unique challenges to delivering optimal nutrition and will be discussed later in this section.

The most commonly encountered viruses causing significant respiratory disease are respiratory syncytial virus (RSV), parainfluenza virus, adenovirus, and influenza. Less commonly described pathogens in children are cytomegalovirus, enterovirus, rhinovirus, measles, and human metapneumovirus.[4,5] Common bacterial pathogens include *Streptococcus pneumoniae*, *Haemophilus influenza*, *Staphylococcus aureus*, and *Mycoplasma pneumonia*.[4] Children with underlying chronic diseases may develop infections from gram-negative or anaerobic bacteria. Children may infrequently develop fungal infections. Immunocompromised children are at risk of opportunistic infections such as invasive pulmonary aspergillosis, pulmonary candidiasis, or *Pneumocystis carinii* pneumonia.[4]

Noninfectious causes of pediatric lung disease leading to respiratory failure include chemical pneumonitis, idiopathic interstitial lung disease, and pulmonary hemorrhage. Chemical pneumonitis can be caused by aspiration of gastric contents or from inhalation or ingestion of toxic substances. Pulmonary hemorrhage in children results from a variety of different causes, many of which require endotracheal intubation and institution of mechanical ventilation with positive end expiratory pressure (PEEP) to help control bleeding.[4]

Acute Lung Injury and Acute Respiratory Distress Syndrome

When reviewing the literature on respiratory failure, the terms acute lung injury (ALI) and acute respiratory distress syndrome (ARDS) are often used. The definitions of ALI and ARDS were developed by a consensus group of expert intensivists from North America and Europe in 1994 to aid researchers and clinicians in comparing patients with similar degrees of lung injury.[6] The definition included (1) acute onset of hypoxia, (2) bilateral infiltrates on chest x-ray, (3) lack of evidence of heart failure as the cause of lung disease (pulmonary artery wedge pressure <18 mm Hg if data available), and (4) $PaO_2/FiO_2 \leq 300$ for ALI and ≤ 200 for ARDS. There is much debate in the literature regarding the imperfections of these definitions, particularly in pediatrics. A consensus group aiming to address some of the shortcomings of the previous definition developed the Berlin definition of acute lung injury in 2011.[7] This definition has been subsequently evaluated in infants and children and appears to be valid in pediatric ARDS.[8,9] These definitions are used to risk-stratify patients in clinical trials for treatment and/or management of respiratory failure due to lung injury.

Acute lung injury and ARDS can have multiple etiologies and do not imply a specific cause of lung disease. The etiology of ARDS is often classified as direct or indirect lung injury, with direct lung injury having a causative agent that directly attacks the lungs, whereas the mechanism for indirect lung injury involves injury to the lungs through a secondary mechanism. Examples of direct lung injury in children include pneumonia, aspiration pneumonitis, traumatic pulmonary contusions, and inhalation injury. Causes of indirect lung injury in children include sepsis, shock, cardiopulmonary bypass, burns, and transfusion-related lung injury.[10]

TYPES OF MECHANICAL VENTILATORY SUPPORT

The type of mechanical ventilation used can have implications for methods of providing children with nutrition. Therefore, these will be discussed briefly along with their nutritional implications.

Noninvasive Ventilation

Noninvasive ventilation is accomplished by use of a mask that may fit either over the patient's mouth and nose or just over the nose. This mask is connected to a machine that delivers a continuous constant positive pressure, in the case of continuous positive airway pressure (CPAP), or a higher pressure at the time of inhalation and lower (but still positive) pressure at the time of exhalation in the case of bilevel positive airway pressure (BiPAP). Bilevel positive airway pressure machines can be set in a similar manner to conventional mechanical ventilation, but with the use of a noninvasive mask as opposed to an invasive endotracheal tube.

When evaluating patients receiving noninvasive ventilation (CPAP or BiPAP) for nutritional support, two important considerations are unique to this form of ventilatory support. The ability of noninvasive ventilation to work effectively depends upon the mask being able to form a reasonably tight seal over the patient's face. Unfortunately, oral and nasal feeding tubes often interfere with forming this seal. However, this can often be overcome by adjustments in the CPAP or BiPAP settings. Therefore, noninvasive ventilation should not be considered an absolute contraindication to nasal or oral tube feeding.

The second consideration in feeding patients on noninvasive ventilation is that the air being delivered by the CPAP or BiPAP machine is not just being delivered to the lungs, as it is during ventilation through an endotracheal tube; some of it is invariably delivered unintentionally into the stomach. Therefore, patients on noninvasive ventilation can develop gaseous distention of their gastrointestinal (GI) tract. This is generally considered a benign problem.[11] However, in individual patients, the increased abdominal distention may impede pulmonary mechanics or cause increased vomiting and/or problems with feeding intolerance. Techniques such as venting of the feeding tube between feedings, preventing constipation, and nasojejunal feedings may help to overcome these problems. Also, if patients are at high risk of vomiting, it may be prudent to choose a mask that fits over their nose and not their mouth so that if they do vomit, it is not trapped in the mask and forced back into their lungs with the airway pressure being used to provide the CPAP or BiPAP. Future studies aimed at evaluating the optimal method of feeding children on noninvasive ventilatory support are desirable.

Mechanical Ventilation Through an Endotracheal Tube

Ventilation using an endotracheal tube placed directly into the trachea and connected to the ventilator eliminates some of the problems encountered when attempting to provide enteral feeding to patients on noninvasive ventilation. In this case, all of the air is delivered directly into the lungs and placement of a nasogastric (NG) or orogastric feeding tube will not interfere with the ability to provide good ventilation. However, mechanical ventilation through an invasive endotracheal tube has its own set of unique problems that may contribute to difficulty tolerating enteral nutrition (EN). We will discuss some of the more common methods of ventilation utilizing an endotracheal tube and their effects on enteral feeding tolerance.

Conventional Mechanical Ventilation

Conventional mechanical ventilation is the most common ventilation strategy used in children with respiratory failure throughout the world.[5] A multitude of different modes can be used with a conventional ventilator. All of these modes deliver ventilator breaths utilizing positive pressure. These different modes share common characteristics that have implications for the ability to provide good nutritional support.

Conventional ventilators deliver air into the lungs, using positive pressure. This differs significantly from the way that healthy people breathe spontaneously. In spontaneous, unassisted breathing, air is drawn into the lungs using negative pressure, much like sucking liquid through a straw. Positive pressure ventilation with continuous PEEP has been shown to contribute to both fluid and sodium retention in both human and animal models.[12-14] Because fluid retention is known to impede ventilator weaning,[15] patients are often fluid restricted and given diuretics to combat fluid retention. The fluid restriction placed on patients can inhibit the ability to deliver adequate calories,[16] and diuretic use can cause electrolyte disturbances such as hyponatremia, hypokalemia, and metabolic alkalosis, particularly from loop diuretics such as furosemide.

Neurally Adjusted Ventilatory Assist

Neurally adjusted ventilatory assist (NAVA) is a form of ventilatory support where an NG tube with a special monitoring device is utilized. Electrodes embedded in this special NG tube are able to detect electrical activity of the diaphragm and transmit it to the ventilator, which then delivers a proportional pressure to support the spontaneous effort. The peak inspiratory pressure is related to amount of electrical activity generated by the diaphragm, and is terminated once the diaphragmatic activity drops below a certain level. The synchrony between the phrenic nerve activation and ventilator breath is thought to be more comfortable for patients, as they have greater ability to trigger ventilator breath effectively than in other forms of ventilation.[17] The important nutritional consideration in this form of ventilation is that the NG tube used for sensing the phrenic nerve can be used as a feeding tube. If it is in the patient's best interest to receive nasojejunal feedings, a second nasal tube may be placed to provide this, and the NG tube needed for NAVA can be used for venting air from the stomach.

High-Frequency Oscillatory Ventilation

High-frequency oscillatory ventilation is quite different from conventional ventilation in that a relatively constant mean airway pressure is set and then ventilation occurs through oscillations in pressure around the set mean airway pressure. Patients on HFOV do not have chest wall movement that appears similar to spontaneous ventilation as they do in conventional mechanical ventilation. Instead, their chest wall moves in a rapid, jiggling motion. Because of this unconventional method of breathing, it is felt to be fairly uncomfortable, and patients need to be heavily sedated and often chemically paralyzed to tolerate it. Many of the drugs used to keep patients comfortable and sedated decrease bowel motility as an unintended side effect[18] and can negatively affect feeding tolerance. In critically ill children requiring an endotracheal tube, it is difficult to avoid the use of these drugs for comfort, which can impede gastrointestinal motility. Patients being supported with HFOV are usually on chemical paralysis and will require deeper sedation and pain control, potentially leading to even greater problems with gastrointestinal motility.

IMPORTANCE OF PROVIDING NUTRITION TO CRITICALLY ILL CHILDREN WITH RESPIRATORY FAILURE

Delivering appropriate nutrition is crucial during respiratory failure in critically ill children. Children who develop critical illness or injury may be malnourished at the time of admission. In fact, in one recent study, 30% of children were malnourished at the time of admission to the pediatric intensive care unit (PICU).[19] A significant proportion of children may be either underweight or overweight or obese at admission.[20,21] Furthermore, during critical illness or injury, the energy needs of children vary greatly, with some needing more than the predicted amount and others needing less than the predicted amount.[22] While standard equations have been developed to predict energy expenditures, these equations may not be accurate during critical illness or injury. Energy expenditure can be measured, but this is not always feasible during critical illness. Thus, critically ill and injured children are at risk for both underfeeding and overfeeding.[23,24] Details of energy requirements and the importance of accurate estimation of these requirements during critical illness are described in chapter 3. We will further discuss techniques utilized to provide appropriate nutrition to critically ill children with pulmonary failure.

Nutrition Goal

Establishing a goal for daily macronutrient delivery and providing a means to achieve this goal are paramount to the success of the nutritional strategy, particularly EN, in critically ill children. A retrospective study recently demonstrated that a documented nutrition goal was significantly associated with achievement of EN.[25] This goal should ideally be established via the use of indirect calorimetry. The use of a feeding protocol for gastric feedings has been shown to be effective in meeting nutritional goals and safe in terms of clinical complications.[26] The use of a feeding protocol for postpyloric feedings has also been shown to be effective in meeting nutritional goals and safe with respect to clinical complications.[27] In one PICU, the establishment of an early enteral feeding protocol resulted in a dramatic reduction in time to reach goal nutrition from a median of 32 hours in the preprotocol group to a median of 14 hours in the protocol group ($p < 0.0001$).[28] Furthermore, the establishment of a nutrition support team has been shown to be associated with increased use of EN, decreased use of parenteral nutrition (PN), and decreased mortality rates in one academic PICU.[29]

Nutritional Strategies in Mechanically Ventilated Patients

Most of the nutritional studies in pediatric critical care have been performed in mechanically ventilated patients. Large, randomized, controlled nutrition trials in critically ill children are lacking. A brief synopsis of feeding strategies in mechanically ventilated patients is presented next. For further details on EN, see chapter 8, and on PN, see chapter 7.

Several studies suggest that trophic enteral feeding (<25% of recommended calories) may be beneficial for critically ill children.[30-35] Also, larger volumes of enteral feeding may be beneficial in critically ill children.[19,36] Conversely, PN has been associated with increased morbidity and mortality.[19,37] It is important to remember that sicker patients are more likely to be deemed unfit to tolerate EN and be provided PN instead. In an adult randomized, controlled trial (RCT), late initiation of PN was associated with faster recovery and fewer complications, as compared with early initiation.[38] In another adult multicenter RCT of patients with relative contraindications to EN and expected ICU stay of over 48 hours, over 1,300 subjects were randomized to either pragmatic nutrition therapy or early PN. In this latter study, there were no significant differences in day-60 mortality between the 2 groups, and the authors concluded that the early PN strategy was not associated with increased harm. Although, the early PN strategy was associated with significantly fewer days of invasive ventilation, there were no differences in ICU or hospital length of stay between the 2 groups.[39] In patients who are not ready for EN, the use of early PN to achieve target calories needs to be balanced against the likelihood of harm associated with PN therapy. Similar studies are required in critically ill children.

Underfeeding and Overfeeding Mechanically Ventilated Patients

The metabolic response to critical illness is characterized by hypermetabolism, hyperglycemia, increased lipolysis, and net protein catabolism.[40] One of the cardinal metabolic features of critical illness is the catabolic response seen in skeletal muscle.[40] Skeletal muscle protein is broken down, and the amino acids are used for gluconeogenesis and protein synthesis. This, along with prolonged immobilization and suboptimal nutrient intake, results in loss of lean body mass. Optimal nutritional support may help decrease the protein imbalance seen in critical illness.[40,41] Underfeeding can be detrimental to maintenance of muscle mass and function. Skeletal muscles need energy for their own intrinsic metabolism in addition to the energy required for motor activity.[42] A lack of energy may compromise energy metabolism of muscle fibers and lead to muscle weakness.[42] When total daily energy expenditure is not matched by the nutrient intake, further catabolism of body energy stores and muscle proteins occurs.[43] The respiratory musculature is not spared, and weakness of the respiratory musculature may lead to prolonged dependence on mechanical ventilation in the face of inadequate nutrition support.

It is equally important to avoid overfeeding mechanically ventilated patients. When overfeeding occurs, the ratio of carbohydrate to fat oxidation increases over time.[44] This leads to proportionately more carbon dioxide (CO_2) production.[44] Under normal circumstances, minute ventilation is increased to rid the body of the CO_2. However, in the ventilated patients, this leads to increased ventilator requirements and can prevent weaning of ventilatory support.[44]

OXIDATIVE STRESS, RESPIRATORY FAILURE, AND SPECIAL NUTRITIONAL CONSIDERATIONS

There is growing evidence that many disease states that lead to respiratory failure, such as sepsis, severe burns, and trauma, are associated with oxidative stress, low levels of antioxidants, and inflammation.[45,46] Because of this association, a number of feeding regimens involving antioxidant supplementation and use of the anti-inflammatory omega-3 fatty acids have been tried in patients with acute lung injury, though the results remain equivocal to date. We will review some of the conflicting evidence for these approaches. A summary of the different adult nutritional trials to date is listed in Table 15-1.

TABLE 15-1. Nutritional Intervention Trials in Critically ill Adults

Author/Year	Patient Population	Type of Study	Supplements	Findings
Beale et al., 2008[51]	55 adult sepsis patients requiring mechanical ventilation	Randomized, controlled	Glutamine, butyrate, beta-carotene, vitamins E and C, Zn, Se	Faster improvement of organ dysfunction in supplement group
Pontes-Arruda 2006[48]	165 adult septic patients requiring mechanical ventilation	Randomized, controlled	Omega-3 fatty acids, alpha-linolenic oil, vitamins E and C, Se	Improved mortality, oxygenation, ventilator-free days, ICU-free days and less new organ dysfunction in supplement group
Berger 2006[52]	41 severely burned adult patients	Randomized, controlled	Cu, Se, Zn	Decreased nosocomial infections in supplement group
Berger 2008[53]	200 adults with organ failure from major trauma, cardiac surgery, or subarachnoid hemorrhage	Randomized, controlled	Vitamins C and B_1, Se, Zn	Decreased CRP levels in supplemented group, no difference in infectious complications; decreased length of hospital stay in supplemented trauma patients
Collier 2008[54]	4,294 adult trauma patients	Retrospective – before and after implementation of protocol for antioxidant supplementation in trauma patients	Ascorbic acid, alpha-tocopherol, Se	Improved mortality, hospital, and ICU length of stay after implementation of supplementation protocol
Angstwurm 1999[55]	42 adult patients with SIRS	Randomized, placebo controlled	Se	Improved Se levels and glutathione peroxidase activity and severity of illness scores in supplemented group
Angstwurm 2007[56]	294 adults with SIRS, sepsis, and septic shock	Randomized, placebo controlled	Se	Improved Se levels and glutathione peroxidase activity and improved 28-day mortality in supplemented group
Forceville 2007[57]	60 adults with severe septic shock	Randomized, placebo controlled	Se	No difference in mortality, hospital length of stay, organ failure rates, or nosocomial infections
Manzanares 2012[63]	2,531 critically ill adults	Meta-analysis of 21 randomized controlled trials 1980-2011	Various antioxidants	Reduced mortality, decreased duration of mechanical ventilation; no effect on hospital or ICU length of stay
Rice 2011[50]	272 critically ill, mechanically ventilated adults	Randomized to study formula with supplements vs. isocaloric formula	Omega-3 fatty acids, alpha-linolenic acid and antioxidants	Study stopped for futility and increased days on mechanical ventilation and in ICU with study formula
Heyland 2013[58]	1,223 critically ill, mechanically ventilated adults	2-by-2 factorial randomization	Antioxidants, glutamine, both, or placebo	Increased in hospital and 6-month mortality and mechanical ventilation in glutamine group; no effect in antioxidant group

Zn, Zinc ; Cu, Copper; Se, Selenium.

Omega-3 Fatty Acids

In 1999, Gadek et al. published the results of a study of 146 adult patients with ARDS randomized to receive either a standard feeding formula or a continuous infusion of a feeding regimen enriched with eicosapentaenoic acid (EPA), GLA, and antioxidants. Patients fed the enriched diet had improved oxygenation, needed less time on the ventilator, and had less development of new organ failure.[47] This led to a similar study by Pontes-Arruda. In this study, 165 septic adult patients requiring mechanical ventilation were randomized to receive continuous feeding of a standard formula or a formula enriched with EPA, GLA, and antioxidants. In this study, the patients randomized to receive the study diet had better outcomes, with less development of organ failure, less time on the ventilator, shorter lengths of stay both in the ICU and the hospital, and decreased mortality.[48] During the same time frame, Singer et al. published the results of their study of 100 adults with ARDS who were randomized to receive either a similar regimen of standard formula or formula enriched with EPA and GLA. This study found that patients receiving the study diet had fewer days on the ventilator, but no difference in survival.[49]

Because of the promising results of the earlier studies, the National Heart, Lung, and Blood Institute (NHLBI) ARDS Clinical Trials Network undertook a similar study where patients were randomized to receive twice-daily enteral supplements of omega-3 fatty acids, GLA, and antioxidants or an isocaloric-isovolemic, carbohydrate-rich control supplement. Patients also had plasma interleukin 6 (IL-6), IL-8, and EPA levels and urine levels of leukotrienes performed. While patients fed the study supplement had increased EPA levels as predicted, they had no difference in leukotriene levels. The supplemented patients had more diarrhea, more days on the ventilator, and longer ICU stays. These results were in direct contrast to previous studies, and the study was stopped for futility by the Data Safety and Monitoring Board after 272 patients were randomized.[50] It is uncertain if the method employed for supplementation in the Rice study was the reason for the different outcome, as they gave their supplements on a twice-daily schedule. The previous studies had mixed their supplements in with the enteral feedings and were, therefore, given on a continuous basis. The fact that there were no clinical effects despite increased plasma levels of EPA seems to suggest that this combination of fatty acids was ineffective. These supplements/formula are not currently recommended outside a clinical trial.

Vitamins and Trace Elements

A number of small clinical trials in adults have shown potential benefit of vitamin and trace-element supplementation in critically ill adults.[48,51-57] However, the combinations of supplements given have been variable, as have the benefits seen. It is difficult to know which supplements are important in which situation and at what dose.

In the largest blinded trial to date, 1,223 mechanically ventilated, critically ill adults with multiorgan failure were enrolled. The subjects were randomized using a 2×2 factorial design to one of 4 groups: (1) glutamine supplements, (2) antioxidant supplements, (3) both, or (4) placebo. The group that received glutamine supplementation showed an increase in in-hospital and 60-day mortality and a trend toward increased 28-day mortality. The glutamine group also had a longer duration of mechanical ventilation. The antioxidant group did not seem to have any harm or benefit from the supplements. Therefore, the best available data do not support the routine use of glutamine or antioxidants in critically ill adults.[58]

Data on supplementation of vitamins and trace elements in children are lacking. In one study from the National Institute of Child Health and Human Development (NICHD) Collaborative Pediatric Critical Care Research Network (CPCCRN), 293 PICU patients were randomized to receive either supplementation with zinc, selenium, glutamine, and metoclopramide or supplementation with whey protein. There were no differences found in infectious complications between the 2 groups, which was the primary endpoint of the study.[59] There was also no difference between groups for ICU length of stay, ventilator days, or survival. In a subgroup of immunocompromised patients, a decreased rate of sepsis and nosocomial infections was reported in the group supplemented with zinc, selenium, glutamine, and metoclopramide. The role of antioxidants and micronutrient supplementation in critically ill children is unclear, and this strategy cannot be recommended based on available evidence. Future studies examining the role of this intervention in immunocompromised patients or those with existing deficiencies of these components are needed.

Future Complementary Nutritional Therapies

Recently, there has been an interest in complementary and alternative therapies in critical illness. Some of these therapies involve nutritional substances such as resveratrol found in red grapes, curcumin found in the common Indian spice turmeric, and ginger.[60,61]

Curcumin is thought to have anti-inflammatory properties through inhibition of nuclear factor-kappa B (NF-κB). In a rat model of sepsis-induced ALI, animals given intraperitoneal curcumin administered 2 and 12 hours after the initiation of sepsis showed significantly less lung inflammation. Rats treated with the curcumin also had down-regulation of the inflammatory cytokines tumor necrosis factor (TNF)-alpha, IL-8, and macrophage migration inhibitory factor.[62] Curcumin has not been studied in humans with ALI, but it has been shown to have beneficial effects in human studies on a variety of other inflammatory diseases, such as atherosclerosis, cancer, neurodegenerative diseases, pancreatitis, and rheumatoid arthritis.[60]

Ginger is also felt to possess anti-inflammatory properties through inhibition of cyclooxygenase and lipooxygenase. In a randomized, placebo-controlled trial involving 32 adult ARDS patients, patients randomized to receive ginger had improved outcomes. The ginger group had lower inflammatory marker levels, including IL-1, IL-6, and TNF-alpha. They also had improved oxygenation, shorter duration of mechanical ventilation, and shorter length of ICU stay.[61] This study was small; therefore, in order for there to be widespread recommendations regarding ginger supplementation in patients with ALI, larger studies need to be done.

CONCLUSIONS

There is much that is unknown regarding optimal nutrition in critically ill children with respiratory failure. What is known is that these patients will require some form of nutrition to recover from their illness. The best available evidence suggests that EN is preferable to parenteral. It is likely that early EN is better than prolonged periods of being without any nutritional intake. Both underfeeding and overfeeding of carbohydrate calories is associated with undesirable effects and must be avoided. However, the exact amount of calories needed, how quickly to advance feedings, and even what type of formula is best in a specific situation is still relatively unknown. These important clinical questions need to be studied in the pediatric population. The importance of nutrition in improving outcomes in this group cannot be ignored. Hippocrates was probably accurate when he said, "Let food be thy medicine and medicine be thy food."

KEY POINTS

- Children with acute and chronic respiratory failure are at risk of worse outcomes due to underfeeding or overfeeding.
- Indirect Calorimetry allows measurement of energy expenditure and must guide energy prescription in mechanically ventilated children.
- Suboptimal energy and protein intake in this population results in depletion of lean body mass, weakness, and potentially prolonged dependence on mechanical ventilation.
- On the other hand, carbohydrate overfeeding may result in increased carbon dioxide burden and further worsening of respiratory status.
- The role of antioxidant and micronutrient supplementation in critically ill children with respiratory failure has not been proven.

REFERENCES

1. Jardine D, Bhutta OJ, Inglis A. Specific diseases of the respiratory system: Upper airway. In: *Pediatric critical care: expert consult premium.* 4th ed. Fuhrman BP, Zimmerman JJ, Eds. Philadelphia, PA: Mosby; 2011:561-573.
2. Miller CK, Willging JP. The implications of upper-airway obstruction on successful infant feeding. *Semin Speech Lang.* 2007;28(3):190-203.
3. Santschi M, Jouvet P, Leclerc F, et al. Acute lung injury in children: Therapeutic practice and feasibility of international clinical trials. *Pediatr Crit Care Med.* 2010;11(6): 681-689.
4. Benson JC, Parakininkas D, Rice TB. Pneumonitis and interstitial disease. In: *Pediatric critical care: Expert consult premium.* 4th ed. Fuhrman BP, Zimmerman JJ, Eds. Philadelphia, PA: Mosby; 2011:609-631.
5. Jartti T, Jartti L, Ruuskanen O, Soderlund-Venermo M. New respiratory viral infections. *Curr Opin Pulm Med.* 2012;18(3):271-278.
6. Bernard GR, Artigas A, Brigham KL, et al. Report of the American-European Consensus Conference on acute respiratory distress syndrome: definitions, mechanisms, relevant outcomes, and clinical trial coordination. *J Crit Care.* 1994;9(1):72-81.
7. ARDS Definition Task Force, Ranieri VM, Rubenfeld GD, et al. Acute respiratory distress syndrome: the Berlin Definition. *JAMA.* 2012;307:2526-2533.
8. Khemani RG, et al. Evaluating the Berlin definition in pediatric ARDS. *Intensive Care Med.* 2013;39(12): 2213-2216.

9. De Luca D, et al. The use of the Berlin definition for acute respiratory distress syndrome during infancy and early childhood: multicenter evaluation and expert consensus. *Intensive Care Med*. 2013;39(12):2083-2091.

10. Ventre K, Arnold J. Acute lung injury and acute respiratory distress syndrome. In: *Roger's Textbook of Pediatric Intensive Care*. 4th ed. Nichols DG, Ed. Philadelphia, PA: Lippincott Williams & Wilkins; 2008:731-732.

11. Havranek T, Madramootoo C, Carver JD. Nasal continuous positive airway pressure affects pre- and postprandial intestinal blood flow velocity in preterm infants. *J Perinatol*. 2007;27(11):704-708.

12. Frass M, Popovic R, Hartter E, Auinger C, Woloszczuk W, Leithner C. Atrial natriuretic peptide decrease during spontaneous breathing with continuous positive airway pressure in volume-expanded healthy volunteers. *Crit Care Med*. 1988;16(9):831-835.

13. Rossaint R, Krebs M, Forther J, Unger V, Falke K, Kaczmarczyk G. Inferior vena caval pressure increase contributes to sodium and water retention during PEEP in awake dogs. *J Appl Physiol*. 1993;75(6):2484-2492.

14. Mackie DP, Spoelder EJ, Paauw RJ, Knape P, Boer C. Mechanical ventilation and fluid retention in burn patients. *J Trauma*. 2009;67(6):1233-8; discussion 1238.

15. National Heart, Lung, and Blood Institute Acute Respiratory Distress Syndrome (ARDS) Clinical Trials Network, Wiedemann HP, Wheeler AP, et al. Comparison of two fluid-management strategies in acute lung injury. *N Engl J Med*. 2006;354(24):2564-2575.

16. Rogers EJ, Gilbertson HR, Heine RG, Henning R. Barriers to adequate nutrition in critically ill children. *Nutrition*. 2003;19(10):865-868.

17. Verbrugghe W, Jorens PG. Neurally adjusted ventilatory assist: a ventilation tool or a ventilation toy? *Respir Care*. 2011;56(3):327-335.

18. Mixides G, Liebl MG, Bloom K. Enteral administration of naloxone for treatment of opioid-associated intragastric feeding intolerance. *Pharmacotherapy*. 2004;24(2):291-294.

19. Mehta NM, Bechard LJ, Cahill N, et al. Nutritional practices and their relationship to clinical outcomes in critically ill children—an international multicenter cohort study. *Crit Care Med*. 2012;40(7):2204-2211.

20. Hulst J, Joosten K, Zimmermann L, et al. Malnutrition in critically ill children: from admission to 6 months after discharge. *Clin Nutr*. 2004;23(2):223-232.

21. Skillman HE, Mehta NM. Nutrition therapy in the critically ill child. *Curr Opin Crit Care*. 2012;18(2):192-198.

22. Alexander E, Susla GM, Burstein AH, Brown DT, Ognibene FP. Retrospective evaluation of commonly used equations to predict energy expenditure in mechanically ventilated, critically ill patients. *Pharmacotherapy*. 2004;24(12):1659-1667.

23. ASPEN Board of Directors and the Clinical Guidelines Task Force. Guidelines for the use of parenteral and enteral nutrition in adult and pediatric patients. *J Parenter Enteral Nutr*. 2002;26(1 Suppl):1SA-138SA.

24. Mehta NM, Bechard LJ, Leavitt K, Duggan C. Cumulative energy imbalance in the pediatric intensive care unit: Role of targeted indirect calorimetry. *J Parenter Enteral Nutr*. 2009;33(3):336-344.

25. Wakeham M, Christensen M, Manzi J, et al. Impact of registered dietitians: early medical record documentation of an estimated caloric requirement in critically ill children is associated with higher daily caloric intake and with use of the enteral route. *JAND*. 2013. In press.

26. Briassoulis GC, Zavras NJ, Hatzis MD TD. Effectiveness and safety of a protocol for promotion of early intragastric feeding in critically ill children. *Pediatr Crit Care Med*. 2001;2(2):113-121.

27. Sánchez C, López-Herce J, Borrego R, Mencía S. Early transpyloric enteral nutrition in critically ill children. *Pediatr Crit Care Med*. 2007;8(1):88.

28. Petrillo-Albarano T, Pettignano R, Asfaw M, Easley K. Use of a feeding protocol to improve nutritional support through early, aggressive, enteral nutrition in the pediatric intensive care unit. *Pediatr Crit Care Med*. 2006;7(4):340-344.

29. Gurgueira GL, Leite HP, Taddei, José Augusto de Aguiar Carrazedo, de Carvalho WB. Outcomes in a pediatric intensive care unit before and after the implementation of a nutrition support team. *J Parenter Enteral Nutr*. 2005;29(3):176-185.

30. Sondheimer JM. A critical perspective on trophic feeding. *J Pediatr Gastroenterol Nutr*. 2004;38(3):237-238.

31. Hernandez G, Velasco N, Wainstein C, et al. Gut mucosal atrophy after a short enteral fasting period in critically ill patients. *J Crit Care*. 1999;14(2):73-77.

32. Buchman AL, Moukarzel AA, Bhuta S, et al. Parenteral nutrition is associated with intestinal morphologic and functional changes in humans. *J Parenter Enteral Nutr*. 1995;19(6):453-460.

33. Tyson JE, Kennedy KA. Minimal enteral nutrition for promoting feeding tolerance and preventing morbidity in parenterally fed infants. *Cochrane Database Syst Rev*. 2000;(2)(2):CD000504.

34. Rubinson L, Diette GB, Song X, Brower RG, Krishnan JA. Low caloric intake is associated with nosocomial bloodstream infections in patients in the medical intensive care unit. *Crit Care Med*. 2004;32(2):350-357.

35. MacFie J, Reddy BS, Gatt M, Jain PK, Sowdi R, Mitchell CJ. Bacterial translocation studied in 927 patients over 13 years. *Br J Surg*. 2006;93(1):87-93.
36. Mikhailov TA, Kuhn EM, Manzi JN, et al. Early entral nutrition is associated with lower mortality in critically ill children. *J Parenter Enteral Nutr*. 2014 Jan 8. [Epub ahead of print]
37. Goday PS, Kuhn EM, Mikhailov TA. Early parenteral nutrition is associated with significantly higher mortality in critically ill children. *J Parenter Enteral Nutr*. 2013. In press.
38. Casaer MP, et al. Early versus late parenteral nutrition in critically ill adults. *N Engl J Med*. 2011;365:506-517.
39. Doig GS, et al. Early parenteral nutrition in critically ill patients with short-term relative contraindications to early enteral nutrition: a randomized controlled trial. *JAMA*. 2013;309:2130-2138.
40. Wray CJ, Mammen JM V, Hasselgren P-O. Catabolic response to stress and potential benefits of nutrition support. *Nutrition*. 2002;18:971-977.
41. Ziegler T, MD, Gatzen C. Strategies for attenuating protein-catabolic responses in the critically ill *Ann Rev Med*. 1994,1:459-480.
42. Volkert D. The role of nutrition in the prevention of sarcopenia. *Wiener Medizinische Wochenschrift*. 2011;161: 409-415.
43. Plank L, Hill G. Energy balance in critical illness. *Proc Nutr Soc*. 2003;62:545552.
44. Liposky JM, Nelson LD. Ventilatory response to high caloric loads in critically ill patients. *Crit Care Med*. 1994;22:796-802.
45. McArthur J, Quasney MW. The role of selenium in sepsis. *Open Inflammation Journal*. 2011;4:115-119.
46. Heidemann SM, Holubkov R, Meert KL, et al. Baseline serum concentrations of zinc, selenium, and prolactin in critically ill children. *Pediatr Crit Care Med* 2013;14(4):202-206.
47. Gadek JE, DeMichele SJ, Karlstad MD, et al. Effect of enteral feeding with eicosapentaenoic acid, gamma-linolenic acid, and antioxidants in patients with acute respiratory distress syndrome. *Crit Care Med*. 1999; 27(8):1409-1420.
48. Pontes-Arruda A, Aragão AMA, Albuquerque JD. Effects of enteral feeding with eicosapentaenoic acid,[gamma]-linolenic acid, and antioxidants in mechanically ventilated patients with severe sepsis and septic shock. *Crit Care Med*. 2006;34(9):2325-2333.
49. Singer P, Theilla M, Fisher H, Gibstein L, Grozovski E, Cohen J. Benefit of an enteral diet enriched with eicosapentaenoic acid and gamma-linolenic acid in ventilated patients with acute lung injury. *Crit Care Med*. 2006;34(4):1033-1038.
50. Rice TW, Wheeler AP, Thompson BT, Steingrub J, Rock P. Enteral omega-3 fatty acid, γ-linolenic acid, and antioxidant supplementation in acute lung injury. *JAMA*. 2011;306(14):1574-1581.
51. Beale RJ, Sherry T, Lei K, et al. Early enteral supplementation with key pharmaconutrients improves sequential organ failure assessment score in critically ill patients with sepsis: Outcome of a randomized, controlled, double-blind trial. *Crit Care Med*. 2008;36(1):131-144.
52. Berger M, Eggimann P, Heyland D, et al. Reduction of nosocomial pneumonia after major burns by trace element supplementation: aggregation of two randomised trials. *Crit Care*. 2006;10(6):R153.
53. Berger M, Soguel L, Shenkin A, et al. Influence of early antioxidant supplements on clinical evolution and organ function in critically ill cardiac surgery, major trauma, and subarachnoid hemorrhage patients. *Crit Care*. 2008;12(4):R101.
54. Collier BR, Giladi A, Dossett LA, Dyer L, Fleming SB, Cotton BA. Impact of high-dose antioxidants on outcomes in acutely injured patients. *J Parenter Enteral Nutr*. 2008;32(4):384-388.
55. Angstwurm MW, Schottdorf J, Schopohl J, Gaertner R. Selenium replacement in patients with severe systemic inflammatory response syndrome improves clinical outcome. *Crit Care Med*. 1999;27(9):1807-1813.
56. Angstwurm MW, Engelmann L, Zimmermann T, et al. Selenium in intensive care (SIC): results of a prospective randomized, placebo-controlled, multiple-center study in patients with severe systemic inflammatory response syndrome, sepsis, and septic shock. *Crit Care Med*. 2007;35(1):118-126.
57. Forceville X, Laviolle B, Annane D, et al. Effects of high doses of selenium, as sodium selenite, in septic shock: a placebo-controlled, randomized, double-blind, phase II study. *Crit Care*. 2007;11(4):R73.
58. Heyland D, Muscedere J, Wischmeyer PE, et al. A randomized trial of glutamine and antioxidants in critically ill patients. *N Engl J Med*. 2013;368(16):1489-1497.
59. Carcillo JA, Dean JM, Holubkov R, et al. The randomized comparative pediatric critical illness stress-induced immune suppression (CRISIS) prevention trial. *Pediatr Crit Care Med*. 2012;13(2):165.
60. Clarke JO, Mullin GE. A review of complementary and alternative approaches to immunomodulation. *Nutr Clin Pract*. 2008;23(1):49-62.

61. Vahdat Shariatpanahi Z, Mokhtari M, Taleban FA, et al. Effect of enteral feeding with ginger extract in acute respiratory distress syndrome. *J Crit Care.* 2013;28(2):217.e1-e6.

62. Xiao X, Yang M, Sun D, Sun S. Curcumin protects against sepsis-induced acute lung injury in rats. *J Surg Res.* 2012;176(1):e31-e39.

63. Manzanares W, Dhaliwal R, Jiang X, Murch L, Heyland DK. Antioxidant micronutrients in the critically ill: a systematic review and meta-analysis. *Crit Care.* 2012;16:R66.

CHAPTER 16

Nutrition in Acute Liver Failure and Acute Pancreatitis

Diana Lerner

Steven Werlin

- LIVER FAILURE
- ACUTE LIVER FAILURE
- PATHOPHYSIOLOGY OF MALNUTRITION
  - Assessment of Nutritional Status
  - Estimating Nutritional Needs
  - Nutrition Support in Liver Failure
  - Fluid and Electrolytes
  - Carbohydrate
  - Protein
  - Lipid
  - Vitamins and Minerals
- PANCREATITIS
  - Acute Pancreatitis
  - Chronic Pancreatitis
  - Pathophysiology
  - Etiology
  - Severity
  - Clinical Management
  - Nutrition
  - Other Nutrition Issues in Acute Pancreatitis
- KEY POINTS
  - References

LIVER FAILURE

Liver failure is a final common pathway for a broad range of diagnoses. In the patient with liver failure, accurate nutritional assessment may be complicated by fluid shifts and organomegaly. Nutrition therapy in this population can be complex due to metabolic and electrolyte derangements. When chronic liver disease (CLD) is present, malabsorption of fats and fat-soluble vitamins may lead to multiple nutritional deficiencies. Liver failure requiring admission to the pediatric intensive care unit (PICU) can be divided into 2 categories: acute liver failure (ALF) and acute-on-chronic liver failure (ACLF). Even during early stages of disease, impaired nutritional status has been associated with poor clinical outcome and higher morbidity and mortality in the posttransplant period.[1-3] This chapter will review some of the underlying causes of malnutrition and provide recommendations for assessment and management of nutrition support for patients with liver disease in the PICU setting.

ACUTE LIVER FAILURE

The Pediatric Acute Liver Failure (PALF) study group defined the following entry criteria for ALF (Table 16-1).[4]

Liver failure has been further classified based on the timing of onset of encephalopathy. Hyperacute liver failure occurs within 1 week of onset, ALF from 1 to 4, weeks and subacute liver failure from 4 to 12 weeks after onset of hepatic disease.[1,2,5] These definitions may be difficult to apply in pediatrics due to the complexity of assessing encephalopathy in young children.

The exact incidence of pediatric ALF is not known. Among all age groups, the incidence of ALF is estimated to be 5.5 per million per year.[3,4] Approximately 675 pediatric liver transplants are done in the United States each year, of which 10% to 13% are done in patients with ALF. These numbers do not include children who recover or die without liver transplantation.[6,7]

The etiology of ALF varies with geographical location and age. Data from 215 consecutive ALF patients who presented to King's College Hospital in London showed a bimodal distribution with the highest prevalence in neonates and infants followed by a smaller peak after 15 years of age.[4,8] In the first month of life, it is prudent to consider metabolic disorders and herpes simplex type 1 and 2. Early intervention in these cases can prevent morbidity and mortality. In adolescents, drug toxicity predominates as the cause of ALF. In the Western world, the etiology of up to half of ALF cases remains undetermined. Toxic exposures and drug toxicity account for 25%, followed by viral infections, metabolic and autoimmune liver diseases, Wilson disease, and hematological malignancies.[4,9,10] In South-East Asia and Latin America, viral hepatitis, predominantly hepatitis A and E, are responsible for the majority of ALF diagnoses.[4,11,12]

Acute-on-chronic liver failure was defined by a working group from the American Association for the Study of Liver Disease (AASLD) and the European Association for the Study of the Liver (EASL) as "acute deterioration of preexisting, chronic liver disease, usually related to a precipitating event and associated with increased mortality at 3 months due to multisystem organ failure."[13]

Without liver transplantation, ACLF is associated with a mortality rate of over 70%.[14] The most common causes of CLD in children leading to liver failure are biliary atresia, alpha-1-antitrypsin deficiency, autoimmune hepatitis, Alagille syndrome, Wilson disease and progressive familial intrahepatic cholestasis (PFIC).

PATHOPHYSIOLOGY OF MALNUTRITION

Protein-energy malnutrition leading to growth delay is reported in up to 60% of patients with CLD.[3] The etiology of malnutrition is multifactorial and includes decreased dietary intake, malabsorption, increased energy expenditure, and disordered substrate use.

Decreased intake is the most common reason for malnutrition. Patients with liver disease suffer from anorexia due to the disease process and prescription of unpalatable formulas. Altered taste perception may occur with zinc deficiency. Congestive gastropathy, dysmotility, and organomegaly can lead to early satiety and vomiting. Malabsorption is most common in cholestatic liver diseases and is due to decreased intraluminal concentration of bile salts, as well as bile salt deconjugation from bacterial overgrowth and from associated pancreatic insufficiency in diseases such as Alagille syndrome and cystic fibrosis. Decreased absorption of long-chain fatty acids manifests as steatorrhea and fat-soluble vitamin deficiencies. The chronic disease state leads to increased utilization of energy. Malnutrition is further exacerbated by major insults, such as variceal hemorrhage, infection, or surgery, and increased respiratory effort from ascites and organomegaly.[11]

TABLE 16-1. Diagnostic Criteria for Acute Liver Failure

1. Hepatic-based coagulopathy not corrected by vitamin K 2. Biochemical evidence of liver injury 3. No known evidence of chronic liver disease (CLD)	Prothrombin time (PT) ≥15 seconds or international normalized ratio (INR) ≥1.5 with hepatic encephalopathy Or: PT ≥20 seconds or INR ≥2.0, regardless of encephalopathy

Assessment of Nutritional Status

Evaluation begins with a detailed nutrition history focusing on intake (volumes and types of foods) and losses (vomiting, diarrhea), as well as recent changes in weight. A pediatric dietitian can be a valuable resource to assess current intake. On physical examination, it is important to assess muscle bulk and presence of subcutaneous fat. Malabsorption of fat-soluble vitamins such as vitamin D and K may manifest as bowed limbs and easy bruising and bleeding. A careful skin evaluation may uncover signs of zinc or essential fatty acid deficiencies.[11]

Standard assessment measures such as body mass index (BMI) and new assessment techniques such as bioelectrical impedance have proven unreliable in adult cirrhotic patients with ascites or edema. Due to impaired linear growth, weight-for-height Z-scores are often misleadingly normal.[11]

In children with CLD, triceps skinfold thickness is superior to weight-for-length Z-scores for assessment of malnutrition.[15] Upper extremities are less likely to be affected by edema and produce more reliable measurements. Subjective global nutritional assessment (SGNA) was shown to be a reliable tool for assessment of malnutrition in young children.[16] Subjective global nutritional assessment includes a history of weight loss during the previous 6 months; changes in dietary intake, gastrointestinal symptoms, functional capacity, and metabolic demands; signs of muscle wasting; and the presence of presacral or pedal edema.[17]

The most accurate technique of nutritional assessment in patients with cirrhosis is the measurement of body cell mass, whether by whole-body potassium count, by stable isotope dilution, or by total-body electrical conductivity, but these techniques are not widely available.[6,8] Subjective global nutrition assessment, anthropometry, and handgrip strength are adequate when performed by experienced personnel.[9-11]

Estimating Nutritional Needs

The liver is a key organ in the production and the distribution of nutrients. Under normal conditions, the liver utilizes 20% to 25% of the body's energy. In ALF, energy demands are increased despite a substantial loss of hepatocyte mass.[18] Increased demands persist despite sedation, analgesia, muscle paralysis, and mechanical ventilation.[7]

In adults with ALF, the recommended energy intake is 35 to 40 kcal/kg body weight per day.[9] Recommendations based on children with biliary atresia and indirect calorimetry studies in children with CLD suggest a starting point of 130% of predicted resting energy expenditure (REE), with some children needing as much as 200% of REE.[3,8,19] These recommendations are based on children who are not critically ill. In the PICU, indirect calorimetry should be utilized whenever possible to assess the energy needs of these children.

Nutrition Support in Liver Failure

There are no well-designed, randomized, controlled studies addressing nutrition in critically ill children with acute or chronic liver failure.[20] A recent Cochrane review concluded that no standard recommendations for parenteral or enteral nutrition (EN) can be made based on currently available evidence.[21] However, an international multicenter cohort study found an improved 60-day survival in ventilated critically ill children who received a higher percentage of their goal EN.[22] Similarly, in critically ill adults, a negative energy balance (determined by indirect calorimetry) while in the ICU was associated with an increase in morbidity, including respiratory distress syndrome, pressure sores, sepsis, renal failure, need for surgery, and total complications.[23]

Implementation of an evidence-based nutrition management protocol increases the likelihood of early initiation of enteral feeding in the ICU setting.[24] On admission, all patients in the PICU should have a nutritional assessment and their caloric requirements should be estimated or preferably measured. Hemodynamically stable, critically ill patients who have a functioning gastrointestinal tract should be fed within 24 hours of admission. Nasogastric tube feedings are well tolerated even in the presence of esophageal varices, but gastrostomy placement in the presence of CLD is associated with a higher risk of complications and is not routinely recommended.[9] For children who do not tolerate bolus feedings, continuous nasogastric or nasojejunal feeds improve nutritional status.[11] Parenteral nutrition (PN) is associated with increased mortality and infection rate in critically ill children and should only be utilized when EN is not possible.[22] However, short-term PN is beneficial when enteral feeding is contraindicated, such as during intra-abdominal sepsis or variceal bleeding. Short-term PN does not increase cholestasis, and standard amino-acid formulations are safe.[3]

The European Society for Clinical Nutrition and Metabolism (ESPEN) recommends initiating PN if fasting is expected past 72 hours in patients with moderate or severe malnutrition.[10] In small, critically ill children with liver disease, PN may need to be started within 24 hours if prolonged fasting is expected.

Fluid and Electrolytes

Accurate assessment and management of fluid balance are paramount to the safety of patients in liver failure. Although more pronounced in ACLF, patients with both ACLF and ALF can become intravascularly volume depleted and have low serum albumin levels. Decreased intravascular volume can compromise end-organ perfusion and increase the risk of hepatorenal syndrome. The Saline versus Albumin Fluid Evaluation (SAFE) study conducted in adults in the intensive care setting demonstrated the safety and efficacy of both albumin and saline as volume expanders. Subgroup analysis suggested possible improvement in mortality in septic patients who received albumin.[25] However, rapid volume expansion with colloids or crystalloids may worsen ascites and increase the risk of cerebral edema and variceal hemorrhage. Limiting fluid therapy to 75% to 80% of maintenance and restricting blood products to active bleeding or prior to invasive procedures decrease those risks. Giving blood products unnecessarily can increase the risk of rebleeding and makes ongoing assessment of liver injury and transplant organ procurement more difficult. Recombinant factor VII (r FVII a) can be used in coagulopathic patients who are volume overloaded.[26] A blood transfusion threshold of hemoglobin <7g/dL(70g/L) is tolerated if tissue hypoperfusion is not present.[13,27] Frequent monitoring of serum sodium, potassium, magnesium, and phosphate is necessary.

Carbohydrate

Children with ALF are at high risk for fasting hypoglycemia due hepatocyte loss and decreased glycogen storage capacity. Blood glucose should be monitored every 1 to 2 hours. When initiating EN or PN, glucose should provide 50% to 60% of nonprotein-energy requirements. Children with ALF are commonly started on a 10% glucose-containing intravenous infusion. If hypoglycemia remains an issue, glucose infusions should provide at least 6 to 8 mg/kg per minute.[28] A serum glucose concentration of 144 to 180 mg/dL (8 to 10 mmol/L) is well tolerated and is recommended in the clinical management of critically ill adult patients, including those with cirrhosis.[13]

Protein

The etiology of protein deficiency in patients with liver disease is multifactorial. There is decreased synthesis, increased degradation, and loss due to bleeding. During acute exacerbations, protein requirements will increase further.[29] Adults with cirrhosis have been shown to shift toward catabolism and begin muscle breakdown after only 12 hours of fasting, 6 times faster than in the healthy adult.[30] Hence, extreme protein restriction is not recommended. Enteral or parenteral administration of amino acids is safe and should be initiated at 0.8 to 1.2 g/kg per day.[9]

Critically ill children have significantly less protein reserve than adults and are more susceptible to the effects of catabolic stress. Protein is routinely given at 3 g/kg per day, but giving up to 4 g/kg per day has been shown not to precipitate encephalopathy in younger children.[11]

An abnormal ratio of aromatic amino acids (AAA) to branched-chain amino acids (BCAA) has been found in adults and children with liver disease and has been postulated to worsen hepatic encephalopathy (HE).[11] Administration of BCAA has been shown to stimulate hepatic protein synthesis in patients with CLD and improve nutritional status.[31] A Cochrane review published in 2003 concluded that BCAA do not affect morbidity or mortality of cirrhotic patients, but the majority of the studies reviewed were small and lacked scientific rigor.[32] Despite these findings, the ESPEN guidelines support the use of a BCAA-enriched formula in adult patients with HE and advanced cirrhosis, and recommend using amino acid solutions high in BCAA. The majority of hepatology units in Europe reported regularly using BCAA solutions.[10] Recent publications suggest possible benefits of long-term administration of BCAA.[33,34] BCAA have fallen out of favor in the United States and are reserved only for HE unresponsive to standard therapy. Development of more palatable and affordable formulations will allow further evaluation of potential benefits of supplementation. Currently, most patients in ALF can be treated safely with standard protein formulations. Frequent monitoring of serum ammonia should guide adjustments in amino acid prescription, with a goal of less than 140 mg/dL (100 mmol/L).[10]

Lipid

Decreased carbohydrate availability leads to increased fat oxidation in children with end-stage liver disease and can rapidly deplete fat stores. In ALF, hepatocytes rely heavily on energy derived from the oxidation of fatty acids and ketogenesis. Thus, adequate provision of lipid is an important supportive measure. Lipid can be safely prescribed at a rate of 0.8 to 1.2 g/kg per day in adults, or 30% to 35% of total caloric intake in children. Most infants with liver disease need 2 to 4 g/kg per day, but requirements of up to 8 g/kg per day (when provided enterally) may be necessary for adequate growth.[3] In the presence of cholestasis, the decreased bile acid pool leads to impaired digestion and absorption of long-chain triglycerides, which include essential fatty acids (linoleic, linolenic acids).[11] If cholestasis is present, at least 30% to 60% of total fat should be provided as medium-chain triglycerides (MCTs), usually provided as MCT oil, which has been shown to decrease steatorrhea and improve growth.[28] The most commonly used infant formulas predominantly containing MCT oil are listed in Table 16-2. Breastfeeding can be safely continued if the child is growing well. Expressed breast milk can be supplemented by powdered formula or added MCT to increase the caloric density.[28] In addition, MCT oil can be supplemented separately in a total daily dose of 1 to 2 mL/kg per day divided in 2 to 4 doses.[17] Commercially available sources of MCT oil are listed in Table 16-2. Care must be taken that the patient receives an adequate amount of essential fatty acids to prevent deficiency, which can manifest as growth impairment; a dry, scaly rash; thrombocytopenia; and impaired immune function. A plasma triene:tetraene ratio above 0.05 can indicate mild deficiency, with much higher values seen with moderate and severe deficiency. Lab turnaround time may limit the usefulness of this test in the PICU setting.[17]

When PN is required, our center uses standard lipid formulations, since other lipid formulations are not easily available in the United States. On the other hand, two-thirds of European liver centers that participated in a survey used parenteral lipid mostly in the form of a long-chain triglyceride (LCT)/MCT emulsion for critically ill patients with liver disease.[18] Care must be taken to decrease the lipid infusion rate when treating patients with ALF and mitochondrial dysfunction or microvesicular steatosis due to impaired hepatic beta-oxidation associated with these disorders.[10]

Vitamins and Minerals

The intestinal absorption of vitamins A, D, E, and K is strongly dependent on adequate hepatic secretion of bile acids.

TABLE 16-2. Formulas and Modular Nutrients Used in Liver Disease

Name (Manufacturer)	MCT Content	Notes
<u>Formulas</u>		
Pregestimil (Mead Johnson)	55% MCT oil	Complete formula
Alimentum (Abbot Nutrition)	33% MCT oil	Complete formula
PediaSure Peptide (Abbot Nutrition)	50% MCT oil	Complete formula
Enfaport (Nestle)	84% MCT oil	Complete formula
Nutren Junior (Nestle)	21% MCT oil	Complete formula
Portagen (Mead Johnson)	87% MCT oil	Incomplete formula
Peptamen Junior (Nestle)	60% MCT oil	Complete formula
<u>Modular nutrients</u>		
MCT Oil (Nestle)	100% MCT oil	7.7 kcal/mL, 8.3 kcal/gram
MCT Procal (VitaFlo)	97% MCT oil	6.5 kcal/gram
Super Soluble Duocal (Nutricia)	35% MCT oil	5 kcal/gram

Vitamin A

Low levels of vitamin A were found in 69% of children with CLD.[11] Chronic deficiency in vitamin A results in night blindness and irreversible damage to the cornea. A role in the modulation of the immune system has been speculated due to decreased morbidity and mortality in patients with infectious diseases treated with vitamin A supplementation. Vitamin A deficiency is diagnosed when retinol:retinol binding protein molar ratio is less than 0.8 or serum retinol is less than 20 mcg/dL (0.7 mmol/L) . Oral supplementation ranges from 5,000 to 25,000 units/day of a water-soluble preparation.[17]

Vitamin D

Up to 25% of children with CLD are vitamin D deficient, and 17% have radiologic evidence of rickets. Breastfed infants are at particularly high risk due to low levels of vitamin D in breast milk. Vitamin D deficiency causes defective bone mineralization. Deficiency is diagnosed when the serum 25-OH-vitamin-D level is below 30 ng/mL (75 nmol/L).[17] Treatment recommendations are outlined in Table 16-3.

Vitamin E

Up to 75% of children with CLD are deficient in vitamin E.[11] Vitamin E deficiency causes peripheral neuropathy and poor nerve conduction. Vitamin E deficiency is present if vitamin E to total lipid ratio is less than 0.6 mg/g under the age of 1 and less than 0.8 mg/g over the age of 1. Treatment consists of oral administration of alpha tocopherol (acetate): 25 to 200 IU/kg per day or tocopherol polyethylene glycol 1000 succinate (TPGS) 15 to 25 IU/kg per day.[17]

Vitamin K

Vitamin K is required for the synthesis of coagulation factors II, VII, IX, and X; protein C; and protein S. Approximately 23% of children with CLD have a coagulopathy due to vitamin K deficiency. In the presence of an elevated INR in the setting of an ICU admission, a trial of intravenous vitamin K of 1 to 5 mg/day for 3 days is standard practice, with monitoring of INR for improvement. Vitamin K doses in adults range from 5 to 10 mg/day. When chronic malabsorption is suspected, the patient should receive 2.5 to 5 mg of oral vitamin 2 to 7 times per week.[17] Adequate dosing can be monitored with coagulation studies.

Trace Elements

Approximately 33% of children with liver failure are iron deficient, and 40% are zinc deficient. Decreased iron levels and increased total iron-binding capacity are diagnostic, and treatment consists of enteral elemental iron up to 5 to 6 mg/kg per day. A plasma zinc level of less than 60 mcg/dL (9 mmol/L) should be treated with oral elemental zinc of 1 mg/kg per day.

PANCREATITIS

Recent publications have documented an increased incidence of acute pancreatitis in children.[35,36 1-3 2-4] The estimated prevalence of acute pancreatitis in adults is between 6 and 45/100,000 person-years.[37] Estimates of the incidence of pancreatitis in children suggest an incidence of between 3.6 and 13.2 cases per 100,000 children.[38,39] The latter number is in the range of the incidence for pancreatitis in adults, confirming that pancreatitis is not as rare a condition in children as previously thought.

Acute Pancreatitis

Pancreatitis is a condition characterized by swelling and inflammation of the pancreas.

Acute pancreatitis (AP) appears suddenly and typically lasts for several days. Complete spontaneous resolution is expected within 5 to 7 days. Acute pancreatitis is the most common disorder of the exocrine pancreas in children.[35,36] Recurrent episodes of AP may lead to chronic pancreatitis (CP).

Acute pancreatitis in children has been recently defined by an expert committee as an episode of abdominal pain suggestive of, or compatible with, AP (i.e., abdominal

TABLE 16-3. Suggested Therapy for Vitamin D Deficiency[11]

25-OH-Vit D level	PO Dose <40 kg	PO Dose >40 kg
<10 ng/mL (<25 nmol/L)	100 IU/kg per day	5000 IU/day
11-19 ng/mL (26-47 nmol/L)	75 IU/kg per day	4000 IU/day
20-29 ng/mL (48-74 nmol/L)	50 IU/kg per day	3000 IU/day

pain of acute onset, especially in the epigastric region) associated with serum lipase and/or amylase activity at least 3 times greater than the upper limit of normal.[40] Lipase is the preferred test because of its higher sensitivity and specificity (lipase 82% to 100%; amylase 85% to 98%).[41] It should be noted that serum lipase returns to normal more slowly than serum amylase. Signs and symptoms of acute pancreatitis are frequently nonspecific and include fever, abdominal pain and tenderness, nausea and vomiting, guarding, and abdominal distension. Abdominal pain in young children may be vague and atypical. While imaging is not required in all patients, a diagnosis of AP can be made when the amylase and lipase are normal if imaging findings characteristic of, or compatible with AP, are present. Imaging is frequently normal in mild pancreatitis.

Chronic Pancreatitis

In contrast, CP is a progressive inflammatory disease of the pancreas, characterized by irreversible morphologic changes and gradual fibrotic replacement of the gland. Loss of exocrine and endocrine function results from fibrosis and parenchymal damage.[40] Therefore, CP is, by definition, a progressive disease. Children can present with features diagnostic of CP without having had a prior diagnosis of AP.

Pathophysiology

Traditionally, it was thought that after an initial insult such as ductal damage or obstruction, there is premature activation of trypsinogen to trypsin within the acinar cell;[42] trypsin then activates other proenzymes, leading to a cascade of enzyme activation, autodigestion, further enzyme activation, and the release of active proteases. More recently, it has been demonstrated that although intracellular trypsin induces local pancreatic injury, local and systemic inflammation may be mediated by pro-inflammatory cytokines such as nuclear factor kappa-light-chain-enhancer of activated B cells (NF-kB), which is then followed by a pro-inflammatory response.[42]

Etiology

In adults, 80% to 90% of cases are due to alcohol abuse and gallstones. The remaining 10% to 20% are caused by trauma—including endoscopic retrograde cholangiopancreatography (ERCP)—drugs, and other less common etiologies. In contrast, in children, trauma, biliary tract disease, drugs, and systemic illness are the etiologies in the majority of cases.[36] Other etiologies include congenital anatomic abnormalities, metabolic disorders, and following solid organ and stem cell transplantation. Between 10% and 20% of cases are considered idiopathic. In recent series, an increasing number of cases are associated with mutations in the PRSS1, SPINK1, CFTR, and CTRC genes.[43] In these patients, CP develops following recurrent episodes of AP.

Severity

The natural history of pancreatitis is variable, with about 20% of adult patients having "severe" episodes.[44] The mortality of severe necrotizing pancreatitis is up to 20%, while the mortality of mild episodes is less than 1%. Because of this difference in mortality and morbidity, in order to provide optimal care, a variety of scoring systems have been devised in order to predict which patients will require intensive care. Unfortunately, these scoring systems are not useful in children because most adult cases are due to chronic alcohol abuse, and a significant negative predictor in most scoring systems is age >65 years. The published pediatric scoring systems have not been validated.[45] In pediatric studies, the mortality of severe pancreatitis is much lower.[46] Severe pediatric pancreatitis requiring PICU admission has been infrequently reported in children; however, the outcome may be better than in adults.

Clinical Management

Clinical management of the patient with pancreatitis in the PICU includes vigorous fluid resuscitation and correction of electrolyte abnormalities. Aggressive hydration has been associated with better outcomes in adult patients. Children are usually given 1.5 to 2 times maintenance requirements, unless cardiovascular and/or renal comorbidities exist. Early aggressive intravenous hydration is most beneficial in the first 12 to 24 hours, and lactated Ringer's solution may be the preferred isotonic crystalloid replacement fluid. The goal of aggressive hydration should be to decrease the blood urea nitrogen. Other measures, such as the treatment of infection and pain management, will not be reviewed here.

Nutrition

Traditionally, the patient with AP has been treated with enteral fasting and PN.[47] It was felt that gut rest allowed the pancreas to rest and thus heal more rapidly. Enteral fasting and PN were justified by the fact that many patients with AP develop increased abdominal pain and rising serum amylase and lipase when enterally fed. However, it is now known that an important feature of pancreatitis is *pancreastasis*, defined in a similar manner as cholestasis—that is, poor flow of pancreatic secretions. Enteral feeding has been shown in a number of conditions to decrease morbidity and mortality in ICU patients and only infrequently exacerbates the pancreatitis episode. Enteral nutrition probably maintains the integrity and function of the intestinal mucosal barrier and increases gut contractility, which prevents bacterial overgrowth and translocation.[48] Enteral nutrition also attenuates the acute-phase response.[49]

A Cochrane review from 2009 concluded that "there is little evidence to support or refute the need to provide nutrition to critically ill children in a paediatric intensive care unit during the first week of their critical illness."[50] The authors found only one relevant randomized, controlled trial (RCT) for this review. In contrast, Mehta et al. reported in 2013 that early nutritional therapy is associated with improved 60-day survival in critically ill children.[22] Patients given early protocolized EN had a lower prevalence of acquired infections. In a review of studies examining protein balance in critically ill children, Bechard et al. demonstrated that a positive protein balance could be achieved in mechanically ventilated children with optimal protein and energy intakes.[51] There are no published guidelines or studies relating to nutritional support of the child with AP. There is a single report of 2 children with severe AP who were treated successfully with nasojejunal feedings in the PICU and switched to oral feeding when discharged to the general ward.[52]

In contrast, there are a number of controlled studies, reviews, and meta-analyses of nutritional therapy of adults with both severe and mild pancreatitis; thus, our recommendations will be based on PICU studies in children without pancreatitis and on these adult studies, which are reviewed next.[47,53-62] This section will consider only the most recent studies and reviews. Various formulas have been used, including elemental, semielemental, polymeric, "immunomodulating," and high MCT. Since no type of formula has been found to be superior, a polymeric formula is usually recommended.

Yi reviewed 8 RCTs including 381 adult patients comparing EN to PN in severe AP.[59] Patients treated with EN had lower mortality, fewer infections, fewer surgical interventions, and less organ failure than patients treated with PN.

Mirtallo et al. reviewed 8 societal reports in order to develop international consensus guidelines for nutrition therapy in AP.[60] They concluded that EN is preferable to PN in patients with AP and should be used first, even in the presence of fistulas, ascites, and pseudocysts. Intragastric feeding is frequently effective, and transpyloric feeding is not always necessary.[53] Continuous feeding is preferred over cyclic feeding. A small, peptide-based, MCT-containing formula was recommended.

In his review of nutrition support for AP, Grant concluded that *early* nutrition support—particularly EN, but also PN—reduces complications and improves survival.[58] Early nutritional therapy decreases the cytokine response and reduces the incidence of gastroparesis and intestinal ileus. To be effective, nutritional support must begin within 72 hours. Since full EN may take days to establish, a combination of EN and PN should be considered at admission to the PICU. Since EN decreases the inflammatory response and decreases infectious complication, hospital stay and mortality EN should be considered "an active therapeutic intervention that improves the outcome of patients with pancreatitis".[57]

Sharma reviewed the use of probiotics and found them to be of no benefit in adults with severe pancreatitis.[62] In one trial, mortality was 8/152 in the probiotic group and 0/144 in the control group.[63] Hence, until further data are available, probiotics are not recommended in the treatment of AP.

Fortunately, most children with AP are otherwise healthy and have no specific nutritional deficits. Some children with CP and pancreatic insufficiency may be malnourished. Since in critically ill children a low weight-for-age is correlated with longer PICU and hospital lengths of stay and higher mortality, nutritional rehabilitation may be required in some patients.[16,64]

Other Nutrition Issues in Acute Pancreatitis

- A rise in serum amylase and lipase is typically associated with enteral feeding, but does not imply worsening of the pancreatitis and is not a reason to stop EN.
- About 4% of patients experience worsening of abdominal pain during EN. These patients should be treated with PN. About 20% of patients have an increase in abdominal pain when transitioned to oral feedings. Specialized enteral nutrition may need to be temporarily resumed in these patients.

KEY POINTS

- Nutritional status in liver failure is linked to pre- and posttransplant morbidity and mortality, and should be assessed on admission to the PICU.
- Hypoglycemia is common in liver failure, and the serum glucose level should be monitored closely.
- Protein demands are increased during liver failure, and enteral or parenteral protein does not need to be restricted in pediatric patients.
- Cholestatic diseases place children at higher risk for steatorrhea and fat-soluble vitamin deficiencies. Enteral feeding is preferred in liver failure and can be done safely with nasogastric tube placement, but when EN is not tolerated, PN should be started in a timely fashion.
- Early institution of nutritional support within 48 to 72 hours of admission to the PICU may reduce complications in patients with AP.
- Enteral nutrition delivered by nasogastric or nasojejunal tube is generally well tolerated and is the nutritional therapy of choice in AP.

REFERENCES

1. Alvares-da-Silva MR, Reverbel da Silveira T. Comparison between handgrip strength, subjective global assessment, and prognostic nutritional index in assessing malnutrition and predicting clinical outcome in cirrhotic outpatients. *Nutrition*. 2005;21(2):113-117.
2. Kondrup J. Nutrition in end stage liver disease. *Best Pract Res Clin Gastroenterol*. 2006;20(3):547-560.
3. Protheroe SM. Feeding the child with chronic liver disease. *Nutrition*. 1998;14(10):796-800.
4. Dhawan A. Acute liver failure in children and adolescents. *Clin Res Hepatol Gastroenterol*. 2012;36(3):278-283.
5. Bernal W, Auzinger G, Dhawan A, Wendon J. Acute liver failure. *Lancet*. 2010;376(9736):190-201.
6. Teran JC. Nutrition and liver diseases. *Curr Gastroenterol Rep*. 1999;1(4):335-340.
7. Cochran JB, Losek JD. Acute liver failure in children. *Pediatr Emerg Care*. 2007;23(2):129-135.
8. Ramaccioni V, Soriano HE, Arumugam R, Klish WJ. Nutritional aspects of chronic liver disease and liver transplantation in children. *J Pediatr Gastroenterol Nutr*. 2000;30(4):361-367.
9. Plauth M, Cabré E, Riggio O, Assis-Camilo M, Pirlich M, Kondrup J, et al. ESPEN Guidelines on Enteral Nutrition: liver disease. *Clin Nutr*. 2006;25(2):285-294.
10. Plauth M, Cabré E, Campillo B, et al. ESPEN Guidelines on Parenteral Nutrition: hepatology. *Clin Nutr*. 2009;28(4):436-444.
11. Nightingale S, Ng VL. Optimizing nutritional management in children with chronic liver disease. *Pediatr Clin North Am*. 2009;56(5):1161-1183.
12. Mouzaki M, Lee Ng V. Acute liver failure in children. *Clin Ped Emerg Med*. 2010;11(3):198-206.
13. Ginès P, Fernández J, Durand F, Saliba F. Management of critically-ill cirrhotic patients. *J Hepatol*. 2012;56 Suppl 1:S13-24.
14. Lal J, Thapa BR, Rawal P, Ratho RK, Singh K. Predictors of outcome in acute-on-chronic liver failure in children. *Hepatol Int*. 2011;5(2):693-697.
15. Sokol RJ, Stall C. Anthropometric evaluation of children with chronic liver disease. *Am J Clin Nutr*. 1990;52(2):203-208.
16. Vermilyea S, Slicker J, El-Chammas K, et al. Subjective global nutritional assessment in critically ill children. *J Parenter Enteral Nutr*. 2013;37(5):659-66.
17. Sultan MI, Leon CDG, Biank VF. Role of nutrition in pediatric chronic liver disease. *Nutr Clin Pract*. 2011;26(4):401-408.
18. Schütz T, Bechstein W-O, Neuhaus P, Lochs H, Plauth M. Clinical practice of nutrition in acute liver failure: a European survey. *Clin Nutr*. 2004;23(5):975-982.
19. Pierro A, Koletzko B, Carnielli V, et al. Resting energy expenditure is increased in infants and children with extrahepatic biliary atresia. *J Ped Surg*. 1989;24(6):534-538.
20. Meyer R, Harrison S, Sargent S, Ramnarayan P, Habibi P, Labadarios D. The impact of enteral feeding protocols on nutritional support in critically ill children. *J Hum Nutr Diet*. 2009;22(5):428-436.
21. Koretz RL, Avenell A, Lipman TO. Nutritional support for liver disease. Cochrane Database Syst Rev. 2012;5:CD008344.
22. Mehta NM, Bechard LJ, Cahill N, et al. Nutritional practices and their relationship to clinical outcomes in critically ill children—an international multicenter cohort study. *Crit Care Med*. 2012;40(7):2204-2211.
23. Fang JC, DeLegge MH. Enteral feeding in the critically ill: the role of the gastroenterologist. *Am J Gastroenterology*. 2011;106(6):1032-1037.
24. Barr J. Outcomes in critically ill patients before and after the implementation of an evidence-based nutritional management protocol. *Chest*. 2004;125(4):1446-1457.

25. Finfer SI, Bellomo R, Boyce N, et al. A comparison of albumin and saline for fluid resuscitation in the intensive care unit. *N Engl J Med.* 2004;350(22):2247-2256.
26. D'Agostino D, Diaz S, Sanchez MC, Boldrini G. Management and prognosis of acute liver failure in children. *Curr Gastroenterol Rep.* 2012;14(3):262-269.
27. Villanueva C, Colomo A, Bosch A, et al. Transfusion strategies for acute upper gastrointestinal bleeding. *N Engl J Med.* 2013;368(1):11-21.
28. Novy MA, Schwarz KB. Nutritional considerations and management of the child with liver disease. *Nutrition.* 1997;13(3):177-184.
29. Tsouka A, McLin VA. Complications of chronic liver disease. *Clin Res Hepatol Gastroenterol.* 2012;36(3):262-267.
30. Owen OE, Reichle FA, Mozzoli MA, et al. Hepatic, gut, and renal substrate flux rates in patients with hepatic cirrhosis. *J Clin Invest.* 1981;68(1):240-252.
31. Khanna S, Gopalan S. Role of branched-chain amino acids in liver disease: the evidence for and against. *Curr Opin Clin Nutr Metab Care.* 2007;10(3):297-303.
32. Als-Nielsen B, Koretz RL, Kjaergard LL, Gluud C. Branched-chain amino acids for hepatic encephalopathy. Cochrane Database Syst Rev. 2003;(2):CD001939.
33. Muto Y, Sato S, Watanabe A, et al. Effects of oral branched-chain amino acid granules on event-free survival in patients with liver cirrhosis. *Clin Gastroenterol Hepatol.* 2005;3(7):705-713.
34. Les I, Doval E, García-Martínez R, et al. Effects of branched-chain amino acids supplementation in patients with cirrhosis and a previous episode of hepatic encephalopathy: a randomized study. *Amer J Gastroenterol.* 2011;106(6):1081-1088.
35. Park A, Latif SU, Shah AU, et al. Changing referral trends of acute pancreatitis in children: a 12-year single-center analysis. *J Pediatr Gastroenterol Nutr.* 2009;49(3): 316-322.
36. Morinville VD, Barmada MM, Lowe ME. Increasing incidence of acute pancreatitis at an American pediatric tertiary care center: is greater awareness among physicians responsible? *Pancreas.* 2010;39(1):5-8.
37. Yadav D, Lowenfels AB. Trends in the epidemiology of the first attack of acute pancreatitis: a systematic review. *Pancreas.* 2006;33(4):323-330. Review. Erratum in: *Pancreas.* 2007;34(1):174.
38. Keim V, Witt H, Bauer N, et al. The course of genetically determined chronic pancreatitis. *JOP.* 2003;4(4):146-154
39. Rebours V, Boutron-Ruault MC, Schnee M, et al. The natural history of hereditary pancreatitis: a national series. *Gut.* 2009;58(1):97-103.
40. Morinville VD, Husain SZ, Bai H, et al. Definitions of pediatric pancreatitis and survey of present clinical practices. *J Pediatr Gastroenterol Nutr.* 2012;55(3):261-265.
41. Lippi G, Valentino M, Cervellin G. Laboratory diagnosis of acute pancreatitis: in search of the Holy Grail. *Crit Rev Clin Lab Sci.* 2012;49(1):18-31.
42. Sah RP, Garg P, Saluja AK. Pathogenic mechanisms of acute pancreatitis. *Curr Opin Gastroenterol.* 2012; 28(5):507-515.
43. Sultan M, Werlin S, Venkatasubramani N. Genetic prevalence and characteristics in children with recurrent pancreatitis. *J Pediatr Gastroenterol Nutr.* 2012; 54(5):645-650.
44. Brisinda G, Vanella S, Crocco A, et al. Severe acute pancreatitis: advances and insights in assessment of severity and management. *Eur J Gastroenterol Hepatol.* 2011; 23(7):541-551.
45. Fabre A, Petit P, Gaudart J, et al. Severity scores in children with acute pancreatitis. *J Pediatr Gastroenterol Nutr.* 2012; 55(3):266-267.
46. Raizner A, Phatak U, Baker, K, Patel M, Husain SZ, Pashankar DS. Acute necrotizing pancreatitis in children. *J Pediatr.* 2013;162(4):788-92
47. Al-Omran M, Groof A, Wilke D. Enteral versus parenteral nutrition for acute pancreatitis. Cochrane Database Syst Rev. 2003;(1):CD002837.
48. Ong JP, Fock KM. Nutritional support in acute pancreatitis. *J Dig Dis.* 2012;13(9):445-452.
49. Windsor AC, Kanwar S, Li AG, et al. Compared with parenteral nutrition, enteral feeding attenuates the acute phase response and improves disease severity in acute pancreatitis. *Gut.* 1998;42(3):431-435.
50. Joffe A, Anton N, Lequier L, et al. Nutritional support for critically ill children. Cochrane Database Syst Rev. 2009; (2):CD005144.
51. Bechard LJ, Parrott JS, Mehta NM. Systematic review of the influence of energy and protein intake on protein balance in critically ill children. *J Pediatr.* 2012; 161(2):333.
52. Carreazo NY, Ugarte K, Bada C. When should we start oral intake in children with severe acute pancreatitis? *Evid Based Med.* 2008;13(1):4-5.
53. Kumar A, Singh N, Prakash S, Saraya A, Joshi YK. Early enteral nutrition in severe acute pancreatitis: a prospective randomized controlled trial comparing nasojejunal and nasogastric routes. *J Clin Gastroenterol.* 2006;40(5):431-434.
54. O'Keefe SJ, Sharma S. Nutrition support in severe acute pancreatitis. *Gastroenterol Clin North Am.* 2007;36(2): 297-312.

55. Petrov MS, van Santvoort HC, Besselink MG, van der Heijden GJ, Windsor JA, Gooszen HG. Enteral nutrition and the risk of mortality and infectious complications in patients with severe acute pancreatitis: a meta-analysis of randomized trials. *Arch Surg.* 2008;143(11):1111-1117.

56. Doley RP, Yadav TD, Wig JD, et al. Enteral nutrition in severe acute pancreatitis. *JOP.* 2009;10(2):157-162.

57. Marik PE. What is the best way to feed patients with pancreatitis? *Curr Opin Crit Care.* 2009;15(2):131-138.

58. Grant JP. Nutritional support in acute and chronic pancreatitis. *Surg Clin North Am.* 2011;91(4):805-820.

59. Yi F, Ge L, Zhao J, et al. Meta-analysis: total parenteral nutrition versus total enteral nutrition in predicted severe acute pancreatitis. *Intern Med.* 2012;51(6):523-530.

60. Mirtallo JM, Forbes A, McClave SA, Jensen GL, Waitzberg DL, Davies AR, International Consensus Guideline Committee Pancreatitis Task Force. International consensus guidelines for nutrition therapy in pancreatitis. *J Parenter Enteral Nutr.* 2012;36(3):284-291.

61. Thomson A, Subramaniam K, Davies A. Nutritional therapy in acute pancreatitis: time to take stock. *Nutrition.* 2012;28(7-8):731-732.

62. Sharma B, Srivastava S, Singh N, Sachdev V, Kapur S, Saraya A. Role of probiotics on gut permeability and endotoxemia in patients with acute pancreatitis: a double-blind randomized controlled trial. *J Clin Gastroenterol.* 2011;45(5):442-448.

63. Bjarnason A, Adler SN, Bjarnason I. Probiotic prophylaxis in predicted severe acute pancreatitis. *Lancet.* 2008;372(9633):114-115.

64. Goday P, Sachdeva R, Mikhailov, T. Does admission weight affect mortality and morbidity in the pediatric intensive care unit? (abstract). *J Parenter Enteral Nutr.* 32:316, 2008.

CHAPTER 17

Nutrition for the Infant or Child in the Cardiac Intensive Care Unit

Nazima Pathan

Luise Marino

■ MALNUTRITION AND FEEDING PROBLEMS IN THE CHILD WITH CONGENITAL HEART DISEASE

Type of Cardiac Lesion
Inadequate Caloric Intake
Prenatal Growth Restriction

■ OPTIMAL NUTRITION FOLLOWING SURGERY FOR CONGENITAL HEART DISEASE

Clinical Consequences of Malnutrition Following Congenital Heart Surgery
The Importance of Monitoring Growth
When Is Enteral Feeding Safe?
Micronutrients, Not Just Calories

■ SPECIAL SITUATIONS

Interstage Feeding and Growth in Children with Hypoplastic Left Heart
Nutritional Management of Protein-Losing Enteropathy
Nutritional Management of Chylothorax

■ KEY POINTS

References

■ MALNUTRITION AND FEEDING PROBLEMS IN THE CHILD WITH CONGENITAL HEART DISEASE

Globally, congenital heart disease (CHD) represents one-third of all major congenital anomalies, affecting between 0.3% and 1.5% of all pregnancies (around 40,000 children are born with CHD per year in the United States).[1] Growth faltering is commonly seen in children with CHD, particularly those with cyanotic disease and univentricular physiology. Children with CHD exhibit early and progressive falls in their growth trajectory in comparison to healthy children, with reductions in weight-for-age Z-score, head circumference, and length-for-age Z-score. The process of surgery and bypass, in addition to the effects of cardiac failure and chronic disease, involve a significant degree of metabolic and nutritional stress, such that postoperative malnutrition presents a further burden on restoring growth toward normal parameters. Early nutrition support is crucial, particularly in those undergoing surgery in the neonatal and infant period, where there is little reserve during what is a critical time for brain development.

A number of factors contribute to malnutrition in children undergoing surgery for congenital heart disease, as the following sections explain.

Type of Cardiac Lesion

Single-ventricle and complex cardiac lesions are associated with a greater risk of malnutrition. These children may also have had restricted feeds preoperatively in the setting of heart failure and fluid restriction. While there is no evidence that enteral feeding increases the risk of necrotizing enterocolitis (NEC), some clinicians withhold feeds if there are concerns about splanchnic perfusion (single-ventricle lesions, severe left ventricular outflow tract, and aortic arch anomalies).

Children with cyanotic lesions usually have symmetrical growth restriction and are shorter and lighter, whereas those with acyanotic lesions tend to have asymmetrical growth retardation with a low weight-for-age and normal height. In addition, children with left-to-right shunts tend to weigh less than cyanotic children do, which may be due to pulmonary hypertension. Where there is pulmonary stenosis and/or coarctation of the aorta, linear growth is usually more affected than weight. The presence of hypoxia and breathlessness is common, and while the duration of the hypoxia may affect growth, the severity does not appear to affect tissue metabolism profoundly.[2]

Inadequate Caloric Intake

Children with CHD often have comorbidities that may affect the ability to swallow or absorb feeds effectively. In addition, prolonged intubation and hospitalization are likely to add to swallowing problems and oral aversion. Gastroesophageal reflux is relatively common in neonates with CHD, and may reduce the success of oral feeds at the volumes needed to restore growth. Other factors that contribute to an inadequate calorie intake include:[3]

1. Fatigue on feeding leading to low intake
2. Fluid restriction
3. Poor absorption
4. Increased metabolic expenditure
5. Early satiety
6. Anorexia
7. Frequent infections
8. Frequent use of antibiotics affecting gut flora

Postoperative fluid restriction will inevitably restrict the volume available to provide feeds. Children with heart failure and chronic disease may also struggle to feed well and achieve their caloric requirements. Some children may have poor enteral feed tolerance, particularly if intestinal mucosal blood supply is reduced or there is hypoxia. Heart disease has been shown to be an independent risk factor for the nonattainment of caloric goal during the pediatric intensive care unit (PICU) stay. De Menezes showed that by the fourth day, 93% of children undergoing congenital heart surgery have yet to meet 90% of their basal metabolic requirements (BMR) and are significantly more likely not to achieve optimal energy intakes compared to noncardiac critically ill children. However, the use of parenteral nutrition (PN) (either exclusively or as a supplement to enteral intake) and the early identification of malnutrition were protective factors for achieving calorie goals.[4]

Prenatal Growth Restriction

It is likely that complex and chronic fetal anomalies result in intrauterine growth restriction. Several case series have reported an association between CHD and intrauterine growth restriction, although when babies with chromosomal and extra cardiac anomalies are excluded, the association is less well defined.[5]

OPTIMAL NUTRITION FOLLOWING SURGERY FOR CONGENITAL HEART DISEASE

Given the multiple contributors to malnutrition in children with CHD, it is vital that these children receive the best possible nutrition support following surgery to mitigate the consequences of malnutrition. The consequences of malnutrition and an approach to providing nutrition post-surgery are discussed in the sections that follow.

Clinical Consequences of Malnutrition Following Congenital Heart Surgery

There is increasing evidence that malnutrition is associated with deficient growth, wound healing, and immune function in children undergoing surgery for CHD. In addition to prolonging the time for recovery from surgery, long-term malnutrition is associated with a range of neurodevelopmental sequelae. Early intervention and close monitoring by specialized dietitians may improve feeding, developmental, and family outcomes.

Malnutrition and growth failure during infancy are associated with impaired executive functioning and poorer scholastic performance in children with CHD.

Stunting or poor linear growth has the greatest influence on neurodevelopment[6] and poor functional outcomes.[7] Poor growth postoperatively in the first few weeks to months is associated with increased risk of mortality.[8]

The Importance of Monitoring Growth

Because growth failure is so common among children with complex CHD—in particular, those with left-to-right shunt lesions—it is imperative that there is a defined nutrition care pathway targeting weight and length gain, ensuring infants grow as well as possible prior to and following palliative/corrective surgery. It is important to establish early on factors that may contribute to and/or affect optimal growth. There are numerous problems with accurate plotting on growth charts, which can lead to growth-monitoring inaccuracies. Ways of overcoming this involve the conversion of weight and height standard deviation or Z-score for length/height, weight, and body mass index.[3] There has been a focus on the need for reliable screening tools and intervention thresholds, aiming to optimize growth in children with CHD.[9,10]

The most common definition for growth faltering in the United Kingdom is weight crossing more than 2 centiles downward during a period of 1 month. This would be equal to –0.68 of a Z-score, indicating that a child may have weight faltering, but is not yet malnourished according to the World Health Organization (WHO) definition (e.g., moderate malnutrition using the WHO definition is ≤–2 Z-scores). There are several different tools with a variety of cutoffs to define these terms (Table 17-1). The WHO defines moderate and severe malnutrition as a weight for height of –2 to –3 Z-scores and >–3 Z-score, respectively.[11] Ideally, an infant should gain 10 g/kg per day,[12] and if this rate of weight gain is not being achieved, the nutrition care plan should be amended.

For infants with chronic disease, anthropometric measurements should be performed more frequently (Table 17-2).

TABLE 17-1. WHO Classification of Malnutrition[11]

Classification	Moderate Malnutrition	Severe Malnutrition
Weight-for-height (acute malnutrition/wasting)	–3 ≤ SD score <2 (70% to 80%)	<–3 (<70%)
Height-for-age (chronic malnutrition/stunting)	–3 ≤ SD score <2 (80% to 85%)	<–3 (<85%)

During a PICU admission, every attempt should be made to perform a length and weight measurement weekly.

The metabolic rate may vary during recovery from congenital heart surgery. Initially, it is likely to be high,[13,14] particularly in prolonged bypass surgery. Underdelivery of calories and proteins may result in catabolism and loss of muscle mass.

Key to adequate nutritional intake during a PICU admission is knowledge of energy requirements. Although a significant amount of research has been performed on exploring energy requirements in nonventilated children with heart disease, limited information is available on energy expenditure in the postsurgical cardiac child that is ventilated and in the PICU.

Only a small number of studies have investigated resting energy expenditure (REE) of postsurgical cardiac patients using indirect calorimetry. Avitzur et al. compared the energy expenditure of cyanotic to noncyanotic cardiac children after open heart surgery and found their energy expenditure to range between 59 kcal/kg per day and 62 kcal/kg per day.[15] Li et al. found that children post-Norwood procedure had an REE ranging from 43 kcal/kg to 41 kcal/kg on different days of admission.[14] We investigated the relationship between measured energy expenditure and delivered energy in a cohort of children

TABLE 17-2. Recommended Frequency for Anthropometrical Review

	Preterm	Term–12 m	12–24 m	2–18 y
Weight	Daily	Daily	3 × week	Weekly
Length	Every 2 weeks	Every 2 months	Every 3 months	Yearly
Head circumference	Every 2 weeks	Monthly	Monthly	—
Mid upper arm circumference	Monthly	Monthly	Monthly	Monthly

undergoing congenital heart surgery.[13] Patients received a mean of 15.9 kcal/kg per day of intravenous or enteral feed on the day of measurement, versus the measured REE of 67.8 kcal/kg per day, leaving a mean energy deficit of 51.1 kcal/kg per day (SD ± 23.83) in the first 48 hours after surgery. Undelivery of calories perioperatively and a decline in weight-for-age Z-score were also documented by Nicholson et al. in 65 infants undergoing congenital heart surgery, where median weight-for-age Z-score declined by −1.3 (IQR −1.7 to −0.7).[16]

Interestingly, cardiopulmonary bypass appears to increase energy requirements in the early postoperative period. In the study of De Wit et al., mean REE of patients requiring bypass was 73.6 kcal/kg per day (SD ± 15.11) in children undergoing bypass and 58.3 kcal/kg per day (SD ± 10.88) in nonbypass cases ($p = 0.022$). An important issue in this study and in others of cardiac and noncardiac critically ill children is that calculation of energy requirements using currently available formulas does not adequately predict caloric expenditure compared to that measured using indirect calorimetry.[13]

However, because only 27% of PICUs within Europe routinely use indirect calorimetry, alternative proxies are required.[17] Predicted energy requirements in children consist of BMR to which energy required for activity, heat loss, and growth is added. In healthy infants, around 30% to 35% of predicted energy requirements are used for growth. In critically ill infants, the anabolic process of growth ceases during the catabolic phase. In addition, infants are maintained in a thermoneutral environment with humidified air and are sedated, and on occasion paralyzed, reducing energy requirements with regard to those attributed to heat loss and activity. C-reactive protein (CRP) is well correlated with severity of disease, and in infants undergoing thoracic or abdominal surgery, a measure of >6 mg/dL is associated with high stress,[18] and it has been suggested that in the absence of indirect calorimetry, measures that predict BMR be used (Food Agricultural Organization/Schofield height and weight equations) until CRP values are ~<2 mg/dL, at which point anabolism will resume.[19]

When Is Enteral Feeding Safe?

While enteral feeds are known to be protective to the gut mucosa and may assist in establishing a normal gut microbiome, concerns about intestinal hypoperfusion and the presence of umbilical catheters mean that some units routinely withhold enteral feeds in babies with prostaglandin-dependent cardiac lesions. In a recent international survey, 44% of U.S. clinicians, compared to 7% of non-U.S. clinicians, reported that they do not give routine preoperative enteral feeds to this patient group. In those who do feed enterally, there appears to be great variation in how attending clinicians assess feed tolerance, some using clinical assessment while others rely on diagnostic tools, including abdominal x-ray, blood lactate levels, and abdominal regional oxygen saturation (measured by near infrared spectroscopy).[20] The lack of consensus suggests that further studies are needed to examine the safety of enteral feeding in this high-risk population.

Vasoactive drugs are used to support cardiac output and blood pressure in patients with cardiac failure.[21] High doses of multiple medications, such as clonidine, and vasoactive drugs have been associated with increased risk of nonocclusive bowel injury.[22,23] Splanchnic perfusion may also be compromised following cardiac surgery due to poor cardiac output. It is, therefore, imperative to monitor for any signs of feeding intolerance and take early corrective measures.[21]

Oral feeding is often difficult to achieve, and a proportion of children continue to require nasogastric/nasojejunal (NG/NJ) tube feeds/gastrostomy feeding to achieve required intake by the time of hospital discharge. Inability to achieve oral feeds is, of course, generally associated with a longer hospital stay (during a crucial time for development) and, therefore, has potential to affect long-term neurocognitive outcome.[24] Of note, the longer the time taken to start oral feeds, the worse the feeding outcomes.

The National Pediatric Cardiology Quality Improvement Collaborative has a focus on achieving optimal nutrition and makes a number of recommendations. The key points are to monitor growth, parental education to help them recognize indicators of hunger in babies with CHD, positioning for feeds, and creating a relaxed feeding environment.[10] A focus on the experience of feeding more than the volume fed in the early stages may help to encourage success in establishing oral feeds. There is a balance to consider in the need to use a feeding tube to improve weight gain versus the risk of delayed oral feeding skills. Early identification and management of comorbidities that might affect oral feeding (vocal cord palsy, gastroesophageal reflux, and cricopharyngeal incoordination) could improve long-term outcomes.

Choice of Feed

Breast milk has been shown to prevent NEC and as such should be the feed of choice in patients at risk,[25] such as babies who are in shock and those with lesions that have a systemic-to-pulmonary shunt or impaired mesenteric blood flow, including hypoplastic left heart, truncus arteriosus, and aortopulmonary window, where the risk of NEC is higher.[26,27] If needed, expressed breast milk (EBM) can be supplemented with breast milk fortifier, which has a negligible effect on gastric emptying.[28] If breast milk is not available and the patient is also on multiple high-dose inotropes and clonidine, then a ready-to-use, sterile, protein hydrolysate should be considered.

Feeding Route

Transpyloric feed using an NJ feed may increase the success of enteral feeding compared to using an NG tube. Caution should be exercised in those infants with cyanotic lesions, as there is some evidence of an increased risk of NEC with NJ feeds.[29] During critical illness, feeds should be given continuously over 20 to 21 hours via an enteral feeding pump, reducing the metabolic and thermic response to feeds, in addition to decreasing the risk of gut ischemia.[30]

Parenteral Nutrition

Although PN is beneficial and life saving in a variety of clinical conditions, it can also result in numerous potentially serious side effects. The risk of such complications can be minimized by carefully monitoring patients and the use of nutrition support teams. Full anthropometry should be undertaken at the start of PN and weight monitored twice weekly during therapy with PN. Renal and liver function, full blood count, and plasma albumin should be measured at the beginning of treatment and weekly. In the early stages, plasma electrolytes (sodium, potassium, calcium, phosphate, magnesium, and chloride) may need to be monitored daily until daily requirements are established and levels appear to be stable. Triglyceride levels should be monitored before therapy and weekly thereafter.[31]

Risks and complications of PN include:[31-34]

- Deficiency:
  - Calorie (resulting in malnutrition, wasting)
  - Micronutrient (these include zinc – hair loss, poor wound healing; iron – anemia; essential fatty acids – scaly dermatitis; other vitamins including thiamine and B vitamins)
- Solution related:
  - Low or elevated electrolyte levels
  - Hypo- or hyperglycemia
  - Hyperlipidemia
  - Hyperbilirubinemia
  - Liver steatosis and cholestasis
  - Micronutrient toxicity (fat-soluble vitamins may not be cleared well in children who are hemofiltered)
- Line related:
  - Sepsis (aseptic techniques using a dedicated PN line are clearly of great importance)
  - Occlusion of the PN line (prevent by flushing the line with heparinized saline and using inline filters)
  - Thrombosis/embolism from the PN line (heparinization or antithrombotic treatment may be needed in children who have a higher risk or history of thrombosis)

Micronutrients, Not Just Calories

The feeding of the critically ill cardiac child should take into account protein and micronutrient requirements in addition to energy deficiency. Deficiencies may result in muscle wasting, poor wound healing, and delayed organ recovery or diseases associated with micronutrient deficiencies.

Protein requirements during critical illness are not well established. A term neonate (first month of life) should receive between 1.5 and 3 g/kg per day, older infants and children require between 1 and 2.5 g/kg per day and 1 to 2 g/kg per day, respectively.[35] In critically ill children, although total energy expenditure is lower than anticipated, they are catabolic, and a negative nitrogen balance has been shown to occur at an intake of <2.1 g/kg per day. Positive nitrogen balance was only achieved with a protein intake of 2.8 g/kg per day.[36,37] Critically ill children may therefore require up to 3 g/kg per day of protein to achieve a positive nitrogen balance.[34] Sterile energy-, protein-, and micronutrient-rich feeds should be used instead of modular additions such as fat and carbohydrate to standard feeds, as this practice is associated with disturbed protein-energy (PE) ratio, increased risk of bacterial contamination, and errors in feed preparation.[38]

An ideal PE ratio for catch-up growth resulting in lean body mass accretion rather than deposition of adipose tissue has been shown to be a PE of 8.9% to 12%.[39,40] Therefore, enriching products with modular additions of fat and carbohydrate alone often results in a PE of 4.5% to 6%, which does not favor optimal catch-up growth in growth-faltering infants.[38,39] In infants with moderate growth faltering, a weight gain of 10 g/kg per day is considered good. In these children, where weight gain averages 5 to 10 g/kg per day, it is important to review whether intake targets are being met and/or whether an infection is being missed.[11]

Micronutrient supplementation has been shown to be effective in promoting catch-up growth in children under the age of 5 years and should be considered a routine supplement in cardiac infants who are growth faltering. This should include a multiple micronutrient formulation that includes folate, and vitamin D.[39]

SPECIAL SITUATIONS

Conditions associated with an even higher risk of nutritional complications following cardiac surgery include hypoplastic left heart syndrome, protein-losing enteropathy, and chylothorax.

Interstage Feeding and Growth in Children with Hypoplastic Left Heart

Growth failure among infants with hypoplastic left heart syndrome (HLHS) is considered to be such a problem in the United States that facilitating better growth has been seen as a key component to improving interstage outcomes, particularly prior to the performance of superior cavopulmonary connection (SCPC).[41] In a cohort of $n = 50$ HLHS infants undergoing the Norwood procedure, their median weight at admission was unchanged at discharge, suggesting a period of growth failure,[42] which is reported among other similar cohorts of infants.[16] In addition, infants with univentricular CHD undergoing surgery during the neonatal period had an average decline in weight-for-age Z-score of $<-1.5 \pm 0.8$, in addition to a significant decline in linear growth (height-for-age Z-scores) from baseline to pre-SCPC, increasing postsurgery complications, which has been corroborated in other studies.[43]

Of interest, in a recent study involving 93 infants, 47% of which had CHD (33% had HLHS), there was no difference in REE between healthy infants and those with CHD or between infants with a single-ventricular or biventricular physiology,[31] which has been corroborated by other groups.[44] At 3 months of age, REE between all of the groups was no different; however, infants with CHD had significant growth faltering and lower percent fat, despite there being no difference in REE. It is likely that diminished fat reserves contribute to growth failure in infants with CHD.[31]

Nutritional Management of Protein-Losing Enteropathy

Protein-losing enteropathy (PLE) is a rare occurrence but is a feature of congestive cardiac heart failure and results in intestinal losses of protein, resulting in hypoproteinemia and malnutrition. Dietary management of PLE includes the provision of a high-protein diet supplemented with fat-soluble vitamins. In those patients with lymphangiectasia, a low-fat diet with medium-chain triglycerides (MCTs) may be appropriate, aiming for a maximum of 5 to 10 g per day of long-chain fat, although in some children it is necessary to stop oral feeds and maintain nutrition status through the provision of PN.[45]

Nutritional Management of Chylothorax

Chylothorax is a relatively common early postoperative complication, with an incidence of 6.6%.[46] The postoperative leakage of lymphatic fluid (protein, fat, lymphocytes) into the pleural space may result from the surgical disruption of the thoracic duct or one of its main tributaries, resulting in increased pressure within the intrathoracic lymph system.[47]

Chylothorax can be defined by the following parameters:

- Triglycerides > .1 mmol/L
- Chylomicrons (+)
- Chylomicrons (−) plus lymphocyte fraction >80% present in the pleural fluid

Chylothorax is usually managed conservatively, with the principal aim of decreasing the thoracic lymph flow. First-line conservative management includes the use of very low long-chain triglyceride (LCT) and high MCT enteral feeding (medium-chain fatty acids [6 – 12 carbon lengths] are absorbed directly into the portal system and do not enter the lymphatic system). Adequate calories, fluid, protein, and electrolytes must be provided, regardless of feeding method.[46]

It is also important to provide enough essential fatty acids (linoleic and linolenic acid) to prevent essential fatty acid (EFA) deficiency. The American Academy of Pediatrics (AAP) recommends that at least 3% of daily calories come from EFAs. Others report adequate EFA if linoleic acid supplies 1% to 2% of total calories and linolenic acid supplies 0.54% of total calories.[48]

The aim is not to give more than 1 g of LCT per year of life, up to a maximum of 4 to 5 g LCT per day,[3] although the efficacy of this has not been studied in a randomized controlled trial.[46] Achieving less than 1 g of LCT in infants under the age of 1 year without compromising optimal nutrition intake is challenging, and supplementary PN should be considered.

If the chylous leak is responsive to a predominantly MCT-based diet, then there should be an improvement in losses within the first week, decreasing to <10 mL/kg per day and ceasing by the end of the second week of treatment. However, if the chylous drainage remains unchanged or increases after the first week, the MCT diet should be discontinued and PN should be commenced. Once chylous drainage has decreased to <5 mL/kg per day, PN can be replaced by an MCT diet, which should continue until drainage has ceased. A normal diet can resume within 2 to 4 weeks.[46]

KEY POINTS

- Children with CHD are at significant risk of nutritional deterioration and failure to thrive.
- Fluid restriction, increased energy expenditure, inability to sustain oral intake, and intolerance to EN are some of the factors that impede optimal nutrient delivery in children with CHD.
- Enteral nutrition is frequently held in high-risk infants due to concerns related to ischemic intestinal injury. Careful monitoring for EN intolerance is necessary to avoid this risk. Breast milk has been shown to prevent NEC and, as such, should be the feed of choice in patients at risk.
- Malnutrition and growth failure during infancy is associated with impaired executive functioning and poorer scholastic performance in children with CHD.
- Chylothorax is a known complication in children with CHD. It is managed with MCT-based enteral formula, or with PN in resistant cases.

REFERENCES

1. Hoffman JI, Kaplan S. The incidence of congenital heart disease. *J Am Coll Cardiol.* 2002;39(12):1890-900.
2. Varan B, Tokel K, Yilmaz G. Malnutrition and growth failure in cyanotic and acyanotic congenital heart disease with and without pulmonary hypertension. *Arch Dis Child.* 1999;81(1):49-52.
3. Shaw V, Lawson M. *Clinical Paediatric Dietetics.* 3rd edition ed. Oxford: Blackwell Publishing; 2007.
4. de Menezes FS, Leite HP, Nogueira PC. What are the factors that influence the attainment of satisfactory energy intake in pediatric intensive care unit patients receiving enteral or parenteral nutrition? *Nutrition.* 2013;29(1):76-80.
5. Wallenstein MB, Harper LM, Odibo AO, et al. Fetal congenital heart disease and intrauterine growth restriction: a retrospective cohort study. *J Matern Fetal Neonatal Med.* 2012;25(6):662-665.
6. Ravishankar C, Zak V, Williams IA, et al. Association of impaired linear growth and worse neurodevelopmental outcome in infants with single ventricle physiology: a report from the pediatric heart network infant single ventricle trial. *J Pediatr.* 2013;162(2):250-256 e2.
7. Cohen MS, Zak V, Atz AM, et al. Anthropometric measures after Fontan procedure: implications for suboptimal functional outcome. *Am Heart J.* 2010;160(6):1092-1098, 8 e1.
8. Eskedal LT, Hagemo PS, Seem E, et al. Impaired weight gain predicts risk of late death after surgery for congenital heart defects. *Arch Dis Child.* 2008;93(6):495-501.
9. Mehta NM, Corkins MR, Lyman B, et al. Defining pediatric malnutrition: a paradigm shift toward etiology-related definitions. *J Parenter Enteral Nutr.* 2013;37(4):460-481.
10. Medoff-Cooper B, Ravishankar C. Nutrition and growth in congenital heart disease: a challenge in children. *Curr Opin Cardiol.* 2013;28(2):122-129.
11. WHO. *Management of Severe Malnutrition: A Manual for Physicians and Other Senior Health Workers.* Geneva; 1999.
12. de Onis M, Onyango A, Borghi E, Siyam A, Blossner M, Lutter C. Worldwide implementation of the WHO Child Growth Standards. *Public Health Nutr.* 2012;15(9):1603-1610.
13. De Wit B, Meyer R, Desai A, Macrae D, Pathan N. Challenge of predicting resting energy expenditure in children undergoing surgery for congenital heart disease. *Pediatri Care Med.* 2010;11(4):496-501.
14. Li J, Zhang G, Herridge J, et al. Energy expenditure and caloric and protein intake in infants following the Norwood procedure. *Pediatri Care Med.* 2008;9(1):55-61.
15. Avitzur Y, Singer P, Dagan O, et al. Resting energy expenditure in children with cyanotic and noncyanotic congenital heart disease before and after open heart surgery. *J Parenter Enteral Nutr.* 2003;27(1):47-51.
16. Nicholson GT, Clabby ML, Kanter KR, Mahle WT. Caloric intake during the perioperative period and growth failure in infants with congenital heart disease. *Pediatr Cardiol.* 2013;34(2):316-321.

17. Hulst JM, Joosten KF, Tibboel D, van Goudoever JB. Causes and consequences of inadequate substrate supply to pediatric ICU patients. *Curr Opin Clin Nutr Metab Care.* 2006;9(3):297-303.

18. Chwals WJ, Letton RW, Jamie A, Charles B. Stratification of injury severity using energy expenditure response in surgical infants. *J Pediatr Surg.*1995;30(8):1161-1164.

19. Letton RW, Chwals WJ, Jamie A, Charles B. Early postoperative alterations in infant energy use increase the risk of overfeeding. *J Pediatr Surg.* 1995;30(7):988-992; discussion 92-93.

20. Howley LW, Kaufman J, Wymore E, et al. Enteral feeding in neonates with prostaglandin-dependent congenital cardiac disease: international survey on current trends and variations in practice. *Cardiol Young.* 2012;22(2):121-127.

21. Byhahn C, Strouhal U, Martens S, Mierdl S, Kessler P, Westphal K. Incidence of gastrointestinal complications in cardiopulmonary bypass patients. *World J Surg.* 2001; 25(9):1140-1144.

22. Frey C, Takala J, Krahenbuhl L. Non-occlusive small bowel necrosis during gastric tube feeding: a case report. *Intensive Care Med.* 2001;27(8):1422-1425.

23. Holzer P, Painsipp E. Differential effects of clonidine, dopamine, dobutamine, and dopexamine on basal and acid-stimulated mucosal blood flow in the rat stomach. *Crit Care Med.* 2001;29(2):335-343.

24. Sables-Baus S, Kaufman J, Cook P, da Cruz EM. Oral feeding outcomes in neonates with congenital cardiac disease undergoing cardiac surgery. *Cardiol Young.* 2012; 22(1):42-48.

25. Lucas A, Cole TJ. Breast milk and neonatal necrotising enterocolitis. *Lancet.* 1990;336(8730):1519-1523.

26. McElhinney DB, Hedrick HL, Bush DM, et al. Necrotizing enterocolitis in neonates with congenital heart disease: risk factors and outcomes. *Pediatrics.* 2000;106(5):1080-1087.

27. Cheung YF, Ho MH, Cheng VY. Mesenteric blood flow response to feeding after systemic-to-pulmonary arterial shunt palliation. *Ann Thorac Surg.* 2003;75(3):947-951.

28. McClure RJ, Newell SJ. Effect of fortifying breast milk on gastric emptying. *Arch Dis Child Fetal Neonatal Ed.* 1996; 74(1):F60-62.

29. Babbitt C. Transpyloric feeding in the pediatric intensive care unit. *J Pediatr Gastroenterol Nutrit.* 2007;44(5): 646-649.

30. Dani C, Pratesi S, Barp J. Continuous milk feeding versus intermittent bolus feeding in preterm infants. *Early Human Dev.* 2013. 89 Suppl 2:S11-2.

31. Irving SY, Medoff-Cooper B, Stouffer NO, et al. Resting energy expenditure at 3 months of age following neonatal surgery for congenital heart disease. *Congenit Heart Dis.* 2013;8(4):343-351.

32. Meyer R, Furlano RI, Sidler MA. *Leitlinien für Pädiatrische Parenterale Ernährung.* Basel: Universitats Kinderspital beider Basel, 2012.

33. Hallum NS, Baxter JP, O'Reilly DS, McKee RF. Home parenteral nutrition in Scotland: frequency of monitoring, adequacy of review and consequence for complication rates. *Nutrition.* 2010;26(11-12):1139-1145.

34. Koletzko B, Goulet O, Hunt J, et al. 1. Guidelines on Paediatric Parenteral Nutrition of the European Society of Paediatric Gastroenterology, Hepatology and Nutrition (ESPGHAN) and the European Society for Clinical Nutrition and Metabolism (ESPEN), Supported by the European Society of Paediatric Research (ESPR). *J Pediatr Gastroenterol Nutr.* 2005; 41 Suppl 2:S1-87.

35. Hart ML, Ceonzo KA, Shaffer LA, et al. Gastrointestinal ischemia-reperfusion injury is lectin complement pathway dependent without involving C1q. *J Immunol.* 2005; 174(10):6373-6380.

36. Powis MR, Smith K, Rennie M, Halliday D, Pierro A. Characteristics of protein and energy metabolism in neonates with necrotizing enterocolitis—a pilot study. *J Pediatr Surg.* 1999;34(1):5-10;

37. Pierro A, Eaton S. Metabolism and nutrition in the surgical neonate. *Semin Pediatr Surg.* 2008;17(4): 276-84.

38. Clarke SE, Evans S, Macdonald A, Davies P, Booth IW. Randomized comparison of a nutrient-dense formula with an energy-supplemented formula for infants with faltering growth. *J Hum Nutr Diet.* 2007;20(4):329-339.

39. Golden MH. Proposed recommended nutrient densities for moderately malnourished children. *Food Nutr Bull.* 2009;30(3 Suppl):S267-342.

40. Pencharz PB. Protein and energy requirements for 'optimal' catch-up growth. *Eur J Clin Nutri.* 2010; 64 Suppl 1: S5-7.

41. Kugler JD, Beekman Iii RH, Rosenthal GL, et al. Development of a pediatric cardiology quality improvement collaborative: from inception to implementation. From the Joint Council on Congenital Heart Disease Quality Improvement Task Force. *Congenit Heart Dis.* 2009;4(5): 318-328.

42. Kelleher DK, Laussen P, Teixeira-Pinto A, Duggan C. Growth and correlates of nutritional status among infants with hypoplastic left heart syndrome (HLHS) after stage 1 Norwood procedure. *Nutrition.* 2006;22(3):237-244.

43. Medoff-Cooper B, Irving SY, Marino BS, et al. Weight change in infants with a functionally univentricular heart:

from surgical intervention to hospital discharge. *Cardiol Young.* 2011;21(2):136-144.

44. Mehta NM, Costello JM, Bechard LJ, et al. Resting energy expenditure after Fontan surgery in children with single-ventricle heart defects. *J Parenter Enteral Nutr.* 2012;36(6):685-692.

45. Braamskamp MJ, Dolman KM, Tabbers MM. Clinical practice. Protein-losing enteropathy in children. *Eur J Pediatr.* 2010;169(10):1179-1185.

46. Panthongviriyakul C, Bines JE. Post-operative chylothorax in children: an evidence-based management algorithm. *J Pediatri Child Health.* 2008;44(12):716-721.

47. Chan EH, Russell JL, Williams WG, Van Arsdell GS, Coles JG, McCrindle BW. Postoperative chylothorax after cardiothoracic surgery in children. *Ann Thorac Surg.* 2005;80(5):1864-1870.

48. Suddaby EC, Schiller S. Management of chylothorax in children. *Pediatr Nurs.* 2004;30(4):290-295.

CHAPTER 18

Nutritional Support of the Pediatric Surgical ICU Patient

Jeremy Fisher
Faraz Khan
Eric Sparks
Tom Jaksic

- INTRODUCTION
- PERIOPERATIVE NUTRITION: AN OVERVIEW
  - When to Support: Preoperative Nutrition
  - Postoperative Nutrition
  - Establishing Nutritional Needs
  - Choice of Route
  - Formula Types
- ABDOMINAL AND GASTROINTESTINAL SURGICAL DISEASE
  - Necrotizing Enterocolitis
  - Intestinal Failure
  - Intestinal Dysmotility
  - Patients with Increased Stoma or Stool Output
  - Chyle Leak
  - Extracorporeal Membrane Oxygenation
- CONCLUSIONS
- KEY POINTS
  - References

INTRODUCTION

Appropriate nutritional support is essential to the care of children undergoing surgery, not only to assure appropriate wound healing and convalescence, but also to ensure normal future growth. The limited lean body mass of neonates and children makes them particularly sensitive to injury-induced catabolism and its associated morbidity and mortality. Despite this catabolic response, a carefully designed nutritional support regimen can spur anabolism. Without question, the advancement of nutritional therapy, including parenteral nutrition, has played a key role in improved survival of a number of neonatal and childhood surgical conditions.

Pediatric surgical intensive care unit (ICU) patients present unique challenges: They are prone to inadequate enteral feeding due to anorexia, enteral nutrition (EN) intolerance, and perioperative ileus. Among other diagnoses, managing critically ill intestinal failure (IF) patients may be particularly complex. Furthermore, pediatric surgical patients may respond differently to the stress of surgery than do adults.

The postoperative increase in energy requirement in neonates is remarkably transient. This adds a degree of complexity in establishing the appropriate nutritional regimen for these patients. While many of the basic principles of critical care nutrition apply to the surgical patient, specific diagnoses and operations warrant special consideration.

PERIOPERATIVE NUTRITION: AN OVERVIEW

As with any patient, the essential questions in providing nutrition to pediatric surgical patients are (1) when to provide nutritional support, (2) how much to give, (3) what route to employ, and finally (4) what formulation to give.

When to Support: Preoperative Nutrition

For malnourished adults undergoing planned operations, a period of 2 to 3 weeks of preoperative EN has been shown to reduce operative complications, including overall hospital length of stay, surgical site infections, anastomotic leak, and renal and hepatic failure.[1] The application of these findings in young children is unclear. The use of perioperative parenteral nutrition (PN) is controversial. A meta-analysis of preoperative PN for mild-to-moderately malnourished patients showed little benefit and potential increase in complications.[2] Patients with severe malnutrition may benefit from 7 to 15 days of preoperative PN and 3 days of postoperative PN, though infection risk is higher in this group.[3] These recommendations may not apply to neonates since they have exceptionally limited nutritional stores.

There is a sizeable body of literature showing the ill effects of preoperative starvation on the metabolic state after surgery. In adult patients, preoperative starvation has been associated with worsening of insulin resistance, which is typically seen after surgery; this is an independent risk factor for an increase in length of stay.[4] Multiple adult studies have shown the reversal of this insulin resistance by providing a carbohydrate load (either orally or intravenously) about 2 hours prior to surgery.[4-7] This concept has not been tested in children.

Postoperative Nutrition

In critically ill adults, early postoperative enteral feeding decreases infection rates.[8,9] The initiation of EN, however, is subject to the patient's tolerance of feeds in the face of postoperative intestinal dysfunction. In these circumstances, a combination of PN and EN is frequently recommended. For postoperative pediatric patients, PN promotes nitrogen balance and increases levels of insulin-like growth factor 1.[10] Postoperative PN has been recommended for patients unable to take oral feeds for several days after the surgery; however, total parenteral nutrition (TPN) may be associated with higher infection rates with minimal benefits in wound-healing rates.[2] Postoperative starvation also places these patients at risk, and thus PN has been recommended for children who will not be able to tolerate EN for 5 to 7 days.[11] Neonates, with even smaller reserves, may require more prompt nutritional intervention.

Establishing Nutritional Needs

Determining the optimal nutrition prescription for a surgical patient is based on preexisting nutritional status, accurate estimation of macronutrient requirement, and attention to the fluid and electrolyte replacement strategy.

Nutritional Status

The first step in addressing the appropriate dietary needs of surgical patients is the same as for others: assessment of baseline nutritional status. Growth and development are the essential objectives of pediatric nutrition. Term neonates grow at a rate of 25 to 30 grams per day for the first 6 months of life, doubling birth weight by 5 months, and tripling it at 12 months. Body length increases by 50% by the end of the first year. Preterm infants, alternatively, tend to lose more weight in the first week of life and gain weight more slowly since they have yet to enter the high-weight-gain period that would have occurred during the third trimester.[12] Nonetheless, once they recover from early prematurity and acute surgical illness, they should demonstrate catch-up growth.

Malnutrition is not uncommon among pediatric surgical patients.[13] Specific tools to quantify nutritional status, including the mini nutrition assessment and subjective global assessment, are described elsewhere in this text. Surgical patients should be evaluated using the same instruments, and thus weight, height, and head circumference should be measured and compared against standardized curves and expressed as Z-scores for age. Additional growth charts are available for those with special health care needs (e.g., cerebral palsy). In the surgical critical care setting, weight is the essential measure, as it is a more accurate index of acute changes, though it can be influenced significantly by fluid volume status. Length, head circumference, and bone age reflect long-term nutritional status. Biochemical markers are less reliable in this population, as they may be substantively altered by stress and inflammation.

Energy Requirements

Though published tables based on consensus may provide gross estimations for recommended intake,[14] establishing an individual child's energy requirements can be challenging. Indirect calorimetry (IC) is a relatively accurate measure of energy expenditure in which carbon dioxide production and oxygen consumption are measured and energy expenditure (EE) can be derived using the Weir equation.[15] Two caveats in its use in ICU patients are that IC may be inaccurate when a significant leak around the endotracheal tube is present or in the setting of high FiO_2 (>0.6). Using this method, a more specific starting point for understanding an individual's caloric needs can be established. However, the physician must account for presumed variation in metabolic rate through changes in clinical course, which adds a degree of imprecision. For example, the evanescent nature of the postsurgical metabolic response in children can result in overestimation of energy needs. In a group of children who underwent cardiac surgery, postoperative EE was reported to be below levels of controls who did not undergo surgery.[16] In premature neonates, preoperative energy requirements appear to be a strong predictor of postoperative needs.[17] Overall, reports from the past decade appear to suggest that the EE after major surgery is comparable to preoperative status in infants and children.

Fluid and Electrolyte Replacement

Careful monitoring and recording of "ins" (enteral and intravenous [IV] provision) and "outs" (urine, emesis, ostomy, and stool outputs) are essential in the successful care of hospitalized surgical patients. While maintaining appropriate volume is a constant concern in ICU patients, specific electrolyte or micronutrient losses because of high ileostomy output, for example, can be overlooked. Care of critically ill surgical patients requires consideration of the individual's specific disease, operation, and postoperative anatomy. These are discussed further in the following sections.

Choice of Route

The issue of whether to provide EN, PN, or both is central to care of ill children. Children undergoing abdominal surgery, with its attendant postoperative dysmotility, frequently require a nuanced use of each route. Thus, this issue is brought to the forefront throughout this chapter. The use of EN promotes intestinal adaptation, reduces infectious complications, and avoids the hepatotoxicity associated with PN.[18] Even in patients on PN, small amounts of luminal nutrients (trophic feeding) can be hepatoprotective. In short, EN should be employed whenever possible, even if it must be augmented with PN.

Formula Types

Each individual surgical patient requires careful consideration in choosing the appropriate EN formulation. Some postoperative pediatric patients, specifically those with IF, may require different types of enteral nutrients over the course of childhood. Thus, in surgical patients, formula selection must be a dynamic, ongoing process. The sections that follow detail disease-specific formula selection.

ABDOMINAL AND GASTROINTESTINAL SURGICAL DISEASE

The challenge of nutritional management of abdominal surgical diseases in neonates is how to appropriately start and advance enteral feeds, while properly supporting growth through PN. There are a few considerations for specific disease entities, but ultimately, those with difficulty advancing to enteral feeds fall within some subset of the IF category. Brief disease-specific concerns are presented here, followed by a detailed discussion of IF.

Necrotizing Enterocolitis

Necrotizing enterocolitis (NEC) is an ischemic disease of the gastrointestinal tract affecting premature neonates. The incidence of NEC among infants of birth weight less than 1500 g is 9%.[19] Mortality is inversely proportional to birth weight and proportional to disease severity. Infants who require operations have a higher mortality (about 31% overall) than those with mild disease that can be managed medically (between 6% and 11%).[20] Though NEC is among the most studied disease in children, the management of feeding in neonates at risk for or with a history of NEC remains widely varied across neonatal intensive care units (NICUs).

Enteral Feeding in Neonates at Risk for Necrotizing Enterocolitis This topic is covered extensively elsewhere in this book. Briefly, there are substantial data regarding feeding in very-low-birth-weight neonates at risk for NEC that have yielded remarkably few data-driven recommendations. The risk of developing NEC is decreased when neonates are enterally fed with breast milk as opposed to formula (quality of evidence I, grade A recommendation).[21] A meta-analysis of 5 studies shows a relative risk for NEC of 2.5 (95% confidence interval 1.2 to 5.1) when evaluating formula versus donor breast milk.[22] (No randomized controlled trials have compared mother's milk to formula.) Furthermore, the protective effects of breast milk are dose dependent; higher proportion of feeds as breast milk result in lower risk of NEC or death.[23,24]

Theoretically, exposure to a small amount of enteral substrate should allow improved development of the gastrointestinal tract in premature neonates. Trophic or minimal enteral feeding is defined as starting on day of life 1 to 3 at 15 to 20 mL/kg per day divided every 2 to 3 hours for the first 7 days of life.[18] A Cochrane review comparing early trophic feeding to fasting until day of life 7 found no difference in risk of developing NEC, time to full feeds, length of stay, or mortality.[25] Minimal enteral feeding may be considered a safe alternative to fasting in this population (quality of evidence IB).[21]

Advancement of enteral feeds before day of life 4 or after 5 to 7 days does not appear to affect the risk of NEC or all-cause mortality.[26] Another meta-analysis found that fast advancement of enteral feeds (30 to 35 mL/kg per day) did not increase risk of NEC over slow advancement (15 to 20 mL/kg per day), though this analysis did not include infants with birth weights less than 750 grams.[27] Early advancement is a safe alternative to fasting or continuing trophic feeds (quality of evidence IB), and fast advancement of feeds is safe, especially in larger very-low-birth-weight neonates.[21]

Most very-low-birth-weight infants require tube feeds since suck and swallow coordination does not develop fully until 32 to 34 weeks gestation. The use of continuous versus bolus feeds, however, is controversial. A Cochrane review found no difference in the incidence of NEC, time to achieve full feeds, or growth when comparing continuous versus intermittent feeds.[28]

The response to feeding intolerance in the premature neonate is probably the most controversial aspect of nutritional management in this population. While sudden increases in gastric residuals appear to be a harbinger of NEC, the presence of any significant residual is not predictive. In the absence of other clinical or radiographic signs of NEC, continuation of trophic feeds may be appropriate.[21]

Further research regarding medication and dietary supplementation to prevent NEC is ongoing. Until then, a standardized feeding plan for very-low-birth-weight (<1,500 g) neonates, based on available evidence and consensus, may reduce NEC rates and improve overall mortality.[29,30]

Intestinal Failure

Though the specific management of children with various abdominal wall and intestinal disorders differs, a number of these can result in some degree of IF. An understanding of the principles of treating children with IF is, therefore, essential to successful management of their nutrition.

Etiology

Necrotizing enterocolitis, intestinal atresia, gastroschisis, and malrotation with volvulus can all lead to IF and are the most common causes. A variety of other conditions make up the remaining few patients, including Hirschsprung disease with small intestinal aganglionosis. Though the management of pediatric IF has evolved and outcomes have improved substantially over the last 20 years, appropriate nutritional provision for these patients remains challenging. The advent of multidisciplinary IF centers has likely been instrumental in improving outcomes. The mortality has improved from almost 50% to about 10% over the last 40 years.[31-33]

Definitions

Pediatric IF represents intrinsic bowel disease, resulting in an inability to sustain growth, hydration, or electrolyte homeostasis. Short-bowel syndrome (SBS) is generally considered a subset of IF created by actual small intestine loss or resection. Other diseases can result in IF without SBS—for example, mucosal enteropathies (microvillus inclusion disease, tufting enteropathy, etc.) and motility disorders (such as chronic intestinal pseudo-obstruction). Some disease processes incur elements of both of these conditions. Necrotizing enterocolitis, for example, can result in both SBS and elements of poor motility and malabsorption.

Though the ability to wean from PN is dependent on the quantity of bowel remaining, SBS cannot be defined by a specific measurement of bowel length. In neonates, 35 cm of small bowel is associated with a 50% probability of weaning from PN.[34] Some patients with much more intestine, however, still fail to wean from PN, as poor absorption or motility likely contributes to their disease. Conversely, those with as little as 10 cm have also successfully weaned from PN (**Fig. 18-1**).[34]

While the effect of bowel length on outcome is confounded by prematurity and measuring technique, residual small intestinal length remains the strongest clinical predictor of ultimate enteral feeding tolerance.[34,35]

The segment of bowel lost has implications for both management strategies and outcomes for patients with SBS. Traditionally, the presence of the ileocecal valve has been thought to be a favorable prognostic factor. More than the effect of the valve itself, its presence is a marker for

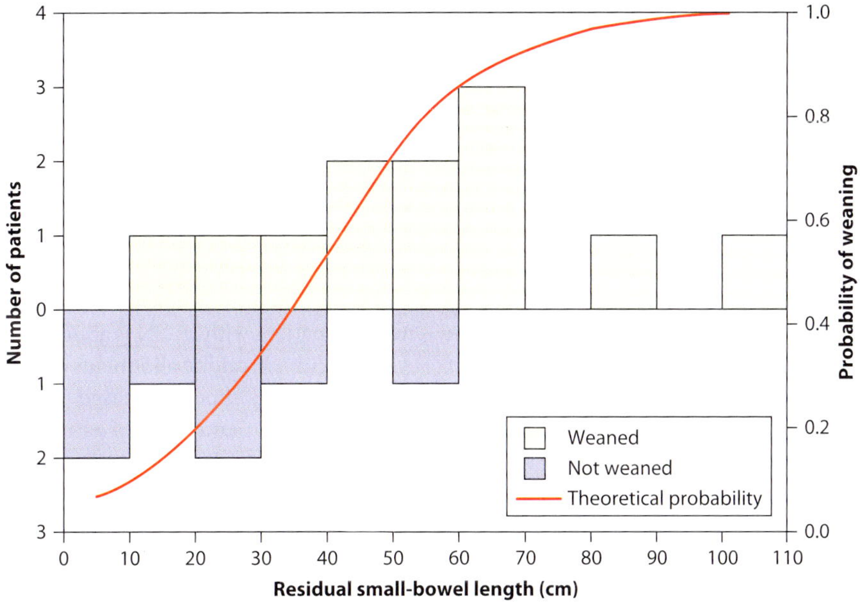

FIGURE 18-1. Residual small-bowel length and enteral nutrition tolerance in children with short bowel syndrome.

Reproduced with permission from Andorsky DJ, Lund DP, Lillehei CW, et al. Nutritional and other postoperative management of neonates with short bowel syndrome correlates with clinical outcomes, J Pediatr 2001;139(1):27-33.

having retained the terminal ileum, which plays essential physiologic roles in both absorption and motility. Colonic loss generally has a modest effect on nutrient absorption, with the notable exception of some short-chain fatty acid transfer. However, the colon effectively absorbs water and electrolytes, and therefore, the conservation of colon and/or the prompt reversal of stomas significantly reduces IV fluid requirements and is associated with improved SBS outcomes.[34]

In the absence of direct measurement of length, or as an adjunct to it, enterocyte mass can also be quantified biochemically. Citrulline is a nonprotein amino acid that is produced by the intestinal mucosal cells. In enterally challenged patients, serum citrulline concentration has been shown to closely correlate with intestinal length and can predict the ability to successfully wean from PN.[36] Functionally, neonatal SBS can be defined as PN dependence of greater than 3 months duration, though more complex definitions have also been employed.[37]

Clinical Presentation and Assessment

Patients with IF are typically treated in the clinical care setting at the time of their initial illness and may return when they encounter severe sequelae of long-term PN, such as sepsis related to indwelling central venous catheters or liver failure related to intestinal failure–associated liver disease (IFALD).

Since most etiologies occur in the neonatal period, patients tend to present with initial IF symptoms in the NICU. While some children with NEC or gastroschisis, for example, may tolerate enteral feeding with relative ease, neonates with typical underlying IF diagnoses will have some degree of difficulty. Feeding intolerance may present as vomiting, abdominal distention, and/or high stool or stoma output. Over time, abdominal radiographs typically show progressively more dilated small intestine. This may be seen even in the absence of obstruction and is part of the physiologic intestinal adaptation.

In both a critical care and outpatient setting, the first step of IF management is an accurate clinical assessment. The patient's surgical history, including what length or which portions of the bowel remain, should be carefully reviewed. Presence or absence of the ileum should be noted, as it is essential for absorption of long-chain fatty acids, fat-soluble vitamins (A, D, E, K), zinc, and vitamin B_{12}. Once the patient's anatomy is clearly understood, the intestinal motility should be evaluated. Such investigation is most important in patients with specific underlying diseases, such as ruling out mechanical obstruction and Hirschsprung disease.

As with any critically ill pediatric patient, obtaining precise body measurements (including weight, length, and head circumference) is essential in evaluating the nutritional status of IF patients. Assessment of body composition, as described in detail elsewhere in this book, is indicated.

In this population, micronutrient and vitamin deficiencies are relatively common, so evaluation must include specific attention to zinc, iron, copper, magnesium, and selenium levels.[38] However, such deficiencies tend to become apparent when PN is stopped, and therefore, they are more likely to present in the outpatient setting than in the ICU. Recent micronutrient shortages, on the other hand, may become problematic in critically ill patients. A small amount of enteral intake may provide adequate micronutrients in ambulatory PN patients, but those on PN in the ICU may not be able to tolerate any EN and hence, may be more susceptible.

Metabolic bone disease is prevalent in SBS patients.[39] It is most likely a result of inadequate parenteral phosphate and calcium, calcium malabsorption, reduced weight-bearing exercise, and inappropriate vitamin D provision. Serum 25-hydroxy vitamin D_3 levels are the most accurate representation of vitamin D status, as it robustly reflects hepatic stores. In outpatient management of IF, some centers utilize dual-energy x-ray absorptiometry (DEXA) to monitor bone mineral density in children older than 5 years. In critically ill children, especially neonates, clinical experience would indicate that a sudden spike of serum alkaline phosphatase may be related to pathologic fractures.

As mentioned earlier, the complete accounting of all outputs (stomal, stool, urine) is paramount in the assessment of any critically ill surgical patient, especially those with IF. High stomal/stool outputs can be caused by impaired absorption, hyperosmolarity of feeds, food allergy/intolerance, infection, or any combination of these. Large stool losses are associated with nonanion gap acidosis from bicarbonate loss, zinc loss and deficiency, and sodium loss. Overall zinc level adequacy can be measured by checking serum levels. Urinary sodium concentrations less than 10 mEq/L better delineate total body sodium depletion than do serum levels, though this measurement may be confounded in the ICU setting by the use of diuretics. Adequate sodium provision in the face of stool losses is essential in this population because total body sodium depletion is associated with growth failure.[40]

Nutritional Management

The goal of nutritional provision in children with IF is similar to others: attaining optimal growth and development. These patients have specific challenges and barriers to these goals, however.

Practically, the objective of an outpatient intestinal rehabilitation program is to attain complete enteral autonomy (wean from PN), preferably providing all calories orally. This process may be completed for some patients while still in the ICU; for many, it will take longer. Nevertheless, the concepts driving advancement of feeds are pertinent in this context.

During the initial hospitalization or later critical illness of a patient with IF, PN is almost uniformly required. Amino acid and caloric allotments of PN for children with IF in this setting should be based on the requirements of healthy children and tailored as needed using the tools described earlier. Both underfeeding and overfeeding (which results in hepatic steatosis, hyperglycemia, and increased CO_2 production) should be avoided.

Parenteral nutrition should be cycled (given over less than 24 hours) as quickly as possible. This prevents persistent hyperinsulinism and theoretically decreases the likelihood of hepatic steatosis and PN cholestasis.[41,42] Serum glucose levels below 60 mg/dL while off PN are a contraindication to cycling. Providing EN while PN is off can counteract hypoglycemia. Since neonates have very high requirements for glucose, cycling off PN for more than 6 hours at a time is not recommended.[43] In older children, PN duration of 12 or fewer hours is ideal. Since PN is often used to maintain volume and regulate acid–base status, cycling may not be feasible in the ICU setting and is not recommended in critically ill neonates and children.

Transitioning off PN is appropriate for those who are able to tolerate an appropriate number of calories enterally while maintaining growth. In the outpatient setting, PN is weaned by first reducing daily calories provided, then by replacing nights with IV fluid only. Some children may require IV hydration after PN has been completely discontinued.

Evidence supports the use of breast milk and amino acid (elemental) formulas for more rapid transition to full EN in neonates with IF.[34] The compromised mucosal barrier in children with SBS places them at higher risk for cell-mediated allergic enteritis, as proteins are able to cross more freely. Amino acid formulas eliminate risk of such peptide-mediated allergies and are thus preferred in this population. Allergies tend to improve over time, and eventually patients tolerate more complex proteins in their diets. Oral nutrition is the ultimate objective. In the absence of oral stimulation, neonates develop oral aversion that may be difficult to overcome later in life. For this reason, oral intake should be encouraged as early as possible in neonates with IF.

To summarize, for IF patients, careful accounting of IV and enteral intake and stoma, stool, and urine output allows for appropriate advancement of enteral feeds while avoiding over- or underfeeding. The ultimate goal is to maintain growth while increasing enteral, and eventually oral, nutrition and weaning PN. This process is usually accomplished in the outpatient setting, but may be started in the ICU.

Complications of Intestinal Failure

Consequences of IF and long-term PN may be discovered while a child is admitted to the ICU, or, more frequently, may be the cause for readmission. Hence, a review of their management is essential.

Intestinal Failure-Associated Liver Disease Also referred to as PN cholestasis or PN-associated liver disease (PNALD), IFALD is more likely to occur in patients with longer duration of PN, who have lower birth weights, were premature, and who have had more septic episodes.[34,44,45] Because these factors are often more closely associated with IF rather than PN exposure alone, IFALD is probably the more accurate term. Classically, the PN-associated cholestasis was seen in 25% to 33% of neonates on PN.[46] Recent therapy has reduced this substantially.[32] The pathophysiology of this phenomenon is not completely understood, but seems to be related to both PN formulation and a number of specific patient factors. While biochemical markers may give an incomplete picture of IFALD, typically, elevated serum transaminases and direct bilirubin are seen initially. This tissue damage results in poor hepatic synthetic function late in disease, reflected in prolonged prothrombin time (PT), international normalized ratio (INR), and hypoalbuminemia. Splenic enlargement and attendant thrombocytopenia may be seen later. Routine liver enzyme and function tests should be mandatory for those on long-term PN. On physical examination, jaundice, scleral icterus, and hepatosplenomegaly may be appreciated. Any signs consistent with portal hypertension should prompt liver ultrasound to evaluate for portal hypertension, including Doppler of liver, spleen, hepatic arteries, portal vein, and hepatic veins. Liver biopsies show cholestasis, bile duct proliferation, periportal inflammation, variable amounts of fibrosis, and ultimately, cirrhosis.[47]

Normalization of serum direct bilirubin is thought to be an initial marker of IFALD resolution. Serum alanine aminotransferase (ALT) levels typically normalize later.[48] Despite improvement in these biochemical markers, significant hepatic damage and even cirrhosis have been seen on subsequent biopsies.[47] Any liver damage short of cirrhosis is thought to be reversible. Additional measures of liver function have been investigated, though are not used routinely, including nonradioactive ^{13}C-methionine stable isotope studies. This test accurately and noninvasively differentiates cirrhotic from noncirrhotic infants with IFALD.[49,50]

Transition to full EN (weaning from PN) is the most effective therapy for IFALD. In a cohort of infants with IFALD and severe cholestasis, institution of enteral feeds decreased the serum bilirubin rapidly in one-quarter of patients, and all patients who were able to attain full EN had complete normalization of serum bilirubin within 3 to 4 months.[51]

Clearly, a quick transition to full enteral feeds is not possible in all patients with IFALD. One alternative therapy is the modification of the lipid portion of PN. It has been clearly demonstrated that the administration of lipids in excess of 1 g/kg per day is associated with the development of IFALD.[52,53] However, the provision of 1g/kg per day of lipid or less helps prevent and treat IFALD in children with IF.[53,54] Though a theoretical risk of essential fatty acid deficiency exists with these low doses of lipids, it is rarely encountered. Some centers provide lipid allotments of 0.5 g/kg per day or less and have seen deficiencies at these doses.[54]

The clinical signs of essential fatty acid deficiency include a dry, scaly rash. Biochemically, an elevated triene-to-tetraene ratio is typically apparent before symptoms. Humans require alpha-linolenic acid and linoleic acid (the "essential fatty acids") as about 2% of their total caloric intake. In neonates, the omega-3 fatty acids (eicosapentaenoic acid and docosahexaenoic acid—EPA and DHA) may also be essential. In patients whose lipid provisions are restricted, monthly lipid profile monitoring is recommended.

In neonates with IF, the provision of parenteral fish oil–based lipids (omega-3 fatty acids) at 1g/kg per day is associated with the reversal of hyperbilirubinemia in 89% of patients.[32,55] In these studies, cholestasis resolved at a mean of 81 days. Protracted use of fish oil emulsions has not been associated with essential fatty acid deficiency in neonates.[56] Omegaven® is a commercially available fish oil formula that has been used for parenteral support. It is not approved by the U.S. Food and Drug Administration (FDA), but it can be obtained on a compassionate-use basis for rescue therapy for patients with established IFALD after approval of an investigational new device (IND) application. The mechanism of Omegaven's® hepatoprotective effects is not completely understood, but may be due in part to the absence of certain compounds and the anti-inflammatory properties of omega-3 fatty acids. Plant-derived phytosterols found in standard soy-based lipids (and not in Omegaven®) have been shown to cause hepatic injury.[57] Omega-3 fatty acids (EPA and DHA) are precursors to cytokines with anti-inflammatory effects, whereas standard soy-based, omega-6 fatty acids have inflammatory metabolites.[58]

In addition to soy-based Intralipid and fish oil–based Omegaven® (Fresenius Kabi, Bad Homburg, Germany), another lipid emulsion is being used widely in Europe. SMOFlipid® (Fresenius Kabi) is a composite of 30% soybean, 20% medium-chain triglycerides (MCTs), 25% olive oil, and 15% fish oil that has been well tolerated in children with IF. Intestinal failure–associated liver disease is a significant problem with even those neonates who are successfully weaned from PN, carrying some degree of fibrosis or cirrhosis on liver biopsy.[47] In light of the currently available data, use of hepatoprotective strategies at the time of initiating PN may be advisable.

When some enteral tolerance can be established, the addition of enteral ursodeoxycholic acid may be helpful in the treatment of IFALD. This medication promotes bile flow with rare side effects. Efficacy has not been well established in IF patients, but the compound does appear to reduce transaminase and bilirubin levels in cholestasis of pregnancy.[59]

Lastly, there is some concern that copper and manganese can accumulate in the liver in the setting of IFALD.[60] For this reason, trace minerals are typically given at half doses, and the levels are followed to prevent deficiency.

Catheter-Associated Bloodstream Infections The presence of the central line required for the provision of PN is a substantial liability for patients with IF. Catheter-associated bloodstream infections (CABSIs) are likely the most common reason for ICU admission in IF patients on home PN, though line sepsis may also develop in neonatal inpatients with IF. Despite the addition of various protocols to improve sterility in handling central lines, the overall infection rate remains in the range of 10 per 1,000 catheter days.[61,62] Intestinal failure patients may be at higher risk, perhaps because of stool contamination or bacterial translocation from the gastrointestinal tract into the bloodstream. Two-thirds of the infections can be attributed to *Staphylococcus* species, while the rest include gram-negative bacteria.[61]

Thorough assessment of a child with a central catheter and symptoms of fever, lethargy, irritability, or ileus (abdominal distention) is essential. Blood cultures (both from the line and peripheral) should be drawn, after which those with fever or significant concern for CABSI should be given broad-spectrum IV antibiotics through the catheter (for example, vancomycin and piperacillin/tazobactam). Antibiotics may be discontinued if blood cultures are negative at 48 hours. A positive blood culture mandates a 14-day course of antibiotics, with coverage dictated by sensitivities. Children with hemodynamic instability or fungal infections should have their catheters removed. Alternatively, persistently positive blood cultures (3 or more consecutive days) in the face of appropriate IV antibiotic therapy may be an indication for catheter removal.

Ethanol locks have been shown to reduce CABSI rates and are indicated for children who have had recurrent infections. A retrospective study of infants with IF on home PN who received 70% ethanol locks 3 times per week showed greater than a fourfold reduction in CABSI (from 9.9 to 2.2 infections per 1,000 catheter days).[61] Ethanol penetrates biofilms that form on catheters, and no pathogens have developed resistance to this compound.

Bacterial Overgrowth Small-bowel bacterial overgrowth (SBBO) is a common problem among children with IF, affecting up to 60% to 70% of patients.[63] Typical symptoms are bloating/distention, excess flatulence, and foul-smelling stools. In addition, SBBO can worsen dysmotility, result in mucosal ulceration with bleeding, deconjugation of bile acids, and the generation of D-lactic acid and other toxic byproducts. Constipation or increased stool output may result.

Given that these complaints are frequent in IF patients, SBBO may be difficult to diagnose. Endoscopy with quantitative duodenal cultures can confirm the diagnosis ($>10^5$ colony-forming units) may guide therapy.[64,65] Typically, the initial treatment for SBBO is empiric, however. First-line therapy is often a schedule of enteral antibiotics given 7 days per month. If necessary, the frequency can be increased (i.e., antibiotic every other week) and/or a second antibiotic may be added. Some children require constant therapy with rotating antibiotic classes. First-choice antibiotic therapy should target anaerobes (i.e., metronidazole) or gram-negative bacteria (ciprofloxacin).

The excess burden of bacteria can also produce harmful amounts of D-lactic acid, which can produce D-lactic acidosis in IF patients. Whereas L-lactate is generated in normal anaerobic metabolism and is easily converted to L-pyruvate in humans, mammalian enzymes cannot process D-lactate, and thus toxic levels can accumulate. In neonates, D-lactic acidosis may present with anion gap acidosis and seizures. Older children demonstrate confusion, slurred speech, and delayed cognition. An elevated serum D-lactate level is diagnostic. Treatment consists of hydration and reduction in bacterial colonization using enteral antibiotics.

Finally, bacterial overgrowth can also render measurement of B_{12} levels inaccurate by producing an analogue that is biochemically inert in humans. Thus, accurate assessment of B_{12} in children with IF requires measurement of methylmalonic acid and homocysteine levels. An elevation of these substrates indicates a deficiency in the cofactor for their degradation, B_{12}.

Intestinal Dysmotility

For the pediatric intensivist caring for surgical patients, intestinal dysmotility is of paramount concern. Such poor motility can occur acutely as postoperative ileus, or chronically in IF patients. Many children with SBS, specifically those with a history of NEC, appear to have a component of disordered motility that potentiates their IF. In others, such as patients with pseudo-obstruction and those with a history of NEC without resection, chronic dysmotility can lead to IF in the absence of anatomically short bowel. Each of these three circumstances is frequently encountered in the ICU.

Despite advances in our understanding of intestinal physiology, many of the nuances of bowel motility remain unclear. For this reason, therapy to enhance motility has not changed appreciably in the last 3 decades.

In the setting of a child without IF with postoperative gastrointestinal dysfunction, the main component of treatment is bowel rest with nasogastric (NG) decompression in certain circumstances. While evidence is mounting that NG tubes are not necessary and may be harmful in adults and older children after intestinal operations,[66,67] their use is clearly still indicated for certain groups of children. Ventilated neonates typically require NG decompression, given the tendency toward aerophagia and the impact of abdominal distention on diaphragmatic excursion. Older children undergoing a Ladd procedure or operations like nephrectomies with significant retroperitoneal dissection tend to have significant postoperative emesis, which can be avoided with prophylactic NG placement. Currently, there are no well-studied pharmacological agents for the treatment of postoperative ileus in pediatric patients. The mu opioid receptor antagonist alvimopan appears to shorten the duration of intestinal dysfunction after surgery in adults,[68] but it has not yet been evaluated for use in children.

Treating chronic dysmotility is difficult, since each of the few prokinetic agents available has significant drawbacks. Erythromycin (and its longer-acting analogue azithromycin) is a motilin-receptor agonist that induces phase III of the migrating motor complex.[69] Unfortunately, both induce mostly gastric (and not small intestinal) motility and rapidly lose their effects due to tachyphylaxis. Octreotide is typically not used because it may accentuate intestinal ischemia. Metoclopramide can induce tardive dyskinesia, which led to an FDA "black box" warning against its prolonged use. Domperidone can treat gastroparesis, but is available only through an IND application through the FDA, given concerns over the potential for cardiac dysrhythmias. The remaining agent, cisapride, appears to improve both gastric and small intestinal motility, and clinically has been shown to improve enteral tolerance.[70] However, it was withdrawn from the U.S. market because it can cause torsades de pointes in certain patients. Despite that action, it can be obtained from the manufacturer for patients who meet specific selection criteria (i.e., normal electrocardiogram) and who will be followed by physicians using a defined protocol and using a regulated dosing regimen. Unfortunately, the numerous contraindications to the use of cisapride all but exclude its use in the ICU.

Patients with Increased Stoma or Stool Output

Precise monitoring of stool/stoma output in children with IF is an essential element in their care. Tolerance of enteral feeding is often determined by its effect on the stool volume. Stoma outputs of less than 2 mL/kg/hr, or about 10 stools per day (with appropriate fluid provision), are typically acceptable in infants. Beyond this threshold, the risk of dehydration, electrolyte abnormalities, and micronutrient deficiencies is significant. In particular, ileostomy effluent typically contains high levels of zinc (17 mg/L) and thus, careful monitoring and replacement are essential. When mechanical, ischemic, and infectious causes of high output can be eliminated, loperamide may be used to decrease stoma or stool volume. It is important to note that loperamide elixir is sometimes dissolved in alcohol, which, when administered, causes a paradoxical increase in output. Crushed pills in water or specially requested nonalcohol elixirs are alternatives.

Chyle Leak

Chylothorax occurs after about 5% of operations to correct congenital heart disease. It results in significant increase in length of stay and morbidity in the forms of worsening restrictive lung disease, increased risk of infection, bleeding or thrombosis, hypovolemia, and severe protein-energy malnutrition. It also increases mortality, especially in children with single-ventricle physiology.

Chyle leak appears to occur as a consequence of direct trauma to the thoracic duct or secondary to increased pressure in the central venous system (e.g., after a Fontan procedure, venous thrombosis, or mediastinal fibrosis). The diagnosis is confirmed if pleural fluid shows triglycerides >110 mg/dL, white blood cells (WBC) >1,000 cells/microL, and lymphocytes >80%.

Surgery is typically reserved for patients who fail a course of medical therapy. The goal of treatment is to reduce the volume through the thoracic duct to less than 10 mL/kg per day to allow it to heal. Though authors differ on the specific medical therapy algorithms, most agree that dietary modification, including low long-chain triglyceride (LCT) formulas and MCT supplementation, should be first-line treatment. Whereas LCTs pass into the lymphatics, MCTs are absorbed directly into the portal system,[71] and thus, this modification leads to decreased flow through the thoracic duct. This intervention alone is effective in up to 71% of cases.[72] Fat-free human breast milk with MCT supplementation is an alternative that allows preservation of immunologic benefits. If limitation of LCTs is unsuccessful, a trial of enteral rest with complete PN is the usual next step.[73]

Octreotide and its long-acting analogue, somatostatin, have been used to treat chyle leak successfully. Though the mechanism is unclear, a decrease in splanchnic blood flow is likely involved. No randomized controlled trials have confirmed its efficacy, but multiple large case studies have shown up to 80% success rates.[74] In those studies, dosing ranged from 10 to 40 mcg/kg per day, given subcutaneously, to 0.3 to 10 mcg/kg per hour as a continuous IV infusion. The effect is typically seen in 5 to 6 days, with a median duration of therapy of 10 to 18 days.

Surgical correction is generally undertaken after 2 to 4 weeks of failed medical therapy. In the largest series, thoracic duct ligation had a >90% success rate.[75] Pleurodesis and pleuroperitoneal shunts have also been employed. Though classically performed as open operations, they can also be accomplished using video-assisted thoracic surgery (VATS). Successful percutaneous embolization of the thoracic duct is also a viable alternative.[76]

Extracorporeal Membrane Oxygenation

Extracorporeal membrane oxygenation (ECMO) is used in the setting of profound cardiopulmonary failure and employs a membrane oxygenator attached to a modified heart–lung machine. Though ECMO has been used in adults and children, neonatal respiratory failure remains the most common indication. This intervention has been shown to improve mortality, however, the metabolic burden while on and after ECMO is substantial. Thus, close attention to nutritional support in such patients is essential.

Energy Requirements During Extracorporeal Membrane Oxygenation Therapy

Extracorporeal membrane oxygenation replaces approximately 80% of cardiopulmonary work and provides additional metabolic relief in the form of thermoregulation. Rather than providing a metabolic "rest state," however, neonates on ECMO have shown some of the highest EE ever recorded, as much as double those of healthy neonates on PN.[77] However, subsequent studies have shown that neonates on ECMO have a mean EE that is similar to age-matched healthy neonates. Thus, resting EE may be highly variable and is difficult to measure in these patients.

In contrast to the variability of EE in patients on ECMO, the effect on protein metabolism is clear: Even with aggressive PN, protein turnover is doubled.[78] As with other critically ill patients, amino acids are redistributed away from skeletal muscle toward healing tissues (wounds) and those involved in the inflammatory response, specifically the liver. Acute-phase protein production increases (including fibrinogen, haptoglobins, alpha-1-antitrypsin, transferrin, alpha-1-acid glycoprotein, C-reactive protein, albumin, and retinol-binding protein). In fact, neonates can lose up to 15% of their lean body mass during a 7-day course of ECMO.[77] A number of strategies have been used to combat this catabolism. Increasing energy supply alone is ineffective and potentially harmful. The addition of high-dose insulin to appropriate protein intake has been shown to decrease catabolism,[79] though this effect is not apparent with clinical doses. An adequate provision of protein is the most effective strategy in protecting lean body mass.

Nutritional Outcomes

The effects of malnutrition while on ECMO are lasting. The catabolic state seen in patients on ECMO may persist for up to 3 weeks after completion.[77] Overall, neonates who undergo ECMO tend to have poor long-term nutritional outcomes. In infants with congenital diaphragmatic hernia (CDH) who survived ECMO, a higher incidence of gastroesophageal reflux and feeding dysfunction were seen in the first year after discharge, with more than a third of this cohort requiring tube feedings. are fully enterally fed at 12 months following ECMO.[80] The resulting growth failure persists to at least 12 to 24 months.[81] These results underscore the importance of a well-designed nutritional regimen in mitigating long-term metabolic effects of ECMO.

The preponderance of literature regarding nutritional interventions in the context of ECMO concerns infants with respiratory failure. The American Society for Parenteral and Enteral Nutrition (A.S.P.E.N.) has published clinical guidelines for nutritional support of neonates on ECMO.[82] Given the small patient populations and difficulty in assessing nutritional parameters in this population, guidelines are based on mostly nonrandomized cohorts with contemporaneous controls (level III evidence).

When to Feed

Optimum weight gain is difficult to achieve in pediatric patients on ECMO, both because reserves may be limited (especially in neonates) and fluid intolerance may limit nutrient infusion. Furthermore, significant catabolic effects are seen within days of initiation of ECMO. Hence, nutritional support should be initiated expeditiously.

Energy Requirements

Despite studies demonstrating variability in EE rates, overall, it appears that energy requirements of neonates treated with ECMO are equivalent to healthy subjects, with mean EE 55 to 57 kcal/kg per day.[82] While increasing caloric provision may be tempting, excess calories do not decrease protein catabolism and can exacerbate respiratory failure by increasing CO_2 production. Establishing EE for an individual patient proves difficult because IC and nitrogen balance are often inaccurate while on ECMO. Stable isotope studies are more reliable, but generally limited to the research realm. The A.S.P.E.N. guidelines recommend that caloric provisions be based on age-matched healthy neonates, about 100 to 120 kcal/kg per day.[82,83]

Protein Requirements

Neonates treated with ECMO have protein requirements up to 3 g/kg per day.[82] The overall goal is to promote nitrogen balance in the face of the markedly increased whole-body protein breakdown associated with inflammation and critical illness. Positive protein nitrogen balance was seen with nonprotein nitrogen calories >60 kcal/kg per day and nitrogen >240 mg/kg per day. The maximum positive balance occurred with nitrogen intake >400 mg/kg per day.[84] Toxicity has been noted with excessive protein, especially in patients with marginal hepatic or renal function. Low-birth-weight infants receiving 6 g/kg per day of protein have shown initial lethargy and pyrexia followed by higher rates of strabismus and low intelligence quotient at 3 years of age.[85,86]

Route of Feeding

Enteral nutrition is preferred when the clinical situation allows, though there are no large-scale studies evaluating the route of feeding for children on ECMO. As discussed at length in chapter 8, EN is preferable in stable ICU patients with normal gastrointestinal function. One small study found that EN is well tolerated in pediatric patients on ECMO,[87] though the team must remain vigilant for signs of feeding intolerance. Because such studies have not been replicated in neonates, caution in starting EN before clinical stability is advised, although provision of EN for these patients is now common practice. Small amounts of EN may be started (in addition to PN), despite intestinal dysfunction, and subsequently titrated up as tolerated. Small studies have shown no adverse effects (mortality or infections) from the addition of EN in neonates on ECMO.[88] Tolerance of EN may be a marker for improved outcome; those who are slow to tolerate EN have 3.6-fold longer hospital length of stay than those feeding optimally by 4 weeks after ECMO.[89]

CONCLUSION

Nutrition provision in the pediatric surgical population in the ICU, especially those with intestinal dysfunction in the form of postoperative ileus or chronic intestinal failure, poses significant challenges. In children with surgical illness with a functioning gastrointestinal tract, EN must be the route of choice, given the risks associated with PN. For those who require PN, even small amounts of luminal nutrients promote intestinal adaptation and are protective against cholestatic liver disease (IFALD or PNALD). Successful nutritional therapy for critically ill pediatric surgical patients requires a nuanced understanding of their specific disease and operative history. Careful attention to energy and protein requirements will allow optimal nutrition prescription in this group. Increased metabolic demands following surgery may be evanescent in children, even in those with significant illness, such as ECMO patients. Careful accounting of outputs and monitoring of electrolyte and micronutrient levels can help prevent acute and chronic sequelae of deficiencies.

KEY POINTS

- Pediatric surgical ICU patients present unique challenges in terms of nutrient delivery, due to increased risk of anorexia, EN intolerance, and perioperative ileus.
- Enteral nutrition is the preferred route in patients with a functional gastrointestinal tract. Postoperative starvation must be avoided, and PN may be recommended for children who will not be able to tolerate EN.
- Intestinal dysmotility is frequently encountered in the pediatric surgical population in the PICU. The use of prokinetics in this group is challenging due to the side effects of these drugs.
- Increased stomal fluid losses need to be monitored and managed appropriately to prevent fluid and electrolyte derangements.
- Estimates of postoperative energy and protein requirements in children are often inaccurate, resulting in suboptimal delivery. Protein intake must be optimized to offset the negative effects of the profound protein catabolism and to achieve protein balance.

REFERENCES

1. Campos AC, Meguid MM. A critical appraisal of the usefulness of perioperative nutritional support. *Am J Clin Nutr.* 1992;55:117-130.
2. Klein S, Kinney J, Jeejeebhoy K, et al. Nutrition support in clinical practice: review of published data and recommendations for future research directions. National Institutes of Health, American Society for Parenteral and Enteral Nutrition, and American Society for Clinical Nutrition. *J Parenter Enteral Nutr.* 1997;21:133-156.
3. Buzby GP, Williford WO, Peterson OL, et al. A randomized clinical trial of total parenteral nutrition in malnourished surgical patients: the rationale and impact of previous clinical trials and pilot study on protocol design. *Am J Clin Nutr.* 1988;47:357-365.
4. Nygren J, Soop M, Thorell A, Sree Nair K, Ljungqvist O. Preoperative oral carbohydrates and postoperative insulin resistance. *Clin Nutr.* 1999;18:117-120.
5. Ljungqvist O, Nygren J, Thorell A. Modulation of postoperative insulin resistance by pre-operative carbohydrate loading. *Proc Nutr Soc.* 2002;61:329-336.
6. Nygren J, Soop M, Thorell A, Efendic S, Nair KS, Ljungqvist O. Preoperative oral carbohydrate administration reduces postoperative insulin resistance. *Clin Nutr.* 1998;17:65-71.
7. Soop M, Nygren J, Myrenfors P, Thorell A, Ljungqvist O. Preoperative oral carbohydrate treatment attenuates immediate postoperative insulin resistance. *Am J Physiol Endocrinol Metab.* 2001;280:E576-583.
8. Koretz RL, Avenell A, Lipman TO, Braunschweig CL, Milne AC. Does enteral nutrition affect clinical outcome? A systematic review of the randomized trials. *Am J Gastroenterol.* 2007;102:412-29; quiz 68.
9. Lewis SJ, Andersen HK, Thomas S. Early enteral nutrition within 24 h of intestinal surgery versus later commencement of feeding: a systematic review and meta-analysis. *J Gastrointes Surg.* 2009;13:569-575.
10. Marin VB, Rebollo MG, Castillo-Duran CD, et al. Controlled study of early postoperative parenteral nutrition in children. *J Pediatr Surg.* 1999;34:1330-1335.
11. Herman R, Btaiche I, Teitelbaum DH. Nutrition support in the pediatric surgical patient. *Surg Clin North Am.* 2011;91(3):511-541.
12. Rose J, Gibbons K, Carlson SE, Koo WW. Nutrient needs of the preterm infant. *Nutr Clin Prac.* 1993;8:226-232.
13. Cooper A, Jakobowski D, Spiker J, Floyd T, Ziegler MM, Koop CE. Nutritional assessment: an integral part of the preoperative pediatric surgical evaluation. *J Pediatr Surg.* 1981;16:554-561.
14. Otten JJ HJ, Meyers LD, eds. *Dietary Reference Intakes: The Essential Guide to Nutrient Requirements.* Washington, DC 2006;The National Academies Press.
15. Weir JB. New methods for calculating metabolic rate with special reference to protein metabolism. 1949. *Nutrition.* 1990;6:213-221.
16. Mitchell IM, Davies PS, Day JM, Pollock JC, Jamieson MP. Energy expenditure in children with congenital heart disease, before and after cardiac surgery. *J Thorac Cardiovasc Surg.* 1994;107:374-380.
17. Garza JJ, Shew SB, Keshen TH, Dzakovic A, Jahoor F, Jaksic T. Energy expenditure in ill premature neonates. *J Pediatr Surg.* 2002;37:289-293.
18. Beath SV, Davies P, Papadopoulou A, et al. Parenteral nutrition-related cholestasis in postsurgical neonates: multivariate analysis of risk factors. *J Pediatr Surg.* 1996;31:604-606.
19. Fitzgibbons SC, Ching Y, Yu D, et al. Mortality of necrotizing enterocolitis expressed by birth weight categories. *J Pediatr Surg.* 2009;44:1072-1075; discussion 5-6.
20. Hull MA, Fisher JG, Gutierrez IM, et al. Mortality and management of surgical necrotizing enterocolitis in very

low birth weight neonates: a prospective cohort study. *J Am Coll Surg*. 2014;218(6):1148-1155.

21. Ramani M, Ambalavanan N. Feeding practices and necrotizing enterocolitis. *Clin Perinatol.* 2013;40(1):1-10.
22. Quigley MA, Henderson G, Anthony MY, McGuire W. Formula milk versus donor breast milk for feeding preterm or low birth weight infants. *Cochrane Database Syst Rev.* 2007:CD002971.
23. Meinzen-Derr J, Poindexter B, Wrage L, Morrow AL, Stoll B, Donovan EF. Role of human milk in extremely low birth weight infants' risk of necrotizing enterocolitis or death. *J Perinatol.* 2009;29:57-62.
24. Sisk PM, Lovelady CA, Dillard RG, Gruber KJ, O'Shea TM. Early human milk feeding is associated with a lower risk of necrotizing enterocolitis in very low birth weight infants. *J Perinatol.* 2007;27:428-433.
25. Bombell S, McGuire W. Early trophic feeding for very low birth weight infants. *Cochrane Database Syst Rev.* 2009:CD000504.
26. Morgan J, Young L, McGuire W. Delayed introduction of progressive enteral feeds to prevent necrotising enterocolitis in very low birth weight infants. *Cochrane Database Syst Rev.* 2011:CD001970.
27. Fau MJ, Young L, McGuire W. Slow advancement of enteral feed volumes to prevent necrotising enterocolitis in very low birth weight infants. *Cochrane Database Syst Rev.* 2013:CD001241.
28. Premji SS, Chessell L. Continuous nasogastric milk feeding versus intermittent bolus milk feeding for premature infants less than 1500 grams. *Cochrane Database Syst Rev.* 2011:CD001819.
29. Butler TJ, Szekely LJ, Grow JL. A standardized nutrition approach for very low birth weight neonates improves outcomes, reduces cost and is not associated with increased rates of necrotizing enterocolitis, sepsis or mortality. *J Perinatol.* 2013.
30. Patole SK, de Klerk N. Impact of standardised feeding regimens on incidence of neonatal necrotising enterocolitis: a systematic review and meta-analysis of observational studies. *Arch Dis Child Fetal Neonatal Ed.* 2005;90:F147-151.
31. Modi BP, Langer M, Ching YA, et al. Improved survival in a multidisciplinary short bowel syndrome program. *J Pediatr Surg.* 2008;43:20-24.
32. Puder M, Valim C, Meisel JA, et al. Parenteral fish oil improves outcomes in patients with parenteral nutrition-associated liver injury. *Ann Surg.* 2009;250:395-402.
33. Wilmore DW. Factors correlating with a successful outcome following extensive intestinal resection in newborn infants. *J Pediatri.* 1972;80:88-95.
34. Andorsky DJ, Lund DP, Lillehei CW, et al. Nutritional and other postoperative management of neonates with short bowel syndrome correlates with clinical outcomes. *J Pediatr.* 2001;139:27-33.
35. Duro D, Kalish LA, Johnston P, et al. Risk factors for intestinal failure in infants with necrotizing enterocolitis: a Glaser Pediatric Research Network study. *J Pediatr.* 2010;157:203-208 e1.
36. Fitzgibbons S, Ching YA, Valim C, et al. Relationship between serum citrulline levels and progression to parenteral nutrition independence in children with short bowel syndrome. *J Pediatr Surg.* 2009;44:928-932.
37. Sigalet DL. Short bowel syndrome in infants and children: an overview. *Semin Pediatr Surg.* 2001;10:49-55.
38. Yang CF, Duro D, Zurakowski D, Lee M, Jaksic T, Duggan C. High prevalence of multiple micronutrient deficiencies in children with intestinal failure: a longitudinal study. *J Pediatr.* 2011;159:39-44 e1.
39. Dellert SF, Farrell MK, Specker BL, Heubi JE. Bone mineral content in children with short bowel syndrome after discontinuation of parental nutrition. *J Pediatr.* 1998;132:516-519.
40. Haycock GB. The influence of sodium on growth in infancy. *Pediatr Nephrol.* 1993;7:871-875.
41. Jensen AR, Goldin AB, Koopmeiners JS, Stevens J, Waldhausen JH, Kim SS. The association of cyclic parenteral nutrition and decreased incidence of cholestatic liver disease in patients with gastroschisis. *J Pediatr Surg.* 2009;44:183-189.
42. Nghiem-Rao TH, Cassidy LD, Polzin EM, Calkins CM, Arca MJ, Goday PS. Risks and benefits of prophylactic cyclic parenteral nutrition in surgical neonates. *Nutr Clin Prac.* 2013;28:745-752.
43. Collier S, Crough J, Hendricks K, Caballero B. Use of cyclic parenteral nutrition in infants less than 6 months of age. *Nutr Clin Prac.* 1994;9:65-68.
44. Christensen RD, Henry E, Wiedmeier SE, Burnett J, Lambert DK. Identifying patients, on the first day of life, at high-risk of developing parenteral nutrition-associated liver disease. *J Perinatol.* 2007;27:284-290.
45. Kelly DA. Liver complications of pediatric parenteral nutrition—epidemiology. *Nutrition.* 1998;14:153-157.
46. Kubota A, Yonekura T, Hoki M, et al. Total parenteral nutrition-associated intrahepatic cholestasis in infants: 25 years' experience. *J Pediatr Surg.* 2000;35:1049-1051.
47. Fitzgibbons SC, Jones BA, Hull MA, et al. Relationship between biopsy-proven parenteral nutrition-associated liver fibrosis and biochemical cholestasis in children with short bowel syndrome. *J Pediatr Surg.* 2010;45:95-99; discussion 9.

48. Yang CF, Lee M, Valim C, et al. Persistent alanine aminotransferase elevations in children with parenteral nutrition-associated liver disease. *J Pediatr Surg.* 2009; 44:1084-1087; discussion 7-8.

49. Duro D, Duggan C, Valim C, et al. Novel intravenous (13) C-methionine breath test as a measure of liver function in children with short bowel syndrome. *J Pediatr Surg.* 2009;44:236-240; discussion 40.

50. Duro D, Fitzgibbons S, Valim C, et al. [13C]Methionine breath test to assess intestinal failure-associated liver disease. *Pediatr Res.* 2010;68:349-354.

51. Javid PJ, Collier S, Richardson D, et al. The role of enteral nutrition in the reversal of parenteral nutrition-associated liver dysfunction in infants. *J Pediatr Surg.* 2005;40: 1015-1018.

52. Cavicchi M, Beau P, Crenn P, Degott C, Messing B. Prevalence of liver disease and contributing factors in patients receiving home parenteral nutrition for permanent intestinal failure. *Ann Intern Med.* 2000;132:525-532.

53. Colomb V, Jobert-Giraud A, Lacaille F, Goulet O, Fournet JC, Ricour C. Role of lipid emulsions in cholestasis associated with long-term parenteral nutrition in children. *J Parenter Enteral Nutr.* 2000;24:345-350.

54. Shin JI, Namgung R, Park MS, Lee C. Could lipid infusion be a risk for parenteral nutrition-associated cholestasis in low birth weight neonates? *Eur J Pediatr.* 2008;167:197-202.

55. Gura KM, Lee S, Valim C, et al. Safety and efficacy of a fish-oil-based fat emulsion in the treatment of parenteral nutrition-associated liver disease. *Pediatrics.* 2008;121:e678-686.

56. de Meijer VE, Le HD, Meisel JA, Gura KM, Puder M. Parenteral fish oil as monotherapy prevents essential fatty acid deficiency in parenteral nutrition-dependent patients. *J Pediatr Gastroenterol Nutr.* 2010;50:212-218.

57. El Kasmi KC1, Anderson AL, Devereaux MW, Vue PM, Zhang W, Setchell KD, Karpen SJ, Sokol RJ. Phytosterols promote liver injury and kupffer cell activation in parenteral nutrition-associated liver disease. *Sci Transl Med.* 2013;5(206):206.

58. Alwayn IP, Gura K, Nose V, et al. Omega-3 fatty acid supplementation prevents hepatic steatosis in a murine model of nonalcoholic fatty liver disease. *Pediatr Res.* 2005;57:445-452.

59. Glantz A, Marschall HU, Lammert F, Mattsson LA. Intrahepatic cholestasis of pregnancy: a randomized controlled trial comparing dexamethasone and ursodeoxycholic acid. *Hepatology.* 2005;42:1399-1405.

60. Soden JS. Clinical assessment of the child with intestinal failure. *Semin Pediatr Surg.* 2010;19:10-19.

61. Jones BA, Hull MA, Richardson DS, et al. Efficacy of ethanol locks in reducing central venous catheter infections in pediatric patients with intestinal failure. *J Pediatr Surg.* 2010;45:1287-1293.

62. Lee OK, Johnston L. A systematic review for effective management of central venous catheters and catheter sites in acute care paediatric patients. *Worldviews on Evidence-Based Nurs.* 2005;2:4-13; discussion 4-5.

63. Kaufman SS, Loseke CA, Lupo JV, et al. Influence of bacterial overgrowth and intestinal inflammation on duration of parenteral nutrition in children with short bowel syndrome. *J Pediatr.*1997;131:356-361.

64. Ching YA, Modi BP, Jaksic T, Duggan C. High diagnostic yield of gastrointestinal endoscopy in children with intestinal failure. *J Pediatr Surg.* 2008;43:906-910.

65. Gutierrez IM, Kang KH, Calvert CE, et al. Risk factors for small bowel bacterial overgrowth and diagnostic yield of duodenal aspirates in children with intestinal failure: a retrospective review. *J Pediatr Surg.* 2012;47:1150-1154.

66. Kehlet H, Williamson R, Buchler MW, Beart RW. A survey of perceptions and attitudes among European surgeons towards the clinical impact and management of postoperative ileus. *Colorectal Dis.* 2005;7:245-250.

67. Nelson R, Edwards S, Tse B. Prophylactic nasogastric decompression after abdominal surgery. *Cochrane Database Syst Rev.* 2005:CD004929.

68. Vaughan-Shaw PG, Fecher IC, Harris S, Knight JS. A meta-analysis of the effectiveness of the opioid receptor antagonist alvimopan in reducing hospital length of stay and time to GI recovery in patients enrolled in a standardized accelerated recovery program after abdominal surgery. *Dis Colon Rectum.* 2012;55(5):611-620.

69. Di Lorenzo C, Lucanto C, Flores AF, Idries S, Hyman PE. Effect of sequential erythromycin and octreotide on antroduodenal manometry. *J Pediatr Gastroenterol Nutr.* 1999;29:293-296.

70. Raphael BP, Nurko S, Jiang H, et al. Cisapride improves enteral tolerance in pediatric short-bowel syndrome with dysmotility. *J Pediatr Gastroenterol Nutr.* 2011;52:590-594.

71. Frazer AC. Differentiation in the absorption of olive oil and oleic acid in the rat. *J Physiol.* 1943;102:306-312.

72. Biewer ES, Zurn C, Arnold R, et al. Chylothorax after surgery on congenital heart disease in newborns and infants: risk factors and efficacy of MCT-diet. *J Cardiothoracic Surg.* 2010;5:127.

73. Chan EH, Russell JL, Williams WG, Van Arsdell GS, Coles JG, McCrindle BW. Postoperative chylothorax after cardiothoracic surgery in children. *Ann Thorac Surg.* 2005; 80(5):1864-1870.

74. Das A, Shah PS. Octreotide for the treatment of chylothorax in neonates. *Cochrane Database Syst Rev*. 2010;(9):CD006388.

75. Nath DS, Savla J, Khemani RG, Nussbaum DP, Greene CL, Wells WJ. Thoracic duct ligation for persistent chylothorax after pediatric cardiothoracic surgery. *Ann Thorac Surg*. 2009;88:246-251; discussion 51-52.

76. Chen E, Itkin M. Thoracic duct embolization for chylous leaks. *Semin Intervent Radiol*. 2011;28:63-74.

77. Keshen TH, Miller RG, Jahoor F, Jaksic T. Stable isotopic quantitation of protein metabolism and energy expenditure in neonates on- and post-extracorporeal life support. *J Pediatr Surg*. 1997;32:958-962; discussion 62-63.

78. Jaksic T, Wagner DA, Burke JF, Young VR. Proline metabolism in adult male burned patients and healthy control subjects. *Am J Clin Nutr*. 1991;54:408-413.

79. Agus MS, Javid PJ, Ryan DP, Jaksic T. Intravenous insulin decreases protein breakdown in infants on extracorporeal membrane oxygenation. *J Pediatr Surg*. 2004;39:839-844; discussion 44.

80. Bernbaum J, Schwartz IP, Gerdes M, D'Agostino JA, Coburn CE, Polin RA. Survivors of extracorporeal membrane oxygenation at 1 year of age: the relationship of primary diagnosis with health and neurodevelopmental sequelae. *Pediatrics*. 1995;96:907-913.

81. Van Meurs Kp Fau - Robbins ST, Robbins St Fau - Reed VL, Reed Vl Fau - Karr SS, et al. Congenital diaphragmatic hernia: long-term outcome in neonates treated with extracorporeal membrane oxygenation. *J Pediatr*. 1993;122(6):893-899.

82. Jaksic T, Hull MA, Modi BP, Ching YA, George D, Compher C. A.S.P.E.N. clinical guidelines: nutrition support of neonates supported with extracorporeal membrane oxygenation. *J Parenter Enteral Nutr*. 2010;34:247-253.

83. Jaksic T, Shew SB, Keshen TH, Dzakovic A, Jahoor F. Do critically ill surgical neonates have increased energy expenditure? *J Pediatr Surg*. 2001;36:63-67.

84. Weber TR, Shah M, Stephens C, Tracy T, Jr. Nitrogen balance in patients treated with extracorporeal membrane oxygenation. *J Pediatr Surg*. 1993;28:906-908.

85. Goldman HI, Freudenthal R, Holland B, Karelitz S. Clinical effects of two different levels of protein intake on low-birth-weight infants. *J Pediatr*. 1969;74:881-889.

86. Goldman HI, Liebman OB, Freudenthal R, Reuben R. Effects of early dietary protein intake on low-birth-weight infants: evaluation at 3 years of age. *J Pediatr*. 1971;78:126-129.

87. Pettignano R, Heard M, Davis R, Labuz M, Hart M. Total enteral nutrition versus total parenteral nutrition during pediatric extracorporeal membrane oxygenation. *Crit Care Med*. 1998;26:358-363.

88. Wertheim HF, Albers MJ, Piena-Spoel M, Tibboel D. The incidence of septic complications in newborns on extracorporeal membrane oxygenation is not affected by feeding route. *J Pediatr Surg*. 2001;36:1485-1489.

89. Jadcherla SR, Berseth CL. Antroduodenal motility and feeding outcome among neonatal extracorporeal membrane oxygenation survivors. *J Pediatr Gastroenterol Nutr*. 2005;41:347-350.

CHAPTER 19

Immunonutrition

Natalie Z. Cvijanovich
William Manzanares

- INTRODUCTION
- IMMUNE RESPONSE TO CRITICAL ILLNESS
  - Innate Immunity
  - Adaptive Immunity
- IMMUNOLOGIC EFFECTS OF NUTRIENTS
  - Macronutrients
  - Micronutrients
- CLINICAL TRIALS OF IMMUNONUTRITION
  - Adult Trials
  - Pediatric Trials
- CONCLUSION
- KEY POINTS
  - References

INTRODUCTION

The body's reaction to critical illness, whether from infection, surgery, or trauma, is complex and multifactorial, and survival from an insult requires the successful coordination of responses to the stress of illness. A functional immune system is essential for survival, but an appropriate balance between the pro-inflammatory and anti-inflammatory responses must be maintained. It has long been known that baseline nutritional status has effects on inflammation, oxidative status, and immune function. More recently, however, providing specific nutrients to manipulate the immune system *independent* of caloric or macronutrient requirements for nutrition per se has evolved as a therapeutic modality. This is the basis for what has come to be known as immunonutrition.

IMMUNE RESPONSE TO CRITICAL ILLNESS

The immune system is the body's secondary defense against invasion, after skin and mucosal barriers, and is required for healing and repair after injury. Generally, this is a protective response, evolved over generations and across species, resulting in the systemic inflammatory response that is designed to make the environment of the body inhospitable for pathogens. This response in itself, however, can be overly exuberant and is primarily responsible for the multiorgan dysfunction that is commonly seen in the critically ill. With improved survival from initial insults and the organ dysfunction that follows, the balance shifts within several days to a more anti-inflammatory response, termed the compensatory anti-inflammatory response syndrome (CARS). Ultimately, if homeostasis is not restored, prolonged organ dysfunction results.[1]

The components of the immune system can be divided into 2 separate but well-integrated and interdependent groups. The first includes cells designed as first defenders that initiate the inflammatory response, comprising the innate immune system, while the second group is composed of cells that modulate the immune response and ultimately provide immune memory, known as the adaptive immune system. These groups act in concert to respond to injury and invasion by pathogens. Both are affected by baseline nutritional status and can be modulated by macro- and micronutrients.

Innate Immunity

The innate immune system is composed of cells that can respond to initial injury or pathogen invasion, inciting the inflammatory cascade within hours to days. These are monocytes, macrophages, polymorphonuclear (PMN) cells, dendritic cells, and natural killer (NK) cells. They can recognize pathogens upon initial contact via constitutively expressed cell surface receptors. They also function as phagocytes, which may directly kill pathogens intracellularly and/or digest proteins into antigenic peptides that are subsequently presented on the cell surface. The cell surface protein–antigen complex is recognized by lymphocytes, activating the adaptive immune system. Innate immune cells also secrete chemokines, which function as chemical attractants to other immune cells, and cytokines, which affect the function of other cells, such as lymphocytes, monocytes, and macrophages.

The cytokines and chemokines expressed by innate immune cells have both pro- and anti-inflammatory properties. Cytokines that are generally pro-inflammatory are interleukin (IL) -1 beta (IL-1β) and tumor necrosis factor-alpha (TNF-α), both secreted by monocytes and macrophages and causing fever and vasodilation; interferon-gamma (IFN-γ); and others. Anti-inflammatory cytokines include IL-10 and transforming growth factor-beta (TGF-β). Chemokines secreted by cells of the innate immune system include IL-8 and monocyte chemotactic protein (MCP)-1, which promote migration and activation of PMNs, monocytes, macrophages, NK cells, and dendritic cells.[1,2] Interleukin-6, secreted by monocytes and macrophages as well as T-cells, induces a strong pro-inflammatory response and is considered a marker of inflammation, but also has some anti-inflammatory properties.[1]

Dysfunction of the innate immune system can be measured by ex vivo stimulation of whole blood with lipopolysaccharide (LPS), a bacterial endotoxin recognized by the Toll-like receptor (TLR)—4 on monocytes and a potent stimulant of inflammation. Studies have shown a correlation between innate immune dysfunction and poor outcome in adult and pediatric intensive care unit (PICU) populations. In a recent study of 70 critically ill children, 34% were found to have immunoparalysis, as demonstrated by markedly decreased production of TNF-α following ex vivo LPS stimulation of whole blood. These patients were at higher risk for hospital-acquired infection (OR 3.3; 95% CI 1.8 to 6.0, $p \leq 0.0002$) and death (OR 5.8; 95% CI 2.1 to 16, $p \leq 0.0002$).[3] In another recent multicenter study of children with life-threatening influenza, a disease in which bacterial coinfection is common and implies a degree of impaired immunity, patients with influenza had significantly lower TNF-α production with ex vivo LPS stimulation than healthy controls ($p<0.0001$). Furthermore, nonsurvivors had strikingly decreased capacity to produce TNF-α compared to survivors ($p<0.0001$), and those patients who presented with *Staphylococcus aureus* coinfection had evidence of significant innate immune dysfunction when compared with those without any coinfection and those with coinfection with bacteria other than *S. aureus* ($p=0.0012$).[4] A variety of nutritional deficiencies affect innate immunity and some of the potential macro- and micronutrients involved will be discussed in subsequent sections of this chapter.

Adaptive Immunity

The adaptive immune system is composed of T- and B-lymphocytes and is responsible for propagation of the immune response and building of immune memory. Lymphocytes require innate immune cells for activation via antigen presentation and secretion of cytokines and chemokines. With each subsequent exposure to the same antigen, the response of adaptive immune cells is faster and more robust. The activation of the adaptive immune response, in contrast to the innate immune response, peaks days to weeks following illness.[1]

The adaptive immune system can be divided into 2 main classes of lymphocytes. Activated B-lymphocytes, or plasma cells, produce antibodies that bind to antigens via the Fc receptor and are then recognized by the innate immune cells, further activating this system. T-lymphocytes function as CD8-positive cytotoxic cells, participating in lysis of target cells, or CD4-positive helper or regulatory cells, which modulate the immune response by secretion of either pro- or anti-inflammatory cytokines. T-helper 1 (T_H1) cells are considered pro-inflammatory, secreting IFN-γ, and granulocyte macrophage colony-stimulating factor (GM-CSF), which activate innate immune cells and promote B-cell antibody production. T-helper 2 (T_H2) cells, on the other hand, are considered more anti-inflammatory, producing cytokines such as IL-10 and TGF-β, which inhibit macrophage and monocyte activation. Regulatory T-cells (T_{reg}) cells are the most pronounced anti-inflammatory cells, secreting large amounts of IL-10 and TGF-β, as well as inhibiting pro inflammatory cells through direct cell contact.[3]

In the setting of critical illness, a variety of disturbances in adaptive immunity may occur. Initially in the septic patient, there is a local inflammatory response, with robust activation of pro-inflammatory innate immune cells and predominance of T_H1 lymphocytes. This is necessary for adequate phagocytosis and killing of pathogens, antigen presentation to lymphocytes, opsonization, and cytokine and chemokine production that result in containment of the offending organism. However, it has been well described that unopposed or overly robust inflammation in itself causes organ damage and leads to multiple organ dysfunction and the systemic inflammatory response syndrome (SIRS). In fact, high systemic IL-6 levels have been correlated with poor outcome in multiple studies in both adults and children.[1,5] Therapies targeting inhibition of this hyperinflammation have not been successful, likely because the complex interaction between inflammatory mediators is incompletely understood, and we have not yet developed the ability to tailor the degree of inhibition of inflammation to prevent overt immunosuppression.

More recently, there has been recognition of the detrimental effects of predominance of the anti-inflammatory component, or CARS, in which there is a predominance of T_H2 cells and, therefore, increased susceptibility to infection. Following traumatic injury or surgery, there seems to be a shift toward T_H2 predominance, and it is known that these patients are at high risk of developing hospital-acquired infections.[6,7] In the patient with sepsis, although the initial response is that of inflammation, as described earlier, there can be subsequent development of CARS in a subpopulation of septic patients. This has been reflected on a genomic level, with children with septic shock exhibiting repression of genes related to adaptive immunity, including T-cell immunity and major histocompatibility complex (MHC) antigen presentation.[8,9] Again, baseline nutritional status of patients, such as the presence or absence of protein-energy malnutrition, can have significant effects on the function of the adaptive immune system, and in the setting of critical illness, there can quickly develop relative nutrient deficiencies that negatively affect the immune system.

IMMUNOLOGIC EFFECTS OF NUTRIENTS

Both macronutrients and micronutrients can exert immunologic effects.

Macronutrients

The predominant macronutrients with immunologic effects include individual amino acids and omega-3 fatty acids.

Glutamine

Glutamine (GLN), the most abundant amino acid (AA) in plasma and the free intracellular AA pool in skeletal muscle, is now regarded as conditionally essential in certain clinical situations where endogenous synthesis becomes insufficient to maintain both pools.[10,11] As a preferred substrate for enterocytes, GLN has been shown to support the normal immunological structure and function of the gastrointestinal tract.[12] In animal studies, GLN deprivation is associated with loss of intestinal epithelial integrity, while GLN supplementation decreases gut mucosal atrophy during parenteral nutrition (PN),[13] preserves both intestinal and extra-intestinal immunoglobulin A (IgA) levels, prevents lymphocyte and glutathione depletion in the Peyer patches, and does not increase nitric oxide production induced by pro-inflammatory cytokines. However, with respect to bacterial translocation in animal models, studies of parenteral or enteral GLN-supplemented formulas show mixed results. Some have shown decreased bacterial translocation; others have demonstrated no such effect. Others have demonstrated that GLN administration in animals can protect against septic shock following endotoxemia. This protection may be mediated via enhanced tissue heat shock protein (HSP) expression and/or attenuated pro-inflammatory cytokine release.[14] Tissue levels of adenosine triphosphate (ATP) and adenosine diphosphate (ADP) are commonly depleted during shock and may lead to cell death or apoptosis. In shock and myocardial injury reperfusion models, GLN supplementation preserves glutathione levels, ATP/ADP ratio, nicotinamide adenine dinucleotide (NAD^+/NADH) content, and reduces lactate accumulation.[15,16] Regardless of the mechanism, several animal studies have demonstrated improved survival associated with GLN supplementation in models of sepsis.

Heat shock protein expression is vital to cellular and tissue protection after stress or injury, and its absence leads to increased cellular apoptosis. Recent animal and human studies have demonstrated that GLN may enhance tissue HSP expression and reduce inflammatory cytokine release, and that these increased levels are correlated with a decreased length of hospital stay and ventilator time in critically ill patients.[16] Emerging evidence also suggests that some of the benefit of GLN supplementation may be as a consequence of its role as an important precursor for the endogenous synthesis of arginine through an intestinal-renal pathway involving interorgan transport of citrulline.[17] In addition, recent studies suggest that GLN may reduce insulin resistance, another mechanism by which it may confer beneficial effects.

In children, there are several clinical trials of GLN supplementation in heterogeneous patient populations, ranging from neonates to adolescents. However, high-quality randomized clinical trials (RCTs) are scarce and have shown conflicting results, likely partly due to different effects of enteral and parenteral GLN supplementation. These trials have included premature infants; infants with gastrointestinal disease; and children with Crohn disease, short-bowel syndrome, malnutrition/diarrhea, different types of cancer, critical illness such as severe sepsis, burns and major trauma, sickle cell anemia, cystic fibrosis, and diabetes. Moreover, methodological issues have been noted in some studies.[18] There is currently insufficient evidence to recommend routine GLN supplementation in children. A better understanding of the mechanisms of GLN will help us to identify the subpopulations of pediatric patients in whom GLN may or may not be beneficial. Given the abundant evidence demonstrating the safety of GLN therapy in all clinical scenarios, eventual evaluation in specific subgroups of children is warranted.

Glutamine in Specific Pediatric Patient Populations

Glutamine has received ample attention in various pediatric populations and conditions.

Premature infants. The fetus in utero receives a large amount of AA nitrogen from the mother, of which GLN is a major component. Glutamine is the most prevalent free AA in milk and in colostrum. The infant is then dependent on endogenous synthesis and an exogenous supply of GLN to meet the high metabolic demands during the first few months of life. Unfortunately, GLN biosynthetic pathways frequently cannot meet the increased demands of the GLN metabolizing tissue. Acutely stressed, low-birth-weight (LBW) infants transiently suppress the rate of whole-body GLN synthesis during the immediate neonatal period. Oral feeding, or enteral nutrition (EN), is limited in the first 2 to 3 weeks of life because of gastrointestinal immaturity and susceptibility to feeding intolerance, as well as necrotizing enterocolitis (NEC), a serious condition that is associated with preterm and very LBW (VLBW) births, hypoxia, or respiratory distress. Therefore, premature infants may not receive adequate amounts of GLN, and parenteral GLN may be necessary to enhance GLN intake.[19]

Glutamine and tolerance to oral feeding. Parenteral nutrition is one of the most important ways to supply nutrition and energy to premature infants; even so, maturation of their gastrointestinal tract to ensure early weaning from PN to oral feeding as soon as possible should be promoted. Small intestinal epithelia are strongly dependent on an external GLN supply because of the relatively small cellular GLN pool compared with liver or skeletal muscle.[20] Providing GLN supplementation to premature infants improves the tolerance to oral feeding, shortens duration of PN, and results in shorter time to full oral feeds. In addition, GLN supplementation increases serum gastrin level and percentage of fast waves in electrogastrography, suggesting GLN supplementation may contribute to improved intestinal cell maturation and nutrient absorption.

In general, comparisons between all the GLN-EN studies may be hampered by the use of different feeding guidelines for both the introduction of and the reduction or withholding of EN. Because tolerance to enteral feeds depends on a number of factors, such as severity of preceding illness, duration of PN, type of EN, perturbations in mesenteric blood flow, and gastrointestinal motility, the data from these heterogeneous studies in infants are inconclusive.

Glutamine, sepsis, severe sepsis, and necrotizing enterocolitis. Three randomized studies of GLN-EN have been performed in preterm infants. Neu et al.[21] and van den Berg et al.[22] conducted single-center trials, and Vaughn et al.[23] reported a large multicenter trial with 20 participating hospitals. A lower incidence of hospital-acquired sepsis in GLN-supplemented VLBW infants was described by Neu et al. and van den Berg et al.[21,22] The multicenter trial, however, did not demonstrate a lower incidence of sepsis among infants treated with GLN-EN.[23]

Glutamine-enteral nutrition may lead to less atopic dermatitis during the first year of life of VLBW infants by enhancing maturation of the immune response, as demonstrated by van den Berg et al.,[22] but there was no effect on the incidence of bronchial hyper-reactivity and infectious diseases. A multicenter, double-blind RCT on extremely LBW infants conducted by Poindexter et al.[24] failed to show any effect from GLN-PN on NEC, and a recent meta-analysis of GLN supplementation in preterm infants did not reveal evidence of benefit on clinically important outcomes.[25]

Dosing of glutamine in children. Infusions of GLN at doses up to 0.48 g/kg per day have been well tolerated in infants without any apparent complications.[26] However, there are no dosing studies on GLN supplementation in different pediatric patient populations. Furthermore, intravenous (IV) GLN is currently not available for use outside research studies in the United States.

Current evidence on glutamine supplementation. Various systematic reviews and meta-analyses of RCTs performed in adult ICU patients have suggested that GLN supplementation may be associated with significant benefit on mortality, length of stay, and infectious morbidity in critical illness. However, in the recently published REducing Deaths due to OXidative Stress (REDOXS) study,[27] a blinded 2 × 2 factorial trial involving 40 ICUs in North America and Europe, 1,223 mechanically ventilated adult patients with multiorgan failure (MOF) were enrolled. High doses (0.35 g/kg per day) of IV GLN, provided as 0.5 g/kg per day of the dipeptide alanyl-glutamine [Dipeptiven, Fresenius Kabi] and an additional 30 g/day by enteral route, were administered in the treatment group and caused worse outcomes. In fact, GLN-supplemented patients exhibited a high hospital mortality (37.2% vs. 31.0%, p=0.02, in supplemented and nonsupplemented patients, respectively). Furthermore, 6-month mortality was significantly higher in patients who received GLN (43.7% vs. 37.2%, p=0.02). Of note, presupplementation GLN levels were within the normal range, which was an unexplained finding in patients with MOF.[27]

Recommendation. Based on the results of the REDOXS study, administration of PN/EN GLN must be avoided in patients with MOF. However, adult patients *without* MOF should receive PN GLN if available, as this strategy has demonstrated improved clinical outcomes in adults. Future research should define whether a baseline measurement of plasma GLN is required to guide exogenous GLN administration, depending on whether the patient admitted to the ICU is GLN deficient or not. Studies specific to pediatrics are required before routine GLN supplementation can be recommended in this patient population.

Arginine

Arginine is a basic AA that can be classified as "conditionally essential," meaning that under certain circumstances, i.e., critical illness, it becomes essential and deficiency can be detrimental. It is, fundamentally, a donor of nitric oxide (NO) and is the sole AA substrate used for its production.[28] It therefore plays an integral part in the pro-inflammatory response. Nitric oxide production by inducible nitric oxide synthase (iNOS) is stimulated by endotoxin and by T_H1 cytokines, such as IL-1, TNF-α, and IFN-γ. Expression of iNOS increases the generation of NO, resulting in vasodilation, as well as enabling the killing of pathogens. The availability of arginine is regulated by the enzyme arginase 1, expressed in myeloid cells. Arginase 1 expression is induced by T_H2 cytokines (IL-4 and IL-13), as well as IL-6, IL-10, TGF-β, catecholamines, and prostaglandins. Arginase is involved in the urea cycle, generating ornithine and urea. Ornithine plays an important role in wound healing and cell proliferation.[2,28] Activation of arginase results in depletion of arginine and effectively suppresses arginine-dependent functions. Cells expressing arginase are therefore termed myeloid suppressor cells (MSCs).[28] It has been found that in the setting of sepsis, iNOS is predominantly expressed, whereas arginase is induced following trauma and in some cancers.

T-lymphocytes require arginine for proliferation and the development of immune memory, though this appears to be through a mechanism distinct from iNOS or arginase induction. With arginine deficiency, the number of T-cell receptors on the cell membrane is decreased via decreased expression of the ζ-chain peptide component of the T-cell receptor complex. Therefore, in states of high arginase 1 expression or depletion of arginine stores by increased iNOS expression, T-cell function is compromised.[28]

Interestingly, neither myeloid cells nor T-lymphocytes utilize arginine under resting conditions. Myeloid cells do not express high-affinity cell membrane arginine transporters, nor do they express iNOS or arginase until stimulated. Likewise, T-lymphocytes have minimal uptake of arginine under normal circumstances, but with activation, there is marked up-regulation of transport mechanisms, resulting in T-cell proliferation.[28] Thus, dietary supplementation with arginine is likely to be beneficial only in the acute phase and under circumstances where the immunosuppression associated with depletion of arginine is detrimental.

Current evidence on arginine supplementation. This principle of differential response of myeloid cells to stimuli leading to either pro- or anti-inflammatory effects based on stimulation of iNOS or arginase expression, depending on the clinical circumstance, has been reflected in clinical trials of arginine supplementation. Trauma and surgery induce a primarily T_H2-dominated response, stimulating production of arginase and, therefore, depletion of arginine, leading to immunosuppression. These patients are at high risk of developing hospital-acquired infection, and supplementation with arginine has been shown to be beneficial in a variety of adult surgical populations. Two recent meta-analyses have demonstrated that immunonutrition with formulas containing arginine resulted in decreased risk of acquired infections (OR 0.49; 95% CI 0.39-0.62, $p<0.0001$), wound complications (OR 0.60; 95% CI 0.40-0.91, $p=0.02$), and length of stay (LOS) (−3.03 days; 95% CI −3.43 to −2.64 days, $p<0.0001$).[6] Arginine supplementation in the context of an immunomodulating formula containing fish oil and antioxidants, +/− nucleotides) is now recommended by both the American Society for Parenteral and Enteral Nutrition (A.S.P.E.N.) and its European counterpart, the European Society for Clinical Nutrition and Metabolism (ESPEN) for treatment of patients undergoing elective surgery, as well as trauma patients.[2] On the other hand, in patients in whom there is already potential overexpression of pro-inflammatory mediators and iNOS is already highly active, such as patients with sepsis or septic shock, arginine supplementation may, in fact, be detrimental. A meta-analysis of adult ICU patients receiving arginine supplementation via an immune-enhancing diet showed no benefit, and perhaps even a potential for causing harm in the nontrauma patients.[29] Since then, other meta-analyses have not borne out this trend, but concerns remain given the potential for arginine supplementation to promote the generation of NO and subsequent production of peroxynitrite.[2]

In the pediatric literature, there are very few studies of arginine supplementation in critically ill children. In one study of 28 children admitted to a burn unit, the arginine-supplemented group had increased mitogen-stimulated lymphocyte proliferation on day 7 of injury. This study was not powered to detect changes in clinically significant outcomes.[30]

Recommendation. At this time, recommendations for supplementing critically ill children with arginine cannot be made, and further studies are needed.

Omega-3 Fatty Acids

Eicosapentaenoic acid (EPA) and docosahexaenoic acid (DHA) are ω-3 polyunsaturated fatty acids (PUFAs) found in fish oil supplements. Immunomodulation with the ω-3 PUFAs, EPA, and DHA is accomplished via modification of leukocyte activity; down-regulation of expression of NF-κB, peroxisome proliferator-activated receptor γ (PPAR-γ), intracellular adhesion molecule 1 (ICAM-1), and E-selectin; and decreasing cytokine production.[31] In a recent systematic review and meta-analysis of studies supplementing IV fat emulsions (IVFEs) rich in fish oils in critically ill adults, it has been demonstrated that these IVFEs may be capable of decreasing mortality and ventilation days.[31] However, so far, few data are available on the role of IVFE in critically ill children. Larsen et al.[32] conducted an RCT of 2 IVFEs in critically ill neonates having open heart surgery with cardiopulmonary bypass. They reported that supplementation with the IVFE containing 50% medium-chain triglycerides (MCTs), 40% long-chain triglycerides (LCTs) from soybean oil, and 10% fish oil (EPA+DHA) decreased plasma TNF-α levels in those neonates who developed severe sepsis in the postoperative period. This finding suggested that lipid emulsions containing EPA and DHA may reduce systemic inflammation in critically ill infants.

Regarding enteral formulas rich in EPA and DHA, there are no clinical trials in critically ill children. In one systematic review and meta-analysis in critically ill adults, the use of an enteral formula supplemented with fish oils (EPA), borage oils (γ-linolenic acid, or GLA), and antioxidants in patients with acute lung injury (ALI) and acute respiratory distress syndrome (ARDS) was associated with a reduction in mortality and the incidence of new organ dysfunction.[33] Subsequently, the INTERSEPT study (Investigating Nutritional Therapy with EPA, GLA and Antioxidants Role in Sepsis Treatment)[34] found that enteral supplementation with EPA/GLA and antioxidants may play a beneficial role in enterally fed patients during the early stages of sepsis, decreasing the progression of sepsis-related organ dysfunction, in particular, hemodynamic and pulmonary dysfunction.

Recommendation. According to current evidence, enteral formulas with EPA+GLA and antioxidants should be considered in adult ARDS patients.[35] However, the supplementation portion of a 2 × 2 factorial trial of early vs. late EN combined with supplementation with ω-3 fatty acids, GLA, and antioxidants in adults with ARDS (EDEN-Omega)[36] was halted for futility, and a planned pediatric follow-up study was not initiated based on these results. Currently, there is no evidence in the critically ill pediatric population that supplementation with fish oil is beneficial and, therefore, cannot be recommended.

Micronutrients

Various micronutrients, including selenium, zinc, and vitamin C, possess immunomodulatory properties.

Selenium

Selenium (Se) is an essential trace element with antioxidant, immunological and anti-inflammatory properties.[37] Evidence suggests that Se affects both the cell-mediated and humoral aspects of immune function that are linked to inflammatory processes involving the production of reactive oxygen species and redox control processes.[38] Selenium exerts its biological role largely through its presence in selenoproteins, where Se is incorporated into selenocysteine.[39] These selenoproteins have numerous biological functions, especially related to redox signaling, the antioxidant defense system, thyroid hormone metabolism, and the immune response.[40]

Selenium has been demonstrated to inhibit the activation of nuclear factor kappa B (NF-KB), thus modulating selenoprotein and pro-inflammatory cytokine gene expression and exhibiting anti-inflammatory properties.[41] Decreased serum selenium levels in patients with SIRS have been associated with high levels of C-reactive protein (CRP). Recently, Valenta et al.[42] have shown that high-dose selenite supplementation is able to reduce CRP levels, demonstrating its anti-inflammatory effect. Selenium also has an important role in thyroid hormone metabolism. Thioredoxin reductases and iodothyronine deiodinases are selenoenzymes also involved in redox reactions, and it has been shown that low plasma Se levels in critically ill patients correlate with low T_3 levels, though the clinical significance of this remains to be determined.[43]

Selenium deficiency. Common clinical presentations of Se deficiency are congestive cardiomyopathy and myositis.[37] Selenium deficiency was first linked to cardiomyopathy in China (Keshan disease), where there is low soil Se content.[44] Arthritis has also been associated with Se deficiency (Kashin-Beck disease). Additional symptoms of Se deficiency include loss of pigmentation in hair and skin and macrocytosis. Increased transaminases and creatine kinase have been noted in patients on long-term PN without Se supplementation. Clinical states that are associated with Se deficiency and can contribute to the onset of related symptoms are cystic fibrosis, some types of cancer, acquired immunodeficiency syndrome, and burns.

Systemic inflammatory response syndrome is associated with redistribution of micronutrients (vitamins and trace elements) from the circulating compartment to the interstitial compartment and different tissues.[45] Trace elements escape into the interstitial compartment via the capillary leakage characteristic of SIRS. Furthermore, low levels of trace elements may be explained by several other causes, such as losses through biological fluids, hemodilution, previous insufficient intake, low levels in enteral formulas and parenteral mixtures, and continuous renal replacement therapies.[46] Heidemann et al.[47] evaluated serum Se concentration in 278 critically ill children within the first 72 hrs after admission to a PICU. In those patients, Se levels in the serum ranged from 26 to 145 ng/mL and were below normal in 56.1% of children. Selenium levels were inversely associated with measures of illness severity, and those children with an admission diagnosis of infection or sepsis were more likely to have low baseline Se levels than those with other diagnoses (63.2% vs. 42.7%, p=0.001). However, the clinical implications of these findings remain unclear. In a recent meta-analysis of studies of 5 RCTs of Se supplementation in septic adult patients, there was no difference in mortality, hospital-acquired pneumonia, or length of ICU stay.[48]

Dosing of selenium supplementation and monitoring guidance. Normal serum Se levels are in the range 46 to 143 mcg/L (0.61 to 1.9 mmol/L), depending on the geographic area around the world. Adequate intakes in infants range from 10 to 15 mcg/d, while 55 mcg/d is the recommended dietary allowance for adults. Estimates of parenteral sodium selenite or selenious acid requirements for infants vary. It has been suggested that up to 3 mcg/kg per day (0.04 mmol/kg per day) is sufficient to optimize plasma levels. Preterm and term infants can be given up to 30 mcg/d if receiving PN for longer than 4 weeks. In VLBW infants, a daily dose of 5 to 7 mcg/kg per day has been recommended.[49] After the sixth month of life, Se requirements are similar to the adult range. Since the major route of Se excretion is via the kidneys, the Se daily dose in PN must be reduced in patients with renal dysfunction.[50]

During short-term PN, serum or plasma Se levels appear to be the best indicator of Se status. However, it is important to realize that these Se levels reflect acute fluxes between body compartments rather than recent dietary intake. Therefore, selenoprotein P and plasma glutathione peroxidase (GPx-3) activities are more accurate than plasma Se concentrations. Glutathione peroxidase accounts for 30% of plasma Se, and erythrocyte GPx reflects long-term Se status.[51,52] In addition, selenoprotein P, which accounts for up to 60% of Se in plasma, has been shown to be responsive to changes in dietary intake.[53]

However, selenoprotein P is difficult to measure and currently it is not easily available.

Selenium toxicity. Toxicity is highly variable between selenocompounds, and selenite (sodium selenite or selenious acid) is recognized as the most pro-oxidative selenocompound. However, current published human data on Se toxicity resulting from chronic Se excess cannot be extrapolated to short-term PN supplementation. So far, there are no reports of Se toxicity from selenium-supplemented PN or EN, nor from high-dose Se regimens in the ICU, where patients are already Se depleted or exhibit low plasma levels and supplementation has not been given for more than 10 to 14 days.

Recommendation. For children on PN, the recommended Se daily dose depends on age. The recommended PN intake for all preterm/term infants and children is 2 mcg/kg per day.[54,55] In addition, preterm and term infants can be given up to 30 mcg/day (0.4 mmol) for long-term PN. By the sixth month of life, requirements begin to enter the adult range of 100 mcg/day.[49]

In critically ill adult patients with SIRS, a loading dose of 2000 mcg as an IV bolus plus a continuous infusion of 1000 mg over 10 to 14 days has been safely provided. However, there are currently insufficient data to routinely recommend PN Se supplementation for adults or children beyond the daily requirements for patients on PN.

Zinc

Zinc is an essential trace element that is required for normal growth and development, neurocognitive function, glucose homeostasis, response to oxidative stress, and immune function. Although it is present in minute quantities in the body (<0.01% of total body weight), its levels are tightly controlled via intestinal absorption and renal and fecal excretion. Zinc is primarily stored in muscle and bone, with the remainder being found in skin and liver, and only a very small proportion (0.1%) is present in plasma.[56]

Intact zinc homeostasis is required for normal function of both the innate and adaptive immune systems. Zinc deficiency results in impaired NK cell and phagocytic cell function, as well as decreased secretion of IFN-γ, TNF-α, and IL-2, all necessary for effective innate immune function. There is decreased production of IL-12 by macrophages and monocytes, and along with decreased IFN-γ this leads to impaired killing of parasites, viruses, and bacteria.[57] The impaired innate immunity is in part secondary to the loss of both T- and B-cell function that is characteristic of zinc deficiency. This loss occurs via increased apoptosis of pre-B and T-cells. Interestingly, most T_H2 cytokines are not affected by zinc deficiency, except IL-10, which may actually be increased. Overall, there is a shift from proinflammatory T_H1 to T_H2 predominance. However, there is also stress and activation of macrophages and monocytes, resulting in increased levels of IL-1β, IL-6, IL-8, and TNF-α. In animal studies, zinc deficiency is associated with increased inflammation, organ damage, and mortality in a murine model of sepsis, and zinc repletion shortly before injury mitigates these effects.[58] The mechanism for this is being elucidated in ongoing studies.

In developing countries, where dietary zinc deficiency is relatively common, oral zinc supplementation has been shown to decrease the incidence of diarrhea and acute lower respiratory tract infections; zinc also decreases the duration and severity of diarrheal illness.[59] Decreased levels of plasma zinc have been shown to be prevalent among the critically ill, and evidence is mounting that supplementation of zinc has the potential for beneficial effects in this population in both adult and pediatric patients. The differential regulation of a large number of genes dependent on intact zinc homeostasis or playing a direct role in zinc homeostasis has been demonstrated on day 1 of illness among children with septic shock.[9] In this population, zinc levels of nonsurvivors were significantly lower than those of survivors ($p<0.05$). A subsequent study of 20 critically ill children confirmed the finding of low zinc levels, with 100% having low levels.[5] Furthermore, there was an inverse correlation between zinc levels and measures of inflammation such as CRP ($r=-0.75$, $p=0.01$) and IL-6 ($r=-0.53$, $p=0.04$). On day 3 of illness, patients with 2 or more organ failures had lower plasma zinc concentrations than those with 1 or no organ failure ($p=0.03$). In the recently completed CRISIS (Critical Illness Stress Induced Immune Suppression) trial, a prospective, randomized trial of Se, zinc, GLN, and metoclopramide supplementation in critically ill children, baseline zinc levels were found to be low in 84% of patients.[60] The trial was halted for futility, and one cannot draw any conclusions about the specific effect of zinc on this patient population since it was part of a "cocktail" of nutrients. In a meta-analysis of 4 trials of zinc supplementation, Heyland et al found no effect of zinc supplementation on length of stay, infections, ventilator days, or mortality.[59] Only one of the studies, however, used zinc as the sole supplement.

Dosing and toxicity of zinc supplementation. Standard parenteral dosing of zinc under normal circumstances is 200 mcg/kg per day. Under conditions of known excess losses, such as those patients with burns or multiple open wounds, additional supplementation can be considered, though appropriate dosing has not been determined. Zinc is generally well tolerated, though nausea and gastrointestinal discomfort are relatively common with enteral administration. Toxicity with PN supplementation has been reported only with very large unintentional ingestions, manifested by fever, anemia, and pancreatitis.[61] Adult trials of supplementation have used over 500 mcg/kg per day parenterally without deleterious effect.[62]

Recommendation. The many biologic roles of zinc in inflammation and immunity provide a rationale for zinc supplementation in critically ill children. To date, however, there have been no published clinical trials of zinc supplementation alone in this patient population. A dose-finding and safety study has recently been completed whose results may guide future interventional trials for this promising therapy, but currently, routine supplementation of zinc beyond standard daily requirements cannot be recommended.

Vitamin C

Vitamin C (ascorbic acid, ascorbate) is a water-soluble, essential micronutrient that serves as a co-factor in many chemical pathways. Its most important biochemical function is to act as a reducing agent.[63] Vitamin C acts as a cofactor for various enzymes, including those involved in collagen hydroxylation, norepinephrine synthesis, metabolism of cholesterol, and hydroxylation of cortisol. Ascorbic acid is well absorbed in the small intestine, and excess amounts of ascorbic acid are excreted in urine. Deficiency of vitamin C leads to scurvy, which has multiple symptoms and signs, including perifollicular petechiae, bruising, gingivitis, glossitis, arthralgia, and impaired wound healing. In addition, in infants, there may be impaired bone growth and/or scurvy, including perifollicular petechiae and ecchymosis.

Vitamin C in the critically ill. Various studies in critically ill adults suggest that patients with sepsis and severe sepsis or following severe trauma exhibit a significant reduction in circulating ascorbate levels and a depletion of antioxidant capacity.[64] In this context, IV high-dose vitamin C inhibits endotoxin-induced endothelial dysfunction in humans and is able to reverse sepsis-induced suppression of microcirculatory control in animal models of septic shock.[65] Vitamin C supports endothelial NO synthase (NOS) activity, inhibiting inflammation-induced inducible NOS activity in endothelium.[66]

Vitamin C in major burns. Severe burns, defined as ≥30% of the body surface area, lead to endothelial dysfunction; severe fluid and protein leakage from the intravascular space to the interstitial space, inducing fluid retention; expansion of the extracellular space; and hypovolemic shock. In thermal injury, there is a significant reduction in plasma ascorbate levels and thus antioxidant capacity. Therefore, burn injury is a scenario in which the requirement for vitamin C is increased.

In animal models of burn injury, high-dose vitamin C treatment attenuates shock and reduces the risk of MOF. Dubick et al.[67] demonstrated a significant reduction in fluid resuscitation volumes following infusion of 250 mg/kg vitamin C in the first 500 mL of fluids and thereafter an IV infusion of vitamin C at 15 mg/kg per hour. This scheme of supplementation was associated with an improvement in antioxidant status.

In a controlled clinical study, Tanaka et al.[68] evaluated patients with ≥30% burns and treated them with vitamin C (66 mg/kg per hour) during the first 24 hrs. The 24-hr total fluid infusion volumes in the vitamin C group was significantly lower ($P<0.1$) when compared with the control group. Furthermore, fluid retention in the second 24 hrs and the length of mechanical ventilation were significantly lower in the intervention group ($P<0.05$ and $P<0.01$, respectively). In the burn population, therefore, it is reasonable to consider vitamin C supplementation, but again, evidence in pediatrics is lacking.

Vitamin C toxicity and adverse events. Excessive vitamin C may act as a pro-oxidant. In addition, vitamin C increases iron (Fe) absorption and free Fe can promote bacterial proliferation and can exacerbate hemochromatosis. Perhaps the most common side effect of excess vitamin C is hyperoxaluria with renal calculus formation, related to high urinary excretion.[69] Furthermore, high-dose administration may cause diarrhea and gastrointestinal intolerance, although it is generally well tolerated during short-term consumption.

Recommendation. Existing evidence seems to suggest that improved antioxidant capacity with vitamin C supplementation could improve the therapeutic strategy in the critically ill patients with SIRS. However, with the exception of patients with burns, vitamin C is not part of standard care in critically ill adult patients. Further research is warranted and should define the best and safe dose, target patient population, optimal timing, and duration of therapy to optimize the effects on underlying systemic inflammation.

CLINICAL TRIALS OF IMMUNONUTRITION

There have been several trials examining the role of immunonutrition in critically ill adults, while such studies have been fewer in critically ill children.

Adult Trials

Currently, the concept of immunonutrition means the administration of immune-modulating nutrients such as arginine, GLN, and ω-3 fatty acids, which are combined together with macronutrients and are provided in so-called immune-enhancing diets (IEDs) via the enteral route. Over the last 2 decades, several clinical trials have evaluated different IEDs in critically ill patients, although results have been controversial and sometimes contradictory. Current evidence suggests that IEDs can be used in major elective surgery, trauma, burns, head and neck cancer, and nonseptic critically ill patients on mechanical ventilation. In 2009, the A.S.P.E.N. guidelines suggested that IEDs may be provided to surgical critically ill patients (grade A) and medical critically ill patients (grade B).[70] These guidelines recommend that these diets be administered with caution in severe sepsis. In contrast, on the basis of 4 level 1 studies and 22 level 2 studies, which have demonstrated potential harm of IEDs in septic patients, the updated version of the Canadian Clinical Practice Guidelines recommends *against* using IEDs enriched with arginine in critically ill patients.[71]

Pediatric Trials

There have been very few clinical trials of immunonutrition in critically ill children. A pediatric version of the EDEN-Omega study from the adult ARDSNet group (see the section on ω-3 fatty acids earlier) was planned pending results of that study. Because it was halted for futility, the pediatric arm was never carried out. Similarly, the recent closure of the REDOXS trial by the Canadian Critical Care Trials group, whose hypothesis was that supplementation of critically ill patients with GLN and/or antioxidants would lead to improved outcomes, was halted for futility; further subgroup analysis showed a signal toward increased harm among the GLN-supplemented group.[27] Although a subsequent pediatric study had been designed and funding had been obtained, because of the results of the adult study, once again, the pediatric study will not be done. Indeed, a systematic review of existing clinical trials of immunonutrition in critically ill children did not find evidence of benefit.[72]

The largest trial of an immunomodulating formula in critically ill children was recently completed by the Collaborative Pediatric Critical Care Research Network (CPCCRN). This was a prospective, randomized trial of supplementation with enteral Se, GLN, and zinc and IV metoclopramide (a prolactin secretagogue with potential immunomodulatory effects) compared to an isonitrogenous whey protein supplement and IV saline. After enrollment of 293 subjects, the trial was halted for futility. There were several limitations to the trial design, however, including the use of enteral supplementation of nutrients in a population of patients whose gastric and small-bowel absorption is likely highly variable. In addition, whey protein, which was used in the control group, can itself be considered a potential pharmaconutrient; hence, the study was deemed a comparative effectiveness trial. Finally, by giving 4 pharmaconutrients at once, the potential beneficial effects of one may have been counteracted by potential harmful effects of another.[73] At this time, there is insufficient evidence to recommend routine immunonutrition in critically ill children.

CONCLUSION

Nutrition as a therapeutic modality is an important aspect of the care of critically ill children. The inflammatory response to and the functional changes in the immune system seen in the setting of trauma, surgery, infection, or other illness are complex and multifactorial. As understanding of the interactions between the nutritional status of the patient and the response to illness grows, not only the timing of feeding, but also the specific composition of nutrients appropriate to the individual patient will become standard of care. As the body of evidence on macro- and micronutrient supplementation increases, the hope is that intensivists will be able to modulate the pro- and anti-inflammatory response of the host and prevent both excessive inflammation and the subsequent immunoparalysis that can lead to hospital-acquired infections, ultimately improving patient outcomes.

KEY POINTS

- A functioning immune system is essential for survival, and an appropriate balance between the pro-inflammatory and anti-inflammatory response must be maintained.
- The provision of specific nutrients to manipulate the immune system, independent of caloric or macronutrient requirements for nutrition per se, has evolved as a therapeutic modality, and is known as immunonutrition.
- The components of the immune system can be modulated by certain macronutrients (GLN, arginine, and omega-3 fatty acids) and micronutrients (Se, zinc, and vitamin C). At this time, there is insufficient evidence to recommend routine immunonutrition in critically ill children.

REFERENCES

1. Hall MW. Immune Dysfunction in Sepsis. In: Rowin ME, ed. *Current Concepts in Pediatric Critical Care*. Mount Prospect, IL: Society of Critical Care Medicine; 2010:109-117.
2. Mizock BA. Immunonutrition and critical illness: an update. *Nutrition*. 2010;26(7-8):701-707.
3. Hall M, Knatz N, Vetterly C, et al. Immunoparalysis and nosocomial infection in children with multiple organ dysfunction syndrome. *Intensive Care Med*. 2011;37(3):525-532.
4. Hall MW, Geyer SM, Guo C-Y, et al. Innate immune function and mortality in critically ill children with influenza: a multicenter study. *Crit Care Med*. 2013;41(1):224-236.
5. Cvijanovich NZ, King JC, Flori HR, Gildengorin G, Wong HR. Zinc homeostasis in pediatric critical illness. *Pediatr Crit Care Med*. 2009;10(1):29-34.
6. Marik PE, Flemmer M. Immunonutrition in the surgical patient. *Minerva Anestesiol*. 2012;78(3):336-342.
7. Marik P, Zaloga G. Immunonutrition in critically ill patients: a systematic review and analysis of the literature. *Intensive Care Med*. 2008;34(11):1980-1990.
8. Wong HR, Cvijanovich N, Allen GL, et al. Genomic expression profiling across the pediatric systemic inflammatory response syndrome, sepsis, and septic shock spectrum. *Crit Care Med*. 2009;37(5):1558-1566.
9. Wong HR, Shanley TP, Sakthivel B, et al. Genome-level expression profiles in pediatric septic shock indicate a role for altered zinc homeostasis in poor outcome. *Physiol Genomics*. 2007;30(2):146-155.
10. Blomqvist BI, Hammarqvist F, von der Decken A, Wernerman J. Glutamine and alpha-ketoglutarate prevent the decrease in muscle free glutamine concentration and influence protein synthesis after total hip replacement. *Metabolism*. 1995;44(9):1215-1222.
11. Bergstrom J, Furst P, Noree LO, Vinnars E. Intracellular free amino acid concentration in human muscle tissue. *J Appl Physiol*. 1974;36(6):693-697.
12. Parry-Billings M, Evans J, Calder PC, Newsholme EA. Does glutamine contribute to immunosuppression after major burns? *Lancet*. 1990;336(8714):523-525.
13. Alverdy JA, Aoys E, Weiss-Carrington P, Burke DA. The effect of glutamine-enriched TPN on gut immune cellularity. *J Surg Res*. 1992;52(1):34-38.
14. Singleton KD, Beckey VE, Wischmeyer PE. Glutamine prevents activation of NF-KAPPAB and stress kinase pathways, attenuates inflammatory cytokine release, and prevents acute respiratory distress syndrome (ARDS) following sepsis. *Shock*. 2005;24(6):583-589.
15. Wischmeyer PE, Kahana M, Wolfson R, Ren H, Musch MM, Chang EB. Glutamine reduces cytokine release, organ damage, and mortality in a rat model of endotoxemia. *Shock*. 2001;16(5):398-402.
16. Zhao YJ, Wang H, Liu X, Sun M, Kazuhiro H. Protective effects of glutamine in a rat model of endotoxemia. *Mol Med Rep*. 2012;6(4):739-744.
17. Vermeulen MA, van de Poll MC, Ligthart-Melis GC, et al. Specific amino acids in the critically ill patient: exogenous glutamine/arginine: a common denominator? *Crit Care Med*. 2007;35(9 Suppl):S568-576.
18. Mok E, Hankard R. Glutamine supplementation in sick children: is it beneficial? *J Nutr Metab*. 2011:617597.
19. Voss M, Moore SW, van der Merwe I, Pieper C. Fulminanting necrotising enterocolitis: outcome and prognostic factors. *Pediatr Surg Int*. 1998;13(8):576-580.
20. Panigrahi P, Gewolb IH, Bamford P, Horvath K. Role of Glutamine in Bacterial Transcytosis and Epithelial Cell Injury. *J Parenter Enteral Nutr*. 1997;21(2):75-80.
21. Neu J. Glutamine in the fetus and critically ill low birth weight neonate: metabolism and mechanism of action. *J Nutr*. 2001;131(9 Suppl):2585S-2589S; discussion 2590S.
22. van den Berg A, van Elburg RM, Westerbeek EA, Twisk JW, Fetter WP. Glutamine-enriched enteral nutrition in very-low-birth-weight infants and effects on feeding tolerance and infectious morbidity: a randomized controlled trial. *Am J Clin Nutr*. 2005;81(6):1397-1404.
23. Vaughn P, Thomas P, Clark R, Neu J. Enteral glutamine supplementation and morbidity in low birth weight infants. *J Pediatr*. 2003;142(6):662-668.

24. Poindexter BB, Ehrenkranz RA, Stoll BJ, et al. Parenteral glutamine supplementation does not reduce the risk of mortality or late-onset sepsis in extremely low birth weight infants. *Pediatrics.* 2004;113(5):1209-1215.
25. Moe-Byrne T, Wagner JV, McGuire W. Glutamine supplementation to prevent morbidity and mortality in preterm infants. *Cochrane Database Syst Rev.* 3:CD001457.
26. Lacey JM, Crouch JB, Benfell K, et al. The effects of glutamine-supplemented parenteral nutrition in premature infants. *J Parenter Enteral Nutr.* 1996;20(1): 74-80.
27. Heyland D, Muscedere J, Wischmeyer PE, et al. A randomized trial of glutamine and antioxidants in critically ill patients. *N Engl J Med.* 2013;368(16):1489-1497.
28. Popovic PJ, Zeh HJ, Ochoa JB. Arginine and Immunity. *J Nutr.* 2007;137(6):1681S-1686S.
29. Heyland DK, Novak F. Immunonutrition in the critically ill patient: more harm than good? *J Parenter Enteral Nutr.* 2001;25(2 Suppl):S51-55; discussion S55-56.
30. Marin VB, Rodriguez-Osiac L, Schlessinger L, Villegas J, Lopez M, Castillo-Duran C. Controlled study of enteral arginine supplementation in burned children: impact on immunologic and metabolic status. *Nutrition.* 2006;22(7-8):705-712.
31. Manzanares W, Dhaliwal R, Jurewitsch B, Stapleton RD, Jeejeebhoy KN, Heyland DK. Parenteral fish oil lipid emulsions in the critically ill: a systematic review and meta-analysis. *J Parenter Enteral Nutr.* 2014;38(1):20-28.
32. Larsen BM, Goonewardene LA, Joffe AR, et al. Pretreatment with an intravenous lipid emulsion containing fish oil (eicosapentaenoic and docosahexaenoic acid) decreases inflammatory markers after open-heart surgery in infants: a randomized, controlled trial. *Clin Nutr.* 2013;31(3):322-329.
33. Pontes-Arruda A, Demichele S, Seth A, Singer P. The use of an inflammation-modulating diet in patients with acute lung injury or acute respiratory distress syndrome: a meta-analysis of outcome data. *J Parenter Enteral Nutr.* 2008;32(6):596-605.
34. Pontes-Arruda A, Martins LF, de Lima SM, et al. Enteral nutrition with eicosapentaenoic acid, gamma-linolenic acid and antioxidants in the early treatment of sepsis: results from a multicenter, prospective, randomized, double-blinded, controlled study: the INTERSEPT study. *Crit Care.* 2011;15(3):R144.
35. Nutrition CC. Immune Enhancing Diets. Section 4.1b(i) Fish Oils, Borage Oils, and Antioxidants. *Canadian Clinical Practice Guidelines*; http://www.criticalcarenutrition.com. Accessed June 28, 2013.
36. Rice TW, Wheeler AP, Thompson BT, deBoisblanc BP, Steingrub J, Rock P. Enteral omega-3 fatty acid, gamma-linolenic acid, and antioxidant supplementation in acute lung injury. *JAMA.* 2011;306(14):1574-1581.
37. Rayman MP. Selenium and human health. *Lancet.* 2012;379(9822):1256-1268.
38. Vincent JL, Forceville X. Critically elucidating the role of selenium. *Curr Opin Anaesthesiol.* 2008;21(2):148-154.
39. Fairweather-Tait SJ, Bao Y, Broadley MR, et al. Selenium in human health and disease. *Antioxid Redox Signal.* 2011;14(7):1337-1383.
40. Hardy G, Hardy I, Manzanares W. Selenium supplementation in the critically ill. *Nutr Clin Pract.* 2009;27(1):21-33.
41. Forceville X, van Antwerpen P. Selenocompounds and selenium:a biochemical approach to sepsis. In: Vincent JL, ed. *2008 Yearbook in Intensive Care and Emergency Medicine.* Berlin: Springer-Verlag; 2008:454-466.
42. Valenta J, Brodska H, Drabek T, Hendl J, Kazda A. High-dose selenium substitution in sepsis: a prospective randomized clinical trial. *Intensive Care Med.* 2011;37(5):808-815.
43. Angstwurm MW, Schopohl J, Gaertner R. Selenium substitution has no direct effect on thyroid hormone metabolism in critically ill patients. *Eur J Endocrinol.* 2004;151(1):47-54.
44. Hardy G, Hardy I. Selenium: the Se-XY nutraceutical. *Nutrition.* 2004;20(6):590-593.
45. Manzanares W, Hardy G. Selenium supplementation in the critically ill: posology and pharmacokinetics. *Curr Opin Clin Nutr Metab Care.* 2009;12(3):273-280.
46. Berger MM, Shenkin A. Update on clinical micronutrient supplementation studies in the critically ill. *Curr Opin Clin Nutr Metab Care.* 2006;9(6):711-716.
47. Heidemann SM, Holubkov R, Meert KL, et al. Baseline serum concentrations of zinc, selenium, and prolactin in critically ill children. *Pediatr Crit Care Med.* 2013;14(4):e202-206.
48. Kong Z, Wang F, Ji S, Deng X, Xia Z. Selenium supplementation for sepsis: a meta-analysis of randomized controlled trials. *Am J Emerg Med.* 2013;31(8):1170-1175.
49. Hardy G, Menendez AM, Manzanares W. Trace element supplementation in parenteral nutrition: pharmacy, posology, and monitoring guidance. *Nutrition.* 2009;25 (11-12):1073-1084.
50. Hardy G, Reilly C. Technical aspects of trace element supplementation. *Curr Opin Clin Nutr Metab Care.* 1999;2(4):277-285.

51. Harrison I, Littlejohn D, Fell GS. Distribution of selenium in human blood plasma and serum. *Analyst.* 1996;121(2):189-194.

52. Gao Y, Liu Y, Deng G, Wang Z. Distribution of selenium-containing proteins in human serum. *Biol Trace Elem Res.* 2004;100(2):105-115.

53. Burk RF, Hill KE. Selenoprotein P: an extracellular protein with unique physical characteristics and a role in selenium homeostasis. *Annu Rev Nutr.* 2005;25:215-235.

54. Shenkin A. Selenium in intravenous nutrition. *Gastroenterology.* 2009;137(5 Suppl):S61-69.

55. Greene HL, Hambidge KM, Schanler R, Tsang RC. Guidelines for the use of vitamins, trace elements, calcium, magnesium, and phosphorus in infants and children receiving total parenteral nutrition: report of the Subcommittee on Pediatric Parenteral Nutrient Requirements from the Committee on Clinical Practice Issues of the American Society for Clinical Nutrition. *Am J Clin Nutr.* 1988;48(5):1324-1342.

56. Cvijanovich N. Nutrition therapy in the pediatric ICU. In: Rowin ME, ed. *Current Concepts in Pediatric Critical Care.* Mount Prospect, IL: Society of Critical Care Medicine; 2010:39-48.

57. Prasad AS. Zinc: role in immunity, oxidative stress and chronic inflammation. *Curr Opin Clin Nutr Metab Care.* 2009;12(6):646-652.

58. Knoell DL, Julian MW, Bao S, et al. Zinc deficiency increases organ damage and mortality in a murine model of polymicrobial sepsis. *Crit Care Med.* 2009;37(4):1380-1388.

59. Heyland DK, Jones N, Cvijanovich NZ, Wong H. Zinc supplementation in critically ill patients: a key pharmaconutrient? *J Parenter Enteral Nutr.* 2008;32(5):509-519.

60. Heidemann SM, Holubkov R, Meert KL, et al. Baseline serum concentrations of zinc, selenium, and prolactin in critically ill children. *Pediatr Crit Care Med.* 2013;14(4):e202-206.

61. Gallery ED, Blomfield J, Dixon SR. Acute zinc toxicity in haemodialysis. *Br Med J.* 1972;4(5836):331-333.

62. Berger MM, Baines M, Raffoul W, et al. Trace element supplementation after major burns modulates antioxidant status and clinical course by way of increased tissue trace element concentrations. *Am J Clin Nutr.* 2007;85(5):1293-1300.

63. Fukushima R, Yamazaki E. Vitamin C requirement in surgical patients. *Curr Opin Clin Nutr Metab Care.* 2010;13(6):669-676.

64. Berger MM. Antioxidant micronutrients in major trauma and burns: evidence and practice. *Nutr Clin Pract.* 2006;21(5):438-449.

65. May JM. How does ascorbic acid prevent endothelial dysfunction? *Free Radic Biol Med.* 2000;28(9):1421-1429.

66. Baker TA, Milstien S, Katusic ZS. Effect of vitamin C on the availability of tetrahydrobiopterin in human endothelial cells. *J Cardiovasc Pharmacol.* 2001;37(3):333-338.

67. Dubick MA, Williams C, Elgjo GI, Kramer GC. High-dose vitamin C infusion reduces fluid requirements in the resuscitation of burn-injured sheep. *Shock.* 2005;24(2):139-144.

68. Tanaka H, Matsuda T, Miyagantani Y, Yukioka T, Matsuda H, Shimazaki S. Reduction of resuscitation fluid volumes in severely burned patients using ascorbic acid administration: a randomized, prospective study. *Arch Surg.* 2000;135(3):326-331.

69. Mashour S, Turner JF, Jr., Merrell R. Acute renal failure, oxalosis, and vitamin C supplementation: a case report and review of the literature. *Chest.* 2000;118(2):561-563.

70. McClave SA, Martindale RG, Vanek VW, et al. Guidelines for the Provision and Assessment of Nutrition Support Therapy in the Adult Critically Ill Patient: Society of Critical Care Medicine (SCCM) and American Society for Parenteral and Enteral Nutrition (A.S.P.E.N.). *J Parenter Enteral Nutr.* 2009;33(3):277-316.

71. Nutrition CC. EN Composition: Diets Supplemented with Arginine and Select Other Nutrients. *Canadian Clinical Practice Guidelines* 2013; http://www.criticalcarenutrition.com. Accessed June 28, 2013.

72. Briassouli E, Briassoulis G. Glutamine randomized studies in early life: the unsolved riddle of experimental and clinical studies. *Clin Dev Immunol.* 2012;2012:749189. Epub 2012 Sep 18.

73. Carcillo JA, Michael Dean J, Holubkov R, et al. The randomized comparative pediatric critical illness stress-induced immune suppression (CRISIS) prevention trial.* *Pediatr Crit Care Med.* 2012;13(2):165-173.

CHAPTER 20

Cancer and Hematopoietic Stem Cell Transplantation

Lori J. Bechard

Terezie Tolar Mosby

- INTRODUCTION
- NUTRITIONAL STATUS
  - Treatment Complications
- NUTRITIONAL ASSESSMENT
  - Assessment Techniques
- NUTRITION INTERVENTION AND MONITORING
  - Oral Intake
  - Artificial Nutrition Support
- CONCLUSIONS
- KEY POINTS
  - References

INTRODUCTION

A child with cancer faces nutritional challenges. The nutritional well-being of that child is a principal concern of parents and caregivers during all phases of treatment. Management of cancer and related diseases generally includes chemotherapy, radiation, and hematopoietic stem cell transplantation (HSCT) for resistant diseases. The disease itself, as well as its treatment, often lead to an immunocompromised state, thus increasing risk for critical illness and morbidity.

A detailed nutrition assessment is imperative to inform an individualized nutrition care plan that considers the unique concerns raised by a critically ill child with cancer. Limitations to the provision of nutrition may be related to organ function—especially gastrointestinal (GI) feeding tolerance—renal function, and cardiovascular status. Endocrine abnormalities, including hyperglycemia and hypertriglyceridemia, often result from steroids or calcineurin inhibitors used in cancer and HSCT treatment, and may be exacerbated by critical illness. Respiratory failure and sepsis are frequent reasons for admission to a pediatric intensive care unit (PICU) for children with oncologic diseases or following HSCT.[1] Multisystem organ failure may further affect adherence to a planned nutritional regimen.

NUTRITIONAL STATUS

Children and adolescents are at higher risk for development of malnutrition than are adults during cancer treatment due to the proportionally higher nutritional requirements during periods of growth and development. It is difficult to estimate the prevalence of malnutrition during treatment due to lack of uniform criteria and adequate studies.[2] Undernutrition at the time of diagnosis is relatively uncommon in high-income countries, but it continues to be a frequent problem in low-income countries.[3] Malnutrition during treatment depends on many factors, such as the specific tumor, extent of the disease, hospital resources, and treatment strategies. It is estimated that the rate of malnutrition in children with cancer is 0% to 10% for leukemia, 20% to 50% for neuroblastoma, and 0% to 30% for other malignancies.[2]

Nutritional status at diagnosis has prognostic implications. Well-nourished children tolerate intensive cancer treatment better than those who are malnourished and thus have better chances of survival and lower relapse rates.[4] Undernutrition is associated with higher rates of death due to abandonment of therapy, treatment failure,[5] and infectious complications.[6] Malnourished children are at an increased risk for treatment-related complications, reduced tolerance to therapy, altered drug metabolism, increased susceptibility to infection, and poorer treatment outcome. The impact of malnutrition may be more severe in younger children.

Obesity is an increasing problem among children undergoing treatment for cancer and related diseases.[7] A detailed account of childhood obesity, its associated morbidities, and nutritional management during critical illness are provided in chapter 21. Childhood obesity may be associated with hyperlipidemia, hypertension, acanthosis nigricans, diabetes and insulin resistance, hepatic steatosis, cholelithiasis, pseudotumor celebri, sleep apnea, and orthopedic abnormalities.[8] Children and adolescents who are obese are at increased risk for coronary heart disease, stroke, high blood pressure, diabetes, and other chronic diseases as they age.[9] These additional problems can complicate the care and management of obese children with cancer who are critically ill. There are few pharmacological studies describing the half-life, volume of distribution, or clearance of drugs in obese patients.[10] Risks of underdosing or overdosing medications in obese patients may result in poorer treatment outcome or greater toxicities.[10] In pediatric acute myeloblastic leukemia, obese patients have greater treatment-related mortality, similar toxicity and relapse rates, and inferior survival compared to those patients who are not obese.[11] Several studies have reported an association between obesity and mortality among children undergoing treatment for cancer, including HSCT.[12-15]

Treatment Complications

There are many nutrition-related side effects for patients who are undergoing chemotherapy, radiation, and HSCT; these side effects can result in poor nutrient intake and associated weight loss, malnutrition, or cachexia. Children may experience any or all of the following side effects: nausea, vomiting, diarrhea, constipation, altered taste, loss of appetite, mucositis, pancreatitis, colitis, and pneumatosis intestinalis. In addition, complications of treatment may include renal disease, infection, pancreatic insufficiency, hemorrhagic cystitis, and others. Patients undergoing HSCT are also at risk for graft-versus-host disease (GVHD) and veno-occlusive disease (VOD). Severe manifestations of these and other complications may lead to critical illness or multiorgan system disease.

Cancer Cachexia

Protein-energy malnutrition occurs in association with cancer as a result of inadequate intake, combined with the increased stress and catabolism that is caused by the disease and side effects of anticancer treatment. Inadequate energy intake is associated with loss of adipose tissue, which may be indicated by a reduction in skinfold thickness. Cancer cachexia, however, is a recognized condition where the cancer patient has experienced wasting of skeletal muscle tissue along with other components of lean body mass. Loss of muscle mass is associated with decreased functional capacity, increased toxicity of antineoplastic treatment, increased length of stay, and increased risk of nosocomial infections.[16] Cachectic patients also experience a disturbance in whole-protein homeostasis with net protein catabolism, negative nitrogen balance, a decrease in blood urea nitrogen (BUN), and a decrease in serum albumin levels. In the pediatric oncology population, cachexia is influenced by several factors, including type of disease, socioeconomic status, and type of treatment received by the patient. Critical illness may worsen cachexia.

According to Bauer, Jürgens, and Frühwald, "despite the well-documented need for adequate nutrition in long-term outcome in children with cancer, there are no applicable management strategies or pharmacotherapeutic options available at this time to successfully prevent or treat undernourishment and its associated disorders in this population."[17] Thus, the entire medical team must be vigilant and collaborate with caregivers to ensure that the child or adolescent on therapy or who has survived cancer receives optimal nutritional support.

Graft-Versus-Host Disease

Graft-versus-host disease is a complication related to an allogeneic HSCT. The immunoregulatory cells of the donor attack the patient's organs. This causes impaired function of the affected organ and increases the patient's susceptibility to infections. The goal of HSCT is to minimize risk of GVHD by increasing the odds of engraftment. To achieve this, the donor and patient are matched as closely as possible based on human leukocyte antigen (HLA) typing. Graft-versus-host disease can be considered acute or chronic, based on the clinical manifestation of the condition. Traditionally, the designation was determined based on number of days post-HSCT, with GVHD after 100 days being considered chronic. This practice is no longer recommended by the National Institutes of Health; instead, they recommend classification according to the clinical manifestation of the condition.[18]

Graft-versus-host disease can affect many different areas of the patient's body, including the skin, the entire GI tract, liver, and the lungs. Symptoms of GI GVHD could include dry mouth, decreased saliva leading to difficulty swallowing, and burning and discomfort when eating acidic foods. Lack of lubrication in glands in the stomach and intestines could interfere with nutrient absorption. Other common symptoms are nausea, vomiting, diarrhea, abdominal pain, and heartburn. Immunosuppressive medications, such as cyclosporine, mycophenolate, and steroids, are commonly used in the treatment of patients with GVHD. Patients with severe GVHD of the gut may experience high stool output and malabsorption of nutrients. It is recommended that a patient with severe GI GVHD follow a low-bacteria, lactose-free, and/or low-residue, bland diet. These patients may require enteral nutrition (EN) with an elemental formula, or parenteral nutrition (PN) support in cases of uncontrolled GVHD.

Veno-occlusive Disease

Veno-occlusive disease is a potentially serious condition of the liver that results from high doses of chemotherapy or radiation therapy given before HSCT; it is also referred to as sinusoidal obstruction syndrome (SOS). In VOD, the affected blood vessels in the liver swell or become obstructed, which impairs the ability of the liver to remove toxins, drugs, and waste products from the bloodstream. Fluid then accumulates in the liver, causing swelling of the liver and tenderness. Veno-occlusive disease commonly presents with tender hepatomegaly, hyperbilirubinemia, and ascites.[19] Signs and symptoms of VOD are most likely encountered within the first 4 weeks after the conditioning/preparative regimen for HSCT. Patients with VOD may experience rapid weight gain due to fluid accumulation and edema.

Treatment for VOD is generally supportive and usually requires aggressive fluid restriction to minimize fluid retention that may lead to respiratory and renal compromise. This fluid restriction often results in limiting the provision of nutrients. The nutritional intervention for VOD generally involves limiting fluid volume to provide only maintenance requirements, or even less to account for fluids provided with medications and colloid solutions. If PN is required, it must be concentrated so that nutrient needs can be approached or achieved within the volume restriction. A calorically dense formula may be indicated for patients with VOD who are enterally fed.

NUTRITIONAL ASSESSMENT

Nutritional assessment is important for the prevention, recognition, and early treatment of malnutrition. Many different techniques can be used to evaluate the nutritional status of adolescents and children. Choice of technique will depend upon the hospital resources, patient diagnosis, type of treatment, and other factors. Special attention should be paid to metabolic derangements of macronutrients leading to protein-energy malnutrition, as well as deficiencies of micronutrients such as vitamin D, vitamin K, zinc, copper, and selenium.

Screening should be performed within 24 hours of hospital admission for every patient and repeated regularly depending on the child's age, diagnosis, treatment, clinical status, and other risk factors. Risk for malnutrition can be identified by medical personnel, other caregivers, or periodic rescreening, using the criteria indicated in Table 20-1. For more details about nutrition screening, please see chapter 2. An in-depth nutritional assessment is indicated for children at risk for malnutrition.

Weight, height or length, and body mass index (BMI), or weight-for-height in children younger than 2 years, should be compared with reference values on age- and sex-specific growth charts. For children living in the United States and above the age of 2, growth charts created by the Centers for Disease Control and Prevention (CDC) should be used.[20] The World Health Organization (WHO) created the growth standard for children 0 to 2 years of age with data from children representing ethnicities and cultures around the world.[21] In the United States and worldwide, these standards

TABLE 20-1. Assessment of Nutritional Risk

Anthropometric Measurements

Weight Loss
- Greater than 5% weight loss over 30 days
- Current percentile for weight or height has fallen by 2 or more channels

Weight-for-Age
- Less than the 5th percentile or greater than the 85th percentile

Length- or Height-for-Age
- Less than the 5th percentile height-for-age (may indicate chronic malnutrition)

Weight-for-Length
- Less than the 5th percentile or greater than the 95th percentile weight-for-length (if less than 2 years of age)
- Less than the 5th percentile—underweight (indicator of inadequate weight gain)
- Greater than the 95th percentile—may be an indicator of obesity

Body Mass Index (BMI)
- Greater than the 95th percentile—obese
- Greater than the 85th percentile—overweight
- Less than the 15th percentile—undernourished
- Less than the 5th percentile—severely undernourished

Ideal Body Weight (IBW) Calculated from Weight-for-Length
- Greater than 110% IBW—overweight
- Eighty-five percent to eighty percent IBW—mild undernutrition
- Greater than 75% to 84% IBW—moderate undernutrition
- Less than 75% IBW—severe undernutrition

IBW Calculated from BMI
- Greater than 120% IBW—overweight
- Eighty percent to eighty-nine percent IBW—mild undernutrition
- Seventy percent IBW—moderate undernutrition
- Less than 70% IBW—severe undernutrition

Head Circumference-for-Age
- Greater than the 95th percentile (may indicate macrocephaly)
- Less than 5th percentile (may indicate microcephaly or chronic malnutrition during fetal development or during early childhood)

Arm Anthropometry
- Triceps skin fold estimation of energy stores—compare to reference values
- Mid-upper arm muscle circumference, indicator of lean body mass—compare to reference values

Nutrient Intake
- Less than 50% of estimated energy needs for up to 3 days
- Less than 80% of estimated energy needs for longer than 3 days

are now recommended for use in this age group. For children from other countries, the WHO charts should be used for children up to the age of 5.[22] Overweight and obesity classifications in the United States are based upon the CDC BMI-for-age growth charts for children and adolescents less than 20 years of age.[23] Using these comparative standards, the nutritional status of critically ill children with cancer can be evaluated as described in Table 20-2.

Both objective and subjective data should be used to complete a nutritional assessment. One marker alone is

TABLE 20-2. Evaluation of Nutritional Status for the Pediatric Oncology Patient (Adapted from Rogers et al.)

	Underweight*	Normal	Overweight	Obese
BMI	<5th percentile	5th to 85th percentile	>85th to 95th percentile	>95th percentile
WT/LT	<10th percentile	10th to 90th percentile	>90th percentile	

*Weight loss/gain may or may not be present.
For age <2 years: Use weight-for-length (Wt/Lt) percentile or corresponding Z-score
For age ≥2 years: Use Body Mass Index (BMI) percentile or corresponding Z-score
Adapted with permisison from Rogers PC, Melnick SJ, Ladas EJ, et al.: Children's Oncology Group (COG) *Nutrition Committee, Pediatr Blood Cancer* 2008;50(2 Suppl):447-450.

not adequate to evaluate nutritional status. A thorough evaluation should be conducted on all patients identified with risk for malnutrition. Nutritional assessment should be performed by a trained clinical nutrition professional, such as a registered dietitian. In hospitals where dietitians are not available, the physician or nurse needs to be trained in nutritional assessment. Nutritional assessment consists of 3 parts: data collection, data evaluation, and interpretation of findings.[24]

Assessment Techniques

Data collection for a nutritional assessment includes diagnosis, medical history, and a nutrition-focused physical examination. An evaluation of dietary intake and adequacy during cancer treatment is paramount. An understanding of the patient's nutritional status prior to hospitalization will provide important information useful in developing a nutrition plan for the acute condition. The nutrition-focused physical examination of an adolescent or child with cancer is an essential part of a nutritional assessment and should never be omitted. This exam should include the patient's general appearance and activity level. In the critical care setting, activity is often limited to cares, but should be considered nonetheless. The clinician should also examine the patient and look for the presence of edema, ascites, cachexia, obesity, skin changes, dry mucous membranes, petechia or ecchymosis, healing of wounds, glossitis, stomatitis, and cheilosis.

There are some important considerations to data evaluation and interpretation for the nutritional assessment of children in critical care settings. Most importantly is that weight is often not a good indicator of the patient's nutritional status due to possible dehydration, fluid overload, and/or tumor burden. It is also difficult to obtain accurate weight measurements in a PICU, even if a bed scale is available. Arm anthropometry, including triceps skinfold measurements, may be inaccurate with steroid therapy and altered fluid status. Mid-upper arm muscle circumference is appropriate in acute care settings, but most providers are not accustomed to performing these measurements routinely. Nutrition-related laboratory values can also be affected by hydration status, the acute phase, or infection process, as well as medications, especially steroids.

Attention should then be paid to the nutrition-focused physical examination. A review of all relevant components, including vital signs; assessment of overall appearance; assessment of wounds and wound healing; signs and symptoms of macronutrient and micronutrient deficiencies; appearance of the skin, nails, and hair; assessment of hydration status; oral and dysphagia assessment; bowel history; and previous feeding and oral intake history, are essential for an accurate interpretation of the nutritional assessment. Interpretation of the findings will inform the development of an individualized nutrition care plan for the critically ill child with cancer.

Anthropometry and Measures of Body Composition

These types of measures can be termed routine, midlevel, or advanced according to the level of resources required for their completion and by their accuracy and precision. Routine measures include weight, height/length, and head circumference (in children <3 years). Weight-for-height/-length and BMI are compared to growth standards or references to assess the degree of underweight or overweight. Midlevel measures that assess body fat and lean body mass include triceps skin fold thickness, mid-upper arm circumference (and the calculation of mid-upper arm muscle area), and waist-to-hip ratio. Advanced measures include bioelectrical impedance methods, dual-energy x-ray absorptiometry (DEXA), air-displacement plethysmography (ADP), total body potassium (TBK) counting, and isotope dilution methods (deuterium oxide dilution).

Collection of anthropometric data, including body weight, height, and assessment of body fat and lean body mass, is suggested with varying frequency and comparative standards.[25] Advanced-level body composition measurements can be difficult to accomplish in the clinical setting, but anthropometry is safe, easy, quick, inexpensive, and may be more accessible in resource-poor areas. Mid-arm circumference is a simple and convenient measurement that requires little training and equipment and performs as well as weight-for-height at predicting death in developing countries.[26] Extremity measurement may be more sensitive to changes in muscle and fat mass and less affected by tumor mass and fluid shifts than body weight.[27] Population-based norms for arm anthropometrics such as mid-arm circumference and calculated mid-arm muscle area provide means to determine the degree of deviation from measurements of healthy children.

Biochemical and Hematological Indices

Biochemical data relevant to nutritional status include measures of visceral proteins (albumin, prealbumin, retinol-binding protein, and transferrin), blood glucose levels, and lipid profiles. Hematological measures include hemoglobin, hematocrit, and total lymphocyte count. White blood cell counts are often depleted as an intended result of myeloablative therapy. Neutrophils are typically the first to reconstitute, indicating resolving neutropenia and early resumption of immune function. Collected laboratory values should be compared with institutional or laboratory reference values. Laboratory values in critically ill children may be altered due to the effect of the acute phase of illness, medications, or both, and are therefore often unreliable indicators of nutritional status.

Energy and Protein

There are a variety of methods for estimating calorie and protein needs. The energy needs of children and adolescents may be increased during therapy due to fever, infections, GVHD, metabolic complications, and growth demands. Therefore, it is important to perform frequent assessments of the patient's caloric requirements to ensure that they are being met. Tables 20-3 and 20-4 can be used by the health care team to estimate energy and protein requirements.

Since energy expenditure in the PICU is variable and unpredictable, a cautious approach to estimating energy needs is needed for critically ill children with cancer. Studies of children awaiting engraftment following HSCT suggest a decline in energy expenditure over time.[28,29] Reliance on standard equations to estimate energy expenditure and use of stress factors may subject this group to unintended

TABLE 20-3. Estimated Energy Requirements for Infants and Children[47]

W = weight in kilograms
BMR = basal metabolic rate

Age	BMR Equations
0-3 months	(89W – 100) + 175
4-6 months	(89W – 100) + 56
7-12 months	(89W – 100) + 22

Age	1-3 years	3-10 years	10-18 years	18-30 years
Male	60.9W – 54	22.7W + 495	17.5W + 651	15.3W + 679
Female	61W – 51	22.5W + 499	12.2W + 746	14.7W + 496

Activity or stress factors may be carefully considered in individual cases.

Energy expenditure may decline after HSCT with a risk of overfeeding from parenteral nutrition.

TABLE 20-4. Minimum Protein Requirements Using Recommended Dietary Intake[48]

Age	Protein g/kg per day
Infants: 0-6 months	1.52
6-12 months	1.2
Children: 1-3 years	1.05
4-8 years	0.95
9-13 years	0.95
14-18 years	0.85
Adults	0.80

overfeeding. Treatment for cancer may be associated with decreased lipid clearance related to a variety of commonly used medications or hepatic dysfunction. Hyperglycemia resulting from stress or medications such as corticosteroids may necessitate a reduction in carbohydrate provision. Matching energy intake to energy expenditure as determined by serial indirect calorimetry measurements avoids overfeeding[30] and may reduce associated costs and complications.

Children and adolescents receiving therapy for cancer have increased protein needs for tissue repair and to decrease depletion of lean body mass. In addition, the patient may have increased protein needs during high-dose corticosteroid therapy or active GVHD. However, it is important to note that protein provision may need to be modified with altered hepatic, renal, or neurologic function. With malnutrition, protein should be increased to 1.5 to 2.0 times the recommended daily allowance (RDA) for age. Critically ill children may require additional protein to approach a balance of intake with ongoing catabolic losses.[31]

NUTRITION INTERVENTION AND MONITORING

The goals of nutrition therapy for critically ill children and adolescents undergoing cancer treatment are to preserve lean body mass and to achieve age-appropriate growth and development after treatment. These goals can be achieved through dietary modification, use of dietary supplements, use of appetite stimulants, or with more invasive nutritional support techniques.

Oral Intake

Special attention must be paid to food safety to reduce the risk for food-borne illnesses during treatment. Food consumed by immunocompromised patients should be prepared in a manner to minimize bacterial growth. Prepackaged, individual-serving items are frequently used to limit food handling by kitchen personnel. The use of appetite stimulants in this patient population is recommended only when all other attempts to increase oral intake (such as oral supplements) have failed. However, it may be beneficial for children or adolescents with specific diagnoses, such as osteosarcoma.[32]

Artificial Nutrition S.upport

Most critically ill children with cancer will require EN or PN support. Enteral nutrition is always preferred because it has many benefits for patients, including avoiding complications associated with parenteral support, such as intestinal atrophy, toxicity, and complications of intravenous infusions.[17] When EN is not feasible, PN should be administered to preserve or improve nutritional status. Parenteral nutrition is indicated when the child or adolescent is unresponsive to dietary supplementation or has a failure of enteral absorption. In any case, it should be limited to short periods.[17]

Planning nutrition support for children undergoing cancer treatment requires attention to route, volume, and efficacy of the feeding regimen. The goals of nutrition intervention for a child being treated for cancer or HSCT are to preserve lean body mass and support immune function. However, provision of nutrition to critically ill children is often complicated by several limitations. Fluid overload is common among HSCT patients,[1] and management of fluid volume must be considered with regard to medications, blood products, and nutritional fluids. Monitoring intake and output closely facilitates achievement of fluid balance. Medications and fluids required for resuscitation and treatment of acute problems may limit and/or change the volume available for nutritional intake. Interruptions in feedings are common, and tolerance may be poor.

Enteral Nutrition

Continuous feedings may be better tolerated than bolus feedings to avoid gastric distention and volume overload. Gastrointestinal manifestations of disease or treatment, such as mucositis and GVHD, frequently limit the tolerance to both the volume and the quality of formula provided. Small-volume, so-called "trophic" feedings may be useful, if tolerated, in combination with PN. Access to the GI tract through nasal tubes or percutaneous gastrostomies are generally convenient methods for providing EN, as well as options for administering medications and fluid to the GI tract. Achieving enteral feeding goals in a timely manner may improve outcomes in critically ill children,[33] though the optimal amount of energy and other nutrients is not precisely known, and likely will vary with stages of critical illness and changes in clinical condition.

Parenteral Nutrition

With GI toxicities resulting from cancer or HSCT treatment, PN is sometimes required to augment or replace enteral feeding. Parenteral feeding may be needed to achieve nutrient goals when accessibility or function of the GI tract is compromised. Benefits to PN include timely provision of energy and nutrients when absorption or volume tolerance of enteral feeding is inadequate. However, important risks associated with PN suggest the need to cautiously consider expectations with regard to optimal nutrient provision. Problems associated with PN include risk for infections, metabolic disturbances, and liver disease, all of which may be complications of the cancer treatment itself. Children undergoing treatment for cancer or HSCT are often severely immunocompromised, and both exposure to PN and to the PICU significantly increase the risk for bacteremia.[34] Parenteral nutrition is also associated with cholestatic liver disease, which presents similarly to VOD, a complication resulting from high-dose chemotherapy. Minimizing exposure to PN while ensuring appropriate provision of nutrients generally requires an individualized approach to nutrition prescriptions, with frequent monitoring and adjustments for changes in clinical status.

Protein

Critically ill patients often have high protein losses due to inflammation, cytokine production, and inadequate substrate supply. Protein intake needed to minimize nitrogen loss and promote protein balance in children with cancer is unknown, and probably varies by age and clinical characteristics. Critically ill children are likely to require a minimum of 1.5 grams protein per kg of body weight, and in some conditions, much higher amounts.[31] While achieving nitrogen balance should be the goal, accurate testing may not be available in clinical settings. During the most acute and severe phases of critical illness, balanced nitrogen intake and output are unlikely to be possible. As a supplemental amino acid, glutamine has been explored in a variety of settings for its potential to improve GI health and function. Several studies have investigated the impact of oral or intravenous glutamine supplementation following HSCT; however, no significant benefits to mucositis or other clinical outcomes have been observed in children.[35,36]

Carbohydrate

Hyperglycemia is common among critically ill children, and those with cancer or following HSCT are often receiving medications, such as steroids and other immunosuppressants, which further contribute to this problem. The use of PN has been linked with hyperglycemia in adult HSCT patients[37] without diabetes or steroid treatment. In children, the prevalence of metabolic syndrome is more common among HSCT recipients than the healthy population,[38] and various endocrine complications are associated with HSCT.[39] Close monitoring of blood glucose and nutrient requirements is recommended throughout intensive care treatment, as well as in long-term survivors.

Lipids

When volume for nutritional intake is limited, lipids contribute balanced and necessary energy without contributing to hyperglycemia or volume constraints. However, PN and lipids contribute to the risk of hyperlipidemia, and children undergoing cancer and HSCT treatment often require medications associated with hyperlipidemia. Since commonly used soybean-based lipid emulsions contain high amounts of omega-6 polyunsaturated fatty acids, a pro-inflammatory and immunosuppressive biochemical pathway may result from their use in excess. Evidence suggests that fish oil intake may improve endothelial function,[40] lower lipid levels,[41] and may the inflammatory response to illness.[42] Fish oil and other omega-3 fatty acid supplements have been used as complementary therapies to treat a variety of conditions, including hyperlipidemia and anorexia associated with cancer treatment. Intravenous fish oil lipid emulsion has been used in conjunction with standard PN and soybean-based lipid emulsions. Studies have demonstrated safety and efficacy of fish oil emulsions as monotherapy in preserving essential fatty acid status,[43] as well as promise in reducing PN-associated liver disease in infants and children on long-term PN.[44,45] Other lipids that have been used safely alongside PN in children with cancer or HSCT include olive oil emulsions and medium-chain triglyceride/long-chain triglyceride emulsions.[46] Only soybean-based emulsions are currently approved for use in the United States.

CONCLUSION

Children in the PICU with oncologic diseases require specialized nutrition care to address preexisting nutritional status, with ongoing attention to the acute signs and symptoms of their critical illness. Frequent reassessment and collaboration among the critical care team members will ensure that the many facets of critical illness are considered in the development and revision of the nutrition care plan. Oral or enteral feeding should be used whenever possible. If PN is required, consideration and discussion of its risks, benefits, and practical implications are necessary at its initiation and throughout the therapy. The goal for nutrition interventions should be to achieve or maintain age-appropriate growth and development, while minimizing risks associated with disease and medical treatment.

KEY POINTS

- Children with cancer are at risk of nutritional deterioration related to the disease as well as its treatment.
- Intolerance to oral feeding or EN, fluid restriction, and organ dysfunction are common barriers to nutrient delivery in immunocompromised children. Gastrointestinal manifestations of disease or treatment, such as GVHD and mucositis, frequently limit the tolerance to EN.
- Parenteral nutrition may be needed to achieve nutrient goals in this group, particularly when the function of the GI tract is compromised.
- Particular attention to energy and protein requirements and judicious use of PN are essential to achieve optimal nutrient delivery in children with cancer.

REFERENCES

1. Demaret P, Pettersen G, Hubert P, Teira P, Emeriaud G. The critically-ill pediatric hemato-oncology patient: epidemiology, management, and strategy of transfer to the pediatric intensive care unit. *Ann Intensive Care.* 2012;2(1):14.
2. Rogers PC, Melnick SJ, Ladas EJ, Halton J, Baillargeon J, Sacks N. Children's Oncology Group (COG) Nutrition Committee. *Pediatr Blood & Cancer.* 2008;50(2 Suppl): 447-450; discussion 451.
3. Sala A, Rossi E, Antillon F, et al. Nutritional status at diagnosis is related to clinical outcomes in children and adolescents with cancer: a perspective from Central America. *Eur J Cancer.* 2012;48(2):243-252.
4. Donaldson S, Wesley M, DeWys W, et al. A study of the nutritional status of pediatric cancer patients. *Am J Dis Child.* 1981;135:1107.
5. Antillon F, de Maselli T, Garcia T, Rossi E, Sala A. Nutritional status of children during treatment for acute lymphoblastic leukemia in the Central American Pediatric Hematology Oncology Association (AHOPCA): preliminary data from Guatemala. *Pediatr Blood & Cancer.* 2008;50(2 Suppl): 502-505; discussion 517.
6. Israels T, Chirambo C, Caron HN, Molyneux EM. Nutritional status at admission of children with cancer in Malawi. *Pediatr Blood & Cancer.* 2008;51(5):626-628.
7. Gelelete CB, Pereira SH, Azevedo AM, et al. Overweight as a prognostic factor in children with acute lymphoblastic leukemia. *Obesity.* 2011;19(9):1908-1911.
8. Dietz WH, Robinson TN. Overweight Children and Adolescents. *N Engl J Med.* 2005;352(20):2100-2109.
9. Reilly JJ, Kelly J. Long-term impact of overweight and obesity in childhood and adolescence on morbidity and premature mortality in adulthood: systematic review. *Int J Obes.* 2011;35(7):891-898.
10. Rogers PC, Meacham LR, Oeffinger KC, Henry DW, Lange BJ. Obesity in pediatric oncology. *Pediatr Blood & Cancer.* 2005;45(7):881-891.
11. Lange BJ, Gerbing RB, Feusner J, et al. Mortality in overweight and underweight children with acute myeloid leukemia. *JAMA.* 2005;293(2):203-211.
12. Barker CC, Agovi MA, Logan B, et al. Childhood obesity and outcomes after bone marrow transplantation for patients with severe aplastic anemia. *Biol Blood Marrow Transplantation.* 2011;17(5):737-744.
13. Bulley S, Gassas A, Dupuis LL, et al. Inferior outcomes for overweight children undergoing allogeneic stem cell transplantation. *Br J Haematol.* 2008;140(2):214-217.
14. Butturini AM, Dorey FJ, Lange BJ, et al. Obesity and outcome in pediatric acute lymphoblastic leukemia. *J Clin Oncol.* 2007;25(15):2063-2069.
15. White M, Murphy AJ, Hallahan A, Ware RS, Fraser C, Davies PS. Survival in overweight and underweight children undergoing hematopoietic stem cell transplantation. *Eur J Clin Nutr.* 2012;66(10):1120-1123.

16. Coronha AL, Camilo ME, Ravasco P. The relevance of body composition in cancer patients: what is the evidence? *Acta Medica Portuguesa.* 2011;24 Suppl 4:769-778.

17. Bauer J, Jurgens H, Fruhwald MC. Important aspects of nutrition in children with cancer. *Adv Nutr.* 2011;2(2): 67-77.

18. Filipovich AH, Weisdorf D, Pavletic S, et al. National Institutes of Health consensus development project on criteria for clinical trials in chronic graft-versus-host disease: I. Diagnosis and staging working group report. *Biol Blood Marrow Transplant.* 2005;11(12):945-956.

19. Helmy A. Review article: updates in the pathogenesis and therapy of hepatic sinusoidal obstruction syndrome. *Alimentary Pharmacol Ther.* 2006;23(1):11-25.

20. Kuczmarski RJ, Ogden CL, Guo SS, et al. 2000 CDC growth charts for the United States: methods and development. National Center for Health Statistics. *Vital Health Statistics.* June 8, 2000. 2002;11(246).

21. World Health Organization. WHO Child Growth Standards: Methods and development: Length/height-for-age, weight-for-age, weight-for-length, weight-for-height and body mass index-for-age. Geneva, Switzerland: World Health Organization; 2006: http://www.who.int/childgrowth/publications/technical_report_pub/en/index.html. Accessed October 14, 2012.

22. de Onis M, Onyango AW, Borghi E, Siyam A, Nishida C, Siekmann J. Development of a WHO growth reference for school-aged children and adolescents. *Bull World Health Organization.* 2007;85:660-667.

23. Barlow SE. Expert committee recommendations regarding the prevention, assessment, and treatment of child and adolescent overweight and obesity: summary report. *Pediatrics.* 2007;120 Suppl 4:S164-192.

24. Mosby TT, Barr RD, Pencharz PB. Nutritional assessment of children with cancer. *J Pediatr Oncology Nurs.* 2009;26(4):186-197.

25. Neumann CG, Jelliffe DB, Zerfas AJ, Jelliffe EF. Nutritional assessment of the child with cancer. *Cancer Res.* 1982;42 (2 Suppl):699s-712s.

26. Sala A, Rossi E, Antillon F. Nutritional status at diagnosis in children and adolescents with cancer in the Asociacion de Hemato-Oncologia Pediatrica de Centro America (AHOPCA) countries: preliminary results from Guatemala. *Pediatr Blood & Cancer.* 2008;50(2 Suppl):499-501; discussion 517.

27. Smith D, Stevens M, Booth I. Malnutrition at diagnosis of malignancy in childhood: common but mostly missed. *Eur J Pediatr.* 1991;150:318-322.

28. Duggan C, Bechard L, Donovan K, et al. Changes in resting energy expenditure among children undergoing allogeneic stem cell transplantation. *Am J Clin Nutr.* 2003;78(1):104-109.

29. Bechard LJ, Feldman HA, Venick R, et al. Attenuation of resting energy expenditure following hematopoietic SCT in children. *Bone Marrow Transplantation.* 2012;47(10):1301-1306.

30. Sharma TS, Bechard LJ, Feldman HA, et al. Effect of titrated parenteral nutrition on body composition after allogeneic hematopoietic stem cell transplantation in children: a double-blind, randomized, multicenter trial. *Am J Clin Nutr.* 2012;95(2):342-351.

31. Bechard LJ, Parrott JS, Mehta NM. Systematic review of the influence of energy and protein intake on protein balance in critically ill children. *J Pediatr.* 2012;161(2): 333-339 e331.

32. Ringwald-Smith K, Surprise H, Billups C, Daw N. Nutrition Management of Children With Osteosarcoma. *ICAN: Infant, Child, & Adolescent Nutr.* 2011;3(3):152-157.

33. Mehta NM, Bechard LJ, Cahill N, et al. Nutritional practices and their relationship to clinical outcomes in critically ill children—an international multicenter cohort study. *Crit Care Med.* 2012;40(7):2204-2211.

34. Advani S, Reich NG, Sengupta A, Gosey L, Milstone AM. Central line-associated bloodstream infection in hospitalized children with peripherally inserted central venous catheters: extending risk analyses outside the intensive care unit. *Clin Infect Dis.* 2011;52(9):1108-1115.

35. Uderzo C, Rebora P, Marrocco E, et al. Glutamine-enriched nutrition does not reduce mucosal morbidity or complications after stem-cell transplantation for childhood malignancies: a prospective randomized study. *Transplantation.* 2011;91(12):1321-1325.

36. Crowther M, Avenell A, Culligan DJ. Systematic review and meta-analyses of studies of glutamine supplementation in haematopoietic stem cell transplantation. *Bone Marrow Transplantation.* 2009;44(7):413-425.

37. Sheean PM, Braunschweig C, Rich E. The incidence of hyperglycemia in hematopoietic stem cell transplant recipients receiving total parenteral nutrition: a pilot study. *J Am Diet Assoc.* 2004;104(9):1352-1360.

38. Paris C, Yates L, Lama P, Zepeda AJ, Gutierrez D, Palma J. Evaluation of metabolic syndrome after hematopoietic stem cell transplantation in children and adolescents. *Pediatric Blood & Cancer.* 2012;59(2):306-310.

39. Ho J, Lewis V, Guilcher GM, Stephure DK, Pacaud D. Endocrine complications following pediatric bone mar-

row transplantation. *J Pediatr Endocrinol Metabol.* 2011;24 (5-6):327-332.

40. Rizza S, Tesauro M, Cardillo C, et al. Fish oil supplementation improves endothelial function in normoglycemic offspring of patients with type 2 diabetes. *Atherosclerosis.* 2009;206(2):569-574.
41. Hartweg J, Perera R, Montori V, Dinneen S, Neil HA, Farmer A. Omega-3 polyunsaturated fatty acids (PUFA) for type 2 diabetes mellitus. *Cochrane Database of Syst Rev.* 2008(1):CD003205.
42. Wanten GJ, Calder PC. Immune modulation by parenteral lipid emulsions. *Am J Clin Nutri.* 2007;85(5):1171-1184.
43. Le HD, de Meijer VE, Robinson EM, et al. Parenteral fish-oil-based lipid emulsion improves fatty acid profiles and lipids in parenteral nutrition-dependent children. *Am J Clin Nutri.* 2011;94(3):749-758.
44. Puder M, Valim C, Meisel JA, et al. Parenteral fish oil improves outcomes in patients with parenteral nutrition-associated liver injury. *Ann Surg.* 2009;250(3): 395-402.
45. Gura KM, Lee S, Valim C, et al. Safety and efficacy of a fish-oil-based fat emulsion in the treatment of parenteral nutrition-associated liver disease. *Pediatrics.* 2008;121(3):e678-686.
46. Hartman C, Ben-Artzi E, Berkowitz D, et al. Olive oil-based intravenous lipid emulsion in pediatric patients undergoing bone marrow transplantation: a short-term prospective controlled trial. *Clin Nutr.* 2009;28(6):631-635.
47. World Health Organization. Energy and protein requirements. Report of a joint FAO/WHO/UNU expert consultation. *WHO Technical Report Series No. 724.* Geneva: World Health Organization; 1985.
48. National Research Council. *Dietary Reference Intakes for Energy, Carbohydrate, Fiber, Fat, Fatty Acids, Cholesterol, Protein, and Amino Acids (Macronutrients).* Washington, DC: The National Academies Press; 2005.

CHAPTER 21

Nutrition in the Critically ill Obese Child

Carol Okada
Heather Skillman
Nancy Krebs

- INTRODUCTION
- DEFINITIONS
- EPIDEMIOLOGY
- PHYSIOLOGIC CHANGES ASSOCIATED WITH OBESITY
  - Adipose Tissue
  - Cardiovascular System
  - Respiratory System
- COMORBIDITIES OF OBESITY
  - Hypertension
  - Sleep-Disordered Breathing
  - Pulmonary Hypertension
  - Asthma
  - Thromboembolic Disease
  - Insulin Resistance
- SPECIAL CHALLENGES AND CONSIDERATIONS IN CARING FOR THE OBESE PATIENT IN THE PEDIATRIC INTENSIVE CARE UNIT
  - Airway Management
  - Mechanical Ventilation
  - Vascular Access
  - Medication Dosing
  - Nursing Care
  - Outcomes: Morbidity and Mortality of Critically ill Obese Children in the Pediatric Intensive Care Unit
- NUTRITION FOR THE HOSPITALIZED CRITICALLY ILL OBESE CHILD
  - Nutrition Assessment
  - Indirect Calorimetry
  - Estimation of Energy Requirements
  - Protein Requirements
  - Nutrition Support
  - High-Protein Hypocaloric Feeding
  - Weight Loss Interventions Following Critical illness
- CONCLUSION
- KEY POINTS
- References

INTRODUCTION

One in 6 children in the United States is obese.[1] While previous studies in adults have demonstrated obesity as an important comorbid condition that can complicate care, obesity is often underrecognized and consequently overlooked as a comorbidity in children.[2] An understanding of how obesity affects children and their care in the pediatric intensive care unit (PICU) is essential.

The chapter starts with obesity definitions and epidemiology. Key physiologic changes seen in obesity that may affect the critically ill pediatric patient are reviewed. Comorbidities seen in obese patients are discussed, and a focused section on the challenges of caring for these patients in the PICU is included. The chapter ends with considerations for nutrition care for the critically ill obese pediatric patient.

DEFINITIONS

Obesity is defined as excess body fat. Body mass index (BMI) is a readily available proxy for body fatness, based on body weight adjusted for height. The formula is weight in kilograms divided by the square of height in meters: BMI = weight (kg)/(height (m))^2. Body mass index is not a direct measure of body fat, but it correlates strongly with percent body fat in adults; the correlation is somewhat less strong in children.[3]

Because of the impact of growth and changing body composition in children, the Centers for Disease Control and Prevention (CDC) define obesity differently for adults and children. Obesity in adults is defined as a BMI greater than 30 kg/m^2, whereas obesity in a patient 2 years to 19 years is defined as a BMI at the 95th percentile or higher, adjusted for age and gender. Of note, there are older adolescent patients where the 95th percentile BMI is greater than a BMI of 30 kg/m^2, so obesity for the older adolescent is defined as a BMI at or above the 95th percentile or a BMI ≥30 kg/m^2, whichever is lower.[3] Of particular relevance to the discussion in this chapter is the issue of severe obesity. Using the BMI cutoff of 95th percentile does not distinguish degree of severity, yet children with BMI Z-score 3 and above have been shown to have strikingly greater risk for cardiovascular and metabolic comorbidities.[4] The Expert Committee thus advocated for a category of "severe obesity" to designate children with BMI ≥99th percentile for age. For children under the age of 2, normative values for BMI have not been established. Weight-for-length values above the 95th percentile are used to define overweight in this age group; the term obesity is not used.[3,5]

EPIDEMIOLOGY

In the United States, the prevalence of overweight for infants and toddlers from birth to 2 years of age is 9.7%.[1] The prevalence of obesity for children in the United States has increased dramatically in the past 40 years. However, the most recent study in the United States showed the overall prevalence of obesity in children and adolescents over the past decade has remained unchanged at 16.9%. Obesity has dispproportionately affected certain racial/ethnic groups. In 2009-2010, 21.2% of Hispanic children and adolescents and 24.3% of non-Hispanic black children and adolescents were obese compared to 14% of non-Hispanic white children and adolescents. National data are not reported for prevalence of BMI ≥99th percentile for age, but most recent U.S. data indicate a prevalence of 12.3% for BMI ≥97th percentile for 2- to 19-year-olds.[1]

Trends of obesity worldwide mimic those in the United States. Developed countries have the highest prevalence rates of obesity, but developing countries are showing an increasing prevalence over time.[6]

The prevalence of obesity in hospitalized pediatric patients varies between 11% and 20%.[2,7] In the PICU, the prevalence of obesity in patients requiring mechanical ventilation is 13%.[8] In the PICU at Children's Hospital Colorado, data from 2010-2011 indicated the obesity prevalence was 13.7%, and severe obesity prevalence was 4.2%. These numbers emphasize the importance of identifying obesity and understanding special considerations and needs of this patient population.

PHYSIOLOGIC CHANGES ASSOCIATED WITH OBESITY

Obesity affects a number of organ systems and physiology. These effects need to be understood when undertaking nutritional prescriptions in this group of patients.

Adipose Tissue

In the obese pediatric patient, adipose tissue is a complex, highly active metabolic and endocrine organ. It has effects on all parts of the body, either by pure mechanical means or by signaling to other tissues and organs. The major factors released by the adipose tissue (see Table 21-1) give insight into how obesity may heighten the inflammatory response to illness, exacerbate metabolic control, affect cardiovascular response to illness, and make a patient susceptible to organ failure.

Cardiovascular System

Obesity can affect the entire cardiovascular system. Cardiac function, vascular tone, and endothelial function can all be altered by obesity, and these changes can affect the response of the cardiovascular system to critical illness.

It was shown over 50 years ago that obese individuals have increased cardiac output and total blood volume.[9]

TABLE 21-1. Biochemical and Metabolic Effects of Obesity[77-80]

Factor	Main Role	Effects	Concentration in Obesity	Physiologic Consequences in Obesity
Leptin	Metabolic signal of energy sufficiency	• Satiety • ↑ Inflammatory response • ↑ Hematopoiesis • ↑ Angiogenesis	Increased, but there is leptin resistance	• ↑ Inflammation • ↑ Red blood cell production • ↑ Vessel formation in adipose tissue
Adiponectin	Insulin sensitivity	• ↑ Insulin sensitivity • Anti-inflammatory effects	Decreased	• Insulin resistance • ↑ Inflammation
Tumor necrosis factor - alpha (TNF-α)	Pro-inflammatory cytokine	• Activates transcription of nuclear factor-kappa B (NF-κB)	Increased	• ↑ Inflammation • Endothelial dysfunction • Insulin resistance
Interleukin 6 (IL-6)	Pro-inflammatory cytokine	• ↑ Inflammation • Insulin resistance • Endothelial dysfunction	Increased	• ↑ Inflammation • Insulin resistance • Endothelial dysfunction
Interleukin 10 (IL-10)	Anti-inflammatory cytokine	• Antagonistic cytokine to TNF-α and IL-6 • Endothelial-protective properties • Insulin sensitivity	Decreased	• ↑ Inflammation • Endothelial dysfunction • Insulin resistance
Plasminogen activator inhibitor 1 (PAI-1)	Inhibits fibrinolysis	• Decreases break-down of clots • Atherogenesis • Angiogenesis	Increased	• Risk of thrombus formation • Risk of atherosclerosis • ↑ Vessel formation in the adipose tissue
Angiotensinogen	Renal sodium and water homeostasis	• ↑ Total body sodium and water • Increased vascular tone • Angiogenesis	Increased	• Hypertension • ↑ Circulating volume • ↑ Vessel formation in the adipose tissue

The amount of adipose tissue is increased in obese subjects, and an extensive capillary system is needed to support it. The body compensates by increasing stroke volume and cardiac output.[10]

Over a long period, obesity has hemodynamic repercussions that ultimately lead to cardiac dysfunction. The Frank-Starling curve is shifted to the left secondary to increased left ventricular (LV) filling and stroke volume. Over time, the pressure and volume loads on the heart lead to dilation of the LV. As this wall stress continues, there is a resultant hypertrophy and associated LV diastolic dysfunction.[11] Hypertension is often associated with obesity and can add to the left-sided cardiac dysfunction. Other common comorbidities associated with obesity, such as obstructive sleep apnea and pulmonary hypertension, also contribute to right-sided cardiac dysfunction.

There are other theorized mechanisms linking obesity to cardiac dysfunction. There is the possibility that fat and lipid deposition around the organ can modify function by simple compression or by release of locally active molecules that incite inflammation and/or cardiac remodeling. Lipid accumulation in myocardial cells may be toxic, leading to cell dysfunction or death.

The summation of all of these changes places the obese patient at risk of heart failure. The patient often is asymptomatic, and signs of failure on physical examination may be difficult to discern due to body habitus. With the stress of surgery or illness, obese patients with cardiac dysfunction may not tolerate the fluid loading often required in the PICU for resuscitation. Anticipation and early recognition are key. Brain natriuretic peptide (BNP) and N-terminal pro-brain natriuretic peptide (NT-proBNP) may be useful markers to assess cardiac dysfunction. An echocardiogram and consultation by a cardiologist may be helpful in the management of these patients.

The cardiac conduction system can be infiltrated with fat, inflammatory cells, and fibrosis. These changes could predispose an obese patient to arrhythmias, and all obese patients should be monitored with telemetry while in the PICU.

Another aspect of the cardiovascular system affected by obesity is endothelial function. The vascular endothelium is responsible for the production of factors. One important factor is nitric oxide (NO), and its actions include maintenance of vascular tone, regulation of vascular permeability, inhibition of platelet adhesion and aggregation, and prevention of smooth muscle cell proliferation.[12] Nitric oxide production and degradation are influenced by obesity and common comorbidities associated with obesity. The decreased availability of NO in obesity leads to an imbalance between relaxation and contraction and ultimately endothelial dysfunction.[12,13]

Endothelial dysfunction is present at baseline for the obese patient. In the setting of critical illness, these patients may have further alterations in their vascular reactivity and endothelial function. Thus, if an obese pediatric patient is not responding to cardiovascular support as predicted, measurement of cardiac output and vascular resistances may be necessary.

Respiratory System

Obesity promotes a multitude of adverse effects on the respiratory system when people are relatively well, and places them at an even higher risk of respiratory failure in times of disease. This section will review the effects of obesity on the respiratory system.

The most commonly reported effect of obesity on lung function is a reduction in functional residual capacity (FRC). There is an altered balance between inspiratory and expiratory forces due to the mass load of adipose tissue around the rib cage and in the abdominal cavity. It follows that the degree of reduction in FRC depends on where fat deposition occurs. Abdominal and thoracic fat will have more effect on FRC than fat distributed elsewhere. Although studies in children have had small sample sizes, the trend of these studies shows an inverse relationship between FRC and degree of obesity.[14-16]

Upper and lower airway resistance can be increased in obesity. Resistance is highly dependent on lung volume and is therefore affected by reduction in FRC. The other contributing factors are unclear, but may be related to increased airway inflammation and fat deposition in and around the airways.

Total respiratory compliance is reduced. The primary factor leading to decreased compliance relates to the chest wall. It is theorized that fat deposition around the chest, abdomen, and diaphragm decreases chest wall compliance. Decreased lung compliance is likely multifactorial. Increased pulmonary blood flow, premature closure of dependent airways and resultant atelectasis, and increased alveolar surface tension due to reductions in FRC all contribute to the overall reduction in lung compliance.

With reduction in FRC, closing capacity can exceed FRC in obese patients. This leads to premature airway closure during normal tidal volume breaths and can alter ventilation. Compounding this alteration in physiology is the change in regional ventilation that occurs in obesity. In an upright normal-weight patient, the distribution of regional ventilation is greatest in the dependent lung zones and decreases as one approaches the nondependent areas of lung. In an obese individual, this ventilation scheme may be reversed, so the areas that are underventilated are receiving the most blood flow; therefore, obese individuals are at risk of ventilation-perfusion (V/Q) mismatch.

Li and colleagues reported diminished diffusion capacity (DL_{co}) in obese pediatric patients.[15] They speculated that it may reflect lipid deposition and structural changes in the interstitium and in the alveoli as possible causes. The impact is altered gas exchange, but the degree to which is unclear.

Obese patients have a higher basal oxygen consumption, carbon dioxide production, and work of breathing.

They try to maintain eucapnia with a higher level of minute ventilation through rapid, shallow breathing as the respiratory muscles must work against a noncompliant chest. A disproportionate amount of oxygen consumption is dedicated to respiratory work when an obese individual is well. In disease states, this work of breathing and other mentioned alterations in pulmonary physiology predispose these patients to respiratory failure when faced with mild pulmonary or systemic insults.

COMORBIDITIES OF OBESITY

Obesity is associated with a number of comorbidities (see Table 21-2). A comorbidity may be the primary reason for admission to the PICU, may indirectly affect the primary disease process, or may increase the risk for certain complications.

TABLE 21-2. Comorbidities Associated with Childhood Obesity[81]

System	Comorbidity
Cardiovascular	• Atherosclerosis • Hypertension • Left ventricular dilation +/- hypertrophy
Respiratory	• Obstructive sleep apnea • Pulmonary hypertension • Asthma
Hematologic	• Venous stasis • Venous thrombosis
Metabolic/endocrine	• Type 2 diabetes/insulin resistance • Metabolic syndrome • Dyslipidemia • Polycystic ovary syndrome
Gastrointestinal	• Nonalcoholic fatty liver disease • Gastroesophageal reflux • Gallbladder disease • Pancreatitis
Renal	• Glomerulopathy
Neurologic	• Idiopathic intracranial hypertension
Orthopedic	• Slipped capital femoral epiphysis • Tibia vara (Blount disease)
Psychosocial	• Depression

Hypertension

Obesity in childhood and adolescence is associated with hypertension. Thirty-seven percent of hypertensive children are overweight or obese. Obese children and adolescents are 2.5 to 3.7 times more likely to have hypertension than a nonobese counterpart.[13]

Blood pressure is a product of cardiac output and systemic vascular resistance. Factors leading to hypertension include the direct effects of obesity on cardiac output and other theorized mechanisms that increase vascular resistance in obesity: endothelial dysfunction, chronic activation of the sympathetic nervous sytem, insulin resistance, chronic inflammation, activation of the renin angiotensin system by adipose tissue, physical compression of the kidneys by adipose tissue, and sleep apnea.[17,18]

In the PICU, these patients may need administration of antihypertensive agents. More importantly, hypertension in an obese patient may be a marker of endothelial and vascular dysfunction. If there are issues with the cardiovascular system and oxygen delivery, echocardiogram and invasive hemodynamic monitoring may be useful in the management of the patient.

Sleep-Disordered Breathing

During normal sleep, airway tone decreases, but pharyngeal dilator activity maintains airway patency. All individuals have occasional pauses during sleep, but airflow is not limited. Sleep-disordered breathing is a spectrum of diseases where partial or complete cessation of airflow occurs multiple times during the night. A proper diagnosis requires evaluation through polysomnography.

There is a strong association between obesity and obstructive sleep apnea (OSA). The mechanisms for increased risk of OSA in obese children are multiple. Airway obstruction from adenotonsillar hypertrophy is common in obese children, and this limits the size of the upper airway. It is not the only factor causing OSA, however, since an adenotonsillectomy only resolves OSA in 50% of cases. Measurements of airway flow in obese children during sleep have shown they have a positive critical closing pressure of the pharynx, which causes airway collapse with mild negative inspiratory pressure.[19,20]

The obese patient may be more prone to desaturations with obstruction. As discussed previously, obese individuals have decreased chest wall compliance, reduction in

FRC, and V/Q mismatch, which places them at baseline at a higher risk of hypoxemia. Many of these patients may utilize noninvasive ventilation (e.g., continuous positive airway pressure/bilevel positive airway pressure) as a baseline therapy at night. In the PICU, noninvasive ventilation may serve as a means of respiratory support during acute illness, postoperatively or immediately after extubation for patients with OSA.

Obesity hypoventilation syndrome (OHS) is a triad of obesity, daytime hypoventilation, and sleep-disordered breathing without an alternative neuromuscular, metabolic, or mechanical cause of hypoventilation. It is distinct from obesity and OSA in that these individuals have daytime hypercapnia. Impaired respiratory mechanics from obesity, altered central respiratory drive possibly due to central leptin resistance, and impaired metabolic ability to compensate for hypercapnia are proposed mechanisms leading to the ventilation derangements in this syndrome.[21]

Pulmonary Hypertension

A multitude of factors contribute to this pathologic state. Obstructive sleep apnea leads to repetitive nocturnal episodes of hypoxemia, hypercapnia, acidosis, increased sympathetic tone, and wide variations in intrathoracic pressure, which lead to pulmonary vasocontriction and arteriolar remodeling. The cardiomyopathy associated with obesity causes chronically elevated LV filling pressures, and these pressures are transmitted to the pulmonary venous system. Other obesity-related factors that likely add to the risk of pulmonary hypertension include inflammation, endothelial dysfunction, oxidative stress, and increased risk of thromboembolic disease.[22]

Clinically in the PICU, measurement of cardiac markers for heart failure, such as BNP and NT-proBNP, and echocardiography may be helpful in the diagnosis. Ultimately, if the diagnosis of pulmonary hypertension is unclear, cardiac catheterization may be necessary to determine its severity, rule out pulmonary vein obstruction, and assess vascular bed reactivity to different interventions and medications.

Asthma

The link between asthma and obesity is controversial. Studies involving children have been mixed on the association between asthma and obesity. Some clinicians believe obese children and adolescents have chronic inflammation that increases their risk of developing asthma. For those patients admitted to the PICU, the severity of an asthma exacerbation does not appear to be worse in the obese pediatric patient compared to the nonobese patient. However, obese patients admitted to the ICU for severe exacerbations have longer hospital length of stays, even after controlling for asthma severity on admission and at baseline.[23] The reason for longer hospitalizations likely relates to baseline physiologic alterations and other comorbidities associated with obesity.

Thromboembolic Disease

Thromboembolic disease is an underrecognized condition in pediatrics, which has a high incidence of associated morbidity and mortality. The underlying mechanisms linking obesity and thrombosis have not been fully elucidated and are likely multifactorial. Altered blood flow based on fat distribution, oxidative stress, adipokines that lead to a prothrombotic state, chronic inflammation, and endothelial dysfunction likely all play roles.

The association between adult obesity and cerebrovascular disease has been characterized. In the pediatric population, the prevalence of having a BMI ≥85th percentile was associated with cerebral sinovenous thrombosis but not with arterial ischemic stroke.[24]

Based on a national administrative database of hospitalized pediatric patients aged 1 to 17 years, the prevalence of deep vein thrombosis (DVT) was 2.4 cases per 1,000 discharges. Obesity was significantly associated with DVT. An obese patient had a prevalence twice that of a nonobese counterpart.[25]

In the critical care setting, there are many factors that increase the risk of clinically significant thrombosis. Reiter and colleagues developed a risk assessment tool for the PICU patient. Twelve equally weighted factors, including obesity, were incorporated into the risk assessment. While 1 risk factor inferred little risk of symptomatic thrombus, 2 to 5 risk factors inferred moderate risk, and more than 6 risk factors inferred high risk. Pharmacologic DVT prophylaxis should be considered in an obese patient if additional factors such as presence of a central venous catheter, immobility for >72 hours, infection (defined as bacteremia, meningitis, pneumonia, or other infection associated with hemodynamic compromise), orthopedic surgery, major trauma with an Injury Severity Score above 15, malignancy, exogenous estrogen use, burns >30% body surface area, acquired or inherited thrombophilia, age <1 year or older than 14 years, or hypercoagulable state are also present.[26]

Insulin Resistance

Glucose concentration is kept under tight control normally and represents a balance between insulin secretion and insulin sensitivity. Initially when a patient develops peripheral insulin resistance, there is a compensatory increase in insulin production. Glucose concentration remains normal. Failure of this response ultimately leads to glucose intolerance and type 2 diabetes.

Insulin resistance is commonly seen in obese patients, and it is likely the composite result of multiple adipokines. Acute illness or stress further disrupts glucose homeostasis, and hyperglycemia develops. Hyperglycemia itself has pro-inflammatory and pro-thrombotic effects, and it can lead to increased oxidative stress and decreased immune response. Insulin appears to counter these effects, and there is more interest in the pediatric population for tighter glucose control during critical illness. Due to insulin resistance, these patients may require higher insulin infusion rates to optimize glucose control. Two studies on critically ill children post-cardiac surgery have not shown any benefit to intensive glucose control.[27,28] Another study showed that tight glucose control significantly decreased morbidity.[29] Based on these studies, tight glucose control should be considered in patients with significant burns and avoided in patients post-cardiac surgery. The role of tight glucose control in other critically ill children is less clear.

Hyperglycemic hyperosmolar syndrome (HHS) is not a common comorbidity, but it is of particular interest in the critical care setting. It has a high morbidity and mortality rate and represents a medical emergency. Hyperglycemic hyperosmolar syndrome is characterized by elevations in serum glucose and hyperosmolality without significant ketosis. Complications of HHS include hypovolemic shock, thromboembolic events, cerebral edema, rhabdomyolysis, cardiac rhythm disturbances, multiorgan failure, and death.

Unlike diabetic ketoacidosis (DKA), the principle objective of early management of HHS is aggressive restoration of circulatory volume. Hypotonic fluids should be administered in order to gradually decrease serum sodium by 0.5 mEq/L per hour. Insulin therapy may not be necessary. Early insulin treatment and lack of recognition of HHS may be associated with increased risk of death.[30] Electrolyte imbalances should be corrected. Of note, some patients have a mixture of HHS and DKA. The goal of treatment is restoration of circulating volume and close observation for complications of both entities.[31]

SPECIAL CHALLENGES AND CONSIDERATIONS IN CARING FOR THE OBESE PATIENT IN THE PEDIATRIC INTENSIVE CARE UNIT

Despite the increase in obesity rates in children over the past 30 years, hospitals often are not prepared to care for obese pediatric patients. In 2006, a survey was performed by Porter and colleagues to assess whether free-standing children's hospitals had appropriate equipment, trained staff, a clinical protocol, and a system for resuscitation of obese pediatric patients. Of the 28 hospitals that responded, 7 hospitals with bariatric programs were prepared for the care of the obese patient. Twenty-one hospitals that responded did not have a bariatric program, and less than 20% of these hospitals had readily available equipment and trained staff for the obese pediatric patient.[32]

At Children's Hospital Colorado, a multidisciplinary group formed a Pediatric Obesity Care Guideline for the patient admitted to the hospital (Figure 21.1). The goals of the guideline were to facilitate the implementation of evidence-based care and ultimately improve outcomes. The guideline addresses many of the challenges associated with the care of the obese pediatric patient. Of those challenges, airway management, medication dosing and pharmacology, equipment, and nursing care will be highlighted in this section.

Airway Management

Obese pediatric patients have altered respiratory physiology and associated comorbidities, which make them more prone to issues related to intubation. In the controlled setting of the operating room, obese pediatric patients have an increased risk of desaturation, multiple attempts at laryngoscopy, difficult mask ventilation, and airway obstruction.[33]

The care team must be prepared for airway difficulties. A good history evaluating for sleep-disordered breathing, pulmonary hypertension, and previous intubation difficulties is essential. A thorough physical examination that includes the Mallampati score and neck mobility should be performed. To reduce the risk of hypoxemia, preoxygenation with 100% oxygen for at least 3 minutes is suggested. Reverse Trendelenburg positioning with the head of the bed elevated 25 degrees can make bag-mask ventilation easier by lowering abdominal pressure on the diaphragm. An oral airway should be available in case of difficult mask ventilation. Difficult mask ventilation can

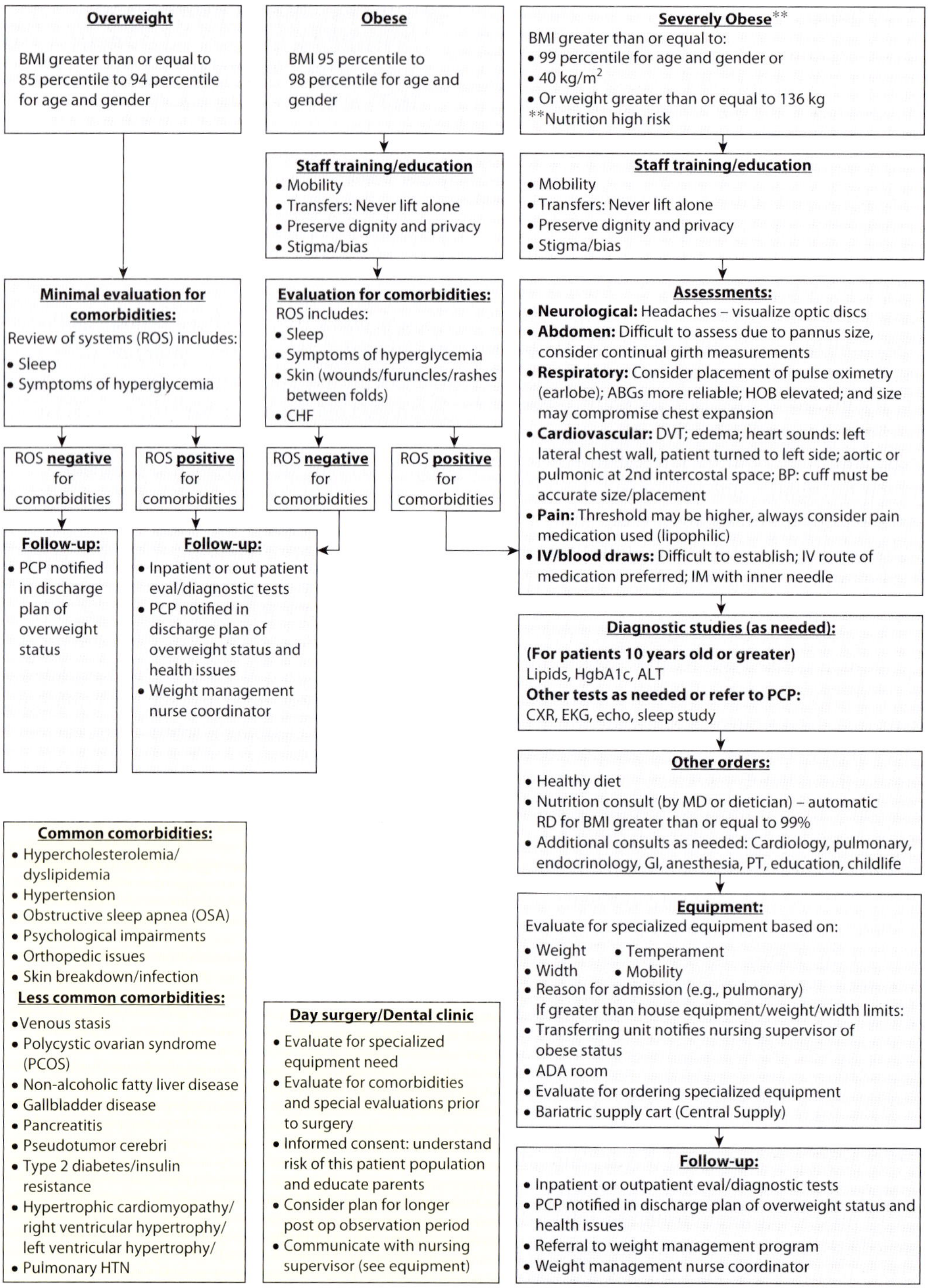

FIGURE 21-1. Obesity care algorithm.

Reproduced with permisison from Porter, R.M., Thrasher J., Krebs, N.F: Pediatric Obesity Clinical Care Guideline. Children's Hospital Colorado, 2012

lead to gastric distention, and placement of a nasogastric tube to decompress the stomach will help with functional residual capacity and ventilation. A laryngeal mask airway should also be available in case of a difficult intubation. Of note, there are no studies evaluating these interventions on outcomes in the pediatric population, and these are expert opinions.[34,35] The risk of aspiration is not increased in obese children compared to their lean counterparts, so rapid sequence induction is not standard of care for the obese patient.[36]

Mechanical Ventilation

The altered physiology of the respiratory system has been reviewed. A multitude of factors can affect weaning from mechanical ventilation, including decreased functional residual capacity, increased chest wall loading, increased airway resistance, and reduced pulmonary compliance. Transition to noninvasive ventilation after extubation has been shown to reduce the postextubation respiratory failure in obese adults.[37] In addition, positioning may be important for respiratory mechanics in the obese patient. The abdominal compartment in obese patients may mechanically load the diaphragm and increase work of breathing. Reverse Trendelenburg positioning decreases the load on the diaphragm, and in adults has shown increased tidal volumes and work of breathing.[38] It should be considered if having difficulties ventilating a patient and during the weaning and periextubation periods.

Vascular Access

Peripheral venous access is more difficult to obtain in obese compared to nonobese children.[39] It is difficult to visualize and to palpate veins under the thicker layer of adipose tissue in obese patients. Similar studies have not been performed evaluating central venous access in obese versus nonobese children. However, one would assume there would be similar difficulties with central access. The use of ultrasound for both peripheral vascular and central vascular catheter placement should be considered if there are difficulties. Another consideration is needle length for vascular access. In some obese patients, standard needles may be too short to clear excessive adipose tissue, and longer needles may be required.

Medication Dosing

Although there have been a number of articles reviewing the influence of obesity on drug disposition, these reviews focus predominatly on adult and animal data. As such, their conclusions may not be applicable to the pediatric patient because changes in fat and fat-free mass occur during periods of growth and development. Many elements of drug disposition are affected by obesity, including drug distribution, metabolism, and clearance. The physiochemical properties of the medication also play a role in how it is metabolized in an obese patient. Consultation with a pediatric pharmacist is recommended because of the numerous factors that affect safe and effective medication dosing in the obese patient.

Most researchers agree that obese children have an excess in whole-body fat mass and lean mass, but the increase in fat mass is substantially higher than in lean mass. Consequently, loading doses of many medications will need adjustment. It has been suggested that loading doses of hydrophilic medications in obese children should be based on ideal body weight (see the "Nutrition Assessment" section) or lean body mass. Partially hydrophilic medications should be based on a percentage of total body weight, and lipophilic medications should be based simply on total body weight. Since maintenance doses rely more on intrinsic metabolic capacity of the liver and kidney, lean body mass is considered the best scalar to use. Regardless of the weight used, it is important to remember that adult maximum doses should not be exceeded.

Obesity results in physiologic changes, such as increased total blood volume, increased cardiac output, alterations in regional blood flow, potential decrease in renal and/or hepatic function, and associated comorbidities. All of these changes can alter the metabolism and elimination of a medication. Each medication needs to be evaluated for an adjustment in dosing frequency based on available information, such as creatinine clearance.

An area of controversy revolves around resuscitation medications.[40,41] Highly water-soluble medications with small volumes of distribution, such as epinephrine, may lead to potentially toxic concentrations if based on actual body weight. Conversely, lipid-soluble medications with larger volumes of distribution, such as amiodarone, could lead to suboptimal concentrations if based on actual body weight. Currently, it is unclear what dosing scalar should be used in resuscitation efforts.

Vasopressors are frequently associated with adverse drug events and are considered high-alert drugs by the Institute of Safe Medication Practices. While few data are available to select an appropriate dosing scalar, the use of ideal body weight for all weight-based dosing strategies is suggested for inotropes (with the exception of milrinone) because these may be associated with severe adverse effects when actual body weight is used in heavier patients. Since these agents are rapidly titrated to clinical response, starting at lower doses based on ideal body weight appears prudent.

Nursing Care

Safety of the patient and of the bedside nurse is an important consideration when dealing with an obese pediatric patient. Weight-appropriate equipment needs to be ordered; protocols for vendors and ordering procedures should be readily accessible by nursing staff. Blood pressure cuffs need to fit appropriately. Children's Hospital Colorado has developed a bariatric supply cart that contains special sized equipment, such as longer intravenous catheters, laryngeal mask airways for patients that weigh greater than 50 kg, and extra-large sequential compression devices.[32] Extra staff to help with patient transfers and patient care may be necessary for the safety of the bedside nurse.

As previously discussed, obese pediatric patients have at least 1 risk factor for development of a DVT. As long as there are no contraindications, there should be consideration for sequential compression devices and possible implementation of prophylactic anticoagulation if the patient has additional risk factors for thrombus formation.

Athough good data are available in adults on the association between pressure ulcer formation and obesity, information is very limited in the pediatric population. In a pediatric trauma study, an increased risk of pressure ulcer formation was noted in obese patients.[42] Routine skin care and assessments, regular and frequent repositioning, and consultation with trained professionals to select appropriate pressure reduction devices are strategies aimed at prevention of pressure ulcers. Adequate nutrition is also an important aspect of pressure ulcer prevention. If a patient develops a pressure ulcer, early identification and treatment by trained personnel improve outcomes.

Outcomes: Morbidity and Mortality of Critically ill Obese Children in the Pediatric Intensive Care Unit

In the adult literature, obesity is not a risk factor for mortality; however, obesity is associated with longer duration of mechanical ventilation and prolonged ICU stays.[43] The mechanical and physiologic impact of obesity on the respiratory system yields a plausible explanation for the increased duration of mechanical ventilation. Obesity influences all of the organ systems and may alter the expected physiologic response to injury and illness, which theoretically complicates care and lengthens stays in the ICU.

In pediatrics, the studies evaluating obesity and risk of morbidity and mortality are mixed.[8, 40, 44-46] Srinivasan and colleagues looked at survival after in-hospital pediatric arrest. Obesity was present in 17% of patients and was associated with a decreased rate of survival to hospital discharge. Theorized reasons for poor outcomes include technical difficulties of cardiopulmonary resuscitation, dosing scalar used for resuscitation medications, and defibrillation dosing in obese patients.[40] In a study evaluating mechanically ventilated pediatric patients, no difference in morbidity or mortality was noted between obese and nonobese counterparts,[8] whereas in another study based in the PICU, an increased risk of mortality was associated with obesity.[44] There is heterogeneity among the studies, which explains the varied results. A systematic review concluded that childhood obesity may be a risk factor for higher mortality in hospitalized children with critical illness, oncologic diagnoses, or transplants.[46] Larger studies to systematically study the effects of obesity on morbidity and mortality in the pediatric population are desirable. It seems likely that duration of mechanical ventilation and PICU length of stay would be longer in the severely obese patient population. In addition, the severely obese pediatric patient may have a higher mortality, although data demonstrating this are currently lacking.

NUTRITION FOR THE HOSPITALIZED CRITICALLY ILL OBESE CHILD

Careful assessment of baseline nutritional status, accurate estimation of macronutrient requirements, and selection of the appropriate route for delivery are important aspects of nutritional therapy in the obese child.

Nutrition Assessment

As with all critically ill children, screening for obesity on admission will help identify those at high nutrition risk requiring detailed nutrition assessment.[47] Children with obesity plus an associated comorbid condition, and those with severe obesity, are considered at high nutrition risk.[48] In addition, critically ill children with obesity who require mechanical ventilation, and those with prolonged inadequate oral intake or significant weight loss are also at high nutrition risk.

Nutrition assessment includes evaluation of weight, height, and BMI; recent and usual dietary intake and physical activity; serum levels of glucose, triglycerides, C-reactive protein, and liver function tests; obesity-related comorbidities; and estimated energy and protein requirements.[49] Weight, height, and BMI are assessed using the CDC 2000 growth charts.[50] No standard exists to identify ideal body weight (IBW) in children; however, it is commonly calculated from the current height in meters squared multiplied by the BMI at the 50th percentile for age.[51] Waist circumference and body composition are rarely assessed in the PICU, due to logistics and inaccuracies caused by abdominal distention and fluid imbalance. Typical methods to evaluate dietary intake such as 24-hour recall, food frequency, and food records are also impractical in the critical care setting. A qualitative or semiquantitative assessment, including questions about frequency of meals and snacks; portion sizes; and consumption of fruits, vegetables, sweetened beverages, and fast food can more quickly reveal useful information.[52] Children with obesity often consume foods with low nutrient density and are at risk for selected vitamin and mineral deficiencies. These should be considered in relation to dietary assessment and disease condition, as well as laboratory assessments, and supplementation initiated as indicated. Micronutrient deficiencies that are commonly seen in obese children include vitamin D and iron; thiamine and folate are commonly low after bariatric surgery.[53,54] With inflammation, serum iron, selenium, zinc, and vitamins A and C are depressed, while ferritin, ceruloplasmin, and copper are increased; therefore, status is more reliably assessed after resolution of the acute stress response.

Indirect Calorimetry

Caloric demands of critically ill obese children are elusive, and measurement of energy expenditure with indirect calorimetry (IC) is the only method to accurately assess requirements.[47,55] Indirect calorimetry determines 24-hour resting energy expenditure with a 10- to 20-minute measurement of oxygen consumption and carbon dioxide production. Inspired and expired gases can be analyzed during spontaneous breathing or mechanical ventilation. Indirect calorimetry measurements are not accurate during mechanical ventilation when the fraction of inspired oxygen is >60%; with air leaks from endotracheal or chest tubes; or with changes in ventilation, energy delivery, or sedation.[56] Where feasible, IC measurements must guide energy prescriptions for obese children to avoid unintended energy imbalance.

Estimation of Energy Requirements

When IC is not available or feasible, energy requirements are typically estimated. Children with obesity have higher fat-free mass as well as fat mass, which produce variable effects on metabolic rate.[57] Standard equations derived from IC measurements in predominantly normal-weight children may overestimate or underestimate the caloric needs of the obese child.[57-60] However, equations developed from measurements in obese children that account for age, sex, and body composition are also not accurate compared to IC.[58-63] In addition, no predictive equation has been evaluated in critically ill children with obesity. Due to a lack of evidence, none of the available methods to estimate energy expenditure can be recommended for obese children during critical illness. However, in clinical practice, 2 or more predictive equations could be compared to help identify an initial calorie target (see Table 21-3), while providing adequate protein and monitoring the patient's response to nutrition support.

Protein Requirements

The suggested protein intake for critically ill children is 1.5 to 2 g/kg, but requirements for those with obesity are unknown.[55] For critically ill obese adults, expert guidelines recommend protein intake of >2 to 2.5 g/kg using IBW while monitoring nitrogen balance, C-reactive protein, and wound healing.[49] This may be an appropriate approach for critically ill children with obesity, but requires further investigation in this population (see Table 21-4).

Nutrition Support

Without nutrition support, the critically ill obese patient is at risk for increased loss of lean body mass due to insulin resistance and poor fuel utilization.[49] Early enteral nutrition positively affects outcomes and is the standard of care for patients with critical illness, regardless of preadmission nutritional status.[49,55] Parenteral nutrition may be required in children who are intolerant to or unable to receive enteral nutrition. An approach to nutrition support therapy that avoids complications associated with underfeeding or overfeeding, such as refeeding syndrome and hyperglycemia, is recommended for hospitalized children with obesity.[47] Critically ill obese children should receive a complete multivitamin, with

TABLE 21-3. Calculation of Resting Energy Expenditure in Children (kcal/d)

Equation	Population Studied	Suggestions[1]
Schofield[82] Males, 3-10 years: (19.59 × Wt) + (1.303 × Ht in cm) + 414.9 Females, 3-10 years: (16.96 × Wt) + (1.618 × Ht in cm) + 371.2 Males, 10-18 years: (16.25 × Wt) + (1.372 × Ht in cm) + 515.5 Females, 10-18 years: (8.365 × Wt) + (4.65 × Ht in cm) + 200.0	Children and adolescents predominantly with normal weight status	May be used for obese children and adolescents, but may underestimate or overestimate requirements
World Health Organization[83] Males, 3-10 years: (22.7 × Wt) + 495 Females, 3-10 years: (22.5 × Wt) + 499 Males, 10-18 years: (17.5 × Wt) + 651 Females, 10-18 years: (12.2 × Wt) + 746	Children and adolescents predominantly with normal weight status	May be used for obese children and adolescents, but may underestimate or overestimate requirements
Maffeis[63] Males: [1287 + (28.6 × Wt) + (23.6 × Ht in cm) – 69.1 × Age)] × 0.239 Females: [1552 + (35.8 × Wt) + (15.6 × Ht in cm) – 36.3 × Age)] × 0.239	Children 6-10 years with obesity and normal weight status	May underestimate energy requirements in obese children Limited age range studied
McDuffie[59] Males, anthropometric parameters: [(0.037 x Wt) – (4.67 × 1 ÷ Ht in cm^2) – (0.159 × Race) + 6.792] × 239 Females, anthropometric parameters: [(0.046 × Wt) – (4.492 × 1 ÷ Ht in cm^2) – (0.151 × Race) + 5.841] × 239 Males, body composition: [(0.078 × FFM) + (0.026 × FM) – (2.646 × 1 ÷ Ht in cm^2) – (0.244 × Race) + 4.8] × 239 Females, body composition: [(0.101 × FFM) + (0.025 × FM) + (0.293 × Ht in cm^3) – (0.185 × Race) + 1.643] × 239	Black and white children 6-11 years with obesity and normal weight status; body composition by DEXA	May overestimate energy requirements in obese children Limited age range studied
Molnar[62] Males: [(50.9 × Wt) + (25.3 × Ht in cm) – (50.3 × Age) + 26.9] × 0.239 Females: [(51.2 × Wt) + (24.5 × Ht in cm) – (207.5 × Age) + 1629.8] × 0.239	Children and adolescents 10-16 years with obesity and normal weight status	Improved accuracy compared to other equations Limited age range studied
Derumeaux-Burel[58] Body composition: [(0.1371 × FFM) – (0.1644 × Age) + 3.3647] × 239	Children and adolescents 3-18 years with obesity; body composition by BIA	Requires BIA
Tverskaya[60] Body composition: 775 + (28.4 × FFM) – (37 × Age) + (3.3 × FM) + (82 × Sex)	Children and adolescents 3-18 years with obesity; body composition by DEXA	Requires DEXA

TABLE 21-3. (Continued)

Equation	Population Studied	Suggestions[1]
Lazzer[61] Anthropometric parameters: [(892.68 × Sex) – (115.93 × Age) + (54.96 × Wt) + (1816.23 × Ht in m) + 1484.50] × 0.239 Body composition: [(909.12 × Sex) – (107.48 × Age) + (68.39 × FFM) + (55.19 × FM) + 3631.23] × 0.239	Caucasian children and adolescents 7-18 years with obesity; body composition by BIA	Improved accuracy compared to other equations Children 6 years and younger not studied

[1]Based on clinical experience.
Age, years; BIA, bioelectrical impedance analysis; DEXA, dual-energy x-ray absorptiometry; FFM, fat-free mass in kg; FM, fat mass in kg; Ht, height; Race, black: 1, white: 0; Sex, male: 1, female: 0; Wt, weight in kg.

TABLE 21-4. Protein Requirements in Critical illness[49,55]

Children 2-18 years	1.5 to 2 g/kg/d
Adults	1.2 to 2 g/kg/d
Adults with obesity	2 to 2.5 g/kg/d using ideal body weight

additional vitamin D and other micronutrients if deficiencies are anticipated or identified. Enteral iron absorption is inhibited by hepatic production of hepcidin during inflammation, and research is needed to study the effects of iron supplementation on oxidant stress and infection in critical pediatric illness.[64] Meanwhile, empiric iron supplementation should be avoided, and delaying iron supplementation until acute phase of illness has subsided is prudent.

High-Protein Hypocaloric Feeding

Providing calories at 60% to 70% of measured or predicted energy expenditure with protein at >2 to 2.5 g/kg using IBW is recommended for critically ill adults with obesity to avoid complications from overfeeding and to improve outcomes.[49] In a retrospective study of critically ill obese adults receiving enteral nutrition, those on hypocaloric, high-protein feedings experienced significantly shorter duration of antibiotic therapy and days in the ICU compared to patients on a eucaloric, high-protein regimen.[65] Positive nitrogen balance or equilibrium was also achieved with hypocaloric enteral and/or parenteral nutrition in approximately half of critically ill obese adults with multiple traumatic injuries prospectively evaluated.[66] Case reports have described improved pulmonary function following rapid weight loss in a morbidly obese child and a young adult with Prader-Willi syndrome and acute respiratory failure treated with very low-calorie diets.[67,68] However, due to a lack of evidence of benefit and at least theoretical risk of harm, hypocaloric nutrition therapy is not recommended for critically ill obese children.[47,55] Although patients are at risk for complications from overfeeding, clinical practices resulting in unintentional underfeeding are prevalent. In an international, multicenter study of PICU nutrition practices, mean daily intake from enteral nutrition compared to goal was 38% for calories and 43% for protein.[69] A strategy that targets hypocaloric feeding for the critically ill obese child may increase the risk of adverse outcomes from underfeeding, particularly when the effects are compounded by delayed initiation and frequent interruptions in nutrition support.

Weight Loss Interventions Following Critical illness

Although no studies have evaluated weight loss interventions in the PICU, some children with severe obesity or associated comorbid conditions may benefit from aggressive weight reduction following recovery from critical illness (see the following section). Behavior change and physical activity are key components to long-term successful weight loss; however, only dietary strategies and bariatric surgery will be discussed here in the context of severe obesity with comorbid conditions.

Dietary Interventions

Several dietary strategies have been researched in children and adolescents with obesity, including macronutrient modification and restriction of energy intake. In an investigation of the so-called "protein-sparing modified fast" (PSMF) diet conducted in a metabolic unit, obese children and adolescents achieved a mean weight loss of 7 kg in 4 weeks.[70] Compared to a low-fat diet, a high-protein, low-carbohydrate (HPLC) diet resulted in significantly greater short-term weight and BMI Z-score reduction in severely obese adolescents.[71,72] Longer-term benefits for weight loss with HPLC diets over caloric restriction have not been demonstrated.[72,73] Of note, the HPLC diet was associated with significant loss of lean body mass, and thus cannot be considered "protein sparing." We have successfully used the HPLC diet in conjunction with an extended in-patient admission to achieve significant weight reduction (5% to 10% of body weight) and improved severe comorbid conditions in severely obese children. Such an intensive intervention, including physical therapy and patient and family education, can lay the groundwork to achieve sustained behavior change and continued weight reduction post-discharge.

Bariatric Surgery

Surgical intervention for weight loss in obese adolescents is controversial due to a lack of long-term studies. Adolescents with severe obesity and comorbid conditions who are unable to maintain weight loss despite organized attempts, have achieved 95% of adult stature, have a stable psychosocial enviroment, and have a commitment to postoperative nutrition management may be appropriate candidates for bariatric surgery.[74] Depending on the type of procedure, nutrition complications can include dehydration; protein malnutrition; and deficiencies of iron, thiamine, folate, and vitamins D, and B_{12}.[75]

CONCLUSIONS

One in 6 children in the United States is obese, which makes it one of the most important epidemics affecting children today. When an obese pediatric patient becomes critically ill, a multitude of factors affects the course of disease and provision of optimal care. Obesity influences all organ systems and may alter the expected physiologic response to injury and illness. In addition, obese pediatric patients have an increased risk of numerous comorbidities that may complicate the PICU course. Care of the obese pediatric patient in the PICU requires a multidisciplinary approach.

Nutrition support is an essential part of optimizing outcomes in critically ill children. If appropriate for the clinical situation, early enteral feeding is preferred and associated with improved outcomes.[19,55] Indirect calorimetry is the only accurate method to determine energy expenditure in critically ill children, especially those with obesity, but if not available or feasible, energy requirements are typically estimated using standard equations derived from IC measurements in predominantly normal-weight children. These may overestimate or underestimate the caloric needs of the obese child. In all cases, regular monitoring of nutritional status, including weight and body composition, should be implemented. Research is needed to identify protein and energy intake targets to optimize outcomes for critically ill obese children.

Although weight loss is the ultimate manner in which physiologic changes and comorbidities may be reversed, reduction of excess weight is not currently recommended during acute critical illness.

Obesity adds a layer of complexity to the critically ill pediatric patient. Care of this special patient population in the PICU requires an understanding of the alterations in physiology and comorbid conditions, a focus on hospital procedures and nursing care, an appreciation for potential adjustments in medication dosing, and nutrition support specific for an obese pediatric patient.

KEY POINTS

- The prevalence of obesity in children has increased dramatically worldwide.
- Severe obesity negatively affects the cardiovascular and respiratory systems, and increases the likelihood of comorbidities and complications in critically ill children.
- Alteration in physiology due to obesity has implications on airway management, respiratory support, venous access, drug dosing, fluid management, and nutrient intake during critical illness.
- Specific nutritional interventions for the critically ill obese child in the PICU need further investigation.

REFERENCES

1. Ogden CL. Prevalence of obesity and trends in body mass index among U.S. children and adolescents, 1999-2010. *JAMA*. 2012;307(5):483.
2. Woo JG, et al. Obesity identified by discharge ICD-9 codes underestimates the true prevalence of obesity in hospitalized children. *J Pediatr.* 2009;154(3):327-331.
3. Krebs NF, et al. Assessment of child and adolescent overweight and obesity. *Pediatrics.* 2007;120(Suppl): S193-S228.

4. Freedman DS, et al. Cardiovascular risk factors and excess adiposity among overweight children and adolescents: the Bogalusa heart study. *J Pediatr.* 2007;150(1):12-17.e2.

5. Barlow SE and Expert C. Expert committee recommendations regarding the prevention, assessment, and treatment of child and adolescent overweight and obesity: summary report. *Pediatrics.* 2007;120 Suppl 4:S164-192.

6. Dehghan M, Akhtar-Danesh N, Merchant AT. Childhood obesity, prevalence and prevention. *Nutr J.* 2005;4(1):24.

7. O'Connor J, et al. Obesity and under-nutrition in a tertiary paediatric hospital. *J Paediatr Child Health.* 2004;40 (5-6):299-304.

8. Goh VL, et al. Obesity is not associated with increased mortality and morbidity in critically ill children. *J Parenter Enteral Nutr.* 2012;37(1):102-108.

9. Alexander JK, et al. Blood volume, cardiac output, and distribution of systemic blood flow in extreme obesity. *Cardiovasc Res Cent Bull.* 1962;1:39-44.

10. de Divitiis O, et al. Obesity and cardiac function. *Circulation.* 1981;64(3):477-482.

11. Berkalp B, et al. Obesity and left ventricular diastolic dysfunction. *Int J Cardiol.* 1995;52(1):23-26.

12. Esper RJ, et al. Endothelial dysfunction: a comprehensive appraisal. *Cardiovasc Diabetol.* 2006;5:4.

13. Herouvi D, et al. Cardiovascular disease in childhood: the role of obesity. *Eur J Pediatr.* 2013;172(6):721-732.

14. Salome CM, King GG, Berend N. Physiology of obesity and effects on lung function. *J Appl Physiol.* 2010;108(1): 206-211.

15. Li AM, et al. The effects of obesity on pulmonary function. *Arch Dis Child.* 2003;88(4):361-363.

16. Lazarus R, et al. Effects of body fat on ventilatory function in children and adolescents: cross-sectional findings from a random population sample of school children. *Pediatr Pulmonol.* 1997;24(3):187-194.

17. Poirier P, et al. Obesity and cardiovascular disease: pathophysiology, evaluation, and effect of weight loss: an update of the 1997 American Heart Association Scientific Statement on Obesity and Heart Disease from the Obesity Committee of the Council on Nutrition, Physical Activity, and Metabolism. *Circulation.* 2006;113(6):898-918.

18. Srivastava T. Nondiabetic consequences of obesity on kidney. *Pediatr Nephrol.* 2006;21(4):463-470.

19. Gleadhill IC, et al. Upper airway collapsibility in snorers and in patients with obstructive hypopnea and apnea. *Am Rev Respir Dis.* 1991;143(6):1300-1303.

20. Narang I and Mathew JL. Childhood obesity and obstructive sleep apnea. *J Nutr Metab.* 2012 (2012). Article ID:134202. (http://dx.doi.org/10.1155/2012/134202).

21. Chau EH, et al. Obesity hypoventilation syndrome: a review of epidemiology, pathophysiology, and perioperative considerations. *Anesthesiology.* 2012;117(1):188-205.

22. Friedman SE and Andrus BW. Obesity and pulmonary hypertension: a review of pathophysiologic mechanisms. *J Obes.* 2012 (2012), Article ID:505274. (http://dx.doi.org/10.1155/2012/505274).

23. Carroll CL, et al. Childhood obesity increases duration of therapy during severe asthma exacerbations. *Pediatr Crit Care Med.* 2006;7(6):527-531.

24. Pearson V1, Ruzas C, Krebs NF, Goldenberg NA, Manco-Johnson MJ, Bernard TJ. Overweight and obesity are increased in childhood-onset cerebrovascular disease. *J Child Neurol.* 2013 Apr;28(4):517-519.

25. Vu LT, et al. Determination of risk factors for deep venous thrombosis in hospitalized children. *J Pediatr Surg.* 2008;43(6):1095-1099.

26. Reiter PD, et al. Thrombosis risk factor assessment and implications for prevention in critically ill children. *Pediatr Crit Care Med.* 2012;13(4):381-386.

27. Agus MS, et al. Tight glycemic control versus standard care after pediatric cardiac surgery. *N Eng J Med.* 2012;367(13):1208-1219.

28. Macrae D, et al. A randomized trial of hyperglycemic control in pediatric intensive care. *N Eng J Med.* 2014;370(2):107-118.

29. Jeschke MG, et al. Glucose control in severely thermally injured pediatric patients: what glucose range should be the target? *Ann Surg.* 2010;252(3):521-527; discussion 527-528.

30. Canarie MF, et al. Decompensated hyperglycemic hyperosmolarity without significant ketoacidosis in the adolescent and young adult population. *J Pediatr Endocrinol Metab.* 2007;20(10):1115-1124.

31. Zeitler P, et al. Hyperglycemic hyperosmolar syndrome in children: pathophysiological considerations and suggested guidelines for treatment. *J Pediatr.* 2011;158(1):9-14, 14 e1-2.

32. Porter RM, Thrasher J, Krebs NF. Implementing a pediatric obesity care guideline in a freestanding children's hospital to improve child safety and hospital preparedness. *J Pediatr Nurs.* 2012;27(6):707-714.

33. Nafiu OO, et al. Obesity and risk of peri-operative complications in children presenting for adenotonsillectomy. *Int J Pediatr Otorhinolaryngol.* 2009;73(1):89-95.

34. Mortensen A, et al. Anesthetizing the obese child. *Pediatr Anesth.* 2011;21(6):623-629.

35. Veyckemans, F., Child obesity and anaesthetic morbidity. *Curr Opin Anaesthesiol.* 2008;21(3):308-312.

36. Tait AR, et al. Incidence and risk factors for perioperative adverse respiratory events in children who are obese. *Anesthesiology*. 2008;108(3):375-380.

37. El-Solh AA, et al. Noninvasive ventilation for prevention of post-extubation respiratory failure in obese patients. *Eur Respir J*. 2006;28(3):588-595.

38. Burns SM, et al. Effect of body position on spontaneous respiratory rate and tidal volume in patients with obesity, abdominal distension and ascites. *Am J Crit Care*. 1994;3(2):102-106.

39. Nafiu OO, et al. Comparing peripheral venous access between obese and normal weight children. *Paediatr Anaesth*. 2010;20(2):172-176.

40. Srinivasan V, et al. Childhood obesity and survival after in-hospital pediatric cardiopulmonary resuscitation. *Pediatrics*. 2010;125(3):e481-e488.

41. Luten R and Zaritsky A. The sophistication of simplicity... optimizing emergency dosing. *Acad Emerg Med*. 2008;15(5):461-465.

42. Rana AR, et al. Childhood obesity: a risk factor for injuries observed at a level-1 trauma center. *J Pediatr Surg*. 2009;44(8):1601-1605.

43. Akinnusi ME, Pineda LA, El Solh AA. Effect of obesity on intensive care morbidity and mortality: a meta-analysis. *Crit Care Med*. 2008;36(1):151-158.

44. Numa A, et al. Extremes of weight centile are associated with increased risk of mortality in pediatric intensive care. *Crit Care*. 2011;15(2):R106.

45. Alselaim N, et al. Does obesity impact the pattern and outcome of trauma in children? *J Pediatr Surg*. 2012;47(7):1404-1409.

46. Bechard LJ, et al. Influence of obesity on clinical outcomes in hospitalized children: a systematic review. *JAMA Pediatr*. 2013;167(5):476-482.

47. Jesuit C, et al. A.S.P.E.N. clinical guidelines: nutrition support of hospitalized pediatric patients with obesity. *J Parenter Enteral Nutr*. 2010;34(1):13-20.

48. Krebs NF, et al. Assessment of child and adolescent overweight and obesity. *Pediatrics*. 2007;120 Suppl 4:S193-S228.

49. McClave SA, et al. Nutrition therapy of the severely obese, critically ill patient: summation of conclusions and recommendations. *J Parenter Enteral Nutr*. 2011;35 (5 Suppl):88S-96S.

50. Kuczmarski RJ, et al. CDC growth charts: United States. *Adv Data*. 2000;(314):1-27.

51. Phillips S, et al. Ideal body weight in children. *Nutr Clin Pract*. 2007;22(2):240-245.

52. Ross MM, et al. Multidisciplinary treatment of pediatric obesity: nutrition evaluation and management. *Nutr Clin Pract*. 2010;25(4):327-334.

53. Fullmer MA, et al. Nutritional strategy for adolescents undergoing bariatric surgery: report of a working group of the Nutrition Committee of NASPGHAN/NACHRI. *J Pediatr Gastroenterol Nutr*. 2012;54(1):125-135.

54. Sacheck J. Pediatric obesity: an inflammatory condition? *J Parenter Enteral Nutr*. 2008;32(6):633-637.

55. Mehta NM, Compher C, A.S.P.E.N. B.o. Directors, A.S.P.E.N. Clinical Guidelines: nutrition support of the critically ill child. *J Parenter Enteral Nutr*. 2009;33(3): 260-276.

56. Haugen HA, Chan LN, Li F. Indirect calorimetry: a practical guide for clinicians. *Nutr Clin Pract*. 2007;22(4):377-388.

57. Lazzer S, et al. Comparison of predictive equations for resting energy expenditure in severely obese Caucasian children and adolescents. *J Endocrinol Invest*. 2007;30(4):313-317.

58. Derumeaux-Burel H, et al. Prediction of resting energy expenditure in a large population of obese children. *Am J Clin Nutr*. 2004;80(6):1544-1550.

59. McDuffie JR, et al. Prediction equations for resting energy expenditure in overweight and normal-weight black and white children. *Am J Clin Nutr*. 2004;80(2):365-373.

60. Tverskaya R, et al. Comparison of several equations and derivation of a new equation for calculating basal metabolic rate in obese children. *J Am Coll Nutr*. 1998;17(4):333-336.

61. Lazzer S, et al. Development and cross-validation of prediction equations for estimating resting energy expenditure in severely obese Caucasian children and adolescents. *Br J Nutr*. 2006;96(5) 973-979.

62. Molnar D, et al. Measured and predicted resting metabolic rate in obese and nonobese adolescents. *J Pediatr*. 1995;127(4):571-577.

63. Maffeis C, et al. Resting metabolic rate in six- to ten-year-old obese and nonobese children. *J Pediatr*. 1993;122(4):556-562.

64. Heming N, Montravers P, Lasocki S. Iron deficiency in critically ill patients: highlighting the role of hepcidin. *Crit Care*. 2011;15(2):210.

65. Dickerson RN, et al. Hypocaloric enteral tube feeding in critically ill obese patients. *Nutrition*. 2002;18(3):241-246.

66. Dickerson RN, et al. Hypocaloric, high-protein nutrition therapy in older vs younger critically ill patients with obesity. *J Parenter Enteral Nutr*. 2013;37(3):342-351.

67. Nishikawa M, et al. Respiratory failure due to morbid obesity in a patient with Prader-Willi syndrome: an

experience of long-term mechanical ventilation. *J Anesth.* 2006;20(4):300-303.

68. Deschildre A, et al. Effects of hypocaloric diet on respiratory manifestations in Willi-Prader syndrome. *Arch Pediatr.* 1995;2(11):1075-1079.
69. Mehta NM, et al. Nutritional practices and their relationship to clinical outcomes in critically ill children: an international multicenter cohort study. *Crit Care Med.* 2012;40(7):2204-2211.
70. Merritt RJ, et al. Consequences of modified fasting in obese pediatric and adolescent patients. I. Protein-sparing modified fast. *J Pediatr.* 1980;96(1):13-19.
71. Sondike SB, Copperman N, Jacobson MS. Effects of a low-carbohydrate diet on weight loss and cardiovascular risk factor in overweight adolescents. *J Pediatr.* 2003;142(3):253-258.
72. Krebs NF, et al. Efficacy and safety of a high protein, low carbohydrate diet for weight loss in severely obese adolescents. *J Pediatr.* 2010;157(2):252-258.
73. Kirk S, et al. Role of carbohydrate modification in weight management among obese children: a randomized clinical trial. *J Pediatr.* 2012;161(2):320-327 e1.
74. Standard I and Safety C. IPEG guidelines for surgical treatment of extremely obese adolescents. *J Laparoendosc Adv Surg Tech A.* 2009;19(1):xiv-xvi.
75. Hsia DS, Fallon SC, Brandt ML. Adolescent bariatric surgery. *Arch Pediatr Adolesc Med.* 2012;166(8):757-766.
76. Porter RM, Thrasher J, Krebs NF. Implementing a pediatric obesity care guideline in a freestanding children's hospital to improve child safety and hospital preparedness. *J Pediatr Nurs.* 2012;27(6):707-14.
77. Kershaw EE. Adipose tissue as an endocrine organ. *J Clin Endocrinol Metab.* 2004;89(6):2548-2556.
78. Diez JJ, Iglesias P. The role of the novel adipocyte-derived hormone adiponectin in human disease. *Eur J Endocrinol.* 2003;148(3):293-300.
79. Chandran M, et al. Adiponectin: more than just another fat cell hormone? *Diabetes Care.* 2003;26(8):2442-2450.
80. Arslan N, Erdur B, Aydin A. Hormones and cytokines in childhood obesity. *Indian Pediatr.* 2010;47(10):829-839.
81. Daniels SR. The consequences of childhood overweight and obesity. *Future Child.* 2006;16(1):47-67.
82. Schofield WN. Predicting basal metabolic rate, new standards and review of previous work. *Hum Nutr Clin Nutr.* 1985;39 Suppl 1:5-41.
83. Energy and protein requirements. Report of a joint FAO/WHO/UNU Expert Consultation. *World Health Organ Tech Rep Ser.* 1985;724:1-206.

CHAPTER 22

Nutritional Support of Critically ill Children in Resource-Limited Settings

Sunit Singhi

- INTRODUCTION
- IN-HOSPITAL MALNUTRITION
- NUTRITIONAL ASSESSMENT
- ENERGY NEEDS
- CONSIDERATIONS IN SEVERE MALNUTRITION
- PROTEIN REQUIREMENTS
  - Albumin
- LIPID REQUIREMENT
- CARBOHYDRTES
- FLUID INTAKE
- TRACE ELEMENTS
  - Zinc
  - Iron
  - Selenium
  - Magnesium
  - Copper
  - Manganese
- VITAMINS
  - Vitamin A
  - Vitamin D
  - Vitamin E
  - Water-Soluble Vitamins
  - Glutamine and Arginine
- ROUTES AND METHODS
- ENTERAL FORMULAS
- PRACTICAL ISSUES
- KEY POINTS
  - References

INTRODUCTION

The provision of optimal nutrition may be challenging in developing countries due to a higher prevalence of malnutrition and scarcity of resources in the pediatric intensive care unit (PICU). Malnutrition affects nearly 50% of hospitalized children and 20% to 70% of critically ill children, more so in resource-limited countries.[1] In a recent international multicenter cohort, over 30% of patients admitted to 31 PICUs had severe malnutrition on admission, with body mass index (BMI) Z-score >2 (13.2%) or <–2 (17.1%) on admission.[2] Malnutrition was associated with greater length of ventilation, higher rate of complications, longer length of hospital stay and increased costs, and increased mortality.[3,4] Furthermore, it is easy to underfeed critically ill children because of poor gut function, fasting for various surgical and nonsurgical procedures, and fluid constraints.[5] Therefore, nutrition may deteriorate further in the hospital, and specifically in the PICU, with resultant poor outcomes, unless specific attention is paid to management of nutritional losses from drains, wound and skin losses, renal dysfunction, dialysis, etc. In the presence of preexisting malnutrition, children are much more susceptible to the deleterious effects of the protracted catabolic stress caused by critical illness. Compared to adults, children have significantly lower nutritional reserves and higher resting energy expenditure (REE) per unit body weight; the quantity of protein as a percentage of body weight, lipid stores, and carbohydrate reserves are reduced. The caloric and protein deficits accumulate quickly in critically ill children. While public health programs have focused on infant and child malnutrition in the general community, the deterioration of nutritional status in the hospital during critical illness is often neglected.

IN-HOSPITAL MALNUTRITION

Critically ill infants and children are susceptible to "in-hospital malnutrition."[6,7] In a recently completed study in our PICU, among critically ill children staying for 1 week, the proportion of undernourished children defined as weight-for-age Z-score <−2 was 54% in infants under 1 year and 27% in children 1 to 12 years. The number of undernourished children increased between admission and discharge to 70% in infants under 1 year and 53% in children 1 to 5 years of age. A trend toward recovery of anthropometric parameters was seen at 3 and 6 months post-hospitalization (*Shrikant, Bhalla, and Singhi personal communication*). Hypoalbuminemia was present in 21% (92 of 435) patients at admission, and 34% (151/435) by end of the first week of stay and in 37% (164/435) at the end of the second week. The hypoalbuminemic patients had prolonged PICU stay (13.8 vs. 6.7 days) and ventilator requirement (28.8% vs. 8.5%) (unpublished data). Hospital malnutrition has been associated with increased morbidity, mortality, hospital stay, and costs.[8,9] However, hospital malnutrition is underrecognized. Its true incidence and impact, particularly in developing countries, may be much higher than presently estimated.[10] Careful nutritional evaluation of children on admission is essential in order to identify those children who are already undernourished and hence at higher risk of further nutritional deterioration during their hospital stay.[11]

NUTRITIONAL ASSESSMENT

All children admitted to the PICU must undergo nutrition screening to identify those who are at risk of malnutrition. A formal nutrition assessment to obtain baseline data to estimate nutritional needs and to formulate a nutrition care plan is required, especially in those with malnutrition prior to the illness. Other socioeconomic and maternal factors may influence the degree of nutritional deterioration in hospitalized children. In a study of hospitalized children in Ethiopia, less than a third of the children were classified as having a normal nutritional state on admission. There were no significant differences in weight-for-age between children from rural and urban settings. Parental occupation and income, as well as maternal age, were significant predictors of nutritional state in the hospital.[12] The degree of malnutrition at admission was associated with increased risk of mortality, especially in those with respiratory disease. An assessment of nutritional status should include all the following, as no single indicator is reliable:

- **Anthropometric:** Weight and height at admission; change in weight.
- **Clinical:** Subjective global assessment and evaluation for signs of micronutrient deficiency.
- **Serum albumin and prealbumin:** While low levels of these proteins have traditionally been considered to reflect malnutrition, they are probably best considered inflammatory markers that decrease with inflammation. It should also be remembered that levels of albumin are normal in marasmus and anorexia nervosa. Serum albumin is an excellent prognostic marker in various critical illness states, as it is an inflammatory marker.

ENERGY NEEDS

The REE of critically ill children in the PICU ranges widely, from 37 to 62 kcal/kg per day.[13-15] The hypermetabolic response apparent in adults is not so evident in critically ill children.[16] Currently available standard equations are not reliable in predicting actual measured energy expenditure and overestimate the energy expenditure.[17] Several factors can alter energy needs. Energy needs vary with the stage of illness and the use of various treatments. They decrease with use of sedation, neuromuscular blockade and mechanical ventilation, and in the presence of multiple organ system failure. The need is higher in neonates with bronchopulmonary dysplasia, in the postoperative period after major surgeries, and in spontaneously breathing patients. Children on ventilators have an REE of approximately 45 kcal/kg per day, while those breathing spontaneously are likely to have a higher energy expenditure.[18,19] Recent studies have shown that a critically ill child does not have exceptionally high energy needs, probably because of transient growth cessation during extreme stress, sedation, and low levels of physical activity. Yet, reports of a high prevalence of critically ill children who are not meeting their recommended levels of protein and energy are not uncommon.[20] Ideally, the estimate of energy requirement should be individualized and measured daily. Indirect calorimetry (IC) allows bedside measurement of energy expenditure and may guide nutrient prescription in critically ill patients. However, IC testing requires resources and expertise, which is lacking in a majority of hospitals, especially in the developing world. In the absence of a direct measure of energy expenditure, estimates derived from published equations may be used with caution. Many reports have shown that the use of standard equations may overestimate the energy needs during critical illness.

Critically ill children in the acute phase of illness have lower energy and nutrient requirements as compared to healthy children. Healthy infants have an energy requirement of 100 to 120 kcal/kg per day of which approximately 50% is basal metabolic rate (BMR), 30% is required for growth, 10% for diet-induced thermogenesis, and the remaining 10% for physical activity.[21] The majority of critically ill children, with the possible exception of severely burned patients in the acute phase, have an energy expenditure that equals or is less than basal metabolic requirements according to predictive equations because of sedation, mechanical ventilation, reduced physical activity, and growth cessation.[16,22]

The initial calorie intake is aimed at attenuating loss due to hypercatabolism without overloading the metabolism and the cardiovascular system. It should be similar to the REE recommended for healthy children. Once metabolic stress has resolved, calories should be added or reduced after careful appraisal of caloric needs. We aim to provide a caloric intake equal to the BMR, and add 10% to account for stress in the catabolic phase (50 to 55 kcals/kg per day in infants and gradually reducing to 25 kcal/kg per day in adolescents). Both underestimates and overestimates are potentially harmful. Enterally fed critically ill children require an additional 10% because of obligate malabsorption. A surfeit of calories does not result in improved protein accretion and often results in significant hyperglycemia.

In a cohort of 116 of 140 patients, mean ± SD age 49.2±44 (range 2-144) months, who stayed in our PICU for more than 5 days, with a PICU stay of 12 to 17 days, mechanical ventilation for 8 to 11 days, and an average BMI of 15.2, a higher percentage of patients (43%) died in the lowest calorie group (Table 22-1). Feeds could be started on day 1 in 47 patients, in an additional 47 patients on day 2, and in 10 patients, feeds could be started after day 3. Seventy-eight (67.2%) patients required mechanical ventilation. Sixty-three (54%) patients had hemodynamic instability and required inotropic agents, and 52 (44.8%) patients needed neurological monitoring. Twenty-six (17.2%) patients died during the study; 11 of them before day 6.

TABLE 22-1. Outcomes of 140 Patients Staying for > 5 Days in Our ICU with Respect to Caloric Intake

Group	Calorie Intake	Survived	Adverse Outcome*	P Value
Total enrolled (n = 140)		**114 (81.4%)**	**26 (17.2%)**	
Group-1 (n = 23)	=<60% of maintenance cal/day	13 (56.5%)	10 (43.4%)	**0.0001**
Group-2 (n = 40)	61% to 90% of maintenance cal/day	37 (92.5%)	3 (7.5%)	
Group-3 (n = 26)	90% to 110% of maintenance cal/day	25 (96.2%)	1 (3.8%)	
Group-4 (n = 27)	>110% of maintenance cal/day	26 (96.3%)	1 (3.7%)	
Total eligible (n = 116)	Total	101 (87.1%)	15 (12.9%)	

Reproduced with permission from Madarkar B, Baranwal A, Singhi S: Dissertation submitted for award of degree of Doctor of Medicine (MD) Postgraduate Institute of Medical Education & Research, Chandigarh, 2011

Critically ill children enter the recovery phase sooner than adults do, usually within a week. Anabolic metabolism often returns, which is presumed to coincide with a gradual increase in prealbumin and a decrease in C-reactive protein (CRP) concentrations. This phase is characterized by a gradual stability in vital parameters. This is presumed to be the time to escalate caloric intake.

CONSIDERATIONS IN SEVERE MALNUTRITION

There is no evidence-based recommendation for critically ill malnourished children. An understanding of the differences and similarities between malnutrition and the catabolism of critical illness, therefore, is important in planning the nutritional support. The metabolic status of critically ill patients is different from that of malnourished children. In the critically ill, there is a catabolic response and elevated BMR, which is usually not reversed by simple nutrition. In contrast, in malnutrition, BMR is depressed; it is reversible, given careful and adequate refeeding. Cortisol is high and insulin is low in children with severe malnutrition, which is similar to what happens during severe stress response. Critical illness in such patients further stretches the already stressed metabolic adjustments. Sustained cortisol elevation is no longer possible due to adrenal exhaustion. Hypoglycemia due to exhausted stores is a common occurrence as compared to stress-induced hyperglycemia, which is in contrast to what happens in normally nourished children. There is a slow breakdown of proteins in edematous malnutrition, resulting in reduced supply of amino acids for synthesis of proteins required for nutrient transport and production of acute-phase reactants.[23] The albumin pool decreases by more than 50%. The amino acid pool is also low, particularly the branched-chain amino acids threonine and tyrosine. Gamma globulins are increased, mainly as alpha-1 globulins (acute-phase reactants); alpha-2 globulins (binding proteins) and beta globulins (transfer proteins) are low.

Fat absorption is impaired due to pancreatic insufficiency in malnourished children. Decreased insulin increases fat utilization, fat deposition in the liver, and the nonessential/essential fatty acid ratio. Increased cortisol

TABLE 22-2. Nutritional Issues in Critically ill Children When There Is Preexisting Malnutrition

Issues	Acute or stabilization phase Week 1 Day 1-2	 Day 3-7	Rehabilitation phase Week 2-6
Hypoglycemia	→ Frequent feeding and monitoring	Frequent feeding and monitoring	
Hypothermia	→		
Hydration	Assess every 6 hours; avoid dehydration → Monitor urine output	Avoid fluid overload	
Electrolytes: sodium, potassium, calcium, magnesium	Manage severe hypokalemia and hyponatremia →	→	
Micronutrients	Mineral mix; no iron →	→	With iron →
Initial feeding	Start at basal level; increase the energy and protein intake gradually →	→	
Feeding to achieve catch-up growth			→

during the initial period of stress increases lipolysis and decreases fatty acid utilization for energy. Fat, therefore, cannot be used as a source of energy in the proportions that are used in normally nourished children.

Malnourished children have a reduced ability to handle substrate, liquids, and solutes because of reduction in cardiac output, glomerular filtration rate, renal blood flow, and renal solute excretion capacity; sodium-potassium pump activity also is lowered. Young children with protein calorie malnutrition are also at increased risk of morbidity and mortality secondary to infections.

In light of all this, it is important to give special attention to the nutrition of undernourished and severity malnourished children right from admission to safeguard against hypoglycemia and hyperglycemia, hypokalemia, dehydration and fluid overload, and to minimize infection-associated morbidity and mortality (Table 22-2). Feeds are introduced gradually to allow for metabolic adaptation to use the energy supply to repair and replenish the stores and for growth.

PROTEIN REQUIREMENTS

In critical illness, there is a high turnover of proteins to allow for the immediate synthesis of mediators of the inflammatory response and tissue repair. Increased proteolysis of skeletal muscle proteins sets in to provide amino acids for the activity of cells involved in the inflammatory response, synthesis of acutely needed enzymes, serum proteins, and glucose and repair of injured tissues. The process requires energy and results in an increase in REE. Several factors enhance protein catabolism, such as bacterial sepsis, postoperative stress, underlying malignancies, and any severely stressed state such as severe burn.

Approximate protein requirements are 2 to 3 g/kg per day in infants and 1.5 to 2.0 g/kg per day in older children. Higher protein use can cause azotemia and acidosis. Currently, there is no specific recommendation regarding special amino acid formulations for nutrition support of critically ill children. Glutamine supplementation remains investigational; it does not result in appreciable benefit over standard amino acid formulations.

Albumin

Low serum albumin is associated with severity of critical illness, but there is no evidence that albumin supplementation improves outcome in burns and in sepsis. On the contrary, all available evidence suggests that albumin supplementation increases mortality.

LIPID REQUIREMENT

The energy needs of critically ill children are met largely by the mobilization and oxidation of free fatty acids. It is the prime source of energy—30% to 40% of the released fatty acids are oxidized for energy. Glycerol released along with free fatty acids may be converted to pyruvate, which in turn is used for gluconeogenesis. Infants and children in the PICU may suffer biochemical essential fatty acid deficiency within 1 week if administered a fat-free diet. Dietary fat should form about 30% to 35% of total calories. A 50:50 blend of medium-chain triglycerides (MCTs) and low-chain triglycerides (LCTs) should be preferred, as it has an even balance of omega-6 and omega-3 fatty acids. Medium-chain triglycerides have a potential advantage, as they are rapidly cleared and oxidized. Omega-3 fatty acids are needed for formation of prostaglandins to maintain regional blood flow and bactericidal activity.

Commercially available lipid solutions for parenteral nutrition obviate the risk of essential fatty acid deficiency, result in improved protein utilization, and do not significantly increase metabolic rate. Lipid supplementation in ill neonates and children should start at 0.5 to 1 g/kg per day and advance over a period of 5 to 7 days to 2 to 4 g/kg per day while closely monitoring triglyceride concentrations to provide 30% to 40% of total calories.

CARBOHYDRATES

Glucose is the major source of energy in critical illness. It should be added to provide the balance of calories after taking into consideration calories from protein and lipids. Glucose is the preferred substrate for the brain, erythrocytes, and the renal medulla and provides an energy source for the repair of injured tissues. In critically ill patients, there is increased glycogenolysis and gluconeogenesis from stored muscle protein and fat stores. Provision of dietary glucose reduces fat oxidation relatively, but it is ineffective in quelling gluconeogenesis in stressed states and can result in significant hyperglycemia and hyperosmolarity because of relative insulin resistance. In severely malnourished children, optimal glycemic status should be ascertained by frequent small feeds and blood glucose monitoring. Malnutrition worsens the prognosis in critically ill children with hypo- or hyperglycemia.[24] The aim should be to maintain glucose between 90 and 150 mg/dL; insulin 0.05 mcg/kg per hour may be used if glucose exceeds 150 mg/dL.

FLUID INTAKE

Hydration status should be assessed using daily weight, obvious edema/puffiness, urine osmolality or specific gravity, urine output, and fluid balance. In the early phase of critical illness, fluid volume should be kept on the lower side of normal to match the caloric utilization and titrated carefully to avoid fluid overload. Fluid overload can trigger multiple organ dysfunction.[25] We usually start with 80% of calculated fluid volume.

TRACE ELEMENTS

Several clinically important trace elements might be deficient in critically ill children. These include zinc, iron, selenium, copper, manganese, iodine and electrolytes, potassium,[26,27] phosphate (refeeding syndromes), magnesium,[28] and calcium.[29] A mineral mix recommended by the World Health Organization (WHO) for malnourished children can meet daily requirements of major trace elements (Table 22-3).

Zinc

Zinc (2 mg/kg per day) should be routinely supplemented in critically ill children in developing countries. Serum zinc levels are low in malnourished patients, in patients with severe pneumonia, and in the critically ill.[30-32] Though zinc, selenium, and glutamine supplementation did not offer any benefit in immune-competent patients,[30,33] in developing countries, zinc supplementation was shown to be beneficial in severe pneumonia in very young children[34]; it was associated with reduced a length of PICU stay and significantly reduced case fatality in children with severe pneumonia,[35] and reduced the risk of treatment failure by 40% in infants aged 7 to 120 days with serious bacterial infection in India.[36] Zinc-losing states such as severe burns need high-dose supplementation: 25 mg/day enterally or 50 mcg/kg per day parenterally.

TABLE 22-3. Composition of Mineral Mix Solution

Substance Amount
Potassium chloride 89.5 g
Tripotassium citrate 32.4 g
Magnesium chloride 30.5 g
Zinc acetate 3.3 g
Copper sulfate 0.56 g
Sodium selenate 10 mg
Potassium iodide 5 mg
Water to make 1000 mL

Adapted with permisison from WHO 2003. Management of a child with serious infection or severe malnutrition, WHO, Geneva. 2003

Iron

Iron deficiency is common in malnourished and hospitalized children in developing countries. But free iron may be detrimental during the acute phase of critical illness and infections. Iron supplementation (3 mg/kg per day) to treat iron deficiency should be started after the acute crisis is over once the child starts gaining weight.

Selenium

Selenium is not recommended in acute infections. Selenium supplementation prevents oxidative stress-induced damage to immune cells and should be given in the recovery phase (30 to 40 mcg/day).

Magnesium

Hypomagnesemia is very common in PICU patients. It is often associated with hypokalemia, hypocalcaemia, hypoalbuminemia, and pH changes. The presence of hypomagnesemia or hypermagnesemia is associated with a significantly higher mortality and longer hospital stay.[28] Therefore, we monitor serum Mg levels and add intravenous Mg SO_4 supplement 0.1 mL/kg per day (0.5 mEq/kg per day).

Copper

Copper deficiency causes depression of the reticuloendothelial system, reduced microbicidal activity of granulocytes, and decreased response of splenic lymphocytes to T-cell and B-cell mitogens. Copper-deficient patients are more susceptible to bronchopneumonia and bacterial sepsis. Copper supplementation (200 to 500 mcg/day) is necessary in malnourished children for optimal recovery of the immune system.

Manganese

There is no role of routine supplementation with manganese in acutely ill children.

VITAMINS

Selected vitamins and trace minerals support immune functions and strengthen epithelial barriers and immune responses.[37] We add a multivitamin preparation to enteral feed or to intravenous fluids to all PICU patients.

Vitamin A

Vitamin A maintains the integrity of epithelial surfaces, lymphocyte proliferation, immunoglobulin production, and T-helper activity. Deficiency causes increased bacterial binding to epithelial cells and reduced thymic weight. In developing countries, vitamin A supplementation has been proven to reduce mortality related to respiratory infections and diarrhea in children. The recommended single dose is 100,000 IU for infants 6 to 12 months and 200,000 U after infancy.

Vitamin D

Vitamin D acts as an immune regulatory and lymphocyte-differentiating hormone. Normal concentrations are needed for proper immune function. However, high-dose vitamin D may also suppress immunity. Though vitamin D deficiency had been associated with greater severity of critical illness and longer PICU stay, the role of targeted vitamin D supplementation in the critically ill child needs further study to make any definitive recommendations.[38] In a prospective study of 124 children treated in our PICU for sepsis, we did not find any relationship between vitamin D status and severity of sepsis (sepsis, n-47; septic shock, n-62; and sepsis with MODS, n-69), frequency of hospital-acquired infections, and outcome of sepsis (unpublished data). However, we administer vitamin D in usual maintenance doses to all PICU patients.

Vitamin E

Currently, there is no study to determine the effects of vitamin E deficiency in critically ill children. Vitamin E, selenium, and zinc increase humoral immune response. Zinc deficiency leads to decreased vitamin E levels.

Water-Soluble Vitamins

Folic acid (5 mg) and vitamins B_1, B_6, B_{12}, and C in therapeutic doses should be supplemented in all critically ill children, as their deficiency sets in early in critical illness. Infections may cause or worsen existing vitamin deficiencies. Concentrations of vitamin A, B_6, and C are low in serum during acute bacterial and viral infections. Reduced concentrations of folic acid occur in infants with diarrhea and acute bacterial infections. Vitamins B_1, B_6, B_{12}, and C have been implicated in regulation of the cellular and humoral immune system. Vitamin B_1 predisposes to tropical pyomyositis. Vitamin C is also an antioxidant and improves phagocytic activity by enhancing microtubular formation.

Glutamine and Arginine

Glutamine and arginine have immune-enhancing properties. Glutamine is the fuel source for lymphocytes, macrophages, and enterocytes. During acute illness, glutamine uptake by small intestine and immune cells exceeds synthesis from skeletal muscle. However, no demonstrable benefit has been shown for glutamine supplementation in pediatric patients. We do not use glutamine and arginine supplements.

ROUTES AND METHODS

Enteral nutrition is preferred to parenteral as long as the gut is available: It could be gastric or transpyloric feeding. Enteral and/or parenteral nutrition should be started as soon as hemodynamic stability is achieved; this also applies to malnourished children. Enteral nutrition has several benefits and a few drawbacks.[39] It reduces length of hospital stay and risk of infection, stimulates gastrointestinal motility, minimizes atrophy of the gastrointestinal mucosa and prevents bacterial translocation by maintaining the integrity of the mucosal membrane, maintains the immune system, and reduces mortality.

We aim to start nasogastric tube feeds within 24 hours of admission to the PICU at 1 mL/kg per feed every 3 hours and gradually advance it over next 2 to 3 days until the desired nutritional target is achieved (Table 22-4). Bolus or intermittent feeding is more physiological and requires less time/equipment with reduced risk of contamination. However, there are more chances of aspiration after such feeds. In children with impaired gut function, continuous feeding (using a peristaltic pump) has the advantage of leaving the smallest residual volume and the least chance of aspiration. It is also beneficial due to lower thermogenic effect and improved substrate utility. When the child can eat orally, both methods of feed delivery can be combined with overnight tube feeds (10 to 12 hrs) and oral intake during the day.

TABLE 22-4. Nutritional Targets for Critically ill Children

Age	Energy kcal/kg per day	Gram/kg per day of various nutrients		
		Protein	Fat	Carbohydrate
1-12 months	100-110	2.5-3	3-4	14-16
1-6 years	90-100	2-3	2-3	14-16
7-12 years	70-90	2-3	2-3	11-13
>12 years	35-70	1-2	2-3	3-9

ENTERAL FORMULAS

Standard enteral formulations that are readily available in North America and Europe are expensive to use in resource-limited settings. Also, parenteral nutrition formulations are not available in pediatric packaging and need compounding. Therefore, we depend on enteral food mix prepared by our dietetics department. Tables 22-5 and 22-6 show various enteral formulas used at our institute. These formulas provide 40% to 55% energy from

TABLE 22-5. Composition of Various Enteral Formulas Prepared by Dietetics Department, Post-Graduate Institute of Medical Education and Research, Chandigarh, India

Type of Formula	Contents		Nutritional Value/100 mL	
Elemental	Proteinex	50 gm	Calories	81.3
	Sugar	100 gm	Proteins	1.6
	Refined oil	30 gm	CHO	10.5
	Water	To make 1000 cc	Fats	3 gm
Polymeric (Milk) (Samolina)	Milk	500 gm	Calories	150
	Sugar	50 gm	Proteins	4 gm
	Samolina	20 gm	CHO	17.5
	Oil	20 gm	Fats	7.5 gm
Enriched milk	Cow's milk (toned)	500 mL	Calories	80
	Oil	30 mL	Proteins	1.75
	Water	To make 1000 cc	CHO	9.82 gm
	Sugar	50 gm	Fats	4.2 gm
Polymeric (Lactose Free)	Rice	50 gm	Calories	62
	Sugar	45 gm	Proteins	0.3
	Oil	30 gm	CHO	8.4 gm
	Water	To make 1000 cc	Fats	3.7 gm
Special Formulas (Renal Formula)	Custard powder	25 gm	Calories	221
	Oil	20 mL	Proteins	3.5 gm
	Sugar	50 gm	CHO	33 gm
	Toned milk	300 mL	Fats	22 gm
Special Formulas (Hepatic Formula)	Milk	250 cc	Calories	100
	Sugar	100 gm	Proteins	1.4 gm
	Rice	75 gm	CHO	2 gm
	Oil	25 mL	Fats	1.5 gm
	Water	To make 1000 cc		

TABLE 22-6. Composition of Various High-Caloric Enteral Formulas Prepared by Dietetics Department, Post-Graduate Institute of Medical Education and Research, Chandigarh, India

Type of Diet	Contents		Nutritional	Value/100 mL
Burn diet A1 (1liter)	Milk	100 mL	Calories	155
	Sugar	60 gm	Proteins	7 gm
	Kidsprot†	50 gm	CHO	18.6 gm
	Skim milk powder	60 gm	Fats	3.15 gm
	Corn flour	5 gm		
	Oil	35 mL		
Burn diet A2* (1liter)	Soyabean	75 gm	Calories	122
	Sugar	60 gm	Proteins	4.66 gm
	Nusowin Child‡	50 gm	CHO	12.8 gm
	Rice	25 gm	Fats	5.9 gm
	Oil	60 mL		

*Lactose free.
† Kidspro: 120 kcal, and 7.2 gm proteins in 30 gm (protein and energy supplement).
‡ Nusowin child: 375 kcal and 46 gm proteins in 100 gm (soy protein isolate powder with docosahexaenoic acid (DHA), calcium, iron, and vitamin D.

carbohydrates, 10% to 15% from proteins, and 30% to 40% from lipids. In the formulation for use in children with cow's milk protein allergy, milk is replaced by soy protein or protein hydrolysate. For malnourished children, initially a milk-based formula with 75 kcal/100 mL and 0.9 g protein/100 mL is usually adequate. Those with persistent diarrhea are given a cereal-based low-lactose and lone osmolality formula. Initially feeding is given every 2 to 3 hours with the feeds being provided through the night. After 2 to 3 days, the child is given formula providing 100 kcal/100 mL and protein 2 to 3 g/100 mL as per tolerance. The feed volume is gradually increased as shown in Table 22-7.

PRACTICAL ISSUES

Children under 2 years of age, those having a prolonged hospital stay, congenital heart disease, extensive burn injuries, and those requiring mechanical ventilation should receive greater attention in initiation and planning of nutrition, as they are at greater risk of developing malnutrition.[4,40,41]

Important barriers to enteral feeding in the PICU that can cause underfeeding include fluid restriction, gastrointestinal intolerance (diarrhea, vomiting, ileus), interruptions because of surgical and diagnostic procedures, and extubation.[5,42] Up to 50% of pediatric patients may be intolerant to enteral feeding using the nasogastric route. In some, gastric emptying is delayed. In these patients, consider the use of prokinetic agents.[43] Transpyloric feeding has been used in postoperative cardiac surgical patients and in PICU patients.[44,45]

Success of enteral feeding requires close coordination with a dietitian. Prior to start of feeds, a written plan should be made that should include fluid, calories, proteins, and electrolyte requirements of the child. Protocol for patient monitoring should be clearly defined (Table 22-8). In a

TABLE 22-7. Frequency and Volume of Feeds in Severely Malnourished Critically ill Children

Days	Frequency	Vol/Kg/Feed	Vol/Kg/Day*
1-2	2 hrly	11 mL	130 mL
3-5	3 hrly	16 mL	130 mL
6 onwards	4 hrly	22 mL	130 mL

Adapted with permission from WHO 2003. Management of a child with serious infection or severe malnutrition, WHO, Geneva. 2004
*Reduce total volume to 80% in ventilated children.

TABLE 22-8. Monitoring Protocol for Patients on Enteral Nutrition

Tolerance	Nutrition and Metabolic	Mechanical
Nausea	Body weight	Confirm tube patency before each use
Vomiting	Serum Na, K, osmolarity	Irrigate feeding tube after intermittent feeds
Diarrhea	Blood glucose, urea, nitrogen	Tablets to be crushed before administration
Constipation	Serum Mg, Ca, PO_4	
Abdominal distension	Urine osmolality/specific gravity	
	Liver function tests	

Reproduced with permission from Singhi S. Basic Pediatric Intensive Care; Fourth edition, New Delhi, Peepee-publishers, 2014

prospective study, with use of a feeding protocol, the nutrition goal was achieved within a mean of 18.5 hours, as compared to 57.8 hours in retrospective controls from the same unit.[46] Patients admitted to units that utilized a feeding protocol had a lower prevalence of acquired infections, independent of the amount of energy or protein intake.[2]

Total parenteral nutrition or mixed nutrition is needed if there is intestinal failure (obstruction, ischemic or severe inflammation, peritonitis, and paralytic ileus), or if there are barriers to deliver optimum energy through the enteral route; for more details, see chapter 7. Enteral nutrition may have trophic effects on the gut and other benefits in such children. However, the evidence base is limited and of poor quality.

KEY POINTS

- Identify malnutrition early on. Malnutrition begets infection and vice versa and worsens the prognosis.
- Set goals for the individual patient; use a protocol.
- Use the gut as long as it is possible. Enteral nutrition is always better than parenteral in reducing infections.
- In critically ill children with malnutrition, resuscitate and treat the underlying condition(s) and prevent hypoglycemia/hyperglycemia, hypokalemia, and hypothermia.
- Zinc has role in respiratory and diarrheal illnesses and patients with burns. Iron and selenium are not recommended in acute infections.
- In malnourished children, start with small amount and gradually increase intake of a cereal-based formula and shift after 2 to 3 days to a formula providing 100 kcal and 2 to 3 g proteins/100 mL, depending on tolerance.
- Immunonutrients improve immune functions in lab and animal studies, but data in children are not sufficient to make recommendations.
- Constantly review and monitor nutritional requirements and intake.

REFERENCES

1. Prieto MB, Cid JL. Malnutrition in the critically ill child: the importance of enteral nutrition. *Int J Environ Res Public Health.* 2011;8(11):4353-4366.
2. Mehta NM, Bechard LJ, Cahill N, et al. Nutritional practices and their relationship to clinical outcomes in critically ill children: an international multicenter cohort study. *Critical Care Med.* 2012;40(7):2204-2211.
3. de Souza Menezes F, Leite HP, Koch Nogueira PC. Malnutrition as an independent predictor of clinical outcome in critically ill children. *Nutrition.* 2012;28(3):267-270.
4. Mehta NM, Duggan CP. Nutritional deficiencies during critical illness. *Pediatr Clin North Am.* 2009;56(5):1143-1160.
5. Rogers EJ, Gilbertson HR, Heine RG, Henning R. Barriers to adequate nutrition in critically ill children. *Nutrition.* 2003;19(10):865-868.
6. Hulst J, Joosten K, Zimmermann L, et al. Malnutrition in critically ill children: from admission to 6 months after discharge. *Clin Nutr.* 2004;23(2):223-232.
7. Joosten KF, Hulst JM. Malnutrition in pediatric hospital patients: current issues. *Nutrition.* 2011;27(2):133-137.
8. Goiburu ME, Goiburu MM, Bianco H, et al. The impact of malnutrition on morbidity, mortality and length of hospital stay in trauma patients. *Nutr Hosp.* 2006;21(5):604-610.

9. Correia MI, Waitzberg DL. The impact of malnutrition on morbidity, mortality, length of hospital stay and costs evaluated through a multivariate model analysis. *Clin Nutr.* 2003;22(3):235-239.

10. Tienboon P. Nutrition problems of hospitalised children in a developing country: Thailand. *Asia Pac J Clin Nutr.* 2002;11(4):258-262.

11. Ozturk Y, Buyukgebiz B, Arslan N, Ellidokuz H. Effects of hospital stay on nutritional anthropometric data in Turkish children. *J Trop Pediatr.* 2003;49(3):189-190.

12. Groenewold WG, Tilahun M. Anthropometric indicators of nutritional status, socioeconomic factors and mortality in hospitalized children in Addis Ababa. *J Biosoc Sci.* Jul 1990;22(3):373-379.

13. Coss-Bu JA, Klish WJ, Walding D, Stein F, Smith EO, Jefferson LS. Energy metabolism, nitrogen balance, and substrate utilization in critically ill children. *Am J Clin Nutr.* 2001;74(5):664-669.

14. Taylor RM, Cheeseman P, Preedy V, Baker AJ, Grimble G. Can energy expenditure be predicted in critically ill children? *Pediatr Crit Care Med.* 2003;4(2):176-180.

15. Vazquez Martinez JL, Martinez-Romillo PD, Diez Sebastian J, Ruza Tarrio F. Predicted versus measured energy expenditure by continuous, online indirect calorimetry in ventilated, critically ill children during the early postinjury period. *Pediatr Crit Care Med.* 2004;5(1):19-27.

16. Framson CM, LeLeiko NS, Dallal GE, Roubenoff R, Snelling LK, Dwyer JT. Energy expenditure in critically ill children. *Pediatr Crit Care Med.* 2007;8(3):264-267.

17. Mehta NM, Bechard LJ, Dolan M, Ariagno K, Jiang H, Duggan C. Energy imbalance and the risk of overfeeding in critically ill children. *Pediatr Crit Care Med.* 2011;12(4):398-405.

18. White MS, Shepherd RW, McEniery JA. Energy expenditure in 100 ventilated, critically ill children: improving the accuracy of predictive equations. *Crit Care Med.* 2000;28(7):2307-2312.

19. Vernon DD, Witte MK. Effect of neuromuscular blockade on oxygen consumption and energy expenditure in sedated, mechanically ventilated children. *Crit Care Med.* May 2000;28(5):1569-1571.

20. Kyle UG, Jaimon N, Coss-Bu JA. Nutrition support in critically ill children: underdelivery of energy and protein compared with current recommendations. *J Acad Nutr Diet.* 2012;112(12):1987-1992.

21. Flaring U, Finkel Y. Nutritional support to patients within the pediatric intensive setting. *Paediatr Anaesth.* 2009;19(4):300-312.

22. van der Kuip M, de Meer K, Oosterveld MJ, Lafeber HN, Gemke RJ. Simple and accurate assessment of energy expenditure in ventilated paediatric intensive care patients. *Clin Nutr.* 2004;23(4):657-663.

23. Jahoor F, Badaloo A, Reid M, Forrester T. Protein metabolism in severe childhood malnutrition. *Ann Trop Paediatr.* 2008;28(2):87-101.

24. Leite HP, de Lima LF, de Oliveira Iglesias SB, Pacheco JC, de Carvalho WB. Malnutrition may worsen the prognosis of critically ill children with hyperglycemia and hypoglycemia. *J Parenter Enteral Nutr.* 2013;37(3):335-341.

25. Favia I, Garisto C, Rossi E, Picardo S, Ricci Z. Fluid management in pediatric intensive care. *Contrib Nephrol.* 2010;164:217-226.

26. Singhi S, Marudkar A. Hypokalemia in a pediatric intensive care unit. *Indian Pediatr.* Jan 1996;33(1):9-14.

27. Maitland K, Pamba A, Newton CR, Lowe B, Levin M. Hypokalemia in children with severe falciparum malaria. *Pediatr Crit Care Med.* 2004;5(1):81-85.

28. Singhi SC, Singh J, Prasad R. Hypo- and hypermagnesemia in an Indian pediatric intensive care unit. *J Trop Pediatr.* 2003;49(2):99-103.

29. Singhi SC, Singh J, Prasad R. Hypocalcaemia in a paediatric intensive care unit. *J Trop Pediatr.* 2003;49(5):298-302.

30. Carcillo JA, Dean JM, Holubkov R, et al. The randomized comparative pediatric critical illness stress-induced immune suppression (CRISIS) prevention trial. *Pediatr Crit Care Med.* 2012;13(2):165-173.

31. Shakur MS, Malek MA, Bano N, Islam K. Zinc status in well nourished Bangladeshi children suffering from acute lower respiratory infection. *Indian Pediatr.* 2004;41(5):478-481.

32. Kumar S, Awasthi S, Jain A, Srivastava RC. Blood zinc levels in children hospitalized with severe pneumonia: a case control study. *Indian Pediatr.* 2004;41(5):486-491.

33. Heyland DK, Jones N, Cvijanovich NZ, Wong H. Zinc supplementation in critically ill patients: a key pharmaconutrient? *J Parenter Enteral Nutr.* 2008;32(5):509-519.

34. Brooks WA, Yunus M, Santosham M, et al. Zinc for severe pneumonia in very young children: double-blind placebo-controlled trial. *Lancet.* 2004;363(9422):1683-1688.

35. Srinivasan MG, Ndeezi G, Mboijana CK, et al. Zinc adjunct therapy reduces case fatality in severe childhood pneumonia: a randomized double blind placebo-controlled trial. *BMC Med.* 2012;10:14.

36. Bhatnagar S, Wadhwa N, Aneja S, et al. Zinc as adjunct treatment in infants aged between 7 and 120 days with probable serious bacterial infection: a randomised,

double-blind, placebo-controlled trial. *Lancet.* 2012; 379(9831):2072-2078.

37. Maggini S, Wintergerst ES, Beveridge S, Hornig DH. Selected vitamins and trace elements support immune function by strengthening epithelial barriers and cellular and humoral immune responses. *Br J Nutr.* 2007;98 Suppl 1:S29-35.
38. Madden K, Feldman HA, Smith EM, et al. Vitamin D deficiency in critically ill children. *Pediatrics.* 2012;130(3): 421-428.
39. Asai T. How should we use prokinetic drugs in patients who are intolerant to enteral feeding? *Crit Care Med.* 2007;35(2):650-651.
40. de Menezes FS, Leite HP, Nogueira PC. What are the factors that influence the attainment of satisfactory energy intake in pediatric intensive care unit patients receiving enteral or parenteral nutrition? *Nutrition.* 2013;29(1):76-80.
41. Zamberlan P, Delgado AF, Leone C, Feferbaum R, Okay TS. Nutrition therapy in a pediatric intensive care unit: indications, monitoring, and complications. *J Parenter Enteral Nutr.* 2011;35(4):523-529.
42. Mehta NM, McAleer D, Hamilton S, et al. Challenges to optimal enteral nutrition in a multidisciplinary pediatric intensive care unit. *J Parenter Enteral Nutr.* 2010;34(1):38-45.
43. Landzinski J, Kiser TH, Fish DN, Wischmeyer PE, MacLaren R. Gastric motility function in critically ill patients tolerant vs intolerant to gastric nutrition. *J Parenter Enteral Nutr.* 2008;32(1):45-50.
44. Sanchez C, Lopez-Herce J, Carrillo A, Bustinza A, Sancho L, Vigil D. Transpyloric enteral feeding in the postoperative of cardiac surgery in children. *J Pediatr Surg.* 2006;41(6):1096-1102.
45. Babbitt C. Transpyloric feeding in the pediatric intensive care unit. *J Pediatr Gastroentero Nutr.* 2007;44(5):646-649.
46. Petrillo-Albarano T, Pettignano R, Asfaw M, Easley K. Use of a feeding protocol to improve nutritional support through early, aggressive, enteral nutrition in the pediatric intensive care unit. *Pediatr Crit Care Med.* 2006;7(4):340-344.

CHAPTER 23

Nursing Considerations in the Provision of Nutrition Support to the Critically ill Child

LYVONNE N. TUME RN RSCN RNT

- INTRODUCTION
- NUTRITION SCREENING AND ASSESSMENT
- NURSING ASSESSMENT
- PLANNING FOR ENTERAL NUTRITION
  - Choosing the Best Route for Providing Enteral Nutrition
  - Trophic Feeds
- DELIVERY OF ENTERAL NUTRITION IN THE CRITICALLY ILL CHILD
  - Interruptions to Enteral Feeding in the Pediatric Intensive Care Unit
  - Feed Intolerance and Gastric Residual Volumes
  - Continuous or Intermittent (Bolus) Enteral Feeding in the Intensive Care Unit
  - Safety Aspects of Delivering Enteral Nutrition
- EVALUATION OF ENTERAL NUTRITION IN THE CRITICALLY ILL CHILD
- THE CRITICAL CARE NURSES' ROLE IN ACHIEVING OPTIMAL NUTRITION
- KEY POINTS
  - References

INTRODUCTION

It is well established that optimal nutrition in the pediatric intensive care unit (PICU) plays an important role in sustaining organ function; preventing further dysfunction of the cardiovascular, respiratory, and immune systems; and improving patient outcomes.[1,2] Good knowledge about nutritional issues is essential for PICU nurses to enable them to effectively contribute to the multidisciplinary team management of critically ill children. The nurse's role entails assessment and problem identification, planning, delivery, and evaluation.[3] The nursing considerations for nutritional support will be discussed in this chapter within these key areas of nursing practice. This chapter will focus on the role of the nursing staff in providing nutritional support and will be supported by best evidence, where available.

NUTRITION SCREENING AND ASSESSMENT

Nutrition screening should be undertaken at the time of admission or within the first 24 hours of admission. Each PICU should have a defined mechanism for having nutrition screening accomplished within this time frame. This screen should identify children who are malnourished or are at risk of malnutrition. No screen has been specifically validated in the PICU, but several pediatric screens are available. Please see chapter 2 for more details on nutrition assessment. Nursing staff must play an important role in nutrition screening. Anthropometric assessments documented on admission by a trained nurse provide crucial information on the nutritional status. Furthermore, the involvement of nursing staff will facilitate safe conduct of anthropometric measurements in critically ill children.

NURSING ASSESSMENT

Assessment of the individual child is a fundamental step in planning care delivery. Each child will have a different underlying injury or illness that has resulted in admission to the PICU and will be at a different stage of physiological maturity; as a result, each child can be expected to have different nutritional requirements and respond differently to nutritional support. A baseline assessment should be undertaken for all children in intensive care at the start of the nurse's shift. First, the pathology or injury that has caused the child's critical care unit admission is fundamental for the nurse to consider. Certain diagnoses may contraindicate enteral feeding, such as necrotizing enterocolitis (NEC), abdominal trauma, or surgery on an acute abdomen; other conditions or therapies are considered to present a high risk for NEC and gut ischemia in neonates, such as coarctation of the aorta (CoA), hypoplastic left heart syndrome (HLHS), having an umbilical artery line, and being on a prostaglandin infusion.[4-8] The pathology may also affect the child's predicted energy requirements (e.g., sepsis, burns, or severe traumatic brain injury); thus, it is essential that the nurse considers the pathology and child's reason for PICU admission, as well as the time point at which the child is currently in the illness/injury timeline. The risk of aspiration, and therefore the safety of commencing enteral feeding, must be considered. Factors known to increase the risk of aspiration are gastrointestinal (GI) reflux and a depressed gag/cough reflex.[9] The child's physiological stability at the time of assessment is also of prime consideration in terms of starting or continuing enteral nutrition (EN). The nurse must consider whether the child's physiological parameters (blood pressure, acid–base balance, and serum lactate) are within the expected targets. If they are not, a discussion with the medical team is essential about whether enteral feeding should start (or indeed if enteral feeding needs to temporarily stop) until physiological stability is achieved. Although there is little evidence within pediatrics to support stopping enteral feeding in children with high lactate levels, a study in adult patients found a high admission serum lactate was highly predictive of gastrointestinal dysfunction.[10] Due to these myriad considerations, many centers have adopted a uniform algorithmic approach for initiating and maintaining nutrition support in the critically ill child. The critical care nurse is often the principal driver of such an algorithmic approach to care in the unit. The role of guidelines for EN support in the ICU is described in more detail in chapter 9.

In addition to the child's illness, the PICU therapies being utilized are an important nursing consideration. Many PICU therapies and drugs affect gut motility and delay gastric emptying time. The gastric emptying rate is reduced in critically ill patients, most commonly from sedative and opiate drugs acting on the visceral smooth muscle of the GI tract, but other factors and drugs can reduce gastric emptying time and impair gastric motility, such as calcium channel blockers, proton pump inhibitors, H_2- receptor antagonists, and vasopressor agents.[11,12] The child's age, weight, and nutritional state are also key considerations when assessing the critically ill child for nutritional support, as this will help determine the type of enteral feed to be used. Parental preferences (for example, the use of expressed breast milk) should be considered, as well as the volume of feed to be given and thus the most practical method to achieve this. Small infants are more commonly fed by intermittent bolus feeds, whereas larger adolescents (who require higher feed volumes) are usually more easily fed by using a feed pump to deliver continuous feeds. The child's nutritional state (whether under- or overweight) on admission to the PICU is also an important factor to consider. These are joint considerations for the dietitian and medical team, but the nurse must take an active role in identifying these issues early on in the child's PICU admission. Other factors for the nurse to consider in the assessment of the child include whether there are any food allergies or intolerances to certain commercial enteral formulas, as well as any particular parental preferences (where appropriate). There are then a number of practical nursing issues to consider at the assessment stage and these include what type (if any) feeding tube or intravenous (IV) access is present for the administration of enteral or parental nutrition. The child's fluid allowance and how much of this is available for nutrition needs to be considered. Following consideration of these factors, the nurse then needs to undertake a clinical assessment of the child to establish a baseline. Inspection should focus on looking at the size and shape of the abdomen (looking for any obvious abdominal distention); the skin color and any shininess of the skin; any scars, lesions, bruising, or trauma; any obvious masses or movements (peristalsis can occasionally be seen); and any asymmetry. Following inspection, the abdomen should be auscultated to establish the presence and frequency of bowel sounds. After auscultation, the abdomen should be percussed to determine any areas of dullness or hyper-resonance. Finally, the abdomen should be gently palpated to detect any areas of tenderness or confirm any masses.[13] If there is any concern over abdominal distention, the abdominal girth should be measured and recorded, with clear markings for where this was done, to determine if girth is increasing. The results of the assessment should always be documented and used to form the baseline for evaluation. Table 23-1 summarizes the nursing assessment aspects of providing EN support.

TABLE 23-1. Summary of Key Nursing Considerations in the Provision of Nutritional Support to the Critically ill Child

NURSING ASSESSMENT
Assess the risk of aspiration
Physiological stability (BP, acid-base, lactate level)
Home therapies (e.g., list of medications and recent dosages)
ICU therapies/drugs in use (e.g., sedation dose)
Known food allergies or feed intolerances of child
Child's nutritional state on ICU admission
Parental feed preferences
Daily fluid allowance; calculate fluid delivered through medications
IV access or Feeding tube in position
Early dietetic referral
Clinical examination of the child's abdomen
Monitoring for other signs of EN intolerance
PLANNING CARE
Consider any planned procedures requiring fasting and clarify duration
Parent involvement in feeds (infants)
Caloric requirements determined and prescribed
Unit guidelines/flowchart to guide enteral feeding
Determine best route for enteral feeding
Equipment for enteral feeding (pump, feed set, pump)
Confirm & document position of feeding tube
Label different catheters and tubes to avoid inadvertent delivery into the wrong site. (e.g., intravenous gastric and postpyloric tubes)
Head of bed elevated 20-30° if possible
DELIVERY OF OPTIMAL NUTRITION
Clear nutritional goal for the day
Minimise or avoid interruptions to feeding
Aware of the factors affecting GRV measurement and its limitations
Use of continuous of intermittent feeds
Hygiene factors for enteral feeding
Safety factors in delivering enteral feeding (tube position confirmation, hygiene)
EVALUATION FOR NUTRITIONAL ADEQUACY AND TOLERANCE
Weight gain, discuss frequency and feasibility of accurate weighing
Head circumference (infants)
Urea and Electrolytes, serum albumin, serum glucose

TABLE 23-1. (Continued)

Absence of nausea and vomiting
Normal frequency and type of bowel movements
Acceptable level of GRV
Bowel sounds present
No abdominal distension
Observant for problems, e.g. NEC, aspiration
Response to feeding
Family support and education
Clinical audit and benchmarking for unit

PLANNING FOR ENTERAL NUTRITION

Once the nurse has assessed the child and established a baseline, then the delivery of care can be planned. In planning the delivery of nutritional support in critically ill children, a number of factors need to be taken into account. The child's care often needs to be planned around specific medical interventions or investigations in a critical care unit and the needs of the family (in terms of involving them in essential cares, e.g., assisting with feeding their child). The goal of the nurse, and the default position in any intensive care unit (ICU), should always be to initiate enteral feeding as early as possible after ICU admission. There is considerable and increasing evidence that early enteral feeding improves outcomes in the critically ill. A systematic review of early enteral nutrition (EEN) (<36 hours after ICU admission) compared to late EN in critically ill adults showed that EEN was associated with significantly lower incidence of infections ($p = <0.0006$) and a reduced length of hospital stay ($p = 0.004$).[14] A meta-analysis demonstrated that even earlier enteral feeding (<24 hour of ICU admission) reduced mortality in critically ill adults,[15] and others have showed that EEN (<6 hours after ICU admission) was possible and improved time to achieve calorie goal.[16]

Once the decision is made to start enteral feeding, the nurse needs to consider the best route of feeding, the dietetic orders for the calorie requirements, and how best to achieve this goal. The use of clinical guidelines and protocols to direct nursing practices in intensive care is very common, and it has been shown that using feeding protocols in PICUs increased the likelihood of patients receiving enteral nutrition closer to their estimated energy requirements.[16,17] Further studies confirm that guidelines help improve calorie delivery in the PICU,[2,16-18] and a recent multicenter cluster randomized controlled trial (RCT) of algorithm-directed EN and parenteral nutrition (PN) in adult critical care found that the algorithm group had significantly more days of EN ($p = 0.042$), a shorter hospital stay ($p = 0.003$), and a trend toward reduced mortality ($p = 0.058$).[19] A recent survey of pediatric intensive care staff in the UK and Ireland found that most PICUs had some written guidance on EN.[20] Thus, the use of an enteral feeding guideline is strongly recommended, as it improves consistency in practice between nurses, reduces confusion and uncertainty, and undoubtedly reduces the time taken to initiate feeding.

Choosing the Best Route for Providing Enteral Nutrition

In almost all PICUs, the default route for starting EN is via the gastric route, with gastric tubes being quick and relatively easy to place and with the majority of critically ill children tolerating feeds administered this way.

The administration of enteral feeds directly into the jejunum or duodenum has been advocated to reduce the problems associated with gastric feed intolerance and reduce the risk of aspiration.[21] Whether transpyloric (TP) feeding should be the first-line route for EN, though, remains questionable, although in some children at high risk for aspiration, it should be a consideration. In many units, the use of TP feeding is advocated in patients who develop feed intolerance via the nasogastric (NG) route, despite the use of prokinetic agents. However, in many ICUs, ensuring accurate placement of postpyloric tubes involves radiographic imaging and may delay the administration of EN, although recently, a new electromagnetic device able to be used in the ICU may help nasojejunal (NJ) tube placement.[22] Some ICUs are very proactive in their use of TP feeding and confident in tube placement, and there is some evidence to support TP feeding in adults. An RCT of NG versus TP feeding in adults with severe traumatic brain injury (n = 104) found the TP route reduced the incidence of pneumonia and improved feed volume delivery and reduced gastric residual volumes (GRVs).[23] However, a systematic review and meta-analysis of 11 trials of TP and gastric feeding in critically ill adults[24] found no difference in mortality and risk of pneumonia in TP compared to NG feeding. They concluded that in considering the difficulties associated with TP tube placement (significantly higher in the TP group), it was not associated with improved clinical outcomes and early use of TP feeding was not justified.

Trophic Feeds

The concept of trophic feeding (giving very small amounts of feed with the goal of stimulating the GI tract) originated in feeding preterm infants and has demonstrated some benefits in this group.[25-27] However, a recent systematic review could not recommend this practice.[28] Despite the uncertainty about whether benefits seen in preterm neonates can be extrapolated to critically ill children, the use of so-called "trophic" feeding is widespread in many PICUs.[20] However, what were considered "trophic" feeds varied considerably. The concept of early "trickle" or "trophic" feeds was recommended in the American Society of Parenteral and Enteral Nutrition (A.S.P.E.N.) adult nutrition guidelines.[29] In an RCT in ventilated adults with respiratory failure,[30] early trophic feeding resulted in clinical outcomes similar to those in the full-energy group, but with fewer episodes of GI intolerance. Despite this, limited evidence supports the theory and practicalities of trophic feed administration in children; however, it remains a widespread practice in PICUs. Table 23-1 summarizes key aspects of planning for nutritional support.

DELIVERY OF ENTERAL NUTRITION IN THE CRITICALLY ILL CHILD

Delivering nutritional support to the critically ill child can be challenging. Enteral feeding is preferred to parenteral feeding in critically ill patients due to the lower risk of infection and to maintain gut integrity.[1,2,31] However, there are many known difficulties to meeting children's nutritional requirements via the enteral route, such as feed intolerance, gastric ileus, periods of cessation of feeds for procedures, and fluid restrictions.

Interruptions to Enteral Feeding in the Pediatric Intensive Care Unit

There is considerable and mounting evidence demonstrating the huge problem of feed interruptions as a significant cause of inadequate calorie delivery in ICUs.[18,32-35] O'Meara et al.[33] found that EN was interrupted 27.3% of the time, with a mean of 6 hours per patient per day. Major reasons for feed stoppage were problems with small-bore feeding tubes (26%), increased gastric residual volumes (13%), and ventilation weaning (12%). This differed from adult trauma patients whose main reasons for stoppage were surgery (27%), diagnostic procedures (15%), and feed intolerance (11%).[32] Critical care literature frequently cites feed interruptions as a major problem for reducing calorie delivery in ICUs.[34] A small study revealed feed interruptions for procedures requiring fasting occurred in 43% of children in one 24-hour period (mean fasting time was 8.9 hours).[18] This is consistent with other pediatric studies[34] and adult ICU studies.[33,34] A recent study found that EN in PICUs was interrupted in nearly one-third of patients due to intolerance to feeds (high GRV, emesis, or diarrhea), blocked/misplaced feeding tubes, or medical procedures requiring fasting.[34] Many of these interruptions were avoidable and affected patient outcomes. The critical care nurse is the only person in a position to be able to coordinate and plan daily care activities with interventions, acting as the child's advocate to be able to reduce the duration of feed interruptions. It is probably one of the most important factors that will facilitate the achievement of the child's calorie goals. It is essential to have a clear consensus among members of the health care team and written guidelines regarding the type of procedures that require fasting and the duration of fasting for each. The nurse should consider the possibility of preprocedure gastric aspiration, rather than fasting, for a procedure or investigation that is often at an unknown exact time. This will not be the case for all procedures, but it is one way to reduce fasting times. Once guidelines are introduced, ongoing monitoring of compliance to guidelines is essential to ensure that practice is changed and interruption times are reduced.

Feed Intolerance and Gastric Residual Volumes

A big challenge associated with enteral feeding in the critically ill child is high GRVs. The use of GRVs as a marker of enteral feeding intolerance is problematic, as there is no evidence regarding the threshold GRV that is indicative of intolerance in critically ill children. The A.S.P.E.N. adult critical care nutrition guidelines[29] recommend a GRV threshold of 500 mL, beyond which feeds may be stopped for intolerance. In children, this becomes less clear, and the A.S.P.E.N. pediatric guidelines suggest that stopping enteral feeds at a GRV of >150 mL or 5 mL/kg may be reasonable; however, this is based on scant evidence.[36] Institutional guidelines on the use of GRV may vary considerably, and in a recent survey of centers in the UK, a maximal GRV of up to 300 mL was tolerated in a large child.[20] Increased GRV is thought to be associated with an increased risk of aspiration of gastric contents and pneumonia. Metheny et al.[37] found this to be common in critically ill patients. However, this level of risk is difficult to quantify, and the risk of aspiration will be different for different patients in the PICU. Using GRV as a sole criteria for feed stoppage is problematic, though, as the measurement of GRV is affected by a number of factors: size of the syringe used to aspirate the feeding tube, the diameter of the feeding tube, the tube position in the stomach, and the individual nurse aspirating the tube.[11] Despite this, it remains the most common method used to assess "feed tolerance."[20,38] Some inaccurate assumptions are commonly made about GRV: one is that the infused feed is the only component of the GRV. However, GRV also includes normal gastric juice and salivary production, which in an adult can amount to a daily volume of around 2,000 to 4,000 mL.[39] Multiple factors affect the gastric emptying rate and thus can increase the GRV in critically ill children.[11,40,41] The direct measurement of gastric emptying is difficult in clinical practice, and the correlation between GRV and gastric emptying remains unclear.[42] Thus, there is on-going debate about the value of using GRV measurement in critically ill patients receiving EN. In a recent RCT of critically ill adults, early EN without any GRV monitoring improved the delivery of EN and was not associated with increased incidence of vomiting or ventilator-associated pneumonia.[42] These findings are supported by a further RCT in critically ill adults, which found that a GRV of 500 mL was not associated with any adverse events or GI complications.[43] Measured GRV is not necessarily accurate, as small lumen feeding tubes, small-size aspirating syringes, and collapsible soft feeding tubes can all produce falsely low GRVs. Gastric residual volume may be erroneous in cases of adherence of the tip of the feeding tube to the gastric mucosa or positioning within the stomach where gastric fluid has not accumulated.[11,44] Larger-volume aspirating syringes produce less suction and are less likely to collapse soft feeding tubes. Two studies (both in critically ill adults) recommend that gastric aspirates be returned and could not demonstrate any higher complication rates in those patients where aspirates were returned compared to those in whom they were not.[45,46] The occlusion of feeding tubes is frequently reported in the literature as a factor causing interruption in enteral feeding. To prevent the occlusion of NG feeding tubes, a small amount of sterile water (just enough to clear the dead space in the feeding tube) may be instilled after NG drug administration (a common cause of blocked tubes). This is also important to ensure the drug actually reaches the patient and does not remain in the feeding tube. The bedside nurse must be aware of the theoretical considerations around GRV, as well as evidence for its use in monitoring for intolerance, and lead the development of sound and evidence-based practice related to GRV monitoring.

Continuous or Intermittent (Bolus) Enteral Feeding in the Intensive Care Unit

There is often debate about whether intermittent (bolus) feeding is superior to continuous NG feeding in critically ill children. In some situations, this is simply a practical issue, for a large adolescent in the ICU, the volume of feeds required for calorie goal attainment precludes intermittent bolus administration; however, for smaller children and infants, this question remains. Only 1 RCT has examined continuous versus bolus feeds in PICU patients, and this showed no difference in GRV between the 2 methods.[47] Studies in preterm infants also found no difference in GRV, although there was a higher GRV in the continuously fed group.[48-51] White et al.[52] found that continuous enteral feeding does not increase total energy expenditure, but bolus feeding does increase the thermic effect of food, thereby increasing energy expenditure. For patients fed via the TP route, continuous feeding is essential to prevent the phenomena of dumping syndrome (presenting as sweating, tachycardia, rebound hypoglycaemia, and diarrhea). This occurs when the sudden influx of a hyperosmolar feed is dumped into the jejunum. Whereas the stomach can distend and contain a large amount of food all at once, the jejunum has limited capacity, and in a normal physiological state will receive small, slow volumes of gastric contents over a longer period of time.[53]

Safety Aspects of Delivering Enteral Nutrition

There are a number of important safety factors for the nurse to consider in delivering EN to critically ill children. The most important safety issue for the nurse to consider is reducing the risk of aspiration and ensuring the correct position of the enteral feeding tube. A number of sentinel events are highlighted in the literature about the risks associated with aspiration, and misplaced NG tubes in particular.[54-56] The nurse is responsible for ensuring the correct position of the feeding tube each shift and before each feed is delivered (if intermittent feeds are used) or regularly if continuous feeds are used. Historically, nurses used a range of methods to confirm NG tube position, such as auscultation of insufflated air if no gastric aspirate could be obtained to test the pH, but the sensitivity of this method to confirm tube position is poor and this is now not recommended.[54] Current recommendations to confirm feeding tube position are first to test the pH of the enteral aspirate with pH paper and achieve a pH of between 1 and 5.5 for confirmation of a gastric position.[55] The second-line tube confirmation test involves x-ray confirmation.[55] However, gastric pH can be affected by a number of factors in critically ill children. A neonate's gastric pH is normally slightly higher than in older children and adults, whose normal gastric pH is 2 to 3.[57] In addition, pH-altering drugs, such as protein pump inhibitors and H_2- receptor blocking agents, and the use of continuous feeds will raise the pH level and make this method of confirming tube position less reliable.[58] In addition, intestinal or esophageal tube position will result in a pH typically greater than 5; thus, the pH method cannot always be relied upon to differentiate between these positions and respiratory tract placement. Children and infants frequently pull at tubes and can dislodge them easily; thus, the nurse needs to be vigilant and check the length of the feeding tube at the nares at the beginning of the shift and before each feed. A combination of methods should always be used to confirm tube placement in children: checking the feeding tube position on x-rays whenever they are taken, noting and marking the tube length at the nares, and aspirating and testing the pH of the gastric contents. The documentation of feeding tube position should also be done every shift. Further important nursing interventions to reduce the risk of aspiration pneumonia include elevation of the head of the bed 20 to 30 degrees (where possible) and meticulous oral care. These are standard practices in many ICUs worldwide, often incorporated into care bundles.[59,60]

Children and neonates on the ICU can be immunocompromised; thus, reducing any sources of bacterial contamination is vital. Enteral feeds are known to be a source of bacterial contamination, and meticulous hand hygiene should be maintained when handling enteral feeds.[61] Many pre-prepared, ready-to-feed enteral formulas are available that are sterile and should be used instead of reconstituted powdered formulas. Where reconstituted powdered formula is deemed appropriate for use, these should ideally be prepared in a designated clean feeds unit, and no additions to feeds should be made outside this unit.[62,63] The ready-to-feed formula can remain hanging in a closed system (if using continuous feeding) for up to 24 hours. Nonsterile feeds, including expressed breast milk, should not be allowed to hang more than 4 hours.[62] There is no evidence for how frequently feed delivery sets should be changed to reduce the risk of infection, but each ICU should have their own policy for this, and this is commonly every 24 hours. Once opened, any feeds not in a closed continuous feeding system should be stored in a refrigerator and discarded after 24 hours.[62] Tables 23-1 and 23-2 summarize key nursing considerations in the delivery of EN.

EVALUATION OF ENTERAL NUTRITION IN THE CRITICALLY ILL CHILD

Once enteral feeding has been initiated, the nurse needs to evaluate the care delivered and reassess the child with a view to changing plans and care delivery as required. On a long-term level, the effectiveness of nutritional support can be assessed by regularly measuring weight gain and head circumference in infants. On a short-term basis, calculating daily the amount of feed (and hence calories) actually delivered compared to the prescribed goal, as well as GRVs used in combination with other clinical assessments such as abdominal assessment, bowel movement frequency and type, bowel sounds, nausea and vomiting, diarrhea, and serum electrolytes, can be used to assess the effectiveness of EN delivery. In addition, in children and infants at risk of gut ischemia or NEC, the nurse must be proactive in looking for signs of this complication. Common signs of NEC include abdominal distention and/or pain or tenderness on palpation, feed intolerance, blood in the stools or gastric aspirates, metabolic acidosis with increasing serum lactate, and hemodynamic instability.[64] Gut ischemia and abdominal compartment syndrome may occur in the older child and present with pain and increasing abdominal distention, accompanied often by

TABLE 23-2. Nursing Recommendations for Optimizing the Delivery of Enteral Nutrition to the Critically ill Child

	Nursing Practice Recommendation
Type of nutritional support	• If enteral nutrition not likely, get parenteral support prescribed and ordered early (to avoid delays)
Timing of enteral nutrition	• Place NG tube as standard and confirm position as soon as possible • If no contraindications, start enteral feeding within 24 hours of PICU admission
Type of enteral feed	• If breast milk not being used, start with standard feeding formula appropriate for child's age and get dietitian review as soon as possible
Ensuring safety in enteral feeding	• Confirm and document feeding tube position at shift baseline and every time a feed is administered or 4-6 hourly if continuous feeds are used • Ensure meticulous hygiene (using aseptic nontouch technique) when preparing feeds and change feeding sets/tubing regularly, and do not leave feeds hanging for more than recommended hang times • Position child with head of the bed elevated 20-30° where possible to reduce the risk of aspiration
Set and review daily nutritional goals	• Know the child's nutritional goal for the day (how many mL of what type of feed and how many kcal this is) • At the end of the 24-hour period calculate and record how much of this goal was achieved and document this • Communicate this progress daily with medical team and dietitian
Reduce feed interruptions	• Ensure written unit consensus on fasting guidelines to improve consistency • Consider the likely medical interventions/investigations for the day and the timing of these and whether they need prior fasting • Coordinate the timing of these interventions where possible to minimize the feed interruption time • Restart feeds as soon as possible after procedure • Avoid NG tube occlusion after drug administration by flushing with sterile water
Be aware of the limitations of GRV	• Use GRV in combination with other clinical assessment parameters in deciding to stop feeds • Use larger syringe sizes when aspirating feeding tubes to avoid falsely low GRVs • Caution in the use of GRV when aspirating fine-bore, soft feeding tubes (likely falsely low GRV) • Consider that GRV is not just the volume of feed delivered but also gastric juice and saliva produced by the patient • Smaller-bore feeding tubes are more likely to produce falsely low GRVs • Using continuous feeds will yield a higher GRV
Observe for complications and feeding problems	• Regular clinical assessment: abdominal distention, pain, vomiting or diarrhea, bowel sounds, GRV • Frequency and type of bowel movements • Acid–base balance, electrolytes, and serum glucose
Consider factors that could reduce feeding problems	• Does the child need prokinetic agents? • Does the child need antiemetics? • Does the child need laxatives? • Could the child's sedation and opiates be reduced?

hypotension, metabolic acidosis, respiratory decompensation, and reduced urine output.[65]

Where possible, it is important to weigh the critically ill child regularly. In some units, this is more easily achieved with special beds/cots that allow weighing without moving the child, whereas in other units, the safety of lifting an invasively ventilated child out of bed onto scales has to be balanced against the risks of this procedure. The child's weight, looked at in combination with the child's overall fluid balance, is an important tool to evaluate nutritional status in the critically ill child. Evaluation of the overall process of optimizing nutrition in a particular critical care unit is best achieved by clinical audit. But it is important that even on a shift-by-shift basis, the care the nurse delivers is evaluated and reflected on (and documented appropriately) in order to optimize the care that children receive. Table 23-1 summarizes the key aspects of the nursing assessment of nutritional support.

THE CRITICAL CARE NURSES' ROLE IN ACHIEVING OPTIMAL NUTRITION

Intensive care nurses are the only constant presence at the child's bedside and play a crucial role in optimizing nutrition with the potential for improving patient outcomes. They also act as the linchpin between different medical and surgical teams and have a key role in the coordination of activities and timing of interventions for the critically ill child. They must "humanize"' the intensive care environment for the families, counsel and support them, and involve the family in decision making. The optimal management for critically ill children can only be achieved by a multidisciplinary team approach, and the intensive care nurse is an integral member of this team; thus, the nurses' role in optimizing nutritional intake in the critically ill child is an important one. The nurse's role is critical in coordinating care to the critically ill child, ensuring that clear nutritional goals are set for the day, and in evaluating the achievement of these goals at the end of each 24-hour period. The bedside nurse must be proactive, acting as the child's advocate to reduce feed interruptions, monitor compliance to institutional nutritional guidelines, and monitor for signs of intolerance to ensure safe EN delivery. Previous research has suggested that nursing practices (especially the variation between individual clinicians) could be contributing to underfeeding in critically ill patients.[66-68] By using feeding guidelines, ensuring compliance to guidelines, and reducing interruptions, the nurse has a key role to play in optimizing the nutritional support provided to critically ill children. The implementation of a nutritional support team or nurse champions around nutrition in an ICU has also shown to contribute to improved unit and patient outcomes related to nutrition.[36]

KEY POINTS

- Critical care nurses play a crucial role in ensuring optimal nutrition practice in the PICU.
- By ensuring timely nutritional assessment and developing safe nutrition delivery practices, nurses can help decrease interruptions to feeding, improve compliance with nutrition guidelines, and help achieve nutrition goals in critically ill children.
- Safe placement of feeding tubes has been led by nursing staff at many centers.

REFERENCES

1. Irving S, Simone S, Hicks F, et al. Nutrition for the critically ill child: enteral and parenteral support. *AACN Clin Issues*. 2000;11:541-558.
2. Briassoulis G, Zavras N, Hatzis T. Effectiveness and safety of a protocol of early intragastric feeding in critically ill children. *Pediatr Crit Care Med*. 2001;2:113-121.
3. Hudak C, Gallo B. *Critical Care Nursing: A Holistic Approach*. Philadelphia, PA: J.B. Lippincott Co;1994.
4. Ho E, Moss A. The syndrome of "mesenteric arteritis" following surgical repair of aortic coarctation. Report of nine cases and review of the literature. *Pediatrics*. 1972;49:40-45.
5. Hasegawa T, Yoshioka Y, Sasaki T, et al. Necrotizing enterocolitis in a term infant with coarctation of the aorta complex. *Pediatr Surg*. 1997;12:57-58.
6. Jeffries H, Wells W, Starnes V, et al. Gastrointestinal morbidity after Norwood Palliation for Hypoplastic Left Heart Syndrome. *Ann Thoracic Surg*. 2006;81:982-987.
7. Willis L, Thureen P, Kaufman J, et al. Enteral feeding in prostaglandin-dependent neonates: is it a safe practice? *J Pediatr*. 2008;867-869.
8. McElhinney D, Hedrick H, Bush D, et al. Necrotizing enterocolitis in neonates with congenital heart disease: risk factors and outcomes. *Pediatrics*. 2000;106(5):1080-1087.
9. Mehta N. Approach to enteral feeding in the PICU. *Nutr Clin Pract*. 2009;24:337-387.
10. Cresci G, Cue J. The patient with circulatory shock: to feed or not to feed? *Nutr Clin Prac*. 2008;23:501-509.

11. Gonzalez J. Gastric residuals: are they important in the management of enteral nutrition? *Clin Nutr*. 2008;4:2-7.
12. Kohm K, Boldt J, Swen P. Motility disorders in the ICU: recent therapeutic options and clinical practice. *Curr Opin Clin Nutr Metabol Care*. 2009;12(2):161-167.
13. Bates B. *A Guide to Physical Examination and History Taking*, 4th ed. Philadelphia, PA: JB Lippincott Co.: 1987.
14. Marik P, Zaloga G. Early enteral nutrition in acutely ill patients: a systematic review. *Crit Care Med*. 2001;29:2264-2270.
15. Doig G, Heighes P, Simpson F, et al. Early nutrition, provided within 24 h of injury or intensive care unit admission, significantly reduces mortality in critically ill patients: a meta-analysis of randomised controlled trials. *Int Care Med*. 2009;35:2018-2027.
16. Petrillo-Albarano T, Pettignano R, Asfaw M, et al. Use of a feeding protocol to improve nutritional support through early, aggressive enteral nutrition in the paediatric intensive care unit. *Pediatr Crit Care Med*. 2006;7:340-344.
17. Mepta N, Bechard L, Cahill N, et al. Nutritional practices and their relationship to clinical outcomes in critically ill children: an international multicentre cohort study. *Crit Care Med*. 2012;40(7):2204-2211.
18. Tume L, Latten L, Darbyshire A. An evaluation of enteral feeding practices in critically ill children. *Nurs Crit Care*. 2010;15:291-299.
19. Martin C, Doig G, Heyland D, et al. Multicentre, cluster-randomized controlled trials of algorithms for critical care enteral and parenteral therapy (ACCEPT). *CMAJ*. 2004;170(2):197-204.
20. Tume L, Carter B, Latten L. A UK and Irish survey of enteral nutrition practices in paediatric intensive care units. *Br J Nutr*. 2012;doi:10.1017/S0007114512003042.
21. Bourgalt A, Ipe L, Swartz S, et al. Development of evidence-based guidelines and critical care nurses' knowledge of enteral feeding. *Crit Care Nurse*. 2007;27(4):17-29.
22. Kline A, Sorce L, Sullivan C, et al. Use of a non-invasive electromagnetic device to place transpyloric feeding tubes in critically ill children. *Am J Crit Care*. 2011;20:453-460.
23. Acosta-Escribano J, Fernandez-Vivas M, Grau Carmona T, et al. Gastric versus trans pyloric feeding in severe traumatic brain injury: a prospective, randomised trial. *Intensive Care Med*. 2010;36:1532-1539.
24. Ho K, Dobb G, Webb S. A comparison of early gastric and post-pyloric feeding in critically ill patients: a meta-analysis. *Intensive Care Med*. 2006;32:639-649.
25. Burrin D, Stoll B, Jiang R, et al. Minimal enteral nutrient requirements for intestinal growth in neonatal piglets: how much is enough? *Am J Clin Nutr*. 2000;71:1603-1610.
26. McClure R, Newell S. Randomised controlled trial of trophic feeding and gut motility. *Arch Dis Child Neonatal*. 1999;80:F54-F58.
27. McClure R, Newell S. Randomised controlled study of clinical outcome following trophic feeding. *Arch Dis Child Neonatal*. 2000;82:F29-F33.
28. Bombell S, McGuire W. Early trophic feeding for very low birth weight infants. *Cochrane Database Syst Rev*. 2009;Issue 3:CD000504.
29. McClave S, Martindale R, Vanek V, et al. Guidelines for the provision and assessment of nutrition support therapy in the adult critically ill patient. *J Parenter Nutr*. 2009;33: 277-316.
30. Rice T, Mogan S, Hays M, et al. Randomized trial of initial trophic versus full-energy enteral nutrition in mechanically ventilated patients with acute respiratory failure. *Crit Care Med*. 2011;39:967-974.
31. Simpson F, Doig G. Parenteral versus enteral nutrition in the critically ill patient: a meta-analysis of trials using the intention to treat principle. *Intensive Care Med*. 2005;31:12-23.
32. Morgan L, Dickerson R, Alexander K, et al. Factors causing interrupted delivery of enteral nutrition in trauma intensive care patients. *Nutr Clin Pract*. 2004;19:511-517.
33. O'Meara D, Mireles-Cabodevila E, Frame F, et al. Evaluation of delivery of enteral nutrition in critically ill patients receiving mechanical ventilation. *Am J Crit Care*. 2008;17:53-61.
34. Mehta N, McAleer D, Hamilton S, et al. Challenges to enteral nutrition in a busy multidisciplinary PICU. *J Parenter Nutr*. 2010;34:38-45.
35. Rogers E, Gilbertson H, Heine R, et al. Barriers to adequate nutrition in critically ill children. *Nutrition*. 2003;19:865-868.
36. Mehta N, Compher C, ASPEN Directors: A.S.P.E.N Clinical Guidelines: Nutrition Support of the Critically Ill Child. *J Parenter Nutr*. 2009;33:260 DOI:10.1177/0148607109333114
37. Metheny N, Clouse R, Chang Y, et al. Tracheobronchial aspiration of gastric contents in critically ill tube-fed patients: frequency, outcomes and risk factors. *Crit Care Med*. 2006;34:1007-1015.
38. Marshall A, West S. Enteral feeding in the critically ill: are nursing practices contributing to hypocaloric feeding? *Intensive Crit Care Nurs*. 2006;22:1-5.
39. Lin H, Citters G. Stopping enteral feeding for arbitrary gastric residual volume may not be physiologically sound: results of a computer simulation model. *J Parenter Nutr*. 1997;21(5):286-289.

40. Deane A, Chapman M, Fraser R, et al. Mechanisms underlying feed intolerance in the critically ill: implications for treatment. *World J Gastroenterol.* 2007;13:3909-3917.
41. Fruhwald S, Holzer P, Metzler H. Gastrointestinal motility in acute illness. *Wien Klin Wochenschr.* 2008;120:6-17.
42. Poulard F, Dimet J, Martin-Lefevre L, et al. Impact of not measuring gastric volume in mechanically ventilated patients receiving early enteral feeding: a prospective study. *J Parenter Nutr.* 2010;34:125-130.
43. Montejo J, Minambres E, Bordeje L, et al. Gastric residual volume during enteral nutrition in ICU patients: the REGANE study. *Int Care Med.* 2010;36:1386-1393.
44. Metheny N. Residual volume measurement should be retained in enteral feeding protocols. *Am J Crit Care.* 2008;17:62-64.
45. Booker K, Niedringhaus L, Eden B, et al. Comparison of 2 methods of managing gastric residual volumes from feeding tubes. *Am J Crit Care.* 2000;9(5):318-324.
46. Juve-Udina M, Carreno-Granero A, Martinez-Estalella G, et al. To return or discard? Randomised trial on gastric residual volume replacement. *Intensive Crit Care Nurs.* 2009;25(5):258-267.
47. Horn D, Chaboyer W, Schluter P. Gastric residual volumes in critically ill paediatric patients: a comparison of feeding regimes. *Aust Crit Care.* 2004;17:98-103.
48. Kocan M, Hickisch S. A comparison of continuous and intermittent enteral nutrition in NICU patients. *J Neurosci Nurs.* 1986;18:333-337.
49. Toce S, Keenan W, Homan S. Enteral feeding in very low birth weight infants. *Arch Ped Adol Med.* 1987;141:439-444.
50. Silvestre M, Marbach C, Brans Y, et al. A prospective randomised controlled trial comparing continuous versus intermittent feeding methods in very low birth weight neonates. *J Pediatr.* 1996;128:748-752.
51. Schanler R, Schulman R, Lau C, et al. Feeding strategies for premature infants: randomised trial of gastrointestinal priming and tube-feeding method. *Pediatrics.* 1999;103:434-439.
52. White M, Shepherd R, McEinery J. Energy expenditure in 100 ventilated critically ill children: improving the accuracy of predicted equations. *Crit Care Med.* 2000;28(7):2307-2312.
53. Niv E, Fireman Z, Vaisman N. Post-pyloric feeding. *World J Gastroenterol.* 2009;15(11):1281-1288.
54. Metheny N. Measures to test placement of nasogastric and nasointestinal feeding tubes: a review. *Nurs Res.* 1988;37(6):324-329.
55. National Patient Safety Agency (NPSA). Reducing the harm caused by misplaced nasogastric feeding tubes in adults, children and infants 2011;NPSA/2011/PSA002. London.
56. Metheny N, Dettenmeier P, Hampton K, et al. Detection of inadvertent respiratory placement of small bore feeding tubes: a report of 10 cases. *Heart Lung J Acute Crit Care.* 1990;19:631-638.
57. MacGregor J. *Introduction to the Anatomy and Physiology of Children:* London: Routledge; 2000.
58. Solana Garcia M, Lopez-Herce Cis J, Sanchez Sanchez C. Gastroesophageal reflux in critically ill children: a review. *ISRN Gastroenterol.* 2013;Article ID 824320, http://dx.doi.org/10.1155/2013/824320.
59. Drakulovic M, Torres A, Bauer T, et al. Supine body position as a risk factor for nosocomial pneumonia in mechanically ventilated patients: a randomised trial. *Lancet.* 1999;354:1851-1858.
60. Aly H, Badawy M, ElKholy A, et al. Randomised controlled trial on tracheal colonization of ventilated infants: can gravity prevent ventilator-associated pneumonia? *Pediatrics.* 2008;122:DOI:10.1542/peds.2007-1826.
61. Patchell C, MacDonald A, George R, et al. Bacterial contamination of enteral feeds. *Arch Dis Child.* 1994;70:327-330.
62. Paediatric Group of the British Dietetic Association: Guidelines for making up special feeds for infants and children in hospital 2007;UK, Food Standards Agency.
63. Anderton A. Microbiological aspects of the preparation and administration of nasogastric and nasoenteric tube feeds in hospitals: a review. *Hum Nutr Appl Nutr.* 1983;37(6):426-440.
64. Lee J, Polin R. Treatment and prevention of necrotizing enterocolitis. *Sem Neonatol.* 2003;8:449-459.
65. Beck R, Halberthal, M, Zonis Z, et al. Abdominal compartment syndrome in children. *Ped Crit Care Med.* 2001;2(1):51-56.
66. Mateo, M. Nursing management of enteral tube feedings. *Heart Lung.* 1996;25:318-323.
67. Fulbrook P, Bongers A, Albarran J. A European survey of enteral nutrition practices and procedures in adult intensive care units. *J Clin Nurs.* 2007;16:2132-2214.
68. Hill S, Nielsen M, Lennard-Jones J. Nutritional support in intensive care units in England and Wales: a survey. *Eur J Clin Nutr.* 1995;49:371-378.

Index

Page references followed by f *indicate figures; those followed by* t *indicate tables.*

A

Abdominal compartment syndrome, 161, 305
Abdominal distension, 130
Abdominal girth, measurement of, 118
Abdominal surgical disease, 229–237
Acid-base physiology and associated disorders
  diagnosis and management of, 80–82, 83t, 84, 84t
  quantification of acid-base status, 79–80
  terminology and mechanisms, 78–79
Acidemia, 78
Acidosis, 76, 78
  metabolic, 81–82
  respiratory, 80–83
Acute Dialysis Quality Initiative, 187
Acute liver failure, 206, 206t
Acute lung injury (ALI), 73
Acute metabolic response to injured children, 3–12
  counter-regulatory hormonal response, 5–10
    AMS-associated anabolic hormone resistance, 6–7
    clinical significance, 10
    energy metabolism associated with acute metabolic stress, 9–10
    metabolic alterations associated with acute metabolic stress, 7–9
  cytokine response in, 5
  neuroendocrine/autonomic nervous system response in, 4–5
  overfeeding associated with acute metabolic stress, 10–12
    hepatic pathophysiology, 11
    immune system pathophysiology, 11–12
    pulmonary pathophysiology, 11
  overview, 3–4, 4f
  serial AMS response assessment, 12
Acute metabolic stress
  anabolic hormone resistance and, 6–7
  energy metabolism associated with, 9–10
Acute metabolic stress (*Cont.*):
  metabolic alterations associated with, 7–9
  overfeeding associated with, 10–12
Acute-on-chronic liver failure (ACLF), 205, 206
Acute pancreatitis, 210–211
Acute Physiology and Chronic Health Evaluation (APACHE) II score, 67
Acute renal failure, 187–191
  energy requirements, 188
  etiology, 187–188
  fluid and electrolyte management in, 189–190
  glucose metabolism and the kidney in, 188–189
  impact of renal replacement therapy in, 190
  lipid metabolism, 189
  metabolic consequences of, 188
  nutrition route in, 190, 191t
  outcome in, 188
  protein metabolism in, 189
Acute respiratory distress syndrome, 73
Acute respiratory failure, 281
Adaptive immune system, 243, 244–245
Adenosine diphosphate (ADP), 245
Adenosine triphosphate (ATP), 245
Adipose tissue, 270
Air displacement plethysmography, 142
Airway management in caring for obese patient in the pediatric intensive care unit, 275, 277
Alagille syndrome, 206
Alanine, 8
Alanine cycle, 8
Albumin for critically ill children in resource-limited setting, 291
Albuterol, 88
Alcohol abuse, 211
Alkalemia, 78
Alkalosis, 78
  metabolic, 82, 83t
  respiratory, 81
Alpha-1-antitrypsin deficiency, 206
American Association for the Study of Liver Disease (AASLD), 206
American Society of Health System Pharmacists, 132
American Society of Parenteral and Enteral Nutrition (ASPEN), 20
  Clinical Guidelines for the Nutrition and Support of the Critically Ill Child, 35, 38, 45, 103, 125, 169, 237, 252, 303
Amino acid requirements in pediatric critical illness, 40–50, 41f, 42t, 43t, 44f, 49f
Aminoglycosoides, 76
Aminosyn PF®, 104
Anemia, 64, 146
  megaloblastic, 67
Anion gap, 80
Anorexia, 6
Antacids, 132
Anthropometry, 21, 23, 261
  in congenital heart disease, 219
  in liver failure, 207
  in malnutrition, 23–24
Anti-infectives, 89, 89t
Antimicrobial drugs, 66
Arginine, 45, 247–248
  for critically ill children in resource-limited setting, 293
  current evidence on supplementation, 247–248
Aromatic amino acids, ratio to branched-chain amino acids, 208
Artificial nutrition support, in cancer and hematopoietic stem cell transplantation, 263–265
Ascites, 175
Ascorbate, 67
Ascorbic acid. *See* Vitamin C (ascorbic acid)
Asthma, 274
Autoimmune hepatitis, 206

B

Bacterial overgrowth, 234–235
Bariatric surgery, 282
Basal metabolic rate (BMR), 34
Best practices in enteral nutrition, 120
Beta agonists, 88
Beta blockers, 76
Biliary atresia, 206
Biochemical testing, 128
Bioelectrical impedance analysis (BIA)
in assessing body composition, 21, 24
in liver failure, 207
Bioelectrical impedance vector analysis (BIVA), 24
Biotin, 67–68
Blind feeding tube placement, 115
Blood glucose, 88
B-lymphocytes, 244
Body composition, 45–46
assessment of, 21, 21–22t, 23–25, 23t
Body length, 23, 142
Body mass index (BMI), 128
in liver failure, 207
Body weight, 23
Bolus feedings in the pediatric intensive care unit, 304
Bone mineral density, 142
Bowel regimen, 131–132
Bowel sounds, 130
Brain injury. *See* Trauma and traumatic brain injury
Brain natriuretic peptide (BNP), 272
Branched-chain amino acids (BCAA), 143, 176
ratio to aromatic amino acids, 208
Breast milk, 148
in chronic heart disease, 220–221
in intestinal failure, 232
Buffers, 78
Burns
enteral nutrition in, 169–170
metabolic response to, 165–166, 166ft
nutritional assessment with, 166, 167t
energy requirements, 168
monitoring nutritional status, 167–168, 167t
protein requirements, 168
status and risk, 166
tools in, 166–167
vitamins and minerals, 168–169
pharmacology and, 171
vitamin C in major, 251

C

Caffeine, 88
Calcium, 76–77
in parenteral nutrition, 107, 147
small-bowel absorption in, 65
Caldwell-Kennedy equation, 187, 188
Caloric deficits, 142
Caloric requirements, estimating, 36–37
Caloric underfeeding, 50
Calorie-to-nitrogen ratio, calculation of, 50
Canadian Clinical Practice Guidelines, 252
Cancer and hematopoietic stem cell transplantation, 257–265
nutritional assessment in, 259–263, 260t, 261t, 262t, 263t
nutritional intervention and monitoring, 263–265
artificial nutrition support, 263–265
oral intake, 263
nutritional status in, 257–259
Cancer cachexia, 258
Carbohydrates
in cancer and hematopoietic stem cell transplantation, 264
for critically ill children in resource-limited setting, 291
in liver failure, 208
in parental nutrition, 103
Carbonic anhydrase, 79
Cardiac intensive care unit, nutrition for infant/child in, 217–223
malnutrition and feeding problems, 217–218
optimal nutrition following surgery for congenital heart disease, 218–222
special situations
chylothorax, 222–223
interstate feeding and growth in children with hypoplastic left heart, 222
protein-losing enteropathy, 222
Cardiac lesions, types of, 218
Cardiopulmonary bypass, energy requirements and, 220
Cardiovascular system in the obese patient, 270–272
Carnitine
in parenteral nutrition, 147
in transport and metabolism of long-chain fatty acids, 106
Caspase-3, 44
Catch-up growth, 177
Catecholamines, 5, 157
Catheter-associated bloodstream infections, 234
Catheter occlusion, 107
Catheter-related blood stream infections (CR-BSI), 107
Chemokines, 243
Cholecalciferol, 65
Cholestasis, 103, 147
chronic, 106
Cholestatic liver diseases, 206
Choline, 68
Chromium, 63–64
in nutritional assessment, 146
in patients with renal dysfunction, 106
Chronic illness, malnutrition and, 39
Chronic liver disease (CLD), 210
Chronic pancreatitis, 211
Chronic renal replacement therapy (CCRT), 39
Chylothorax, 235–236
nutritional mangement of, 222–223
Chylous leak, 222–223, 235–236
Cirrhosis, 207
Citrate, 76
Citrulline, 45, 231
Clostridum-associated diarrhea, 159
Clostridum difficile, 118
Collaborative Pediatric Critical Care Research Network (CPCCRN), 252
Compensatory anti-inflammatory response syndrome (CARS), 243, 245
Complementary nutritional therapies, 199–200
Computed tomography scanning, 25, 46
Congenital disphragmatic hernia, 236
Congenital heart disease, nutrition following surgery for, 218–222
Congestive gastropathy, 206
Constipation, 130, 131
opioid-related, 118
preventive agents for, 131–132
Continuous feedings
in critically ill neonates, 149
in the pediatric intensive care unit, 304
Continuous renal replacement therapy (CRRT), 67, 189, 190
Continuous venovenous hemodiafiltration (CVVHDF), 64
Continuous venovenous hemofiltration (CVVH), 64
Conventional mechanical ventilation, 195–196
Copper, 64
for critically ill children in resource-limited setting, 292
in nutritional assessment, 146
in parenteral nutrition, 106, 147
Cori cycle, 5, 8
Corticosteroids, systemic, 88
Cortisol, 5, 156
Counter-regulatory hormonal response, 5–10, 11
AMS-associated anabolic hormone resistance, 6–7
clinical significance, 10
energy metabolism associated with acute metabolic stress, 9–10
metabolic alterations associated with acute metabolic stress, 7–9

C-reactive protein (CRP), 26, 62
in chronic heart disease, 220
in the critically ill, 128
Critical assessment of injury severity, 10
Critical care nurse, role of, in achieving optimal nutrition, 307
Critical Illness Stress Induced Immune Suppression (CRISIS), 250
Critically ill children
acid-base physiology and associated disorders in
diagnosis and management of acid-base disorders, 80–82, 83t, 84, 84t
quantification of acid-base status, 79–80
terminology and mechanisms, 78–79
electrolyte composition for parenteral formulations in
calcium, 76–77
magnesium, 77
phosphorus, 77–78
potassium, 75–76
sodium, 73–75
energy and macronutrient requirements in, 33–50
energetic derangements during critical illness, 33–34
energy provision in the critically ill, 37–40
enteral nutrition, 37–38
hypermetabolism and hypometabolism, 39–40
malnutrition and chronic illness, 39
nutritional support in the obese child, 39
parenteral nutrition, 38
targeted indirect calorimetry, 38–39, 38t
estimating caloric requirements, 36
correction factors, 36
predictive equations, 37, 37t
reference values for pediatric patients, 36
measuring energy needs, 34–36
gas exchange measurement—indirect calorimetry, 34–35
reversed Fick equation, 36
tracer methodology, 35–36
protein and amino acid requirements in, 40–50, 41f, 42t, 43t, 44f, 49f
enteral nutrition in, 111–121
benefits of early, 112, 112t
best practices in, 120
evaluation and maintenance of
barriers to optimal, 119, 120t
strategies to optimize, 119–120, 120t
tolerance, 118–119
formula selection
Critically ill children, enteral nutrition in, formula selection (*Cont.*):
high-calorie and/or high-protein, 116–118
high-carbohydrate, 118
infant and pediatric, 116
postpyloric feeding tube placement
blind feeding tube placement, 115
elecytromagnetic feeding tube placement, 115–116
fluroscopic feeding tube placement, 115
risks of early, 112–113, 112t
route for
advantages and disadvantages of gastric feeding, 114
advantages and disadvantages of postpyloric feeding, 114–115
gastric versus postpyloric feeding, 113–114, 113t
fluid management in
body water distribution and the intracellular and extracellular compartments, 72
fluid homeostasis, 71
maintenance parental fluid requirements, 72–73
guidelines and algorithms for feeding, 125–134
common components, 126, 127f
development and implementation of enteral nutrition, 132–134
enteral nutrition intolerance, 129–130
enteral nutrition maintenance and adjuncts, 130–132
initiation and advancement of enternal nutrition, 129
preinitation, 128–129
lipid turnover in, 106
micronutrient requirements in the, 59–68
trace elements, 60–64, 60t, 61t, 62t
chromium, 63–64, 106, 146
copper, 64, 106, 146, 147, 292
iron, 64, 106, 146, 210, 292
manganese, 64, 106, 146, 147, 292
selenium, 59, 63, 106, 249–250, 292
zinc, 60–63
vitamins, 64–65, 65–66
ascorbic acid (vitamin C), 60, 67, 190, 251–252
biotin, 67–68
choline, 68
cyanocobalamin (vitamin B_{12}), 67, 190
folic acid, 67, 190
niacin, 66
pantothenic acid (vitamin B_5), 66
pyridoxine (vitamin B_6), 67, 190
riboflavin (vitamin B_2), 66
Critically ill children, micronutrient requirements in the, vitamins (*Cont.*):
thiamine (vitamin B_1), 66, 106–107
vitamin A, 65, 146, 190, 210, 293
vitamin D, 65, 89, 146, 190, 207, 210, 293
vitamin E, 60, 66, 146, 210, 293
vitamin K, 66, 146, 207
nursing considerations in providing nutrition support to, 299–307
delivery of enteral nutrition, 303–305
evaluation of enteral nutrition, 305–307
nursing assessment, 300–301, 301–302t
nutrition screening and assessment, 299–300
planning for enteral nutrition, 302–303
role of the critical care nurse in, 307
nutritional assessment of, 19–30
assessment and screening for malnutrition using clinical and laboratory parameters, 20–21
assessment of body composition, 21, 21–22t, 23–25, 23t
energy requirements, 28, 28t
general evaluation, 21
laboratory assessment, 25–26t, 25–27
severity of illness assessment and risk for malnutrition assessment, 21
challenges and strategies to defining malnutrition, 20
implications for clinical practice, 28, 29f, 30
malnutrition in the critically ill child, 19–20
principles of nutritional assessment, 20
nutritional support of, in resource-limited settings, 287–296
carbohydrates, 291
considerations in severe malnutrition, 290–291
energy needs, 288–290, 289t
enteral formulas, 294–295, 294t, 295t
fluid intake, 292
in-hospital malnutrition, 288
lipid requirements, 291
nutitional assessment, 288
practical issues, 295–296
protein requirements, 291
routes and methods, 293, 294t
trace elements, 292
vitamins, 293
parenteral nutrition support in, 99–108
carbohydrates in, 103
complications in, 107–108
fats in, 106
fluids and electrolytes in, 102–103, 102t
indications for, 100–101, 100t
micronutrients in, 106–107

Critically ill children, parenteral nutrition support in (*Cont.*):
proteins in, 103–106, 104t, 105t
requirements in, 101–102
transition to enteral nutrition, 108
with respiratory failure, 196–197
Critically ill neonate, nutritional support of, 141–150
enteral nutrition in, 147–149
formulas, 148–149, 149f
human milk, 148
intermittent bolus feedings, 149
pasteurized donor human milk, 148
goals for growth and nutrition assessmet
assessment of neonatal nutritional status, 142
clinical assessment tools, 142
energy, 142, 143t
lipids, 144–145, 144f
protein, 143–144
special disease considerations, 143
micronutrients in, 145–146
trace elements, 146
vitamins, 146
parenteral nutrition in, 146–147
vitamins/minerals, 147
Crohn disease, 65
Crystalline amino acids, 104–105
Cuccumin, 200
Cyanocobalamin (vitamin B_{12}), 67, 190
Cyanotic lesions, 218
Cystic fibrosis, 206
Cytochrome P450, 64
Cytokines, 5, 77, 243

D

Deep vein thrombosis (DVT), 274
Dendritic cells, 243
Dermatitis, 146
Diabetic ketoacidosis, 275
Diarrhea, 118, 130
clostridum-associated, 159
Dietary fatty acid intake, 145
Diet-induced thermogenesis (DIT), 34–35
DiGeorge syndrome, 76
Digestive intolerance, 157
Dilutional acidosis, 82
D-lactic acidosis, 234–235
Docosahexaenoic acid (DHA), 144–145, 248
Doubly labeled water (DLW), 28, 35
Drug-nutrient interactions, 65, 87–93
anti-infectives, 89, 89t
defined, 87
electrolyte metabolism, 92–93, 93t
glucose homeostasis, 92, 92t
parenteral nutrition, 90, 91–92t, 92
respiratory distress, 88
seizures, 89, 89t
Dual-energy x-ray absorptiometry (DEXA), 21, 24, 46, 142, 232
Duodenal hematoma, 161–162
Dysmotility, 206
Dysnatremias, 73

E

Early-onset obesity, 156
Eicosatrienoic acid, 145, 248
Electrolytes
abnormalities in, 87
in acute renal failure, 189–190
in liver failure, 208
metabolism, 92–93, 93t
in parenteral nutrition, 102–103, 102t, 147
calcium, 76–77
magnesium, 77
phosphorus, 77–78
potassium, 75–76
sodium, 73–75
Electromagnetic feeding tube placement, 115–116
Elevated AG acidosis, 81–82
Emesis, 130
Encephalopathy, 175
Endothelial dysfunction, 272
Endotracheal tube, mechanical ventilation through, 195
End-stage renal disease, 187
Enemas, 132
Energy
in acute renal failure, 188
in critically ill children, 33–50
energetic derangements during critical illness, 33–34
energy provision in the critically ill, 37–40
enteral nutrition, 37–38
hypermetabolism and hypometabolism, 39–40
malnutrition and chronic illness, 39
nutritional support in the obese child, 39
parenteral nutrition, 38
targeted indirect calorimetry, 38–39, 38t
estimating caloric requirements, 36–37, 37t
measuring energy needs, 34–36
gas exchange measurement—indirect calorimetry, 34–35
reversed Fick equation, 36
tracer methodology, 35–36
protein and amino acid requirements in, 40–50, 41f, 42t, 43t, 44f, 49f
in resource-limited setting, 288–290, 289t
in nutritional assessment, 142, 143t
Energy expenditure (EE)
estimating, 28, 28t
measurement of, 28, 156
Energy metabolism associated with acute metabolic stress, 9–10
Enteral nutrition, 37–38
for burn patients, 169–170
in cancer and hematopoietic stem cell transplantation, 264
for children on extracorporeal membrane oxygenation, 237
contraindications for, 129
in critically ill children, 111–121
benefits of early, 112, 112t
best practices in, 120
evaluation and maintenance of
barriers to optimal, 119, 120t
strategies to optimize, 119–120, 120t
tolerance, 118–119
formula selection
high-calorie and/or high-protein, 116–118
high-carbohydrate, 118
infant and pediatric, 116
gastric feeding route, 114
gastric versus postpyloric feeding, 113–114, 113t
postpyloric feeding route, 114–115
postpyloric feeding tube placement
blind feeding tube placement, 115
elecytromagnetic feeding tube placement, 115–116
fluroscopic feeding tube placement, 115
in resource-limited setting, 293, 294–295, 294t, 295t
risks of early, 112–113, 112t
for critically ill neonates, 147–149
initiation and advancement of, 129
intolerance of, 129
in liver failure, 207
maintenance and adjuncts of, 130–132
fasting guidelines, 131, 131t
feeding tube management, 131
ongoing nutrition surveillance, 131
for nursing of critical ill children
delivery of, 303–305
evaluation of, 305–307
planning for, 302–303
safety aspects of delivering, 301–302t, 305, 306t
in pancreatatis, 212
recommendation over parental nutrition, 128
safety of, in chronic heart disease, 220
toleration of, 125
transition from parenteral nutrition to, 108

Enteral nutrition (*Cont.*):
in trauma and traumatic brain injury, 155, 158–159
benefits, 158
enteral access, 159
indications and contraindications, 158
timing and amount, 158–159
Enteral protein delivery, 48
Enterocutaneous fisula, 162
Epigenetics, 50
Ergocalciferol, 65
Erythrocyte selenium concentration, 63
Erythromycin, 132
Essential fatty acid deficiency (EFAD), 106
clinical signs of, 233
preventing, 222
Estimated energy requirements (EER), 128
of the hospitalized critically ill obese child, 279, 280–281t
Ethanol locks, 234
Ethylene diamine, 77
European Association for the Study of the Liver (EASL), 206
European Society for Clinical Nutrition and Metabolism (ESPEN), 157, 169
Euthyroid sick syndrome, 27
Extracellular fluid (ECF) compartment, 72
Extracorporeal membrane oxygenation, 236–237
energy requirements during, 236
nutritional outcomes and, 236–237
protein requirements in, 237
route of feeding in, 237
timing of feeding, 237
Ex-vivo bioinactivation, 87

F

Failure to thrive, 146
Fat-free mass (FFM), 24
Fat mass (FM), 24
Fats in parental nutrition, 106
Fat-soluble vitamins, 65–66
in nutritional assessment, 146
vitamin A, 65, 146, 190, 210, 293
vitamin D, 65, 89, 146, 190, 207, 210, 293
vitamin E, 60, 66, 146, 210, 293
vitamin K, 66, 146, 207
Feed intolerance, in delivering enteral nutrition, 303–304
Ferritin synthesis, 64
Fluid homeostasis, 71
Fluid management in, in acute renal failure, 189–190
Fluids
in acute renal failure, 189–190
body water distribution and the intracellular and extracellular compartments, 72
Fluids (*Cont.*):
for critically ill children in resource-limited setting, 292
fluid homeostasis, 71
in liver failure, 208
maintenance parental fluid requirements, 72–73
in parental nutrition, 92, 102–103, 102t
Fluoroscopic feeding tube placement, 115
Folic acid, 67, 190
Frank-Starling curve, 271
Free fatty acid production rates, 8–9
Free radicals, inflammation and the generation of, 59
Functional residual capacity, 272
Furosemide, 88

G

Gallstones, 211
Gas exchange measurement, 34
Gastric feeding
advantages and disadvantages of, 114
complications in, 159
versus postpyloric feeding, 113–114, 113t
Gastric residuals, 119
Gastric residual volumes, 129–130
in delivery of enteral nutrition, 303–304
Gastric stress ulcers, 132
Gastroesophageal reflux, 130, 218, 236
Gastrointestinal surgical disease, 229–237
GI motility, diagnostic tests of poor, 129
Ginger, 200
Glasgow coma score, 160
Glomerular filtration rate (GER), 179
Glucagon, 5, 156
Glucocorticoids, 5
Gluconeogenesis, 3, 5, 8, 103, 156
Glucose, medications affecting response, 92t
Glucose homeostasis, 92, 92t
alterations in, 8
Glucose infusion rate (GIR), 103
Glucose metabolism and the kidney, 188–189
Glutamine, 45, 103–104, 245–247
for burn injuries, 171
for critically ill children in resource-limited setting, 293
current evidence on supplementation, 247
dosing of, in children, 246–247
loss of, 156
in premature infants, 246
tolerance to oral feeding, 246
Glutathione peroxidase, selenium in, 63
Glycogenolysis, 157
Glycolysis, 5, 156
peripheral, 8
Graft-versus-host disease (GVHD), 258, 259
Growth failure in congenital heart disease, 219
Growth faltering, in congenital heart disease, 217
Gut ischemia, 305

H

Haldane transformation, 34
Hand-grip strength in liver failure, 207
Harris-Benedict equation, 36, 156
Head circumference, 142
measurement of, 24
Heart rate monitoring, 28
Heat shock protein expression, 245
Heel-to-knee measurement (knemometry), 23–24
Height-for-age (HFA) criteria, 23
Hematoma, duodenal, 161–162
Hematopoietic stem cell transplantation. *See* Cancer and hematopoietic stem cell transplantation
Hemoglobin, 64
Hepatic pathophysiology, 11
Hepatic protein synthesis, 8
Hepatic steatosis, 103
Hepatic tumors, 171
High-calorie and/or high-protein enteral formulas, 116–118
High-carbohydrate enteral formulas, 118
High-frequency oscillatory ventilation, 196
High-protein hypocaloric feeding, 281–282
Hirschsprung disease, 230, 231
Holliday Segar method, as assessing fluid requirements in children, 102, 102t
HOMA method for assessing *B*-cell function, 27
Human milk, 148
pasteurized donor, 148
Human Milk Banking Association of North America (HMBANA), 148
Hyperacute liver failure, 206
Hypercalcemia, 76–77
Hyperglycemia, 6, 11–12, 27, 88, 103, 107–108, 156, 157, 171, 257, 264
Hyperglycemic hyperosmolar syndrome, 275
Hyperinflammatory response, 5
Hyperkalemia, 75–76
Hyperlipidemia, 179
Hypermagnesemia, 77
Hypermetabolism, 39–40
Hypernatremia, 74–75
Hyperphosphatemia, 78
Hypertension, 179, 273
Hypertridemia, 257
Hypertriglyceridemia, 106, 107–108, 147, 189, 257
Hypervolemic hypo-osmolar hypotremia, 74
Hypocalcemia, 65, 76
Hypoglycemia, 290
Hypokalemia, 75, 79, 88

Hypomagnesemia, 76, 77
Hypometabolism, 39–40
Hyponatremia, 73–74
Hypo-osmolar hyponatremia, 73
Hypophosphatemia, 77–78
Hypoplastic left heart syndrome (HLHS), interstage feeding and growth in children with, 222
Hypoviteminosis D, 65
Hypovolemic hypo-osmolar hyponatremia, 73
Hypoxemia, 81

I

Immune system pathophysiology, 11–12
Immunomodulation, 65
Immunonutrition, 243–253
 clinical trials of, 252
 immune response to critical illness, 243–245
  adaptive immunity, 244–245
  innate immunity, 244
 immunologic effects of nutrients, 245–252
  macronutrients, 245–248
  micronutrients, 248–252
Indicator AA technique, 47
Indicible nitric oxide synthase, 247
Indirect calorimetry, 9, 28, 30, 34, 101, 188
 of the hospitalized critically ill child, 279
 in immediate posttransplant period, 180–181
 for measured energy expenditure, 160
 in measuring energy expenditure, 229
Infectious complications in parental nutrition, 107
Innate immune system, 243, 244
Inspissated feedings, 159
Insulin, 6–7, 44–45
 for burn injuries, 171
Insulin-like growth factor (IGF-1), 27
Insulin resistance, 275
Insulin sensitivity, 27
Intensive care unit, nutrient requirements within the, 181–182
Interleukin-6 (IL-6), 77, 128
Intermittent bolus feedings, 149
Intermittent hemodialysis, 190
Intestinal dysmotility, 235
Intestinal failure, 230–235
 complications of, 233–235
Intestinal failure-associated liver disease (IFALD), 231, 233–234
Intestinal obstruction, 159
Intra-abdominal abscess, 159
Intracellular fluid compartment, 72
Intracellular protein turnover in critical illness, 43–44
Intrauterine growth rates, 142
Intravenous fat emulsion (IVFE), 106
 assessing tolerance to, 106
Iodine in parenteral nutrition, 106
Iron, 64
 in chronic liver disease, 210
 for critically ill children in resource-limited setting, 292
 in nutritional assessment, 146
 in parenteral nutrition, 106
Isotope studies, 25

J

Jejunal feeds, 159
Jejunostomy, 159

K

Kashin-Beck disease, 249
Kidney, glucose metabolism and, 188–189
Kidney disease-improving global outcomes (KDIGO), 189
Knemometry, 23–24
Krebs cycle, 8, 66
K+ sparing diuretics, 75

L

Lactic acidosis, 82
Laxatives, 132
Lean body mass, 40, 176
 risk of loss of, 99
Left-to-right shunts, 218
Length-for-age (LFA) criteria, 23, 128
Leucine, 45
Lipids
 in acute renal failure, 189
 in cancer and hematopoietic stem cell transplantation, 264–265
 for critically ill children in resource-limited setting, 291
 in injury-induced alterations in metabolism, 8–9
 in liver failure, 209, 209t
 in nutritional assessment, 144–145, 144f
 turnover, during critical illness, 106
Lipogenesis, 11
Lipolysis, 5, 157
Liver failure, 205–210
 acute, 206, 206t
 hyperacute, 206
 nutritional support in
  carbohydrates, 208
  fluid and electrolytes, 208
  lipids, 209, 209t
  protein, 208
  vitamins and minerals, 209–210
 pathophysiology of malnutrition in, 206–210
  estimating nutritional needs, 207
  nutritional status in, 207
  nutritional support in, 207–208
 subacute, 206
Liver transplantation, 206
 morbidity and mortality following, 175
 nutrition management after, 175–179
Long-chain polyunsaturated fatty acids (LCPUFA), 144
 biosynthesis of, 145
Long-chain triglyceride, 11
Loop diuretics, 76
Low-birth-weight infants, protein requirements for, 237
Low T_3 syndrome, 27
L-pyruvate, 234
Lymphocytes, classes of, 244
Lymphopenia, low plasma zinc in, 61

M

Macronutrients
 in the critically ill child, 33–50
  energetic derangements during critical illness, 33–34
  energy provision in the critically ill, 37–40
   enteral nutrition, 37–38
   hypermetabolism and hypometabolism, 39–40
   malnutrition and chronic illness, 39
   nutritional support in the obese child, 39
   parenteral nutrition, 38
   targeted indirect calorimetry, 38–39, 38t
  estimating caloric requirements, 36
   correction factors, 36
   predictive equations, 37, 37t
   reference values for pediatric patients, 36
  measuring energy needs, 34–36
   gas exchange measurement—indirect calorimetry, 34–35
   reversed Fick equation, 36
   tracer methodology, 35–36
  protein and amino acid requirements in, 40–50, 41f, 42t, 43t, 44f, 49f
 immunological effects of, 245–248
Macrophages, 243
Magnesium, 77
 for critically ill children in resource-limited setting, 292
 in parenteral nutrition, 147
Magnetic resonance imaging, 25, 46
Malabsorption, 118, 146
Malabsorption syndrome, 65
Malnutrition, 125
 acute effects of, 19–20
 assessment and screening for, using clinical and laboratory parameters, 20–21
  assessment of body composition, 21, 21–22t, 23–25, 23t

Malnutrition, assessment and screening for, using clinical and laboratory parameters (*Cont.*):
general evaluation, 21
severity of illness assessment and risk for malnutrition assessment, 21
challenges and strategies in defining, 20
chronic illness and, 39
clinical consequences of, following congenital heart surgery, 218–219
considerations in severe, 290–291
in the critically ill child, 19–20
diagnostic criteria for, using anthropometry, 23–24
in hospitalized children, 287, 288
pathophysiology of, 206–210
in pediatric surgical patients, 228–229
prevalence of acute and chronic in critically ill children, 99
protein-energy, 175
WHO classication of, 219, 219t
Manganese, 64
for critically ill children in resource-limited setting, 292
in nutritional assessment, 146
in parenteral nutrition, 106, 147
Measured energy expenditure (MEE), 9
indirect calorimetry for, 160
Mechanical ventilation
in caring for obese patient in the pediatric intensive care unit, 277
conventional, 195–196
noninvasive, 195
nutritional strategies in, 197
overfeeding, 197
through endotracheal tube, 195
underfeeding, 197
Medication dosing, in caring for obese patient in the pediatric intensive care unit, 277–278
Medium-chain triglyceride, 11, 176
Megaloblastic anemia, 67
Metabolic acidosis, 81–82
Metabolic alkalosis, 82, 83t
Metabolic alterations associated with acute metabolic stress, 7–9
Metabolic bone disease, 232
Metabolic compensation and nonvolatile acids/strong ion difference, 79
Metabolic response
to burn injury, 165–166, 166ft
to trauma, 156–157
Metabolomics, 50
Metallothionein, 61
3-methylhistidine (3MH), 46
Methylnaltrexone, 132
Metoclopramide, 132
Micronutrients, 27
in chronic heart disease, 221–222
in the critical ill child, 59–68
fat-soluble vitamins, 65–66
vitamin A, 65, 146, 190, 210, 293
vitamin D, 65, 89, 146, 190, 207, 210, 293
vitamin E, 60, 66, 146, 210, 293
vitamin K, 66, 146, 207
trace elements, 60–64, 60t, 61t, 62t
chromium, 63–64, 106, 146
copper, 64, 106, 146, 147, 292
iron, 64, 106, 146, 210, 292
manganese, 64, 106, 146, 147, 292
selenium, 59, 63, 106, 249–250, 292
zinc, 60–63
vitamins, 64–65
water-soluble vitamins
ascorbic acid (vitamin C), 60, 67, 190, 251–252
biotin, 67–68
choline, 68
cyanocobalamin (vitamin B_{12}), 67, 190
folic acid, 67, 190
niacin, 66
pantothenic acid (vitamin B_5), 66
pyridoxine (vitamin B_6), 67, 190
riboflavin (vitamin B_2), 66
thiamine (vitamin B_1), 66, 106–107
immunological effects of, 248–252
in nutritional assessment, 145–146
in parental nutrition, 106–107
Mid-upper arm circumference (MUAC), 24, 128, 176
Minerals. *See also specific*
in liver failure, 209–210
in parenteral nutrition, 147
Mixed acid-base disorders, 84
Molybedum, in parenteral nutrition, 106
Monocytes, 243
Mucosal ischemia, 156
Multidisciplinary IF centers, 230
Multiple organ dysfunction syndrome (MODS), 187, 188
Multisystem organ failure, 206
Muscle function tests, 25
Myeloid suppressor cells, 247
Myoglobin, 64

N

Naloxone, 132
Nasoduodeal/nasojejunal access, 159
National Institute of Child Health and uman Development Collaborative Pediatric Critical Care Research Network, 199
National Pediatric Cardiology Quality Improvement Collaborative, 220
Natural killer cells, 243
Necrotizing entercolitis, 229–230, 246
enteral feeding in neonates at risk for, 229–230
risk of, 218
Neonatal nutritional status, assessment of, 142
Nephrotoxicity, 179
Neurally adjusted ventilatory assist, 196
Neuroendocrine/autonomic nervous system response, 4–5
Neutron activation analysis, 25
Neutropenia, 146
Niacin, 66
Nicotinamide, 66
Nicotinamide adenine dinucleotide, 245
Nitric oxide, 247, 272
Nitrogen balance, 46–47
Nitrogen shuttle and metabolic partitioning, 41–43, 41f, 42t
Non-AG acidosis, 82
Noninvasive ventilation, 195
Nonthyroidal illness, 27
Nonvolatile acids, 79
Nonvolatile weak acid buffers, 79
N-terminal pro-brain natriuretic peptide, 272
Nursing care
for obese patient in pediatric intensive care unit, 278
in providing nutrition support to critically ill children, 299–307
delivery of enteral nutrition, 303–305
evaluation of enteral nutrition, 305–307
nursing assessment, 300–301, 301–302t
nutrition screening and assessment, 299–300
planning for enteral nutrition, 302–303
role of the critical care nurse in, 307
Nutrients, interactions with drugs. *See* Drug-nutrient interactions
Nutriogenomics, 50
Nutrition. *See also* Enteral nutrition; Parenteral nutrition
after liver transplantation, 175–179
after small intestinal transplantation, 179–183
in cardiac intensive care unit, 217–223
malnutrition and feeding problems, 217–218
optimal nutrition following surgery for congenital heart disease, 218–222
special situations
chylothorax, 222–223
interstate feeding and growth in children with hypoplastic left heart, 222
protein-losing enteropathy, 222
estimating needs, in liver failure, 207
route for, in acute renal failure, 190. 191t

Nutritional assessment of the critically ill child, 19–30
assessment and screening for malnutrition using clinical and laboratory parameters, 20–21
assessment of body composition, 21, 21–22t, 23–25, 23t
energy requirements, 28, 28t
general evaluation, 21
laboratory assessment, 25–26t, 25–27
severity of illness assessment and risk for malnutrition assessment, 21
challenges and strategies to defining malnutrition, 20
in the hospital, 278–279
implications for clinical practice, 28, 29f, 30
malnutrition in the critically ill child, 19–20
principles of nutritional assessment, 20
Nutritional support
of critically ill children
in resource-limited settings, 287–296
carbohydrates, 291
considerations in severe malnutrition, 290–291
energy needs, 288–290, 289t
enteral formulas, 294–295, 294t, 295t
fluid intake, 292
in-hospital malnutrition, 288
lipid requirements, 291
nutitional assessment, 288
practical issues, 295–296
protein requirements, 291
routes and methods, 293, 294t
trace elements, 292
vitamins, 293
of critically ill neonates, 141–150
enteral nutrition in, 147–149
formulas, 148–149, 149f
human milk, 148
intermittent bolus feedings, 149
pasteurized donor human milk, 148
goals for growth and nutrition assessmet
assessment of neonatal nutritional status, 142
clinical assessment tools, 142
energy, 142, 143t
lipids, 144–145, 144f
protein, 143–144
special disease considerations, 143
micronutrients in, 145–146
trace elements, 146
vitamins, 146
parenteral nutrition in, 146–147
vitamins/minerals, 147
in liver failure, 207–208
Nutritional support (*Cont.*):
of the pediatric surgical ICU patient, 227–238
abdominal and gastrointestinal surgical disease
chyle leak, 235–236
extracorporeal membrane oxygenation, 236–237
increased stoma or stool output, 235
intestinal dysmotility, 235
intestinal failure, 230–235
necrotizing enterocolitis, 229–230
perioperative nutrition, 228–229
postoperative nutrition, 228
Nutrition Risk Score (NRS), 20
Nutrition support
for the hospitalized critically ill obese child, 279, 281
nursing considerations in providing to critically ill children, 299–307
delivery of enteral nutrition, 303–305
evaluation of enteral nutrition, 305–307
nursing assessment, 300–301, 301–302t
nutrition screening and assessment, 299–300
planning for enteral nutrition, 302–303
role of the critical care nurse in, 307
in pancreatitis, 211–212

O

Obesity, 269–283
after liver transplantation, 179
in cancer and related diseases, 258
challenges and considerations in caring for patient in pediatric intensive care unit, 275–278, 276f
airway management, 275, 277
mediation dosing, 277–278
nursing care, 278
outcomes, 278
vascular access, 277
comorbidities of, 273–275, 273t
asthma, 274
hypertension, 273
insulin resistance, 275
pulmonary hypertension, 274
sleep-disordered breathing, 273–274
thromboembolic disease, 274
epidemiology in, 270
nutritional support in, 39, 161
nutrition for the hospitalized critically ill child, 278–282
estimation of energy requirements, 279, 280–281t
high-protein hypocaloric feeding, 281
indirect calorimetry, 279
nutrition assessment, 278–279
nutrition support, 279, 281
Obesity, nutrition for the hospitalized critically ill child (*Cont.*):
protein requirements, 279, 281t
weight loss interventions following critical illness, 281–282
physiologic changes associated with, 270–273, 271t
adipose tissue, 270
cardiovascular system, 270–272
respiratory system, 272–273
Obesity hypoventilation syndrome (OHS), 274
Obstructive sleep apnea, 273
Octreotide, 236
Omega-3 fatty acids, 248
as anti-inflammatory agent, 106
respiratory failure and, 199
Open abdomen, 161
Opioid-related constipation, 118
Oral feeding, tolerance of glutamine to, 246
Oral intake in cancer and hematopoietic stem cell transplantation, 263
Organomegaly, 206
Ornithine, 247
Osteomalacia, 65
Osteopenia of prematurity, 146
Overfeeding, 155, 156, 188, 196
acute metabolic stress and, 10–12
hepatic pathophysiology, 11
immune system pathophysiology, 11–12
pulmonary pathophysiology, 11
mechanically ventilated patients, 197
Oxandrolone for burn injuries, 171
Oxidative stress, 197, 198t

P

Paediatric Logistic Organ Dysfunction (PELOD), 21
Paediatric Yorkhill Malnutrition Score (PYMS), 21
Pancreatasis, 212
Pancreatic insufficiency, 290
Pancreatitis, 210–212
acute, 210–211
chronic, 211
clinical management of, 211
etiology of, 211
nutrition for, 211–212
pathophysiology, 211
severity of, 211
Pantothenic acid (vitamin B_5), 66
Paracetamol absorption test, 129
Parenteral branched-chain AA, 45
Parenteral fluid requirements, maintenance of, 72–73, 72t
Parenteral nutrition, 11–12, 38
calcium in, 76–77, 147
in cancer and hematopoietic stem cell transplantation, 264

Parenteral nutrition (*Cont.*):
carbohydrates in, 103
carnitine in, 147
complications in, 107–108
copper in, 147
for critically ill neonate, 146–147
electrolytes in, 102–103, 102t, 147
fats in, 106
fluids in, 92, 102–103, 102t
indications for, 100–101, 100t
in liver failure, 207–208
magnesium in, 77, 147
manganese in, 147
medication compatibility with, 90–92t
micronutrients in, 106–107
minerals in, 147
in pancreatitis, 212
perioperative, 228
phosphorus in, 77–78
in PICU, 90, 92
postoperative, 228
potassium in, 75–76
proteins in, 103–106, 104t, 105t
requirements in, 101–102
risks and complications of, 221
sodium in, 73–75
total, 228
transition to enteral nutrition, 108
in trauma and traumatic brain injury, 155, 157–158
vitamins in, 147
zinc in, 147
Parenteral nutrition-associated liver disease (PNALD), 11
Parenteral protein delivery, 48, 49f
Pasteurized donor human milk, 148
Pathophysiology of malnutrition, 206–210
Pediatric Acute Liver Failure (PALF) study group, 206
Pediatric Index of Mortality (PIM), 21
Pediatric intensive care unit (PICU)
blood glucose abnormalities in, 92
caring for obese patient in, 275–278, 276f
airway management, 275, 277
mechanical ventilation, 277
medication dosing, 277–278
nursing care, 278
outcomes, 278
vascular access, 277
continuous or intermittent (bolus) enteral feedings in, 304
electrolyte abnormalities, glucose intolerance and protein malnutrition in, 87
energy expenditure in, 262
enteral feeding in, 111
interruptions to, 303
liver failure in, 205
Pediatric intensive care unit (*Cont.*):
malnutrition in, 125
nutrition state of children admitted to, 19, 20
parental nutrition for patients in, 90, 91–92t, 92, 101
respiratory distress in, 88
sepsis in, 89
Pediatric nutritional risk score (PNRS), 20
Pediatric Risk of Mortality Score (PRISM), 21
Pediatric surgical ICU patient
nutritional support of the, 227–238
abdominal and gastrointestinal surgical disease
chyle leak, 235–236
extracorporeal membrane oxygenation, 236–237
increased stoma or stool output, 235
intestinal dysmotility, 235
intestinal failure, 230–235
necrotizing enterocolitis, 229–230
perioperative nutrition, 228–229
postoperative nutrition, 228
Peliosis hepatitis, 171
Percutaneous endoscopic gastrosomy (PEG), 159
Perioperative parenteral nutrition, 228
Peripheral acting mu-opioid receptor antagonists (PAMORAs), 132
Peripheral glycolysis, 8
Phenobarbital, 89
Phenytoin, 89
oral absorption of, 89
Phosphate in parenteral nutrition, 107
Phosphorus, 77–78
Phylloquinone, 66
Plasma C-reactive protein, 46
Plasma zinc in the critically ill, 60–62
Platelet dysfunction, 145
Polymorphonuclear cells, 243
Postburn ileus, 170
Postnatal growth rate goals, for preterm infants, 142
Postoperative starvation, 228
Postpyloric feeding
advantages and disadvantages of, 114–115
versus gastric feeding, 113–114, 113t
tube placement for, 115–116
Posttransplant diabetes mellitus, 179
Potassium, 75–76
Prader-Willi syndrome, 281
Premasol®, 104
Preterm infants
formula for, 148–149, 149f
glutamine in, 246
postnatal growth rate goals for, 142
Pretransplant nutritional care, 180
Procalcitonin, 128
Progressive familial intrahepatic cholestasis (PFIC), 206
Prokinctics, 132
Propranolol for burn injuries, 171
Protein
in acute renal failure, 189
in cancer and hematopoietic stem cell transplantation, 264
for critically ill children, 40–50, 41f, 42t, 43t, 44f, 49f
hospitalized obese, 279, 281t
in resource-limited setting, 291
in liver failure, 208
measurement of status, 25
in nutritional assessment, 142–143
in parental nutrition, 103–106, 104t, 105t
Protein catabolism and anabolic resistance, 44–45
Protein-energy interactions, 48, 50
Protein-energy malnutrition, 175
Protein-energy wasting, 188
Protein kinetics, 118
Protein-losing enteropathy, nutritional management of, 222
Protein-sparing modified fast (PSMF) diet, 281–282
Protein underfeeding, 50
Proteolysis, prevention of, 143
Proteostasis in the critical ill child, 50
Pruritus, 175
Pulmonary hypertension, 274
Pulmonary pathophysiology, 11
Pyridoxal-5-phosphate, 67
Pyridoxine (vitamin B_6), 67, 190

Q

QT prolongation, 132

R

Reference values for pediatric patients, 36
Renal dysfunction, 106
Renal outer medullary potassium channel (ROMK) function, 75
Renal replacement therapy, 190
Renal tubular acidosis, 82
Resource-limited settings
nutritional support of critically ill children in, 287–296
carbohydrates, 291
considerations in severe malnutrition, 290–291
energy needs, 288–290, 289t
enteral formulas, 294–295, 294t, 295t
fluid intake, 292
in-hospital malnutrition, 288
lipid requirements, 291

Resource-limited settings, nutritional support of critically ill children in (*Cont.*):
nutitional assessment, 288
practical issues, 295–296
protein requirements, 291
routes and methods, 293, 294t
trace elements, 292
vitamins, 293
Respiratory acidosis, 80–83
Respiratory alkalosis, 81
Respiratory compensation, 79
Respiratory distress, 88
Respiratory failure, 193–200
acute lung injury in, 194–195
acute respiratory distress syndrome in, 194–195
importance of providing nutrition to critically ill children with, 196–197
mechanical ventilation in, 196–196
conventional, 195–196
endotracheal tube in, 195
high-frequency oscillatory ventilation, 196
neurally adjusted ventilatory assist, 196
noninvasive, 195
parenchymal lung disease and, 194
upper airway obstruction and, 193–194
Respiratory quotient (RQ), 28, 34
Respiratory system in the obese patient, 272–273
Resting energy expenditure
in congenital heart disease, 219–220
in critically ill neonates, 142, 143
in renal failure, 188
Resveratrol, 199–200
Retinol, 65
in nutritional assessment, 146
Reversed Fick equation, 36
Riboflavin (vitamin B_2), 66
RIFEE, 187, 188t

S

Safety in delivering enteral nutrition, 301–302, 305, 306t
Salicylate ingestations, 84
Scaly dermatitis, 145
Schofield equations, 36, 128, 156
Scientific Registry of Transplant Recipients (SRTR), 179–180
Screening Tool for the Assessment of Malnutrition in Paediatrics (STAMP), 20–21
Scurvy, 67
Seizures, 89, 89t
Selenium, 59, 63
for critically ill children in resource-limited setting, 292
deficiency of, 249
dosing of supplementation and monitoring guidance, 249–250
in patients with renal dysfunction, 106
toxicity of, 250
Sepsis, 89, 246
severe, 63
Septic shock, 63
Serial AMS response assessment, 12
Severe sepsis, 63
Severe symptomatic hyponatremia (AMS), 74
Short-bowel syndrome (SBS), 230–231
Siggard-Andersen nomogram, 80
Single-ventricle lesions, 218
Skeletal muscle synthesis, promotion of, 143–144
Skinfold measurements, 45, 128
Sleep-disordered breathing, 273–274
Small-bowel bacterial overgrowth, 234
Small-bowel feeding, 159
Small intestinal transplantation, nutrition management after, 179–183
Small-volume feedings, 264
Sodium, 73–75
Sodium bicarbonate, in treating acute respiratory acidosis, 80–81
Sodium-dependent glucose transporters (SGLTs), 189
Somatostatin, 236
Splanchnic perfusion, 220
Stable isotope measurement, 142
Steatosis, 106
Stoma, patients with increased, 235
Stool output, patients with increased, 235
Stool softeners, 132
$STRONG_{kids}$ tool, 21
Subacute liver failure, 206
Subjective global nutrition assessment (SGNA), 21, 128
in liver failure, 207
Superior cavopulmonary connection (SCPC), 222
Surviving Sepsis Guidelines, 72
Syndrome of inappropriate antidiuretic hormone (SIADH), 73–74
Systemic corticosteroids, 88
Systemic inflammatory response syndrome (SIRS), 63, 67, 107, 245, 249

T

Tachycardia, 102
Talbott method, 36
Tetany, 76
T-helper 1 cells, 244
T-helper 2 cells, 244
Theophylline, 88
Thermic effect of food assessment, 28
Thermogenesis, 34
Thiamine (vitamin B_1), 66
deficiency of, 88, 106–107
Thromboembolic disease, 274
Thrombotic occlusions, 107
Thyroid hormones, 27
T-lymphocytes, 244, 247
Tocopherol, 66
in nutritional assessment, 146
Total body potassium, 25
Total body water (TBW), 25, 72
Total energy expenditure (TEE), 34
components of, 101
Total parenteral nutrition (TPN), 11–12, 38, 228
Total respiratory compliane, 272
Total urinary nitrogen and nitrogen balance, 26–27
Trace elements, 60–64, 60t, 61t, 62t
chromium, 63–64, 106, 146
in chronic liver disease, 210
copper, 64, 106, 146, 147, 292
iron, 64, 106, 146, 210, 292
manganese, 64, 106, 146, 147, 292
in nutritional assessment, 146
respiratory failure and, 199
selenium, 59, 63, 106, 249–250, 292
zinc, 60–63
Tracer methodologies, 47
Transpyloric feeding, enteral feeding and, 221
Trauma and traumatic brain injury, 155–162
enteral nutrition in, 155, 158–159
benefits, 158
enteral access, 159
indications and contraindications, 158
timing and amount, 158–159
metabolic response to trauma, 156–157
hormones, hyperglycemia, and protein catabolism in, 156–157
measurement of energy expenditure, 156
parenteral nutrition in, 155, 157–158
complications in, 158
merits of, 157–158
specific injuries, 159–162
duodenal hematoma, 161–162
enterocutaneous fistula, 162
obese trauma patient, 161
open abdomen, 161
traumatic brain injury, 160, 160f
Triceps skinfold (TSF) thickness, 24, 261
in liver failure, 207
Triene-to-tetraene ratio, 145
TrophAmine®, 104

Trophic feedings, 159, 264, 303
Tumor lysis syndrome, 76
Turmeric, 200
Type 2 diabetes mellitus, 156

U

Ulcers, gastric stress, 132
Underfeeding, 155, 196
  mechanically ventilated patients, 197

V

Valproic acid (VPA), 89
Vascular access in caring for obese patient in the pediatric intensive care unit, 277
Vasoactive drugs, 220
Vasopressors, 277–278
VCO_2/VO_2 ratio, 34
Veno-occlusive disease (VOD), 258, 259
Ventilation-perfusion (V/Q) mismatch, 272
Video-assisted thoracic surgery, 236
Visceral proteins, 25–26, 46, 48
Vitamin A, 65, 190
  in chronic liver disease, 210
  for critically ill children in resource-limited setting, 293
  in nutritional assessment, 146
Vitamin B_1 (thiamine), 66, 106–107
Vitamin B_2 (riboflavin), 66
Vitamin B_5 (pantothenic acid), 66
Vitamin B_6 (pyridoxine), 67, 190
Vitamin B_{12} (cyanocobalamin), 67, 190
Vitamin C (ascorbic acid), 60, 67, 190, 251–252
  in the critically ill, 251
  in major burns, 251
  toxicity and adverse events, 251
Vitamin D, 65, 89, 190
  in chronic liver disease, 207, 210
  in nutritional assessment, 146
Vitamin D (*Cont.*):
  in resource-limited setting, 293
Vitamin E, 60, 66
  in chronic liver disease, 210
  for critically ill children in resource-limited setting, 293
  in nutritional assessment, 146
Vitamin K, 66
  in chronic liver disease, 207
  in nutritional assessment, 146
Vitamins, 64–65
  fat-soluble, 65–66
    vitamin A, 65, 190
      in chronic liver disease, 210
      for critically ill children in resource-limited setting, 293
      in nutritional assessment, 146
    vitamin D, 65, 89, 146, 190, 207, 210, 293
    vitamin E, 60, 66, 146, 210, 293
    vitamin K, 66, 146, 207
  in liver failure, 209–210
  in nutritional assessment, 146
  in parenteral nutrition, 147
  respiratory failure and, 199
  water-soluble
    ascorbic acid (vitamin C), 60, 67, 190, 251–252
    biotin, 67–68
    choline, 68
    cyanocobalamin (vitamin B_{12}), 67, 190
    folic acid, 67, 190
    niacin, 66
    pantothenic acid (vitamin B_5), 66
    pyridoxine (vitamin B_6), 67, 190
    riboflavin (vitamin B_2), 66
    thiamine (vitamin B_1), 66, 106–107
Volatile acids, 79
volvulus with bowel infarction, 159
Vomiting, 119

W

Waterlow criteria, 23
Water-soluble vitamins, 107
  ascorbic acid (vitamin C), 60, 67, 190, 251–252
  biotin, 67–68
  choline, 68
  for critically ill children in resource-limited setting, 293
  cyanocobalamin (vitamin B_{12}), 67, 190
  folic acid, 67, 190
  niacin, 66
  in nutritional assessment, 146
  pantothenic acid (vitamin B_5), 66
  pyridoxine (vitamin B_6), 67, 190
  riboflavin (vitamin B_2), 66
  thiamine (vitamin B_1), 66, 106–107
Weight, 142
Weight-for-age (WEA) criteria, 23, 128
Weight-for-height (WFH) criteria, 23
Weight-for-length-for-age, 128
Weight loss interventions following critical illness, 281=282
White equations, 128, 156
Whole-body calorimetry, 28
Wilson disease, 206
World Health Organization (WHO) criteria, 23, 128, 156, 219, 219t

Z

Zinc, 60–63, 250–251
  in chronic liver disease, 210
  for critically ill children in resource-limited setting, 292
  deficiency of, 107
  in nutritional assessment, 146
  in parenteral nutrition, 106, 107, 147
Zinc deficiency dermatitis, 107
Z-scores, 128